Textbook on
Fibroids

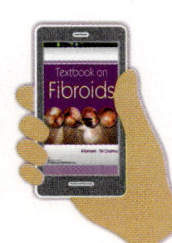

**Surgical Videos
accompanying this book
are available free on
CBSiCentral App**

Textbook on Fibroids

B Ramesh MD (BOM), DGO, FCPS, DFP
Diploma in Gynae Endoscopy (USA)
Fellowship in Assisted Reproduction (UK, Finland)
Consultant Gynae Endoscopic Surgeon
Infertility, ART Specialist and Urogynaecologist
Medical Director, Altius Hospital
Bengaluru, Karnataka, India

Chaithra TM MS, OBG, DNB
Fellowship Programme in Minimal Invasive Surgery (Gynaecology) (Altius Hospital)
Laparoscopic Surgeon and Infertility Specialist
Kochi, Kerala, India

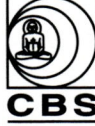

CBS

CBS Publishers & Distributors Pvt Ltd

New Delhi • Bengaluru • Chennai • Kochi • Kolkata • Mumbai
Bhubaneswar • Hyderabad • Jharkhand • Nagpur • Patna • Pune • Uttarakhand

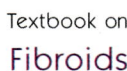

Textbook on
Fibroids

ISBN: 978-93-87085-13-8

First Edition: 2018

Published by Satish Kumar Jain and produced by Varun Jain for
CBS Publishers & Distributors Pvt Ltd
4819/XI Prahlad Street, 24 Ansari Road, Daryaganj, New Delhi 110 002, India.
Ph: 23289259, 23266861, 23266867   Fax: 011-23243014   Website: www.cbspd.com
e-mail: delhi@cbspd.com; cbspubs@airtelmail.in.
Corporate Office: 204 FIE, Industrial Area, Patparganj, Delhi 110 092
Ph: 4934 4934   Fax: 4934 4935   e-mail: publishing@cbspd.com; publicity@cbspd.com

Branches

- **Bengaluru:** Seema House 2975, 17th Cross, K.R. Road, Banasankari 2nd Stage, Bengaluru 560 070, Karnataka
  Ph: +91-80-26771678/79   Fax: +91-80-26771680   e-mail: bangalore@cbspd.com
- **Chennai:** 7, Subbaraya Street, Shenoy Nagar, Chennai 600 030, Tamil Nadu
  Ph: +91-44-26680620, 26681266   Fax: +91-44-42032115   e-mail: chennai@cbspd.com
- **Kochi:** Ashana House, 39/1904, AM Thomas Road, Valanjambalam, Ernakulam 682 016, Kochi, Kerala
  Ph: +91-484-4059061–65,67   Fax: +91-484-4059065   e-mail: kochi@cbspd.com
- **Kolkata:** 6/B, Ground Floor, Rameswar Shaw Road, Kolkata-700014 (West Bengal), India
  Ph: +91-33-2289-1126, 2289-1127, 2289-1128   e-mail: kolkata@cbspd.com
- **Mumbai:** 83-C, Dr E Moses Road, Worli, Mumbai-400018, Maharashtra
  Ph: +91-22-24902340/41   Fax: +91-22-24902342   e-mail: mumbai@cbspd.com

Representatives

- **Bhubaneswar** 0-9911037372
- **Hyderabad** 0-9885175004
- **Jharkhand** 0-9811541605
- **Nagpur** 0-9021734563
- **Patna** 0-9334159340
- **Pune** 0-9623451994
- **Uttarakhand** 0-9716462459

Printed at Magic International Pvt. Ltd., Greater Noida, UP, India

Contributors

Aswath Kumar R MBBS, MD, FICOG
Professor
Jubilee Mission Medical College and
Research Centre, Thrissur

Alphy S Puthiyidom MBBS, MD, FMIS (Laparoscopy)
International Modern Hospital, Dubai, UAE

B Ramesh MD (BOM), DGO, FCPS, DFP
Diploma in Gynaec Endoscopy (USA)
Fellowship in Assisted Reproduction (UK, Finland)
Consultant Gynae Endoscopic Surgeon
Infertility, ART Specialist and Urogynaecologist
Medical Director, Altius Hospital
Bengaluru, Karnataka

Bhaskar Pai DGO, MD, DNBE, FICOG, FRCOG
Senior Consultant, Obstetrician and Gynaecologist
Apollo Gleneagles Hospital, Kolkata

Chaithra TM MS.OBG, DNB
Fellowship Programme in Minimal Invasive Surgery (Gynaecology) (Altius Hospital)
Laparoscopic Surgeon and Infertility Specialist
Specialist, Kochi, Kerala

Chandana Anantha Rama Reddy MBBS, MS OBG, FMIS
Dr Chandana Health Care Clinic
Wilson Garden, Bengaluru

Dipti Gunge MBBS, OBG, DNB
Laparoscopic Surgeon and Infertility Specialist
Navjeevan Super Specialty Hospital
Karad

Dipanwita Banerjee
Specialist, Department of Gynaecological Oncology
Chittaranjan National Cancer Institute
Kolkata

L Fahmida Banu MD, DGO, DNBE, FRCOG, FICOG
Minimally Invasive Surgeon
Consultant Obstetrician and Gynaecologist
FehmiCare Hospital, Hyderabad

Geeta Bharat (Uttur) MS (OBG), MRCOG (UK), DNB, FIGE
Obstetrician, Gynaecologist
Laparoscopic Surgeon, Reproductive
Medicine, IVF Consultant (NUH, Singapore)
Sarvodaya Women's Hospital and Fertility
Center, Dharwad

Haritha Desai MBBS, MS OBG, PGDHL
Consultant Obstetrician and Gynaecologist
Mumbai

Indusekhar Subbanna MBBS, DMRD, MD (Radiology)
Consultant Interventional Radiologist,
HCG Hospital, Colombia Asia Hospital, Bengaluru

K Jayakrishnan MD, DGO, DNB
KJK Fertility and Research Centre
Nalanchira, Trivandrum, Kerala

Jnaneswari TL MBBS, MD, DNB, DNB (Obstetrics and Gynaecology),
Fellowship in Gynaecological Endoscopy
BL Hospital, Bengaluru

Lola Ramachandran MBBS, DNB (Obstetrics and Gynaecology)
Jubilee Mission Medical College and
Research Centre, Thrissur

Madhuri Vidyashankar MBBS, MS, OBG
Fellowship in Minimal Invasive Surgery
Gynaec Endoscopy Surgeon
Milann Fertility Center, Bengaluru

Meenakshi Sundaram MD, DNB (Obstetrics and Gynecology)
Fellowship in Gynaecological Endoscopy
Robotic Surgery Training (USA)
Apollo Hospital, Chennai

Manjula Anagani MD, FICOG
Padmashree Awardee
Maxcure Suyosha Hospitals
Hitech City, Madhapur
Hyderabad, Telangana

Nirmala Sadasivam
Genesis Fertility Research Centre
Maaruthi Medical Centre and Hospitals
Erode, Tamil Nadu

Niranjana Jayakrishnan MD, DNB, OBG
Consultant in Reproduction Medicine
KJK Hospital, Trivandrum

Pooja Sharma Dimri MD DNB FMIS
Consultant, Gynaecologic Endoscopic Surgeon
Bellevue and Cloudnine Hospital, Mumbai

MK Pathanjali Prasanna MBBS, FCARCSI, FRCA, FFICM
Manor Hospital, Walsall, United Kingdom

Reshu Saraogi MS, FMIS
Cogent Care, Bengaluru

Ramachandra C Raghunatha Rao FRCR, DNB, DMRD
Medall-Clumax Diagnostics
Sadashivanagar, Bengaluru

Rajesh V Helavar MD, PDCC (Gastroradiology)
Consultant, Diagnostic and Interventional Radiology
Columbia Asia Referral Hospital
Yeshwanthpur, Bengaluru

Rachana Ghanti MBBS, MS (OBGYN)
Fellowship in Laparoscopy (Altius Hospital)
Behind Gujarat Bhavan
Deshpande Nagar, Hubballi

Sandip Datta Roy MBBS, MS (OBGYN), FICS, FICMCH
FMIS (Fellowship in Gynaecological Endoscopy)
RGUHS, Bangalore
New Alma Hospital, Mannarkkad, Palakkad
Raji Nursing Home, Thrissur, Kerala

Sanjay Patel MD, Diploma in Endoscopy (Germany)
Gynec-Endoscopic Surgeon, Infertility and IVF Specialist
Director, Mayflower Women's Hospital, Ahmedabad

T Shanthala Thuppanna MS (OBG), FIGE (RGUHS), Diploma in
Gynaecological Endoscopy (Germany)
Consultant Gynecological Endoscopic Surgeon
Apollo Spectra and Motherhood, Bengaluru

Sudhir Kale DNB (RD), MNAMS
Lead Consultant Radiologist and Head
Department of Radiology and Imaging Sciences
Aster CMI Hospital, Bengaluru

Shraddha Daksha MBBS, MS, FMIS
Apollo Hospital, Delhi

Shraddha N Kurkuri MBBS, MS, FMIS
Dharwad

Shwetha Pramodh MBBS, DGO, DNB, FIRM
Fellowship in Gynaec Endoscopy (ICOG, Mumbai)
Fellow in Reproductive Medicine
Chief Consultant, Obstetrician and Gynecologist
IVF Specialist and Laparoscopic Surgeon, Tamara Hospital and
IVF Centre, Bengaluru, and
Medical Director
Blossom Infertility and Women Care Centre, Bengaluru

Shyjus Puliyathinkal MBBS, MS (OBG, JIMPER), FMAS, DMAS
Consultant Laparoscopic Surgeon
Associate Professor
Department of Obstetrics and Gynaecology
Kerala

Sabhyata Gupta MD (Gynaecology)
Director and Head
Department of Gynaecology and Gynaec Oncology
Medanta, The Medicity
Gurgaon

Satwik B Metgud MS (OBG), FMAS
Consultant, Gynaec Endoscopy Surgeon
Centre for Assisted Reproduction and Endoscopy
Kasbekar Metgud Clinic
Shivaji Nagar, Belagavi

Vijaya V Mysorekar MBBS, MD (Pathology)
Senior Professor
Department of Pathology
Ramaiah Medical College
MSR Nagar, MSRIT post
Bengaluru

Varsha Rangaraj MS, FMAS, PGDHHM
Fellow in Minimal Access Surgery and
Reproductive Medicine
Consultant Gynaecologist and Laparoscopic Surgeon
Milann-The Fertility Center
#82, CMH Road, Indira Nagar 2nd Stage
Bengaluru

Vivek Salunke MD, DGO
Lilavati Hospital—Bandra, Fortis—Vashi, MGM—Vashi,
Jupiter—Thane, Seven Hills—Andheri, Cloud 9—Malad,
Oyster Hospital—Goregaon
Mumbai

Vidya V Bhat MD, DNB (OBG) MNAMS, FICOG
Obstetrician and Gynaecologist
Sonologist and Laparoscopic Surgeon
Medical Director
Radhakrishna Multispeciality
Hospital and IVF Centre
Bengaluru

Preface

We are pleased to publish this book on Fibroids. It is a comprehensive feast on everything about fibroids. The colour Atlas is a carefully selected collection of original images, very useful for all those undergraduates, gynaecology residents, practising gynaecologists and laparoscopic surgeons to understand the pathophysiology and treatment of fibroids.

We hope this book will provide learners and practitioners to give up-to-date evidence-based care to the patients. We would like to acknowledge all of the contributors for their time and expertise in making this edition possible. A special thanks to our OT staff for their constant support in collecting salient images for colour Atlas.

Recent advances like uterine artery embolization and HIFU are dealt in detail. The technique of laparoscopic myomectomy, selection of patients, complications, fertility following myomectomy are dealt with recent advances in the field. The chapter on various methods of hysterectomy for fibroids is described in detail. We are confident that this book will fulfil all the required information on the topic.

We hope you enjoy the book *Textbook on Fibroids* and useful to all the clinicians dealing with fibroids.

B Ramesh
Chaithra TM

Contents

SECTION 1

Basics of Fibroids

CHAPTER 1

History and Introduction to Uterine Fibroids

● Shraddha Daksha

Uterine fibroids (Fig. 1.1) are the most common pelvic tumour in women, also known as uterine leiomyoma/myoma/fibromyoma/fibroleiomyoma. They are benign smooth muscle tumours of the uterus. They are estimated to be present in a high percentage of all women of reproductive age and also may be discovered incidentally during routine annual examination. Asymptomatic fibroids may be present in 40%–50% of women older than 35 years of age[1]. Using ultrasonography screening, other authors have estimated a cumulative incidence by the age 50, of greater than 80% in African-American women and nearly 70% in white women[2].

Leiomyomas may occur singly or often multiple. They may be subserosal, intramural, or submucosal in location within the uterus or located in the cervix, in the broad ligament, or suspended from a pedicle. Most fibroids start in the muscular wall of the uterus. With further growth, some lesions may develop towards the outside of the uterus or towards the internal cavity. Secondary change may develop within fibroids such as haemorrhage, necrosis, calcification or cystic degenerations.

If the uterus contains too many fibroids to count, it is referred to as diffuse uterine leiomyomatosis.

In the period of Hippocrates in 460–375 B.C., this lesion was known as 'uterine stone'. Galen called this finding as 'scleromas' during the second century of the Christian period. The term fibroid was coined and introduced in 1860 by Rokitansky and in 1863 by Klob[3] (Table 1.1)

In 1854, a German pathologist named Virchow demonstrated that these neoplasms (fibroids) were composed of smooth muscle cells. It was Virchow who introduced the word 'myoma'[4].

Table 1.1: Contribution of surgeons

No.	Surgery	Year	Surgeon
1.	Laparotomy for fibroid	2003	Danville USA5
2.	Open myomectomy	1840	Jean Zulema Amussat, PARIS[7]
3.	Vaginal myomectomy	1845	Atlee, Pensylvania[8]
4.	Hysterectomy for fibroid	1853	Gilman Kimbal, Massachusetts[9]
5.	Abdominal multiple myomectomy	1898	Alexander, Liverpool[3]
6.	Laparoscopic myomectomy	1970	Kurt Semm, Germany[11]
7.	Hysteroscopic myoma resection	1976	Neuwirth[10]
8.	Myolysis	1981	Goldfarb[14]
9.	Uterine artery embolisation	1995	Goodwin[15]
10.	MRgFUS	2003	Tempany CM et al[21]

In 1809, Donville (USA) performed the first laparotomy consequent to an indication of myoma[5]. Mrs. Jane Todd Crawford, President Abraham Lincoln's cousin, was 56 years old when she had an abdominal distention and appeared as if she was pregnant with twins. Laxatives, enemas and phytotherapy were first given as treatments to relieve the distention and volume in the abdomen[3]. A surgeon named Ephraim Mcdowell performed a laparotomy to remove the ovarian cyst containing complex content and when it was analysed, it was known to be a pediculate leiomyoma.[6]

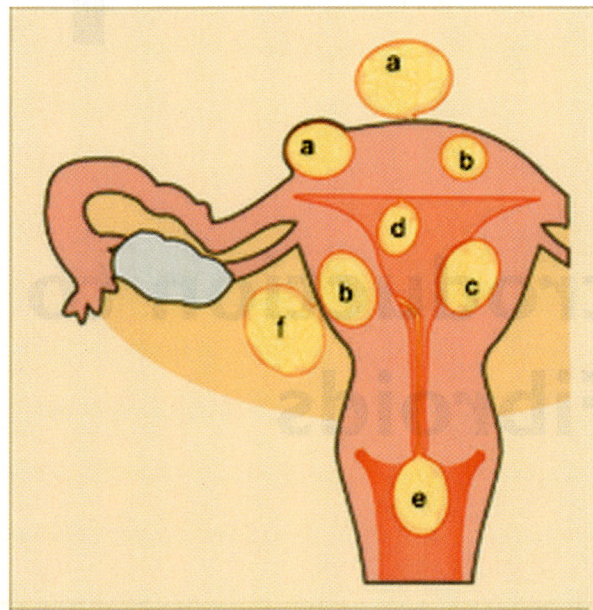

Fig. 1.1: Schematic representation of various types of uterine fibroids. **A.** Subserosal fibroids; **B.** Intramural fibroids, **C.** Submucosal fibroid, **D.** Pedunculated submucosal fibroid, **E.** Pedunculated cervical fibroid, **F.** Fibroid of the broad ligament.

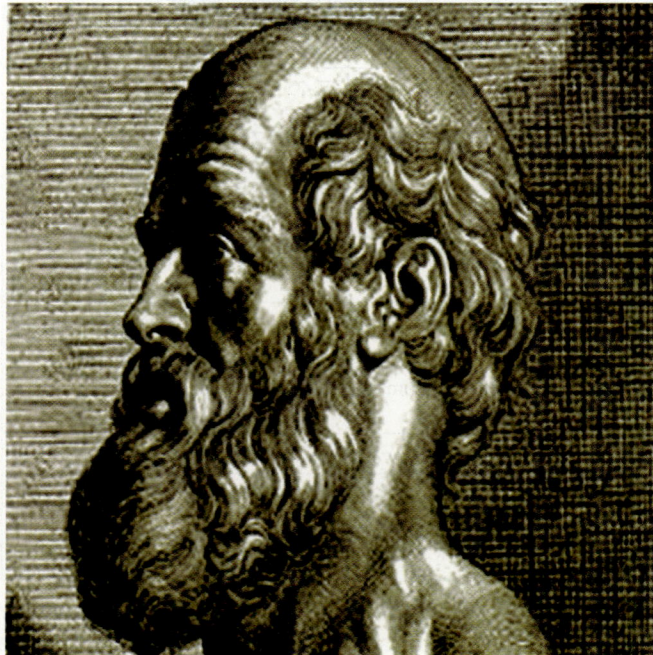

Fig. 1.2: Hippocrates

The first successful operation of uterine fibroids through myomectomy was performed in 1840 by Jean Zuléma Amussat of Paris. In 1842, Amussat reported two submucous fibromyoma cases in which vaginal myomectomies were performed[7]. In 1845, Atlee performed the first successful vaginal myomectomy on a patient with a submucous

pedunculated myoma. Later, Dr Washington Atlee from Pennsylvania was recognized as the first who performed a successful abdominal myomectomy operation that appeared in the American Journal of Medical Science in 1845.

In 1853, Gilman Kimball of Massachusetts conducted the first deliberate myomectomy after diagnosing his patient with uterine fibroids[7]. He is also the first doctor who successfully performed a hysterectomy for the purpose of removing uterine fibroids.[9]

The first abdominal multiple myomectomy was performed by W Alexander of Liverpool in 1898. In the early part of the 20th century, the technique of abdominal myomectomy was refined by many notable gynecologic surgeons, including Kelly, Cullen, Mayo, Rubin, Bonney and others.

In the 1920s, British surgeon Victor Bonney (Fig. 1.3) introduced a specially designed clamp for myomectomy that was placed around the uterine vessels and the round ligaments in an attempt to decrease intraoperative bleeding (Fig. 1.4). By 1930, Victor reported 403 myomectomy cases with minimal fatalities.[3]

Hysteroscopic resection of submucous myomata was first reported by Neuwirth and Amin in 1976 and was reported again by Neuwirth in 1978[10]. The first description of endoscopy is attributed to Phillip Bozzini in 1805, as he

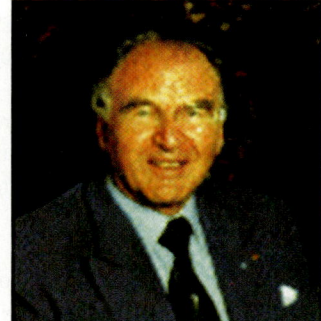

Fig. 1.3: Victor Bonney

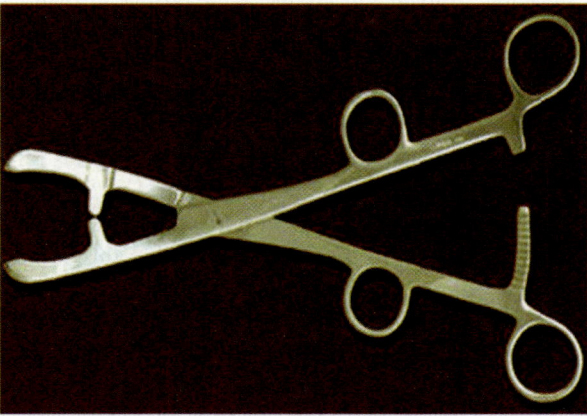

Fig. 1.4: Bonney's myomectomy clamp

attempted to view the urethral mucosa with a simple tube and candlelight. Hysteroscopy was the first gynecologic endoscopic procedure performed when Pantaleoni used a cystoscope to identify uterine polyps in 1869. Laparoscopy was first performed by Jacobaeus of Sweden in 1910, wherein a Nitze cystoscope, composed of a candle and a hollow tube, was used to illuminate the peritoneal cavity. Kalk of Germany was instrumental in developing laparoscopy into a diagnostic and surgical procedure in the early 1930s.[8]

Dr Kurt Semm (Fig. 1.5), a German gynecologist who specialised in infertility, was perhaps the most influential early advocate of modern operative laparoscopy[11]. In the 1960s and 1970s, Dr Semm invented the automatic insufflator, and hundreds of laparoscopic instruments, including a thermocoagulator, loop ligature and devices for extracorporeal and intracorporeal endoscopic knot tying. He was one of the first proponents of video monitoring for laparoscopy, using a series of lenses and mirrors in an articulated arm to connect the laparoscope to a ceiling-mounted video camera. He developed laparoscopic techniques for ovarian cystectomy, myomectomy, treatment of ectopic pregnancy, appendectomy and hysterectomy.

A hand-activated device for laparoscopic tissue removal was developed as early as 1973 and by 1993, the Steiner electromechanical morcellator was introduced.[12] The advent of electromechanical morcellation allowed for marked improvements in ease and speed of specimen retrieval with minimally invasive approaches.[13] As the field of minimally invasive gynecologic surgery has evolved to encompass increasingly challenging procedures, a number of power morcellation devices have been marketed to allow removal of large pathology via small incisions and avoid the morbidity associated with laparotomy.

Another technical innovation called myolysis has been described by Goldfarb and is based on earlier experience in

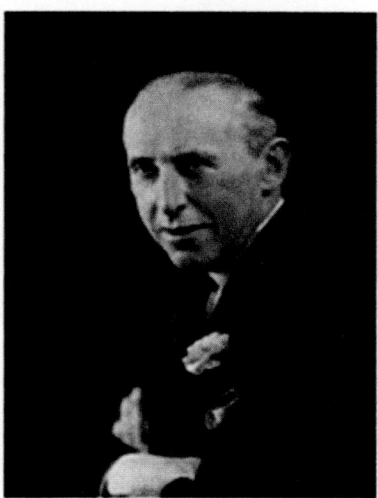

Fig. 1.5: Kurt Semm

Europe. Either neodymium-doped yttrium aluminum garnet (Nd:YAG) laser or bipolar needles are used laparoscopically to penetrate the myomata at multiple sites at a 90° angle to the uterus.[14]

UAE for leiomyomas was first performed in the United States by Goodwin and colleagues in 1995.[15]

Sampson in 1913 was the first to study the blood supply of uterine leiomyomata and its effect on uterine bleeding.[16]

An unusual benign form of leiomyomata uteri, intravenous leiomyomatosis, was first recognized at the turn of the 20th century and has been reported sporadically since then. Before 1982, about 50 cases had been reported, according to Bahary and coworkers[17]. Marshall and Morris presented the first detailed report of this entity in the American literature in 1959. The characteristic feature of this peculiar smooth muscle tumour is the extension of the polypoid intravascular projections into the veins of the parametrium and broad ligaments.

In 1994, the first United States (US) Food and Drug Administration (FDA) approved robotic surgical device called AESOP (automatic endoscopic system for optimal positioning, computer motion, Inc.) was introduced. With this system, the surgeon can control the orientation of the laparoscope through voice commands[18]. In April 2005, the da Vinci Surgical System (Intuitive Surgical, Inc., Sunnyvale, CA) was the first robot approved by the US FDA for gynecologic applications.[19] The da Vinci Robotic Surgical System (Intuitive Surgical) and Zeus Robotic Surgical System (Computer Motion) allow the surgeon to operate from a remote station with hand controls that can provide increased dexterity and minimize fatigue, tremors or incidental hand movement. These systems are being used in surgical centres, but have not gained universal adoption because of technical training and cost limitations. The optimal application for these devices is continuing to be defined.

Prior to the advent of modern minimally invasive surgery techniques, the primary surgical management of symptomatic leiomyomata for women desiring future fertility or uterine conservation was through laparotomy.

Recently, there is an increasing trend for minimal access surgery (MAS) for treatment of uterine myomas. Laparoscopic myomectomy has provided minimal invasive alternative to laparotomy for subserosal and intramural myomas. It is associated with faster postoperative recovery and potentially less postoperative adhesions. Main concerns are however subsequent fertility, reproductive outcome and long-term recurrence. Other alternatives are laparoscopic assisted myomectomy, laparoscopic ultraminilaparotomic embolised myomectomy, laparoscopically-assisted transvaginal myomectomy, myolysis and cryosurgery. Hysteroscopic access is required for submucous myomas.

Interest in non-surgical management also appears to be increasing with more data available regarding minimally invasive procedures, including UAE, radiofrequency ablation and MRgFUS.[19] These procedure has emerged from an investigational realm to common clinical practice.

■ REFERENCES

1. Marshall LM, Spiegelman D, Barbieri RL, et al. Variation in the incidence of uterine leiomyoma among premenopausal women by age and race. Obstet Gynecol. 1997;90:967-73.

2. Day Baird D, Dunson DB, Hill MC, et al. High cumulative incidence of uterine leiomyoma in black and white women: ultrasound evidence. Am J Obstet Gynecol. 2003;188:101-07.

3. Nilo Bozini, Edmund C Baracat. Division of Gynecology - Medical School of University of São Paulo. The history of myomectomy at the Medical School of University of São Paulo Clinics vol.62 no.3 São Paulo 2007.

4. Siskin G. Interventional Radiology in Women's Health.New York: Thieme Medical Publishers Inc.;2009. 27.

5. Hysterectomy: A historical perspective Bailliere's Clinical Obstetrics and Gynaecology. 1997;11:1-22.

6. Drife J, Magowan B. Clinical obstetrics and gynaecology. 2004. p. 10.

7. Leda J. Stacy, M.D. The Treatment of Uterine Fibromyomas. Radiological Society of North America: February 1934 Radiology, 22, 212-218.

8. American Journal of the Medical Sciences: Case of successful Extirpation of a Fibrous Tumour of the peritoneal surface of the Uterus by the large peritoneal section. 1845;18:309-35.

9. Rutkow I. The History of Surgery in the United States. 1775-1900, Vol II p. 102.

10. Neuwirth RS. Hysteroscopic management of symptomatic submucous fibroids. Obstet Gynecol. 1983;62:509.

11. Mettler L, Semm K, Shive K. Endoscopic management of adnexal masses. J Soc Laparoendosc Surg. 1997;1(2):103-12.

12. Steiner R A, Wight E, Tadir Y, et al. Electrical cutting device for laparoscopic removal of tissue from abdominal cavity. Obstet Gynecol. 1993;81(3);471-74.

13. Wang CJ, Yuen LT, Lee CL, et al. A prospective comparison of morcellator and culdotomy for extracting uterine myomas laparoscopically in nullipara.J Minim Invasive Gynecol. 2006;13(5):463-66.

14. Goldfarb H. Laparoscopic coagulation of myoma (myolysis). Obstet Gynecol Clin North Am. 1995;22:807.

15. Goodwin SC, Vedantham S, McLucas B, et al. Uterine artery embolization for uterine fibroids: results of a pilot study. J Vasc Interv Radiol. 1997;8:517.

16. Sampson JA. The influence of myomata on the blood supply of the uterus with special reference to abnormal uterine bleeding. Surg Gynecol Obstet. 1913;16:144.

17. Bahary CM, Gorodeski IG, Nilly M, et al. Intravascular leiomyomatosis.Obstet Gynecol. 1982;59:735.

18. Mettler L, IbrahamM, Jonat W. One year of experience working with the aid of robotic assistant (the voice-controlled optic holder AESOP) in gynaecologic endoscopic surgery. Human reprod. 1998;13:2748-50.

19. Tempany CM, Stewart EA, McDannold N, et al. MR imaging-guided focused ultrasound surgery of uterine leiomyomas: a feasibility study. Radiology. 2003;226(3):897-905.

CHAPTER 2

Aetiology of Uterine Leiomyoma

● Shraddha N Daksha

DEFINITION

Fibroids (various terms are leiomyoma, fibromyoma, myofibroma, leiomyofibroma, fibroleiomyoma, myoma and fibroma) are benign, monoclonal tumours of the smooth muscle cells of the myometrium. They contain large aggregations of extracellular matrix composed of collagen, elastin, fibronectin and proteoglycan (Fig. 2.1).[1]

INCIDENCE

The majority of these monoclonal oestrogen-dependent uterine neoformations afflict mostly women during reproductive age and 80% of the total suffer from this condition during their whole lifetime.[2]

AETIOLOGY

Leiomyoma are benign uterine tumour of unknown aetiology. Although precise aetiology is unknown, advances have been made in understanding the epidemiology, molecular biology, their hormonal, genetic factors and also role of growth factors (Table 2.1).[3]

In considering the development of uterine leiomyoma, it is convenient to subdivide the factors that may be related to tumour genesis into four categories.[3] There are as follows (Figs 2.2 and 2.3):

1. Risk factors.
2. Initiators.
3. Growth promoters.
4. Growth effectors.

Risk Factors

Risk factors are characteristics associated with a condition, generally identified by epidemiological studies. Knowledge of

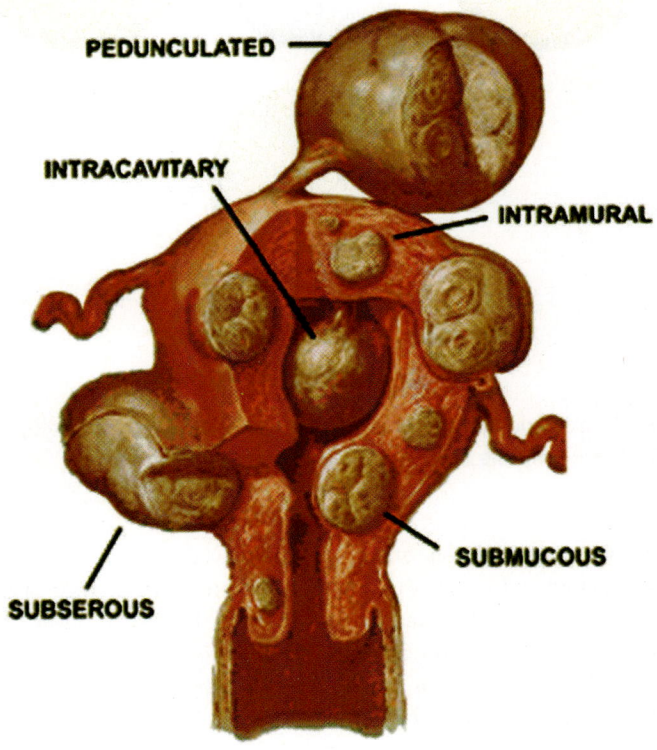

Fig. 2.1: Multiple uterine leiomyomas

Fig. 2.2: Aetiology of uterine leiomyoma

Risk factors	Initiators	Growth promoters	Growth effectors

• Early menarche reproductive age group
• Nulliparity
• Late menopause
• Obesity
• Fatty diet
• Less exercise
• African-american race
• Geographical location
• Smoking
• Ocp
• HRT
• Tamoxifene, xenoestrogens
	Genetic factors:
	• Heritability
	• Clonality
	• Cytogenetics
		Estrogen progesterone
		Estrogen receptor
		Progesterone receptor
		Related enzymes:
		  • 17-beta hydroxysteroid
		    dehydrogenase
		  • Estradiol 14-hydroxylase
		  • 5-alpha reductase
			• TGF-beta
			• bFGF
			• EGF
			• PDGF
			• VEGF
			• IGF
			• PRL

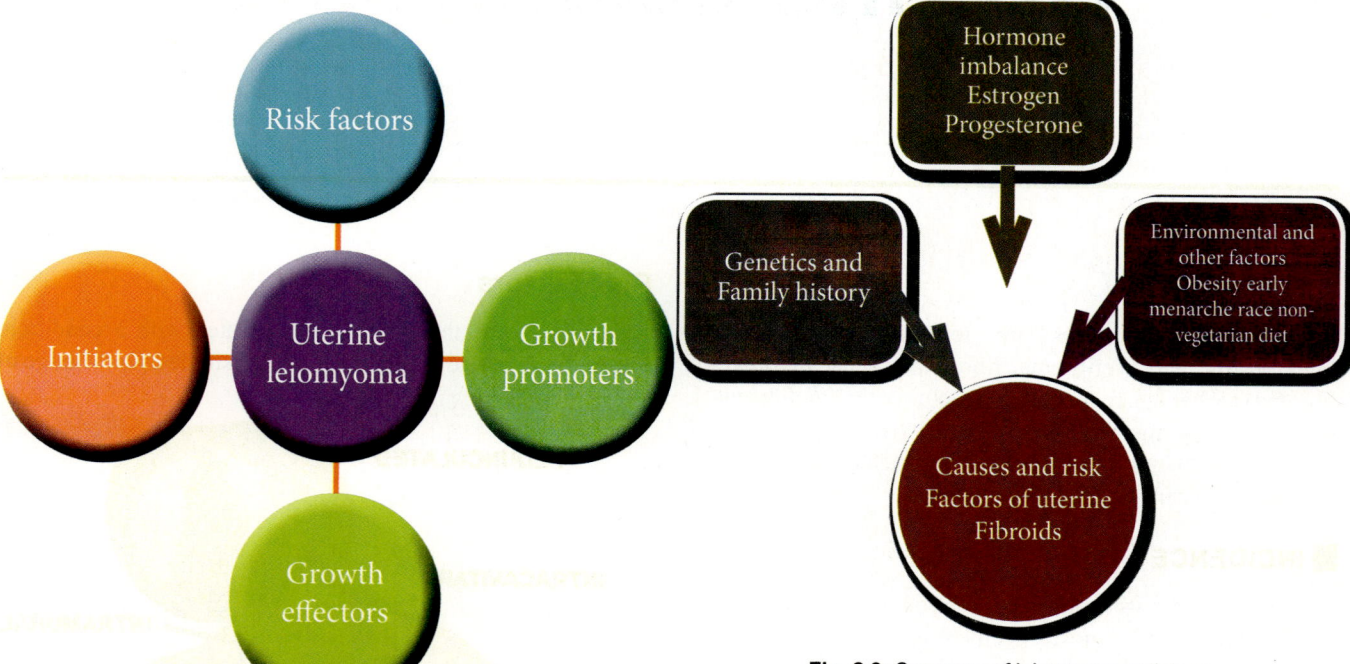

Fig. 2.2: Aetiology of uterine leiomyoma

Fig. 2.3: Summary of leiomyoma aetiology

such predisposing factors may provide clues to the aetiology of these tumours as well as to preventive measures.

Menarche

There is an opinion of slightly increased risk of fibroids associated with early menarche, although the risk has often not been statistically significant.[4–6] The early onset of menstrual cycles may increase the number of cell divisions that the myometrium undergoes during the reproductive years, resulting in an increased chance of mutation in genes controlling myometrial proliferation.[7]

Age

An increase in the prevalence of fibroids with age during the reproductive years has been demonstrated by several epidemiologic studies.[8–11] If the likelihood of fibroid development and growth actually accelerates during the late reproductive years, hormonal factors associated with perimenopause may be important modulators; alternatively, the apparent increase in the late reproductive years may simply represent the cumulative culmination of 20–30 years of stimulation by oestrogen and progesterone.

Parity

Several studies have shown an inverse relationship between parity and the risk of fibroids.[6,9,11,12] An explanation that has been sometimes cited in the literature[9,12] for these findings is that pregnancy reduces the time of exposure to unopposed oestrogens, whereas nulliparity or reduced fertility may be associated with anovulatory cycles characterized by long-term unopposed oestrogens. The alternative possibility exists that uterine fibroids are actually the cause of infertility, rather than the consequence of it; however, the diminished relative risk of fibroids associated with parity remains essentially the same after exclusion of women with a history of infertility.[13]

Menopause

A reduced risk of fibroids requiring surgery in postmenopausal patients could be due to tumour shrinkage in the absence of hormonal stimulus following menopause.[5,6,9]

Obesity

Several studies have found an association between obesity and an increased incidence of uterine leiomyomas. In a prospective study, the risk of fibroids increased approximately 21% for each 10 kg increase in body weight; similar results were obtained when the body mass index (BMI) was analysed rather than weight.[9]

This apparent association between obesity and an increased risk of fibroids may be related to hormonal factors associated with obesity, but other pathologic pathways might also be involved.

Several relevant hormonal associations with obesity are known. A significant increase occurs in the conversion of circulating adrenal androgens to estrone by excess adipose tissue. The hepatic production of sex hormone-binding globulin is decreased, resulting in more unbound physiologically active oestrogen. Because almost all circulating oestrogens postmenopausally are derived from metabolism of circulating androgens by peripheral tissues, including fat, these two mechanisms probably have more impact in postmenopausal than premenopausal women.[14]

In obese premenopausal women, decreased metabolism of estradiol by the 2-hydroxylation route reduces the conversion of estradiol to inactive metabolites, which could result in a relatively hyperoestrogenic state.[15]

Diet

A moderate association was found between the risk of uterine myomas and the consumption of beef, other red meat, and ham, whereas a high intake of green vegetables seemed to have a protective effect[16]. Unfortunately, no estimate of the total caloric intake was obtained, and no attempt was made to estimate the amount of fat in the diet for cases and controls, although one might assume that a higher intake of beef would be associated with a greater amount of fat in the diet (Fig. 2.4A to D).

There are several possible explanations for the greater fecal excretion of oestrogens in vegetarians, including:

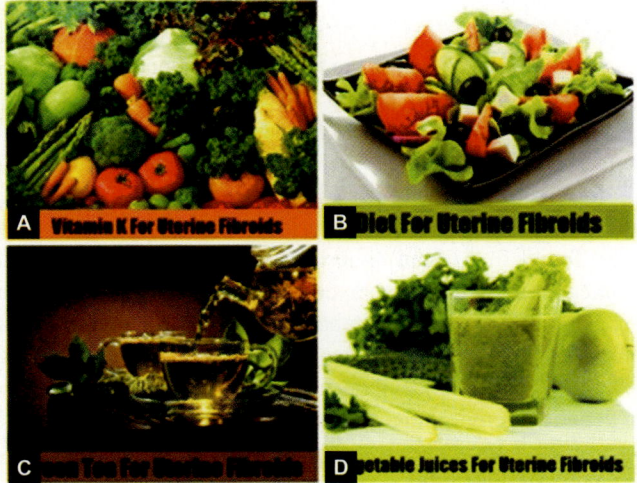

Figs 2.4A to D: Dietary factors that reduce the incidence of leiomyoma. **A.** Vitamin K for uterine fibroids; **B.** Diet for uterine fibroids; **C.** Green tea for uterine fibroids; **D.** Vegetables juices for uterine fibroids.

a. The greater bulk of undigested and nonabsorbed fibre that may shield the oestrogens from bacterial deconjugation and reabsorption.
b. Some characteristic of the vegetarian diet that decreases the ability of the intestinal flora to deconjugate biliary oestrogen conjugates, a necessary step for their reabsorption.
c. An effect related to lower dietary fat levels that might diminish oestrogen absorption.[17,18]

Prediction of the effects of phytoestrogens is uncertain because there are so many variables involved. Despite their weak oestrogenic activity, however, phytoestrogens could conceivably have a significant clinical impact, as their concentrations in the body may exceed those of the endogenous oestrogens.[19]

Exercise

Women in the highest category of physical activity (approximately 7 hours per week) are significantly less likely to have fibroids than women in lowest category (< 2 hours per week).[20] Former nonathletic were found to be 1.4 times more likely than former athletes to develop benign uterine tumours. In addition to differences in the degree of physical activity, however, an athletic lifestyle may have been associated with long-term differences in diet and relative leanness and, in turn, with reduced conversion of androgens to oestrogens in adipose tissue.[21,22]

Racial Differences

The prevalence is relatively higher among African Americans than other ethnic groups based upon ultrasound data, and, more importantly, the clinical prevalence (symptomatic cases) is higher among African Americans because of a higher frequency of multiple lesions and greater size of the fibroids.[8,23]

Although the basis for the higher prevalence among black women is unknown, ethnic differences have been found in circulating oestrogen levels, while on control diets and differences in oestrogen metabolism have been noted. In addition, significantly lower 2-hydroxyestrone (2-OHE1)/16α-hydroxyestrone (16α-OHE1) urinary metabolite ratios have been found in African-American women than in caucasian women, which could also contribute to greater oestrogen exposure, as 2-OHE1 metabolites are devoid of peripheral biological activity, whereas 16α-OHE1 is oestrogenic. Whether the difference in oestrogen metabolism might be due to genetic or environmental factors is unknown (Table 2.2).[24]

Table 2.2: Incidence of leiomyoma in different races[8]

Race	Incidence (per thousand)
Black	30.6
White	8.9
Asian	8
Hispanic	11
American Indian/Alaskan Native	Not determined

Geographical Variation

Knowledge of the prevalence of uterine fibroids in other countries could provide clues to the importance of diet, environmental factors and ethnicity, but unfortunately, few such studies exist in the literature. Although no firm statistical conclusions can be drawn, many reports suggest that uterine fibroids occur commonly in women in many parts of the world.

Smoking

Several studies have revealed a reduced risk of fibroids associated with current smoking but not past smoking.[5,6,9,11,22,25] Several derangements of steroid metabolism have been identified in smokers. Increased 2-hydroxylation of estradiol occurs in smokers, resulting in decreased bioavailability at oestrogen target tissues.[26] Nicotine inhibition of aromatase reduces the conversion of androgens to estrone.[27] Significantly higher serum levels of sex hormone-binding globulin have been found, resulting in less unbound physiologically active oestrogen.[28] Increased androstenedione and cortisol levels have been noted in postmenopausal smokers, suggestive of increased adrenal activity; elevated androgens may be significant, as some evidence exists that androgens can inhibit oestrogen-mediated effects in the rat uterus.[29,30] These studies indicate that the hormonal metabolic effects of smoking are probably multifactorial. In addition, smokers as a group consistently exhibit lower body weights than non-smokers,

possibly because of a lower efficiency of calorie storage and/or an increased metabolic rate.[31]

Oral Contraceptive Pills

Reports in the literature present inconsistencies with regard to the effect of oral contraceptive (OC) use upon the growth of myomas. No conclusions could be drawn regarding the oestrogens present, it has been found that higher the dose of the progestogen norethisterone acetate, lower the incidence of fibroids, in preparations containing the same quantity of the oestrogen ethinylestradiol.[9] In contrast, all preparations containing the progestogen ethynodiol diacetate were associated with an increased incidence of fibroids, regardless of the quantity present, or the type or amount of the accompanying oestrogen.

A significantly elevated risk of fibroids has been reported among women who first used OCs in their early teenage years (13–16 years of age) compared with those who had never used them.[13]

Hormone Replacement Therapy

Fibroids are expected to shrink after menopause, but hormone replacement therapy (HRT) may prevent this shrinkage and may even stimulate growth. The effect of HRT on fibroids in postmenopausal women is obviously a complicated issue resolvable only by future well-controlled studies. Further emphasizing this point is the assertion that an increase in volume or number of uterine myomas during HRT in postmenopause is mostly not related solely to the dose and route of administration of the oestrogen, but also to the type and dosage of progestogen.[32]

Tamoxifen

Tamoxifen is a partial oestrogen agonist that binds to ERs in receptive cells, thereby antagonizing the effects of oestrogen by competitively binding to target organ receptors. Because tamoxifen is effective adjuvant therapy for ER positive breast cancer, it might be expected to induce regression of oestrogen-responsive uterine fibroids. The biologic actions of tamoxifen are complex, and the information gained from animal models and tissue culture is not necessarily directly transferable to humans. The disparate effects of tamoxifen in the breast and uterus exemplify the mixed agonist/antagonist activity of SERMs, which is apparently dictated by the type and the promoter context of the ERs for a given cell type.[33]

Xenoestrogens

A diverse group of exogenous compounds, xenoestrogens, possesses the potential to disrupt normal oestrogenic function as a result of either oestrogenic agonist or antagonistic effects.[34] No common chemical structure is predictive of oestrogenic activity and such substances may originate from dietary, industrial or pharmaceutical sources. The pesticide dichlorodiphenyltrichloroethane (DDT) and its analogs have been shown to be oestrogenic.[35] Also of interest is the finding that the more recently recognized ER-β binds two xenoestrogens, methoxychlor and bisphenol A, with considerably higher affinity than the classic ER, ER-α.[36] In view of the widespread use and exposure to the organochlorine pesticides and other environmental oestrogens, there is a need clearly exists for further investigation of a possible link to fibroid pathogenesis. Studies with the potent synthetic oestrogen diethylstilbestrol have clearly indicated that exogenous oestrogen exposure during critical stages of development can result in permanent cellular and molecular alterations, including the formation of uterine leiomyomas.[37,38]

Initiators

The initiators of fibroids are unknown; however, a few of the theories of initiation have been discussed below. The occurrence of genetic aberrations in fibroid tumour is considered. Despite the abundance of cytogenetic investigations, uncertainty remains as to the primary or secondary nature of these genetic changes and their impact on the initiation and/or promotion of these tumours.

Theories of Initiation

The most important aspect of the aetiology of fibroids are the initiator(s) that remains unknown. Several theories have been advanced.

One hypothesis states that increased levels of oestrogen and progesterone result in an increased mitotic rate that may contribute to myoma formation by increasing the likelihood of somatic mutations.[39] Another favours an inherent abnormality in the myometrium of those who develop fibroids, based upon the finding of significantly increased levels of ER in the myometrium of fibroid uteri.[40] A predisposing genetic factor has been suggested by others on the basis of ethnic and familial predilections.[8,41]

Another interesting theory postulates that the pathogenesis of uterine leiomyomas might be similar to a response to injury[42] in a manner analogous to the development of keloids (hypertrophic scars) following surgery. One avenue of potential injury might be ischemia associated with the release of increased vasoconstrictive substances at the time of menses. Increased secretion of prostaglandins and vasopressin by the endometrium has been noted in patients with dysmenorrhoea, which occurs in up to 70% of women by the 5th year after menarche.[43,44] After vascular injury, basic fibroblast growth factor (b-FGF) is critical to smooth muscle proliferation, and this factor is also overexpressed in leiomyomas.[45,46] Finally, injury related to menses is worthy of consideration in view of the universality of menstruation and the commonality of

fibroids. When we consider the various risk factors, including those that have been attributed in the literature to increased exposure to 'unopposed oestrogens', such as early menarche and nulliparity, we observe that such patients also experience more menstrual cycles than their counterparts.

Of equal uncertainty in the genesis of fibroids is the role of genetic and/or epigenetic changes. The possibility of hereditary genetic predisposition to fibroids cannot be excluded at this time. On the other hand, evidence has been presented, though limited in scope that karyotypic changes may occur secondarily[47] during the evolution or aging of some fibroids. Regardless of whether acquired karyotypic changes occur ab initio or during clonal evolution of fibroids, we can assume that preceding stimuli, conditions, or injuries must be responsible for the induction of genetic or epigenetic changes, and in this sense acquired genetic changes may be regarded as secondary. These changes are therefore discussed in this section, not from the standpoint of purported initiators, but as possible potentiators or effectors of currently unrecognized initiating conditions.

Genetic Findings

There have been numerous studies and reviews of the clonality and cytogenetics of uterine leiomyomas (Fig. 2.5).

Heritability

Is there evidence of a genetic predisposition to fibroids? This question has been approached from four perspectives in ethnic predisposition, twin studies, familial aggregation and

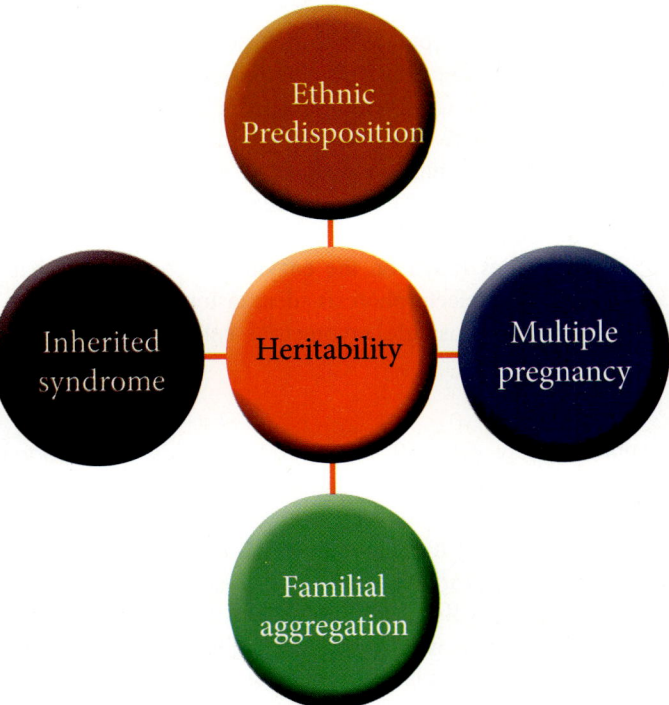

Fig. 2.5: Genetic predisposition to leiomyoma

association with an inherited syndrome. The higher incidence of clinically significant fibroids among African-American women (2.9 times increased risk)[48] has been discussed above.

First degree relatives of women with fibroids have a 2.5 times increased risk of developing fibroids[49]. Monozygous twins are reportedly hospitalised for treatment of fibroids more often than heterozygous twins, but these findings may be the result of reporting bias.[50]

Finally, a rare inherited disorder known as Reed's Syndrome,[51,52,53] or multiple leiomyomatosis, is characterized by the appearance of multiple leiomyomas in the skin, uterus, or both. The family histories in these cases suggest an autosomal dominant inheritance with incomplete penetrance. A subset of these with papillary renal cell carcinoma, have independently linked this disorder to a predisposition gene in the region of chromosome 1q42.3-q43.[54,55,56] In follow-up studies of this chromosomal region, mutations were detected only in the fumarate hydratase gene[57]—a surprising finding, as this enzyme is a component of the essential energy-producing tricarboxylic acid cycle.[58] Furthermore, the gene appears to act as a classic tumour suppressor in that loss of the wildtype allele was observed frequently in the leiomyomata and renal cell cancers.[54] Although this hereditary syndrome is itself rare, the association with inactivation of the fumarate hydratase gene is of interest, as it is possible that other mechanisms of transcriptional silencing of this gene such as promoter hypermethylation could be involved in the development of sporadic leiomyomas.[55]

Clonality

There is general acceptance in the literature that these tumours are monoclonal. The underlying premise of these studies has been based on the Lyon hypothesis, which assumes that only one X chromosome is active in any female cell, the other X chromosome remaining in an inactive state as a Barr body, and that the X chromosome that is inactivated (methylated) is determined randomly.

Early studies based on the enzyme glucose-6-phosphate dehydrogenase electrophoresis demonstrated that fibroids are derived from single myometrial cell, i.e. fibroids are monoclonal.[48]

Cytogenetics

Approximately 40%–50% of uterine fibroids are reported to have non-random chromosomal abnormalities. These include t(12;14)—frequency about 20%, del(7) (q22–q32)—about 17%, trisomy 12—about 12%, 6p21 (deletion, inversion, translocation and insertions—about < 5%.[59] Others chromosomes involved are 3q(del) and 10q. Critical region involved affecting in chromosome[7] appears on long arm. Cellular, atypical and large fibroids are mostly likely to show chromosomal abnormalities.[60]

Growth Promoters

The role of growth promoters of fibroids seems to belong in large part to the ovarian hormones, i.e. oestrogen and progesterone, as discussed below.

Oestrogen has been traditionally proposed as the primary promoter of uterine leiomyoma growth. This supposition has been based in part upon the clinical observations that fibroids occur only after menarche, develop during the reproductive years, may enlarge during pregnancy, and frequently regress following menopause.

Furthermore, because the risk of fibroids is greater in nulliparous women who might be subject to a higher frequency of anovulatory cycles and obese women with greater aromatization of androgens to estrone in the fat, the concept of unopposed oestrogens as an underlying cause of uterine fibroids has sometimes been proposed in the literature[9,12,61,62]. Increased growth of myomas among women taking tamoxifen or receiving transdermal or injected oestrogen replacement therapy further supports the importance of oestrogen. The oestrogen hypothesis has also been supported by clinical trials evaluating the medical treatment of myomas with GnRH agonists, the effective result of which is hypoestrogenism accompanied by regression of the fibroids.[63]

As noted by Rein,[64] however, distinguishing the relative importance of oestrogen versus progesterone is difficult, as progesterone levels, in a manner similar to those of oestrogen, are also cyclically elevated during the reproductive years, are significantly elevated during pregnancy, and are suppressed after menopause. Furthermore, regression of uterine leiomyomata has been induced by treatment with the antiprogesterone drug RU 486, accompanied by reduction in the progesterone receptor (PR) but not the ER in the tumours, suggesting that the regression was attained through a direct antiprogesterone effect.[65] In addition, patients treated with leuprolide (a GnRH agonist, capable of reducing the size of fibroids) who were concomitantly given medroxyprogesterone acetate demonstrated no significant reduction in myoma or uterine volume[66,67]. Indeed, clinical and laboratory evidence to date would appear to indicate that oestrogen and progesterone may both be important as promoters of myoma growth.

The evidence available suggests that during the follicular phase, oestrogen upregulates ER and PR, thus setting the stage for the luteal phase progesterone surge associated with a heightened mitogenic effect and subsequent downregulation of ER and PR.

17β-Hydroxysteroid Dehydrogenase

Regardless of the phase of the cycle, the proliferative index of leiomyomas is significantly higher than that of the myometrium.[68,69,70] This finding is not surprising in view of the elevated levels of both ERs and PRs in leiomyomas throughout the menstrual cycle. Because estradiol up-regulates both of these receptors, there is increased concentration of estradiol in these tumours compared with that in the myometrium (Fig. 2.6).[71]

The demonstration of reduced activity in leiomyomas of the enzyme 17β-hydroxysteroid dehydrogenase,[72,73] the enzyme responsible for the conversion of estradiol to estrone, would seem to provide a plausible explanation for the accumulation of estradiol in these tumours. Although estrone is weakly oestrogenic, it exhibits a lower binding affinity for ERs than estradiol, and it diffuses out of the cell more rapidly than estradiol.

In the myometrium, the activity of this enzyme is maximal during the early secretory phase because of upregulation by progesterone,[74] resulting in a diminished estradiol effect during the second half of the cycle. In leiomyomas, on the other hand, the reduced activity of 17β-hydroxysteroid dehydrogenase may allow for the accumulation of estradiol in the cells during the secretory as well as the proliferative phase of the cycle, thus resulting in continual stimulation by oestrogen, with upregulation of both the ERs and PRs, accompanied the associated growth-promoting effects. Whether the enzymatic deficiency is a quantitative or qualitative one, and regardless of whether it is a primary or secondary development in the genesis of fibroids, the reduced activity of this enzyme could play a significant role in the pathogenesis of these tumours.

Estradiol 4-hydroxylase

4-hydroxylation of estradiol is 8-fold higher than that of 2-hydroxylation in myomas and further more it is substantially elevated in myomas compared with surrounding myometrial tissue.[75] Because the dissociation rate of 4-hydroxyestradiol

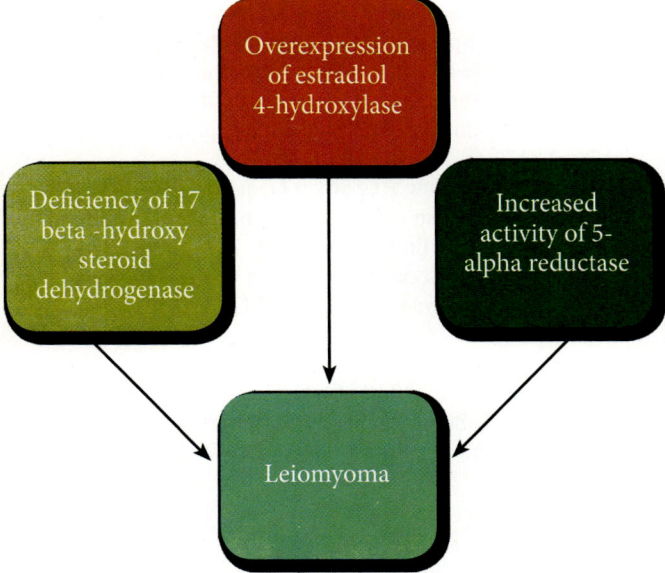

Fig. 2.6: Enzymatic derangements in leiomyoma

from the ER complex is also reduced compared with estradiol,[76] this catechol metabolite may also function as a long-acting oestrogen, and suggesting over expressed 4-hydroxylase activity may play a role in the aetiology of uterine fibroids.[75]

5-alpha Reductase

5-alpha reduced androgens may play a role in the pathophysiology of leiomyoma, because a significant increase in 5-alpha reductase activity in leiomyoma as compared to normal myometrium and endometrium.[77]

Oestrogen and progesterone appear to be promoters of fibroid growth, acting in concert. Thus oestrogen upregulates both ERs and PRs during the follicular phase, followed by progesterone-induced mitogenesis during the luteal phase. The deficiency of the oestrogen-metabolizing enzyme 17β-hydroxysteroid dehydrogenase in fibroids may be responsible for the accumulation of estradiol in these tumours and its consequent growth promoting effects. Likewise, the overexpression of estradiol 4-hydroxylase seems highly significant, as the resulting metabolite possesses long-acting oestrogenic activity.[3]

Effectors (Growth Factors and their Receptors)

The growth promoting effects of oestrogen and progesterone upon the myometrium and uterine myomas may be mediated through the mitogenic effects of growth factors produced locally by smooth muscle cells and fibroblasts.[46,78] Following growth factors/hormones are associated fibroid genesis:
1. Transforming growth factor- beta (TGF-β).
2. Basic fibroblast growth factor (bFGF).
3. Epidermal growth factor (EGF).
4. Pplatelet-derived growth factor (PDGF).
5. Vascular endothelial growth factor (VEGF).
6. Insulin-like growth factor (IGF).
7. Prolactin (PRL).

The levels of several growth factors and their receptors are increased in fibroids. TGF-β3 and bFGF may be especially important in the pathogenesis of these tumours in view of their combined mitogenic effect and promotion of extracellular matrix production. EGF appears to be significant, as it is the only characterized factor, other than TGF-β3, with elevated expression during the luteal phase, when leiomyoma mitotic activity is maximal.[3]

The PDGF is a potent mitogen for vascular smooth muscle cells and another of the heparin-binding growth factors along with bFGF and VEGF. Because of the capacity of these factors to bind to heparin, they may become sequestered in the extracellular matrix, which is typically abundant in fibroids and may therefore serve as a reservoir for these growth factors. The mRNA for PDGF is expressed in leiomyomas, but the levels are similar to those found in the myometrium. On the other hand, significantly more PDGF receptor sites per cell are seen in leiomyomas than in the myometrium, although the PDGF receptor binding affinity in the tumour cells is lower than that of the myometrium. Perhaps the most interesting aspect of PDGF in leiomyomas, however, may not be its growth factor role, acting in isolation, but rather its action in conjunction with other growth factors such as EGF and IGFs.[3]

The IGF-I almost certainly plays an important role because of its potent mitogenic capacity and the overexpression of both the peptide and its receptor in leiomyomas. Growth factors may be the mediators or effectors of sex steroid upregulation, but a primary dysregulation of one or more growth factors must also be considered.[3]

The significance of prolactin production in leiomyomas is not yet well defined; however, interest in this hormone has been stimulated by the finding that prolactin acts as a mitogen for vascular smooth muscle.[79] However, in a recent study, treatment of leiomyoma and myometrial cell cultures with a prolactin-neutralizing antibody inhibited cell proliferation, leading to conclusion that prolactin may be an autocrine or paracrine growth factor for both leiomyoma and myometrial.[80] At this date, it would seem that the prolactin story is unfinished, evolving and of further study.

■ CONCLUSION

Uterine leiomyomas, or fibroids, represent a major public health problem. It becomes symptomatic in one-third of these women. Although the initiator or initiators of fibroids are unknown, several predisposing factors have been identified, including age (late reproductive years), African-American ethnicity, nulliparity, and obesity. Nonrandom cytogenetic abnormalities have been found in about 40% of tumours examined. Oestrogen and progesterone are recognized as promoters of tumour growth, and the potential role of environmental oestrogens has only recently been explored. Growth factors with mitogenic activity, such as transforming growth factor-β3, basic fibroblast growth factor, epidermal growth factor, and insulin-like growth factor-I, are elevated in fibroids and may be the effectors of oestrogen and progesterone promotion.

On the basis of our current state of knowledge, we can only speculate upon the initiators of this common condition. Future research efforts may provide a better understanding, however, of the causes and mechanisms of uterine fibroid tumourigenesis. Insights resulting from elucidation of the basic biology of these tumours might then be successfully translated into preventative strategies that will reduce the incidence and/or morbidity of this disease.

■ REFERENCES

1. Leppert PC, Catherino WH, Segars JH. A new hypothesis about the origin of uterine fibroids based on gene expression profiling with microarrays. Am J Obstet Gynecol 2006; 195: 415-420.
2. Laughlin SK, Schroeder JC, Baird DD. New directions in the epidemiology of uterine fibroids. Seminars in Reproductive Medicine. 2010;28(3):204-210.
3. Flake GP, Andersen J, Dixon D. Etiology and pathogenesis of uterine leiomyomas: a review. Environ Health Perspect. 2003;111:1037-54.
4. Cramer SF, Horiszny JA, Leppert P. Epidemiology of uterine leiomyomas. With an etiologic hypothesis. J Reprod Med. 1995;40:595-600.
5. Parazzini F, La Vecchia C, Negri E, et al. Epidemiologic characteristics of women with uterine fibroids: a case-control study. Obstet Gynecol. 1988;72:853-57.
6. Samadi AR, Lee NC, Flanders WD, et al. Risk factors for self-reported uterine fibroids: a case-control study. Am J Public Health. 1996;86:858-62.
7. Marshall LM, Spiegelman D, Goldman MB, et al. A prospective study of reproductive factors and oral contraceptive use in relation to the risk of uterine leiomyomata. Fertil Steril 1998a;70:432-39.
8. Marshall LM, Spiegelman D, Barbieri RL, et al. Variation in the incidence of uterine leiomyoma among premenopausal women by age and race. Obstet Gynecol 1997;90:967-73.
9. Ross RK, Pike MC, Vessey MP, et al. Risk factors for uterine fibroids: reduced risk associated with oral contraceptives. Br Med J (Clin Res Ed). 1986;293:359-62.
10. Velebil P, Wingo PA, Xia Z, et al. Rate of hospitalization for gynecologic disorders among reproductive-age women in the United States. Obstet Gynecol. 1995;86:764-69.
11. Lumbiganon P, Rugpao S, Phandhu-fung S, et al. Protective effect of depot-medroxyprogesterone acetate on surgically treated uterine leiomyomas: a multicentre case-control study. Br J Obstet Gynaecol. 1996;103:909-14.
12. Parazzini F, Negri E, La Vecchia C, et al. Reproductive factors and risk of uterine fibroids. Epidemiology. 1996;7:440-42.
13. Marshall LM, Spiegelman D, Goldman MB, et al. A prospective study of reproductive factors and oral contraceptive use in relation to the risk of uterine leiomyomata. Fertil Steril. 1998;70:432-39.
14. Glass AR. Endocrine aspects of obesity. Med Clin North Am. 1989;73:139-60.
15. Schneider J, Bradlow HL, Strain G, et al. Effects of obesity on estradiol metabolism: decreased formation of nonuterotropic metabolites. J Clin Endocrinol Metab. 1983;56:973-78.
16. Chiaffarino F, Parazzini F, La Vecchia C, et al. Diet and uterine myomas. Obstet Gynecol. 1999;94:395-98.
17. Goldin BR, Adlercreutz H, Gorbach SL, et al. Estrogen excretion patterns and plasma levels in vegetarian and omnivorous women. N Engl J Med. 1982;307:1542-47.
18. Gorbach SL, Goldin BR. Diet and the excretion and enterohepatic cycling of estrogens. Prev Med. 1987;16:525-31.
19. Adlercreutz H, Fotsis T, Heikkinen R, et al. Excretion of the lignans enterolactone and enterodiol and of equol in omnivorous

and vegetarian postmenopausal women and in women with breast cancer. Lancet 1982;2:1295-99.

20. Baird D, Dunson D, Hill M, et al. Association of physical activity with development of uterine leiomyoma. Am J Epidemiol. 2007;165:157-63.

21. Frisch RE, Wyshak G, Albright NL, et al. Lower prevalence of breast cancer and cancers of the reproductive system among former college athletes compared to non-athletes. Br J Cancer. 1985;52:885-91.

22. Wyshak G, Frisch RE, Albright NL, et al. Lower prevalence of benign diseases of the breast and benign tumours of the reproductive system among former college athletes compared to non-athletes. Br J Cancer. 1986;54:841-45.

23. Baird DD, Schectman JM, Dixon D, et al. African Americans at higher risk than whites for uterine fibroids: ultrasound evidence. Am J Epidemiol. 1998;147:90.

24. Taioli E, Garte SJ, Trachman J, et al. Ethnic differences in estrogen metabolism in healthy women [correspondence]. J Natl Cancer Inst. 1996;88:617.

25. Parazzini F, Negri E, La Vecchia C, et al. Uterine myomas and smoking. Results from an Italian study. J Reprod Med. 1996;41:316-20.

26. Michnovicz JJ, Hershcopf RJ, Naganuma H, et al. Increased 2-hydroxylation of estradiol as a possible mechanism for the anti-estrogenic effect of cigarette smoking. N Engl J Med. 1986;315:1305-09.

27. Barbieri RL, McShane PM, Ryan KJ. Constituents of cigarette smoke inhibit human granulosa cell aromatase. Fertil Steril. 1986;46:232-36.

28. Daniel M, Martin AD, Faiman C. Sex hormones and adipose tissue distribution in premenopausal cigarette smokers. Int J Obes Relat Metab Disord. 1992;16:245-54.

29. Cassidenti DL, Pike MC, Vijod AG, et al. A reevaluation of estrogen status in postmenopausal women who smoke. Am J Obstet Gynecol. 1992;166:1444-48.

30. Hung TT, Gibbons WE. Evaluation of androgen antagonism of estrogen effect by dihydrotestosterone. J Steroid Biochem. 1983.19:1513-20.

31. Wack JT, Rodin J. Smoking and its effects on body weight and the systems of caloric regulation. Am J Clin Nutr. 1982;35:366-80.

32. Polatti F, Viazzo F, Colleoni R, et al. Uterine myoma in postmenopause: a comparison between two therapeutic schedules of HRT. Maturitas. 2000;37:27-32.

33. Hall JM, Couse JF, Korach KS. The multifaceted mechanisms of estradiol and estrogen receptor signaling. J Biol Chem. 2001;276:36869-72.

34. Houston KD, Hunter DS, Hodges LC, et al. Uterine leiomyomas: mechanisms of tumorigenesis. Toxicol Pathol. 2001;29:100-4.

35. Cecil HC, Bitman J, Harris SJ. Estrogenicity of -DDT in rats. J Agric Food Chem. 1971;19:61-5.

36. Enmark E, Pelto-Huikko M, Grandien K, et al. Human estrogen receptor beta-gene structure, chromosomal localization, and expression pattern. J Clin Endocrinol Metab. 1997;82:4258-65.

37. Newbold R. Cellular and molecular effects of developmental exposure to diethylstilbestrol: implications for other environmental estrogens. Environ Health Perspect. 1995; 103(7):83-7.

38. Newbold RR, Moore AB, Dixon D. Characterization of uterine leiomyomas in CD-1 mice following developmental exposure to diethylstilbestrol (DES). Toxicol Pathol. 2002;30:611-16.

39. Rein MS. Advances in uterine leiomyoma research: the progesterone hypothesis. Environ Health Perspect. 2000;108(5):791-3.

40. Richards PA, Tiltman AJ. Anatomical variation of the oestrogen receptor in the non-neoplastic myometrium of fibromyomatous uteri. Virchows Arch. 1996;428:347-51.

41. Schwartz SM, Voigt L, Tickman E, et al. Familial aggregation of uterine leiomyomata. Am J Epidemiol. 2000;151:10.

42. Stewart EA, Nowak RA. Leiomyoma-related bleeding: a classic hypothesis updated for the molecular era. Hum Reprod Update 1996;2:295-306.

43. Emans SJ, Laufer MR, Goldstein DP. Pediatric and Adolescent Gynecology. Philadelphia:Williams and Wilkins. 1998.

44. Coupey S. Primary Care of Adolescent Girls. Philadelphia:Hanley and Belfus. 2000.

45. Lindner V, Reidy MA. Proliferation of smooth muscle cells after vascular injury is inhibited by an antibody against basic fibroblast growth factor.Proc Natl Acad Sci USA. 1991;88:3739-43.

46. Mangrulkar RS, Ono M, Ishikawa M, Takashima S, Klagsbrun M, Nowak RA. Isolation and characterization of heparin-binding growth factors in human leiomyomas and normal myometrium. Biol Reprod. 1995;53:636-46.

47. Mashal RD, Fejzo MLS, Friedman AJ, et al. Analysis of androgen receptor DNA reveals the independent clonal origins of uterine leiomyomata and the secondary nature of cytogenetic aberrations in the development of leiomyomata. Genes Chromosomes Cancer. 1994;11:1-6.

48. Townsend DE, Sparkes RS, Baluda MC, et al. Unicellular histogenesis of uterine leiomyomas as determined by electrophoresis of glucose-6-phosphate dehydrogenase. Am J Obstet Gynecol. 1970;107:1168-73.

49. Vikhlyaeva EM, Khodzhaeva ZS, Fantschenko ND. Familial predisposition to uterine leiomyomas. Int J Gynaecol Obstet. 1995;51:127-31.

50. Treloar SA, Martin NG, Dennerstein L, et al. Pathways to hysterectomy: insights from longitudinal twin research. Am J Obstet Gynaecol. 1992;167:82-8.

51. Thyresson HN, Su WP. Familial cutaneous leiomyomatosis. J Am Acad Dermatol 1981;4:430–434.

52. Fisher WC, Helwig EB. Leiomyomas of the skin. Arch Dermatol. 1963;88:510-20.

53. Reed WB, Walker R, Horowitz R. Cutaneous leiomyomata with uterine leiomyomata. Acta Derm Venereol. 1973;53:409-16.

54. Alam NA, Bevan S, Churchman M, et al. Localization of a gene (MCUL1) for multiple cutaneous leiomyomata anduterine fibroids to chromosome 1q42.3-q43. Am J Hum Genet. 2001;68:1264-69.

55. Kiuru M, Launonen V, Hietala M, et al. Familial cutaneous leiomyomatosis is a two-hit condition associated with renal cell cancer of characteristic histopathology. Am J Pathol. 2001;159:825-29.

56. Launonen V, Vierimaa O, Kiuru M, Isola J, Roth S, Pukkala E, et al. Inherited susceptibility to uterine leiomyomas and renal cell cancer. Proc Natl Acad Sci USA 2001;98:3387–3392.

57. Tomlinson IP, Alam NA, Rowan AJ, et al. Germline mutations in FH predispose to dominantly inherited uterine fibroids, skin leiomyomata and papillary renal cell cancer. Nat Genet. 2002;30:406-10.

58. Rustin P, Bourgeron T, Parfait B, et al. Inborn errors of the Krebs cycle: a group of unusual mitochondrial diseases in human. Biochim Biophys Acta. 1997;1361:185-97.

59. Ligon AH, Morton CC. Genetics of uterine leiomyomata. Genes Chromosomes. Cancer. 2000;28:235-45.

60. Lee EJ, Kong G, Lee SH, et al. Profiling of differentially expressed genes in human uterine leiomyomas. Inj J Gynaecol Cancer. 2005;15:146-154.

61. Cramer DW. Epidemiology of myomas. Semin Reprod Endocrinol. 1992;10:320-24.

62. Romieu I, Walker AM, Jick S. Determinants of uterine fibroids. Post Market Surveill. 1991;5:119-33.

63. Friedman AJ, Harrison-Atlas D, Barbieri RL, et al. A randomized, placebo-controlled, double-blind study evaluating the efficacy of leuprolide acetate depot in the treatment of uterine leiomyomata. Fertil Steril. 1989;51:251-6.

64. Rein MS, Barbieri RL, Friedman AJ. Progesterone: a critical role in the pathogenesis of uterine myomas. Am J Obstet Gynecol. 1995;172:14-8.

65. Murphy AA, Kettel LM, Morales AJ, et al. Regression of uterine leiomyomata in response to the antiprogesterone RU 486. J Clin Endocrinol Metab. 1993;76:513-7.

66. Carr BR, Marshburn PB, Weatherall PT, et al. An evaluation of the effect of gonadotropin-releasing hormone analogs and medroxyprogesterone acetate on uterine leiomyomata volume by magnetic resonance imaging: a prospective, randomized, double blind, placebo-controlled, crossover trial. J Clin Endocrinol Metab. 1993;76:1217-23.

67. Friedman AJ, Barbieri RL, Doubilet PM, et al. A randomized, double-blind trial of a gonadotropin releasing- hormone agonist (leuprolide) with or without medroxyprogesterone acetate in the treatment of leiomyomata uteri. Fertil Steril. 1988;49:404-9.

68. Dixon D, Flake GP, Moore AB, et al. Cell proliferation and apoptosis in human uterine leiomyomas and myometria. Virchows Arch. 2002;441:53-62.

69. Kawaguchi K, Fujii S, Konishi I, et al. Immunohistochemical analysis of oestrogen receptors, progesterone receptors and Ki-67 in leiomyoma and myometrium during the menstrual cycle and pregnancy. Virchows Arch A Pathol Anat Histopathol. 1991;419:309-15.

70. Maruo T, Matsuo H, Samoto T, et al. Effects of progesterone on uterine leiomyoma growth and apoptosis. Steroids. 2000;65:585-92.

71. Otubu JA, Buttram VC, Besch NF, et al. Unconjugated steroids in leiomyomas and tumor-bearing myometrium. Am J Obstet Gynecol. 1982;143:130-3.

72. Eiletz J, Genz T, Pollow K, et al. Sex steroid levels in serum, myometrium, and fibromyomata in correlation with cytoplasmic receptors and 17 beta-HSD activity in different age-groups and phases of the menstrual cycle. Arch Gynecol. 1980;229:13-28.

73. Pollow K, Sinnecker G, Boquoi E, et al. In vitro conversion of estradiol-17 beta into estrone in normal human myometrium and leiomyoma. J Clin Chem Clin Biochem. 1978;16:493-502.

74. Tseng L, Gurpide E. Induction of human endometrial estradiol dehydrogenase by progestins. Endocrinology. 1973;97:825.

75. Liehr JG, Ricci MJ, Jefcoate CR, et al. 4-Hydroxylation of estradiol by human uterine myometrium and myoma microsomes: implications for the mechanism of uterine tumorigenesis. Proc Natl Acad Sci USA. 1995;92:9220-4.

76. Zhu BT, Conney AH. Functional role of estrogen metabolism in target cells: review and perspectives. Carcinogenesis. 1998;19:1-27.

77. Reddy VV, Rose LI. Delta-3-Ketosteroid 5 alpha-oxidoreductase in human uterine leiomyoma. Am J Obstet Gynecol. 1979;135:415.

78. Rein MS, Nowak RA. Biology of uterine myomas and myometrium in vitro. Semin Reprod Endocrinol. 1992;10:310-9.

79. Sauro MD, Zorn NE. Prolactin induces proliferation of vascular smooth muscle cells through a protein kinase C-dependent mechanism. J Cell Physiol. 1991;148:133-8.

80. Nowak RA, Mora S, Diehl T, et al. Prolactin is an autocrine or paracrine growth factor for human myometrial and leiomyoma cells. Gynecol Obstet Invest. 1999;48:127-32.

CHAPTER 3

Pathophysiology of Fibroids

● Vijaya V Mysorekar

Uterine leiomyoma is a benign smooth muscle tumour of the uterus. Fibroids are typically found during the middle and later reproductive years. They are clinically evident in 20%–30% of women over 30 years of age, and are found in about 70% in women less than 50 years of age. After menopause they usually decrease in size.[1]

■ CAUSE

The exact cause of fibroids is unclear. Certain risk factors for fibroids have been noted.[2,3]

Race and Genetic Factors

Fibroids run in families, and with identical twins, it is more likely that both have fibroids, than with non-identical twins. The first-degree relatives of affected women have a 2.5 times increased risk of developing fibroids. Black women are more likely to have fibroids than women of other racial groups. Wei et al[4] found ethnic differences in expression of the dysregulated proteins in uterine fibroids.

Obesity

Fibroids are more common in obese women due to increased effect of oestrogen, as the adipose tissue converts adrenal and ovarian androgens into oestrogens.

Hormones

Fibroids are dependent on oestrogen and progesterone for their growth and are, therefore, common during the reproductive years. Fibroids contain more oestrogen and progesterone receptors than normal uterine muscle cells do. Early menarche, late menopause, nulliparity are associated with a higher risk of developing fibroids due to the unopposed effect of oestrogen. Fibroids are rare before puberty. They show rapid growth during pregnancy and on treatment with exogenous oestrogen. They tend to shrink after menopause due to a decrease in hormone production.

Other Factors

It is not clear whether diet habits, such as consuming red meat, lack of green vegetables and fruit or fibre, and drinking alcohol could influence the growth of fibroids.

Other suggested risk factors are diabetes mellitus and hypertension. Interestingly, it has been suggested that smoking tobacco has a protective effect on the development of uterine fibroids. Nicotine inhibits aromatase and reduces the conversion of androgens to estrone.[5]

■ PATHOGENESIS

The pathogenesis of fibroids is not well understood. Research has shown that uterine fibroids are monoclonal in origin, i.e. they develop from a single mutated myocyte. Several pathogenetic factors such as genetics, gonadal steroid hormones, growth factors, cytokines, chemokines, disorganized extracellular matrix components and angiogenesis have been suggested to play a role in the development and growth of a fibroid. The disease is heterogeneous and different fibroids may have varying etiologies; many may have multifactorial pathogenesis.[5]

Genetics

Cytogenetic anomalies are observed in about 40% of uterine fibroids.[6] These include rearrangements of 6p21 (involving HMGA1 gene, i.e. high-mobility group AT-hook 1 protein gene), t(12;14)(q14–15;q23–24) (involving HMGA2 gene), trisomy 12 (involving HMGA2 gene), del(7)(q22q32), rearrangements of 10q22, and deletions of 3q and 1p.[6-9] Rearrangements involving these genes HMGA1 and HMGA2 disrupt the normal chromatin regulation, initiate unregulated cell proliferation of myometrial stem cells, and thus contribute to the development of uterine fibroids. Specific mutations in the MED12 gene (MED12, mediator subunit complex 12 gene) have been noted in 70% of fibroids.[10,11] The MED12 gene encodes a component of Mediator, a transcriptional regulator complex. Pérot et al state that MED12 seems to be specific to uterine smooth muscle tumours.[12] Tumours with chromosomal rearrangements are generally larger and often within the uterine wall.[8] In addition, some aberrations are associated with specific variants of uterine leiomyomas.[13]

Hereditary Leiomyomatosis and Renal Cell Cancer

An extremely rare autosomal dominant syndrome, the Reed syndrome, is characterized by a predisposition to cutaneous and uterine leiomyomas as well as early-onset renal cell carcinoma. This syndrome is associated with a mutation in the gene located on the long arm of chromosome 1 (1q42.3-43), resulting in inactivation of fumarate hydratase, an enzyme of the Kreb's cycle, responsible for conversion of fumarate to malate.[8,14-16]

Alport syndrome, an X-linked progressive nephropathy, is associated with leiomyomas due to defect in COL4A5 and COL4A6 genes.[17]

Further research will be needed to identify specific genes responsible for the development of leiomyomas, so that those particular genes can be directly targeted for prevention.

Hormones

The normal myometrium of fibroid-containing uteri has been shown to express substantially higher levels of oestrogen receptors.[9] It is believed that oestrogen and progesterone have a mitogenic effect on leiomyoma cells and also act by directly or indirectly influencing a large number of growth factors, cytokines and apoptotic factors as well as other hormones. Increased levels of oestrogens and progesterone could result in an augmentation of mitotic rate that could be responsible for somatic mutation.[5]

Aromatase and 17 beta-hydroxysteroid dehydrogenase are aberrantly expressed in fibroids, indicating that fibroids can convert circulating androstenedione into estradiol.[18]

Aromatase inhibitors are currently being considered for treatment, at doses adjusted such that they would completely inhibit oestrogen production in the fibroid, while not significantly affecting ovarian production of oestrogen and the systemic levels of oestrogen. Aromatase overexpression is particularly pronounced in fibroid tissues of Afro-American women.[19]

Growth Factors

Several growth factors, such as vascular endothelial growth factor (VEGF), epidermal growth factor (EGF), platelet-derived growth factor (PDGF), transforming growth factor (TGF-α and TGF-β) and their respective receptors have been demonstrated to play a role in the growth of fibroids.[5,20] In particular, VEGF, EGF and PDGF promote angiogenesis in fibroids[21]. EGF and PDGF seem to increase deoxyribonucleic acid DNA synthesis and polyploidisation in leiomyoma cells through transient activation of kinase pathways.[5,22] PDGF also regulates the rate of cell proliferation in myometrium and leiomyoma cells.[23]

Recently, higher expression levels of activin and myostatin have been identified in fibroids compared to those in adjacent myometrium. Ciarmela et al[24,25] have hypothesized that activin-A and myostatin play a role in regulating myometrial cell proliferation.

Cytokines and Chemokines

Many cytokines, including tumour necrosis factor α, erythropoietin, interleukin-1 (IL-1), and IL-6, have been implicated in the development of uterine fibroids.[5] A state of excess inflammation, increased endothelial nitric oxide synthesis with influx of inflammatory cytokines such as IL-1 and TNFα, could be one mechanism contributing to fibroid development.

The 'endometrial-subendometrial myometrium unit disruption disease' refers to a pathological thickening or abnormality of the subendometrial myometrium that is the possible site of origin of submucosal and intramural fibroids.[26] In response to mechanical injury such as endometrial ablation or caesarean delivery, where there is an involvement of the subendometrial myometrium, there could be an alteration of endometrial microvascular blood flow with endometrial atrophy and abnormal activation of cytokines and chemokines, which might have an important role in the pathogenesis and growth of uterine fibroids.

Extracellular Matrix Components

Disorganized extracellular matrix (ECM), mainly consisting of collagen subtypes, fibronectin and proteoglycans, is a peculiar feature of fibroids. Matrix metalloproteinases

(MMPs) have been implicated in fibroid remodeling.[5] The β3 subunit of TGF-β3, a growth factor with profibrotic activity, is overexpressed in fibroids compared to normal myometrium.[27] The viscoelastic properties of the ECM contribute substantially to the increased tissue stiffness of fibroids.

Angiogenic Factors

There is strong evidence to show that disordered angiogenesis and altered smooth muscle cell proliferation play a critical role in the pathophysiology of fibroids. Multiple growth factors involved in angiogenesis are over expressed in leiomyoma tissue, as compared to normal myometrium. These include EGF, heparin-binding-EGF, vascular endothelial growth factor, basic fibroblast growth factor, platelet-derived growth factor, transforming growth factor β and adrenomedullin.[21] Angiogenic growth factors play an important role in fibroid growth and survival.

Interplay of Factors

It has been proposed that periodic hypoxia/ischemia, could be linked to cyclic menstrual contractions of the myometrium and the release of increased vasoconstrictive substances at the time of the menses. The resulting ischaemic damage may lead to differentiation of myometrial stem cells into smooth muscle cells. Continued uncontrolled proliferation of mutated stem cell-derived smooth muscle cells would result in foci of myometrial hyperplasia. The effects of gonadal steroids in combination with the chronic hypoxia associated with the rapidly expanding myometrial cell mass stimulate local angiogenic growth factor expression, to provide a vascular support to the growing myometrial cell mass. These, in turn, would promote continued cell proliferation. Smooth muscle cells of the myometrium could also react to injury with the synthesis of extracellular fibrous matrix. After vascular damage, basic fibroblast growth factors are overexpressed in fibroids. Expansion of uterine fibroids is by a slow rate of cell proliferation combined with an increase in the vasculature and the production of excessive amounts of extracellular matrix.[5,21]

The aberrant hypoxic and angiogenic response of the fibroid may make it especially vulnerable to disruption of its vascular supply, a feature that could be exploited for treatment purposes.[21]

■ PATHOLOGY

In strictly pathological terms, the word 'fibroid' is a misnomer, as in reality, the origin of this tumour is from the smooth muscle of the uterine myometrium, and not from fibrous tissue. Hence, the term 'leiomyoma' which is the much preferred term will be used instead of 'fibroid' while describing the pathology of this tumour in the subsequent discussion.

Uterine leiomyomas arise from the myometrial layer of the uterine body or, less commonly, the lower uterine segment, or cervix. Infrequently, a leiomyoma may involve the uterine ligaments.

■ GROSS APPEARANCE

Leiomyomas grossly appear as round, discrete, firm, rubbery, solid nodules that are gray white or tan in colour. They usually appear paler than the surrounding myometrium. They are not truly encapsulated but are sharply circumscribed and compress the surrounding myometrium. This forms a plane of cleavage that enables the leiomyoma to be shelled out at myomectomy. The size varies, from very small to masses of considerable size, sometimes filling the pelvis. Leiomyomas may be single or multiple. If numerous or large, they can grossly distort the uterus (Fig. 3.1). Based on the location in the uterus, leiomyomas can be classified into three types.

Intramural Leiomyomas

Intramural leiomyomas are the most common and are located within the myometrium (Fig. 3.2). They begin as small nodules which, over time, may expand outwards or grow inwards causing distortion of the uterine cavity.

Submucosal Leiomyomas

Submucosal leiomyomas are located just beneath the endometrium and bulge into the uterine cavity (Figure 3.3). They may lead to atrophy or erosion of the endometrium. As the muscular action of the uterus acts to expel the mass, the leiomyoma becomes pedunculated, giving rise to a polyp which hangs into the uterine cavity. With further traction by isthmic contractions, it may appear at the external cervical os (Fig. 3.4), often with an infarcted tip.[8] It may also get ulcerated or infected.

Subserosal Leiomyomas

Subserosal leiomyomas bulge from the serosal surface of the uterus and can become very large (Figs 3.5A and B). They can also grow outwards and become pedunculated, and hang into the peritoneal cavity. A pedunculated subserosal leiomyoma may rarely establish a blood supply from an adjacent structure, such as the omentum, bowel, peritoneum or pelvic wall. Eventually, if there is torsion and necrosis of the pedicle, it may detach from the uterus to become a 'parasitic leiomyoma', surviving only because of its vascular connections with the adjacent tissue.[1,6,9,28-31]

On cut section, leiomyomas typically show a whorled appearance or swirling pattern of smooth muscle bundles (Fig. 3.6). The cut surface tends to bulge due to the release

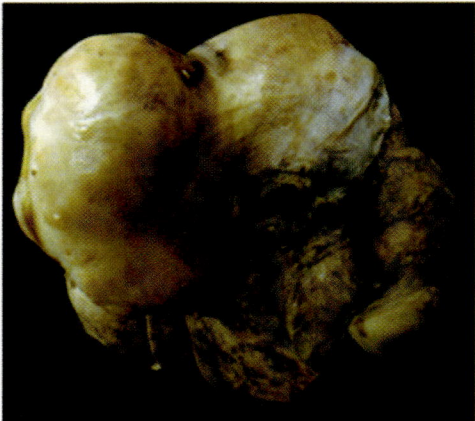

Fig. 3.1: External surface of a uterus, which has been distorted by multiple large leiomyomas. The cervix is identifiable (right).

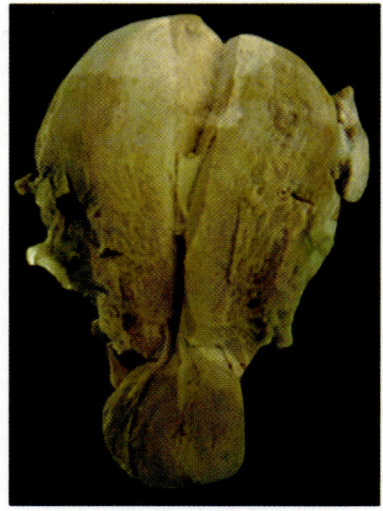

Fig. 3.4: Cervical fibroid

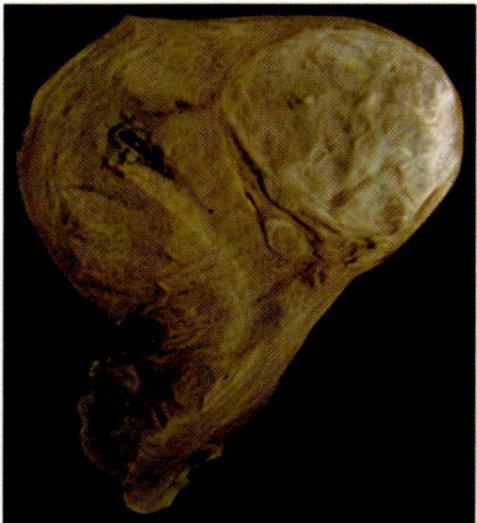

Fig. 3.2: An intramural leiomyoma

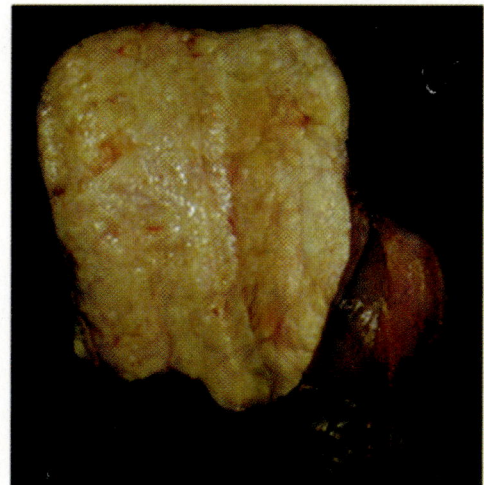

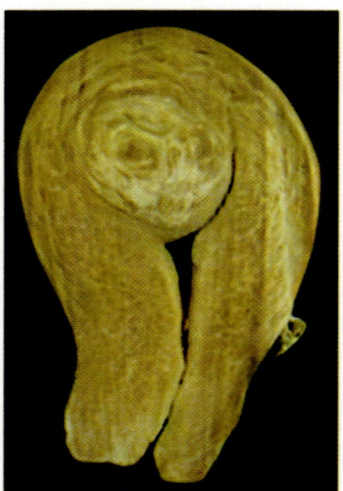

Fig. 3.3: Submucosal fibroid

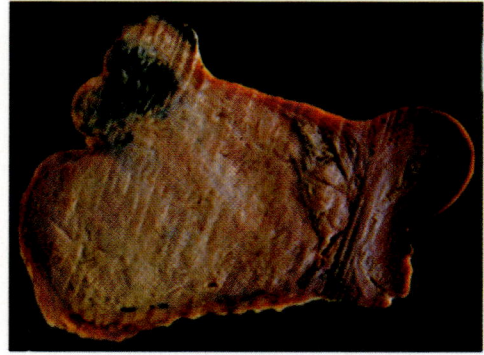

Figs 3.5A and B: Large subserosal fibroids

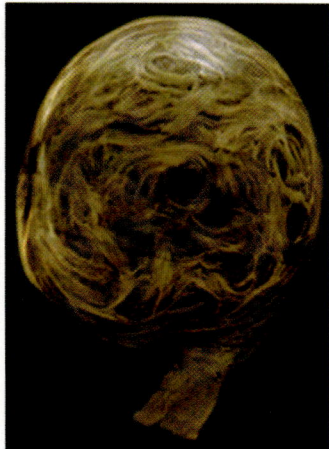

Fig. 3.6: Whorled appearance of fibroid cross section

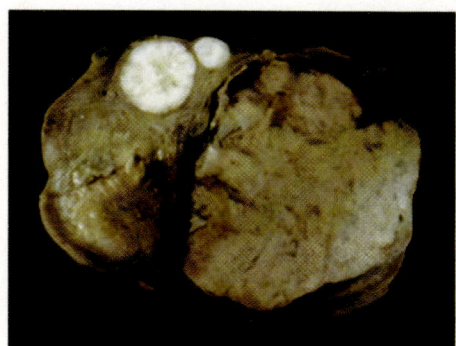

Fig. 3.7: Bulging of cut surface

of intratumoral pressure (Fig. 3.7). Large tumours may show yellow brown or red areas of softening.[1,6,9, 28–31]

■ MICROSCOPY

Microscopically, the tumour is composed of closely packed bundles of smooth muscle cells that resemble normal myometrial cells. The smooth muscle bundles are seen in different directions (whorled), and some bundles appear in transverse section (Fig. 3.8). These smooth muscle bundles are separated by vascular fibrous tissue. Individual tumour cells are elongated, spindle shaped, with a cigar-shaped (blunt ended) nucleus having finely dispersed chromatin and small nucleoli. They have abundant fibrillar eosinophilic cytoplasm and long, slender, bipolar cytoplasmic processes. These cells are uniform in size and shape, with scarce mitoses (Fig. 3.9). The stroma shows lymphocytes and plasma cells. The absence of coagulative necrosis, significant atypia or increased mitotic activity differentiate a leiomyoma from a leiomyosarcoma.[1,6,9,28-31]

High cellularity, prominent blood vessels, multinucleation and nuclear atypia with the appearance of prominent red or orange nucleoli having perinucleolar halos should alert the pathologist to investigate the possibility of the hereditary leiomyomatosis and renal cell cancer (Reed syndrome).[28,32]

Immunohistochemically, uterine leiomyomas characteristically express smooth muscle actin (SMA), muscle-specific actin, desmin, h-caldesmon, and vimentin.[28-30]

■ SECONDARY CHANGES IN A LEIOMYOMA

Secondary changes that may develop within a leiomyoma are as follows.[1,6,9, 28-31]

Hyaline Change

It may be localised or it may affect extensive areas of the tumour. Occasionally even the whole tumour may be hyalinised. The areas of hyaline change have a pale homogeneous eosinophilic, ground-glass appearance (Fig. 3.10).

Cystic Degeneration

It results from liquefaction of degenerated areas of the tumour. The cysts may contain gelatinous material.

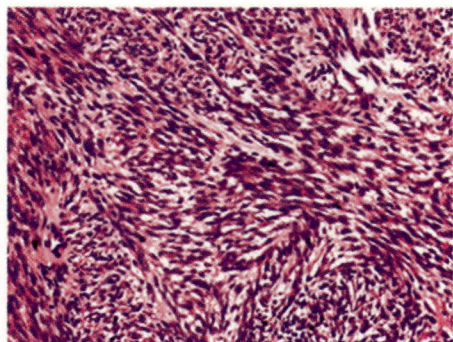

Fig. 3.8: whorled appearance of smooth muscle bundles

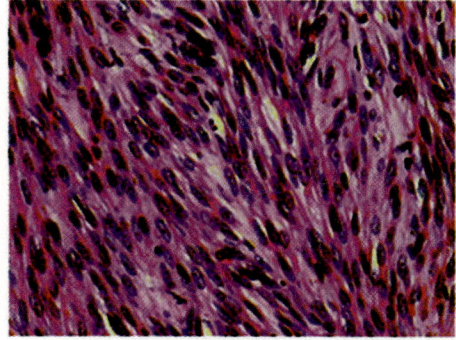

Fig. 3.9: Tumour cells with uniform size and shaper and scarce mitoses

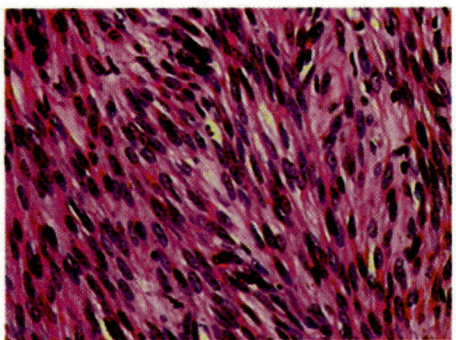

Fig. 3.10: Hyaline degeneration

Myxoid Degeneration

Portions of the tumour show an amorphous, slightly amphophilic matrix within which the tumour cells are embedded.

Red Degeneration (Necrobiosis)

It occurs due to inadequate blood supply to the centre of the leiomyoma, leading to necrosis. This is especially common in pregnancy on account of the rapid growth of the tumour, and is associated with abdominal pain, vomiting and fever. The cut surface becomes more homogeneous and bulging, with loss of the whorled appearance (Fig. 3.11). The colour of the leiomyoma becomes dark red due to staining by fresh blood and the consistency becomes softer. The microscopic appearance in red degeneration shows extensive coagulative necrosis with only ghosts of the muscle cells and their nuclei.

Necrosis

Rarely, even in the non-pregnant state, a leiomyoma may undergo necrosis, resulting in a soft, structureless, pale gray mass. This change is seen most often in submucous leiomyomas that protrude into the uterine cavity.

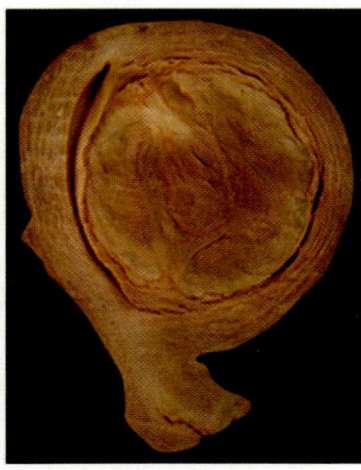

Fig. 3.11: Red degeneration

Torsion and infarction

It may occur in case of a large pedunculated subserosal leiomyoma.

Calcific Degeneration

Calcification in the leiomyoma is seen more often in women after menopause.

Fatty Degeneration

Lipid is deposited in the smooth muscle cells themselves or in histiocytes.

Hydropic Degeneration

There is accumulation of edema fluid within the tumour, in diffuse or perinodular pattern. It is often associated with collagen deposition.

Haemorrhage

It may occur within the tumour.

■ VARIANTS OF LEIOMYOMA

There are a number of variants of benign leiomyoma characterized either by increased mitotic activity or by deviation from the typical histological picture. These variants account for 10% of cases[28] and have been described below.

Cellular Leiomyoma

A cellular leiomyoma is a benign smooth muscle tumour that has a markedly increased number of cells per unit area as compared to the surrounding myometrium and the usual leiomyomas. Grossly, the tumour is soft in consistency, the characteristic whorled pattern may be lacking and the colour appears tan or creamy yellow rather than grayish white. Microscopically, the tumour is very cellular and the cells are closely packed. A fascicular pattern is present in some areas. Palisading (parallel arrangement) of nuclei is present in some cellular leiomyomas[1] (Fig. 3.12). The blood vessels are typically large with thick muscular walls and cleft-like spaces are often seen, possibly representing compressed vessels or edema. Unlike the usual leiomyoma, cellular leiomyomas are less demarcated, and often show focal extensions into the adjacent myometrium. The mitotic count is not higher than 5 per 10 high power fields (HPFs). Nuclear atypia and coagulative necrosis are absent. Cytogenetically, the cellular leiomyoma may be associated with chromosomal aberrations, especially deletion of almost the entire 1p, and rearranged 10q22.[1,6,8,9, 28–3]

Leiomyoma with Bizarre Nuclei

Atypical leiomyoma, bizarre leiomyoma, symplastic leiomyoma and pleomorphic leiomyoma are synonyms

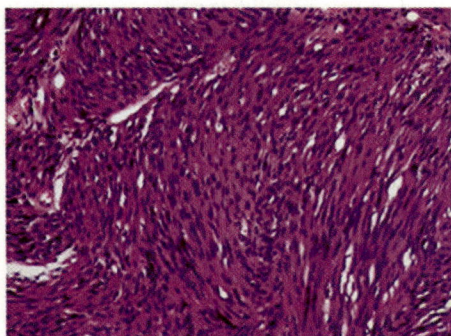

Fig. 3.12: Cellular leiomyoma

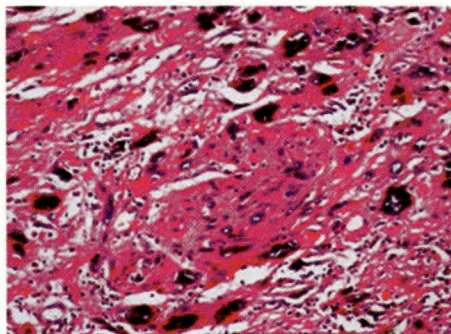

Fig. 3.13: Leiomyoma with bizarre nuclei

for this tumour. The characteristic feature is the presence of bizarre, pleomorphic tumour cells with atypical, hyperchromatic nuclei (Fig. 3.13). The bizarre cells, which constitute more than 25% of the tumour may be focal or diffuse and are multinucleated or have multilobed nuclei. Large, hyperchromatic mononuclear cells are also seen. The nuclei often show degenerative changes such as smudged chromatin, vacuolation, karyorrhexis, and pyknosis. Although atypical leiomyomas show cellular atypia, they have a low mitotic index, generally averaging < 2 mitoses per 10 HPFs, distinguishing them from leiomyosarcomas. Infarct-type necrosis may be seen, but geographic coagulative tumour cell necrosis, sometimes a prominent feature of leiomyosarcomas, is absent in an atypical leiomyoma[28]. Occasionally, an atypical leiomyoma may show increased proliferative activity, but this is characteristically focal. These tumours may show secondary changes such as edema and hyaline change. Cytogenetically, nearly 50% of atypical leiomyomas show loss of almost the entire short arm of chromosome 1 (1p–).[1,6,8,9, 28–31]

Mitotically Active Leiomyoma

A benign smooth muscle tumour, usually of a size less than 8 cm with an increased mitotic rate is labeled as a mitotically active leiomyoma. These leiomyomas have 5 to 15 mitotic figures per 10 HPFs in the most active area. This increased proliferative rate is frequently, but not always, diffusely distributed. Atypical mitotic figures (e.g. multipolarity or extreme polyploidy) are not characteristic of mitotically active leiomyomas. As a rule, coagulative tumour necrosis and cytologic atypia must not be present, otherwise the tumour would be classified as a leiomyosarcoma or atypical leiomyoma.[1,6,8,9, 28-31]

Hydropic Leiomyoma

This type of leiomyoma shows extensive zonal edema with a characteristic perinodular distribution.[29] Areas of hyalinisation are also seen. Due to the edema and hyalinisation, the tumour

cells grow in thin, delicate cords. The tumour may also show high vascularity.[28]

Apoplectic Leiomyoma

This variant occurs in pregnancy and during oral contraceptive treatment, and exhibits haemorrhage and cystic change. Microscopically, the tumour shows stellate zones of recent haemorrhage with nodules of densely cellular smooth muscle. Hence this tumour is also known as haemorrhagic cellular leiomyoma. Mitotic activity is not increased or only focally increased and there is no cellular atypia[9,28].

Lipomatous Leiomyoma (Lipoleiomyoma)

This benign tumour shows a close admixture of smooth muscle cells and mature adipose tissue[9,28] (Fig. 3.14). Other heterologous elements that may very rarely be seen in a leiomyoma are bone, cartilage, skeletal muscle, haematopoietic or lymphoid cells.

Epithelioid Leiomyoma

This is a smooth muscle tumour which has received its name due to the 'epithelial-like' morphology of the tumour cells. The cells are predominantly round or polygonal rather than the spindle-shaped cells of the usual leiomyoma. Grossly, this

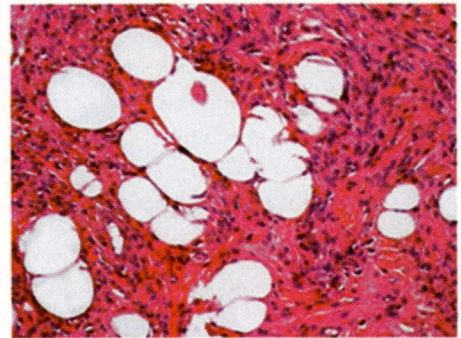

Fig. 3.14: Lipomatous leiomyoma

variant is often not appreciably different from the ordinary leiomyoma. The tumours are less than 6 cm in size, well circumscribed and may be softer and more tan or yellow than the usual leiomyoma.[8,9,28,29] Microscopically, there is no fascicular pattern of growth. Instead, the cells are arranged in sheets, cords, trabeculae or nests. The tumour cells contain rounded nuclei with finely stippled chromatin and a single nucleolus, and their cytoplasm is clear or eosinophilic. The clear appearance of the cytoplasm is due to the presence of glycogen, lipid or both. The mitotic count is < 5 per 10 HPFs, there is no necrosis, and atypia is absent or minimal. A variant of epithelioid leiomyoma is the plexiform tumourlet, which is usually less than 1 cm in size and composed of cells arranged in a more prominent pattern of interwoven islands, ribbons or cords of polygonal or rounded cells. The cells are smaller and darker than those of the other epithelioid leiomyomas, and are often separated by abundant extracellular matrix. [8,9,28–30]

Epithelioid leiomyomas may display a transition to a typical smooth muscle tumour. Immunohistochemically, the tumour cells are positive to antibodies for desmin, smooth muscle actin and h-caldesmon. The commonest cytogenetic abnormality seen is del(7).[29]

Myxoid Leiomyoma

This is a leiomyoma, which is hypocellular with extensive myxoid change. The myxoid stroma is composed of acid mucin that arises from the myxoid degeneration of collagen between bundles of smooth muscle. This stroma typically shows positive staining with alcian blue. The tumour also has large, thick-walled vessels. A myxoid leiomyoma can be differentiated from a myxoid leiomyosarcoma by the absence of pleomorphism, necrosis or infiltration and mitotic index < 2 per 10 HPFs.[9,28,29,31]

Dissecting (Cotyledonoid) Leiomyoma

This variant of leiomyoma grossly resembles placental tissue, due to prominent edema and congestion[1]. The tumour is exophytic, bulky and extends from the uterine wall into the broad ligament and pelvic cavity. It may show bulbous protrusions due to hydropic change. Microscopically, the histological features are of a leiomyoma with extensive degenerative changes. Tongues of bland smooth muscle cells can be seen irregularly dissecting or infiltrating the myometrium. This tumour is benign.[9,28]

Vascular Leiomyoma (Angioleiomyoma)

This variant histologically shows numerous large-caliber vessels with muscular walls and swirling of the spindle cells around the vessels.[1,9]

Unusual Growth Patterns of Leiomyomas

Leiomyomas may have a number of special and unusual growth patterns as described below.

Diffuse (Intrauterine) Leiomyomatosis

This is a rare condition in which there are innumerable ill-defined leiomyomatous nodules in the uterus. Grossly, the uterus is symmetrically enlarged and may reach large dimensions, weighing even 1 kg. The serosal surface is bosselated (irregularly nodular). The nodules, which range from microscopic to 2–3 cm in diameter, are paler than the surrounding myometrium and often present a whorled or trabeculated appearance. Microscopically, the nodules consist of uniform benign cellular smooth muscle bundles that are not as well defined as in the usual uterine leiomyomas. They tend to merge with each other and with the surrounding less cellular myometrium. Clusters of capillaries may be present in the centre of the nodules and are surrounded by hyalinized stroma. Mitotic figures are rare and atypia is lacking.[8,9,28–31]

Intravascular Leiomyomatosis

This is an uncommon condition in which mature smooth muscle is present within the lumina of the uterine and pelvic veins. Intravenous leiomyomatosis involves extension of the leiomyoma beyond the confines of the uterus, along the vessels in the broad ligament, into the uterine and iliac veins and, occasionally, along the inferior vena cava and into the chambers of the heart. Grossly, the uterus is enlarged and the intravenous components appear as nodules or worm-like coils of firm, rubbery tissue. Microscopically, the intravascular components appear similar to the usual leiomyoma. When an adjacent uterine leiomyoma is present, continuity can sometimes be demonstrated between the extravascular and intravascular components. The tumour behaves in a benign fashion with no risk of recurrence or distant metastasis. The long-term prognosis is good; however, involvement of the heart can be fatal.[8,9,28-31]

Benign Metastasizing Leiomyoma

This is a very rare phenomenon in which a histologically typical uterine leiomyoma spreads hematogenously, and grows in more distant sites such as the lungs and regional lymph nodes. Often, the seeding of the blood vessels occurs subsequent to a prior surgical procedure such as dilatation and curettage, myomectomy or hysterectomy. The metastatic nodules may be multiple, with an average size of about 2 cm. The metastatic tumour is usually still hormone dependent; oestrogen receptors and a response to hormone treatment have been demonstrated in the benign metastasizing leiomyoma.

The tumour has low proliferative activity and progression is slow, but pulmonary involvement may cause life-threatening complications and can even be fatal.[6,8,9,28–31] The metastatic tumour may overexpress p53 or show chromosomal aberrations such as deletion of 19q or 22q.[9]

Disseminated Peritoneal Leiomyomatosis

In this exceedingly rare condition, multiple small, nodular deposits of histologically benign smooth muscle are found over the peritoneum, including the serosa of the uterus, tubes and ovaries as well as the omentum, with uterine leiomyomas as their source. The condition affects women of reproductive age and there is a strong association with hormonal stimulation, as in pregnancy, puerperium or use of oral contraceptives. The tumorous lesions of peritoneal leiomyomatosis may be up to 10 cm, but most tumorlets are less than 1 cm. They are well circumscribed, firm nodules with a tan to slightly pink, often whorled cut surface as in the uterine leiomyoma. Each tumorlet consists of histologically bland fascicles of smooth muscle. Some of the lesions may be only microscopic. This condition is an incidental finding and can grossly simulate a malignant tumour, but behaves in a benign manner.[6,8,28–31]

Leiomyosarcoma

Leiomyosarcoma is the malignant counterpart of the leiomyoma. It is a sarcoma composed entirely of smooth muscle. Only a small number of leiomyosarcomas arise from a pre-existing leiomyoma; majority of them arise de novo (on their own).[6,9] The age of women with leiomyosarcoma is about 10 years older than those with leiomyoma, most being over 40 years of age.[8] Apart from this difference in the age of the patient, a number of histopathological features, both gross and microscopic, help in differentiating leiomyomas from leiomyosarcomas. A clear-cut distinction is easily possible in case of typical leiomyomas. However, difficulties may be encountered when the leiomyoma has variant morphology as described earlier. The histopathological features of typical leiomyomas and leiomyosarcomas are summarized in Table 3.1.[8,30]

Smooth Muscle Tumours of Uncertain Malignant Potential (Stump)

Some smooth muscle tumours of the uterus do not fulfill the histological criteria for leiomyoma or leiomyosarcoma. These tumours may exhibit moderate cytologic atypia with a mitotic index of 5 to 10 per 10 HPFs, along with zonal necrosis. Sometimes the tumours may not exhibit cytologic atypia, but may have a mitotic index ≥10 mitotic figures per 10 HPFs, along with zonal necrosis, or they may show a large number of epithelioid cells. Other tumours may lack tumour cell necrosis, have moderate-to-severe atypia, a mitotic index around 10 mitotic figures per 10 HPFs, and have structures that could be regarded either as abnormal mitotic figures or smudged karyorrhectic nuclei. In such cases, it may be impossible to determine with certainty, whether the tumour is benign or malignant. These tumours are placed under a separate category termed as 'smooth muscle tumour of uncertain malignant potential' (STUMP).[1,6,8,28] Such tumours usually occur de novo, rather than from a pre-existing leiomyoma.[6]

■ CLINICAL FEATURES AND COMPLICATIONS

Many fibroids, even large ones, may remain asymptomatic. Submucosal fibroids, even when small, may cause distortin of the endometrial lining, and may ulcerate, leading to menorrhagia.[9] Fibroids that cause heavy bleeding lead to anaemia and iron deficiency. Uterine fibroids that obstruct menstrual flow can cause dysmenorrhoea. Large fibroids may give rise to a feeling of abdominal heaviness or fullness. Fibroids can outstrip their blood supply and cause acute or chronic pain as they degenerate. Sudden pain may also be a presenting feature when there is torsion in case of a pedunculated fibroid. Pedunculated submucous uterine fibroids can dilate the uterine cervix and prolapse into the vagina where they can become infected.

Fibroids can cause infertility or spontaneous abortion. Submucosal fibroids may prevent implantation and growth of an embryo. Distortion of the uterine cavity can cause recurrent second trimester loss. Larger fibroids may even distort or obstruct the fallopian tubes, preventing fertilisation. Fetal malpresentation may occur if the fibroid is occupying the uterine cavity. A large fibroid may obstruct delivery. Premature rupture of membranes or uterine inversion may also occur at the time of delivery[1]. Postpartum haemorrhage could be a complication of fibroids, due to inefficient uterine contraction.[6]

Large uterine fibroids, especially subserosal fibroids, can cause pressure effects on contiguous organs such as the bowel and bladder. Gastrointestinal symptoms such as constipation or abdominal distension may occur. Mesenteric vein thrombosis and thromboembolism, and intestinal gangrene can be serious complications in case of compression caused by a large fibroid. Compression of the ureter may lead to hydronephrosis, and cause symptoms of urinary frequency, urgency and incontinence.[9] Urinary retention may occur in some cases, leading to renal failure. Pelvic vein compression can lead to edema of the legs. Fibroids may rarely be associated with polycythemia, which regresses after excision of the tumour. This is due to the production of erythropoietin by the tumour (myomatous erythrocytosis syndrome).[9,31]

Table 3.1: Histopathological features of typical leiomyomas and leiomyosarcomas

	Feature	Leiomyoma	Leiomyosarcoma
Gross	Number of tumours	May be single or multiple	More likely to be a solitary, dominant mass.
	Size	Variable	Bulky, often greater than 10 cm at presentation.
	Colour	Gray white or tan	Yellowish, pink or gray
	Margins	Well circumscribed. A sharp line of demarcation separates the tumour from the normal myometrium. The tumour does not invade the adjacent myometrium.	Margin is not well defined. The tumour irregularly invades the adjacent myometrium at the margin of the tumour.
	Consistency	Firm and rubbery; cannot indent the cut surface with a finger.	Soft, fleshy and less resilient; can push the examining finger into the tumour.
	Bulging of the cut surface	The cut surface tends to bulge due to the release of intratumoral pressure	The cut surface does not bulge
	Whorled pattern of cut surface	Striking, characteristic feature	Absent
	Haemorrhage	Not a common feature	Commonly present, often irregular in shape and colour
	Necrosis	Absent	Present
	Invasion of adjacent structures or organs	Absent	May be seen in advanced cases
Microscopy	Cellularity	Less cellular than leiomyosarcomas	More densely cellular
	Differentiation	The tumour is composed of smooth muscle cells that resemble normal myometrial cells	Well-differentiated leiomyosarcomas consist of smooth muscle cells similar to those of leiomyoma. At the other end of the spectrum, a poorly differentiated leiomyosarcoma is composed of rounded and pleomorphic cells that have virtually no resemblance to normal smooth muscle cells, with only rare tumour cells demonstrating smooth muscle differentiation.
	Nuclear and cellular atypia	Absence of atypia. Tumour cells are uniform in size and shape.	Atypia is present. Nuclear-to-cytoplasmic ratio is increased. Marked irregularity of cells is seen in high grade tumours.
	Nuclear hyperchromasia	Absent	Present
	Cytoplasm	Abundant fibrillar eosinophilic cytoplasm	Ill-defined cytoplasm
	Mitotic activity	Mitotic index is less than 5 mitotic figures per 10 HPFs	A mitotic index greater than 10 mitotic figures per 10 HPFs is diagnostic. If there is cellular atypia, even a mitotic index of 5–10 per 10 HPFs indicates leiomyosarcoma
	Atypical mitotic figures	Absent	Present
	Tumour giant cells	Absent	Multinucleated tumour giant cells are present
	Haemorrhage	Not a common feature	Commonly present
	Coagulative tumour cell necrosis	Absent	Present and there are sharp lines of demarcation between the areas of necrosis and the viable areas within the tumour.
	Invasion of the surrounding myometrium	Absent	Destructive invasion of the adjacent myometrial tissue. The tumour may even spread through the serosal surface of the uterus and involve other pelvic organs.
	Vascular invasion	Absent	Present in 10%–22% of cases

In very rare cases, malignant transformation of a fibroid to a leiomyosarcoma of the myometrium can develop.[33] In extremely rare cases, uterine fibroids may present as part or early symptom of the hereditary leiomyomatosis and renal cell carcinoma syndrome.[14-16]

KEYNOTES

Uterine fibroid, also known as uterine leiomyoma, is a benign smooth muscle tumour of the uterus.

Fibroids are dependent on oestrogen and progesterone for their growth and are, therefore, common during the reproductive years. Early menarche, late menopause, nulliparity and obesity are associated with a higher risk of developing fibroids.

Cytogenetic anomalies are observed in about 40% of uterine fibroids, the most consistent being rearrangements of 6p21 (involving *HMGA1* gene), t(12;14) (involving *HMGA2* gene), trisomy 12 (involving *HMGA2* gene), and del(7)(q22q32).

Under hypoxic conditions, gonadal steroid hormones, growth factors, cytokines, chemokines, disorganized extracellular matrix components and angiogenesis have been suggested to play a role in the development and growth of a fibroid.

Leiomyomas grossly appear as round, discrete, firm, rubbery, solid nodules that are gray white or tan in colour, and appear whorled on cut section. Based on the location in the uterus, leiomyomas can be classified into three types, i.e. intramural, submucosal and subserosal leiomyomas.

Microscopically, the leiomyoma is composed of closely packed bundles of smooth muscle cells that resemble normal myometrial cells. These cells are uniform in size and shape, with scarce mitoses.

Secondary changes that may develop within a leiomyoma are hyaline change, cystic degeneration, myxoid degeneration, red degeneration, necrosis, calcification, hydropic degeneration and haemorrhage.

Variants account for 10% of cases. These include the cellular, bizarre, mitotically active, hydropic, apoplectic, lipomatous, epithelioid, myxoid, dissecting (cotyledonoid) and vascular variants.

Leiomyomas may show unusual growth patterns including diffuse leiomyomatosis, intravascular leiomyomatosis, benign metastasizing leiomyoma, and disseminated peritoneal leiomyomatosis.

Smooth muscle tumours of the uterus that do not fulfill the histological criteria for leiomyoma or leiomyosarcoma are placed under a separate category termed as 'smooth muscle tumour of uncertain malignant potential'.

The clinical presentations of fibroids are bleeding, pain, abdominal fullness, pregnancy complications, and pressure effects on adjacent organs.

REFERENCES

1. Zaloudek CJ, Hendrickson MR, Soslow RA. Mesenchymal Tumors of the Uterus. In: Kurman RJ, Ellenson LH, Ronnett BM (eds). Blaustein's Pathology of the Female Genital Tract, 6th edn. New York:Springer; 2011. pp. 455-527.
2. Hodge JC, Morton CC. Genetic heterogeneity among uterine leiomyomata: insights into malignant progression. Hum Mol Genet. 2007;16 Spec No 1:R7–13.
3. Okolo S. Incidence, aetiology and epidemiology of uterine fibroids. Best Pract Res Clin Obstet Gynaecol. 2008;22:571-88.
4. Wei JJ, Chiriboga L, Arslan AA, et al. Ethnic differences in expression of the dysregulated proteins in uterine leiomyoma ta. Hum Reprod. 2006;21:57-67.
5. Ciavattini A, Di Giuseppe J, Stortoni P, et al. Uterine fibroids: Pathogenesis and interactions with endometrium and endomyometrial junction. Obstetrics and Gynecology International. 2013;2013:11. http://dx.doi.org/10.1155/2013/173184.
6. Ellenson LH, Pirog EC. The Female Genital Tract. In:Kumar V, Abbas AK, Aster JC (Eds). Robbins and Cotran Pathologic Basis of Disease, South Asia edn. India:Reed Elsevier; 2014. pp. 991-1042.
7. Stewart EA, Morton CC. The genetics of uterine leiomyomata: what clinicians need to know. Obstet Gynecol. 2006;107:917-21.
8. Quade BJ, Robboy SJ. Uterine smooth muscle tumors. In: Robboy SJ, Mutter GL, Prat J, Bentley RC, Russell P, Anderson MC (Eds). Robboy's Pathology of the Female Reproductive tract, 2nd edn. US: Churchill Livingstone Elsevier;2009. pp. 457-84.
9. Rosai J. Female Reproductive System—Uterus:corpus. Rosai and Ackerman's Surgical Pathology, 10th edn. St. Louis: Mosby Elsevier; 2011. pp. 1477-1540.
10. Mäkinen N, Mehine M, Tolvanen J, et al. MED12, the mediator complex subunit 12 gene, is mutated at high frequency in uterine leiomyomas. Science. 2011;334:252-5.
11. Je EM, Kim MR, Min KO, et al. Mutational analysis of MED12 exon 2 in uterine leiomyoma and other common tumors. Int J Cancer. 2012;131:E1044-7.
12. Pérot G, Croce S, Ribeiro A, et al. MED12 alterations in both human benign and malignant uterine soft tissue tumors. PLoS One. 2012;7:e40015.
13. Christacos NC, Quade BJ, Dal Cin P, et al. Uterine leiomyomata with deletions of 1p represent a distinct cytogenetic subgroup associated with unusual histologic features. Genes Chromosomes Cancer. 2006;45:304-12.
14. Tolvanen J, Uimari O, Ryynänen M, et al. Strong family history of uterine leiomyomatosis warrants fumarate hydratase mutation screening. Hum Reprod. 2012;27:1865-9.
15. Sanz-Ortega J, Vocke C, Stratton P, et al. Morphologic and molecular characteristics of uterine leiomyomas in hereditary leiomyomatosis and renal cancer (HLRCC) syndrome. Am J Surg Pathol. 2013;37:74-80.
16. Sudarshan S, Pinto PA, Neckers L, et al. Mechanisms of disease: hereditary leiomyomatosis and renal cell cancer—a distinct form of hereditary kidney cancer. Nat Clin Pract Urol. 2007;4:104-10.
17. Uliana V, Marcocci E, Mucciolo M, et al. Alport syndrome and leiomyomatosis: the first deletion extending beyond COL4A6 intron 2. Pediatr Nephrol. 2011;26:717-24.

18. Shozu M, Murakami K, Inoue M. Aromatase and leiomyoma of the uterus. Semin Reprod Med. 2004;22:51-60.

19. Ishikawa H, Reierstad S, Demura M, et al. High aromatase expression in uterine leiomyoma tissues of African-American women. J Clin Endocrinol Metab. 2009;94:1752-6.

20. Ciarmela P, Islam MS, Reis FM, et al. Growth factors and myometrium: biological effects in uterine fibroid and possible clinical implications. Hum Reprod Update. 2011;17:772-90.

21. Tal R, Segars JH. The role of angiogenic factors in fibroid pathogenesis: potential implications for future therapy. Hum Reprod Update. 2014;20:194-216.

22. Ren Y, Yin H, Tian R, et al. Different effects of epidermal growth factor on smooth muscle cells derived from human myometrium and from leiomyoma. Fertil Steril. 2011;96:1015-20.

23. Suo G, Jiang Y, Cowan B, et al. Platelet-derived growth factor C is upregulated in human uterine fibroids and regulates uterine smooth muscle cell growth. Biol Reprod. 2009;81:749-58.

24. Ciarmela P, Wiater E, Vale W. Activin-A in myometrium: characterization of the actions on myometrial cells. Endocrinology. 2008;149:2506-16.

25. Ciarmela P, Wiater E, Smith SM, et al. Presence, actions, and regulation of myostatin in rat uterus and myometrial cells. Endocrinology. 2009;150:906-14.

26. Tocci A, Greco E, Ubaldi FM. Adenomyosis and 'endometrial-subendometrial myometrium unit disruption disease' are two different entities. Reprod Biomed Online. 2008;17:281-91.

27. Norian JM, Malik M, Parker CY, et al. Transforming growth factor beta3 regulates the versican variants in the extracellular matrix-rich uterine leiomyomas. Reprod Sci. 2009;16:1153-64.

28. Kurman RJ, Carcangiu ML, Herrington CS, Young RH (Eds). Tumours of the uterine corpus. In: WHO classification of tumours of female reproductive organs, 4th edn. Lyon: International Agency for Research on Cancer (IARC); 2014. pp. 122-54.

29. Nucci MR. Tumors of the female genital tract – Myometrium. In: Fletcher CDM (Ed). Diagnostic Histopathology of Tumors, 3rd edn. Philadelphia: Churchill Livingstone Elsevier; 2007. pp. 683-96.

30. Longacre TA, Atkins KA, Kempson RL, et al. Female reproductive system and peritoneum—The uterine corpus. In: Mills SE (Ed). Sternberg's Diagnostic Surgical Pathology, 5th edn. Philadelphia: Wolters Kluwer-Lippincott Williams & Wilkins; 2010. pp. 2184-277.

31. Bhardwaj JR, Deb P (Eds). Female reproductive system. In: Boyd's textbook of Pathology, 10th edn. India: Wolters Kluwer; 2013, pp. 1152-216.

32. Garg K, Tickoo SK, Soslow RA, et al. Morphologic features of uterine leiomyomas associated with hereditary leiomyomatosis and renal cell carcinoma syndrome: a case report. Am J Surg Pathol. 2011;35:1235-7.

33. Bukar M, Audu BM, Mustapha Z, et al. Uterine leiomyosarcoma arising from a fibroid. J Obstet Gynaecol. 2009;29:169-70.

CHAPTER 4

Genetics of Fibroids

● Reshu Saraogi

Uterine leiomyoma (UL) is the most common solid pelvic tumour in the female affecting up to 60% of reproductive aged women and 80% of women during their lifetime.[1] They are benign masses arising from the myometrium and comprises predominantly of smooth muscle and also extracellular matrix (collagen, proteoglycan an d fibronectin).[2]

■ GENESIS OF FIBROIDS

Despite the huge public healthcare burden of uterine leiomyomas, the molecular aetiology of leiomyomas is incompletely understood.

There are two components to myoma development; first the transformation of normal myocytes to abnormal myocytes and then their growth into clinically apparent tumours.[3]

Despite their tumorgenic potential, leiomyomas are morphologically similar to normal myometrial smooth-muscle cells at the cellular level. On microscopic examination, they are seen as interlacing bundles of spindle shaped or stellate smooth muscle cells with little cellular pleomorphism or mitotic activity.[4]

The steroid hormones, estrogen and progesterone are considered the most important regulators of leiomyoma growth. Evidence exists supporting the involvement of genomic instability influencing genes such as estrogen and progesterone receptors. Several genomic and proteomic studies have also provided evidence for altered molecular environment of leiomyomas compared to the normal myometrium, as a possible biomarker in their proliferation and regression.[5]

■ THEORIES FOR FIBROID FORMATION

1. High levels of oestrogen and progesterone increases the mitotic rate of smooth muscle cells and hence the likelihood of somatic mutations followed by fibroid formation.[6]
2. Inherent abnormality in the myometrium exhibiting high levels of estrogen receptors.[7]
3. Growth factors, proteins/polypeptides produced locally by smooth muscle cells and fibroblasts mediate the growth-promoting effects of oestrogen by controlling the proliferation of cells and primarily by increasing the extracellular matrix.[8] Some of the identified myoma-related growth factors are transforming growth factor-β (TGF-β), basic fibroblast growth factor (bFGF), epidermal growth factor (EGF), platelet-derived growth factor (PDGF), vascular endothelial growth factor (VEGF), insulin-like growth factor (IGF), and prolactin.

■ RISK FACTORS

There is enough evidence that fibroid grows in the presence of high estrogen and regresses when oestrogens are low.[7] Thus, several factors predispose women to develop uterine leiomyoma, which include early menarche, late menopause, increasing age, nulliparity, unhealthy diet, lack of exercise, obesity, hyperinsulinemia, oral contraceptives, hormone replacement therapy.

LEIOMYOMAS ARE MONOCLONAL LESIONS

Chromosomal and molecular analyses have shown that development of each leiomyoma is an independent monoclonal process.[9] Analysis of multiple fibroids from the same patient revealed that each fibroid developed independently, as each one showed different chromosomal abnormality.[10,11]

If two fibroids (arising from the same uterus) showed similar chromosomal abnormality, they were either due to recurrent chromosomal aberration in the smooth muscle or just coincidental. Cytogenetically mosaic tumours were also reported to be clonal.[9]

This chromosomal heterogeneity, thus supports the multistep hypothesis of fibroid development, and also explains the clinicopathologic differences seen in fibroids, including variation in size or response to hormonal treatments.[12]

GENETICS OF FIBROIDS

Genetic liability of uterine leiomyomas has been evidenced by a variety of epidemiological, molecular and cytogenetic studies. Evidence for heritability of fibroids further comes from studies analysing ethnic predisposition,[13,14] twin studies,[15] familial aggregation,[16] as well as genetic linkage studies in families with uterine leiomyomata-associated heritable syndromes.

ETHNICITY

Black women are disproportionately affected by uterine fibroids—the incidence and prevalence rates being at least three times greater than those for white women even after other known risk factors are controlled.[13,14] Moreover, Black women are diagnosed more commonly with multiple fibroids, larger fibroids and at an earlier age.

FAMILIAL PREDISPOSITION

First-degree relatives of affected women have a fold higher risk of developing UL.[2,5] The concordance of fibroid diagnosis in monozygotic twins is almost twice that of dizygotic twins. Similarly, a study of a Finnish cohort found that monozygotic twins' concordance for being hospitalised for UL was twice that of dizygotic twins.[17]

SYNDROMES ASSOCIATED WITH FIBROIDS

Although benign, UL have been linked to malignancy through two genomic regions on chromosome1:
1. Hereditary leiomyomatosis and renal cell cancer (HLRCC): This autosomal dominant syndrome predisposes patients to benign leiomyomas of skin and uterus and early-onset renal cell carcinoma. The responsible gene was identified as fumarate hydratase (FH) that encodes a Kreb's cycle enzyme responsible for conversion of fumarate to malate.[18]

   The occurrence of leiomyomas as part of a heritable cancer syndrome is under appreciated and the finding of cutaneous leiomyomas (the mostcommon finding in HLRCC) warrants familial screening.[19]
2. Alport syndrome: It is a progressive nephropathy, the most common mode of inheritance being X-linked transmission. It is associated withuterine leiomyomas due to defect in COL4A5 and COL 4A6 genes.[20]

CYTOGENETIC STUDIES

Standard karyotyping detects chromosomal aberrations such as deletions, duplications and translocations, whereas comparative genome hybridisation detects deletions and amplifications. With further advancements in sequencing technology, small submicroscopic chromosomal abnormalities such as point mutations or epigenetic changes such as methylations have been diagnosed.[7,21,22]

The variety of chromosomal rearrangements, including but not limited to translocation, deletion and trisomy, predict different molecular genetic mechanisms for UL formation and growth.

CHROMOSOMAL ABERRATIONS

Although majority of leiomyomas (60%) are believed to be chromosomally stable, approximately 40% of leiomyomas have detectable cytogenetic rearrangements, such as deletions of 7q and rearrangements involving 12q15 or 6p21. The most common chromosomal aberration in leiomyoma, seen in approximately 20% of karyotypically abnormal leiomyomas, is the characteristic translocation, t(12;14) (q15;q24), specifically associated with leiomyoma.[23] An interstitial deletion of chromosome 7, del(7) (q22q32) is observed with a frequency of about 17% in karyotypically abnormal leiomyomas.

Leiomyomas with chromosome 7 deletions or translocations are usually found in the mosaic state with 46 XX cells. Rearrangements of 6p21 in leiomyoma occur with a frequency of 5% and include t(1;6)(q23;p21), t(6;14) (p21;q24), and t(6;10) (p21;q22), as well as inversions and translocations with other chromosomes.[3]

Other cytogenetic abnormalities of lower frequency include changes of the Xchromosome, including del(X)(p11.2), t(X;12)(p22.3;q15), -X, del(5)t(X;5)(p11;p15), del(X)(q12), del(X)t(X;3) (p22.3;q11.2) and inv(X)(p22q13).

In addition to chromosomal changes, point mutations in MED12 contribute to the development of leiomyomas. A study recently discovered mutations in MED12 exon 2 in 70% of 225 unselected uterine leiomyomas.[24]

Epigenetic changes have also been implicated in leiomyoma formation. Studies directed at identifying epigenetic abnormalities in fibroids demonstrated abnormally hypo- methylated estrogen receptor.[25] Follow-up studies demonstrated globally abnormal genomic methylation in leiomyomas compared to myometrium,[26] implicating possible epigenetic contributions to genetic susceptibility of leiomyoma development.

GENES INVOLVED

1. *HMGA2* (encoding high mobility group AT-hook 2) is the driver gene for tumours carrying 12q15 rearrangements. Chromosomal band 14q24 is almost always the HMGA2-targeted translocation partner in leiomyomas.[27]

2. *HMGA1* (encoding high mobility group AT-hook 1) at 6p21 are also observed and involve 14q24 in some cases.[28,29]

3. The 14q24 breakpoint maps to the RAD51B locus.11 RAD51 homologue B (Saccharomyces cerevisiae) has a role in the repair of deoxyribonucleic acid (DNA) double-strand breaks by homologous recombination.[30]

4. MED12 is a subunit of the mediator complex, a multiprotein complex thought to regulate global as well as gene-specific transcription.[31]

Advances in sequencing technology have allowed genome wide screening studies to identify genes associated with leiomyoma susceptibility. Cha and colleagues[32] genotyped 1607 individuals with uterine fibroids and identified three susceptibility loci associated with uterine fibroids, i.e. 10q24.33, 22q13.1 and 11p15.5. Chromosome 10q24.[33] was found to have the most significant association with leiomyomas and the region was mapped to the 5' region of the *SLK* gene encoding STE20-like kinase. STE20-like kinase is expressed in proliferating myoblasts and is activated by epithelial disruption. STE20-like kinase has a role in myogenic differentiation and cell motility and is activated by scratch wounding.[32] Another gene product located in the region is A-kinase anchor protein-13 (AKAP13). AKAP13 is associated with cytoskeletal filaments in leiomyoma cells. These cells abnormally respond to mechanical stress and this is accompanied by abnormal extracellular matrix deposition.[33] Dysregulation of these processes through mutation may be responsible for the fibrotic phenotype of leiomyomas.

Genome-wide screening by microarray experiments support the conclusion that uterine leiomyomas are a fibrotic disease. Genes involved in fibrosis and extracellular matrix (ECM) production and maintenance accounted for 30% of altered gene expression between leiomyomas and myometrium.[34] The search for the aetiology of abnormal ECM in fibroids implicated transforming growth factor β (TGFβ). TGFβ is a growth factor with profibrotic activity and TGFβ3 is the major isoform expressed in the female reproductive tract.[35] Its receptors are found in leiomyomas and normal myometrium. TGFβ3 and its downstream signaling molecules were overexpressed in leiomyomas compared to myometrium and treatment of rats and human leiomyoma cells with TGFβ pathway inhibitors resulted in decreased production of ECM proteins and an in vivo reduction in the number of fibroids in rats.[36,37] Furthermore, downregulation of the TGFβ pathway decreased messenger ribonucleic acid (RNA) expression of multiple *ECM* genes in uterine leiomyomas.[38] Therapy directed at disruption of this fibrotic process holds promise as a future therapeutic method.

CONCLUSION

Further molecular analysis would help to identify putative candidate genes in uterine leiomyomata formation. Identification of genes involved may aid in the genetic diagnosis of the condition, prediction of genetic risks and management of the condition by appropriate therapeutic measures.

Studying affected women and their first-degree relatives who also have uterine fibroids through cytogenetic and molecular studies is crucial to dissecting and defining the genetic loci that contributes to the development of uterine leiomyomas.

REFERENCES

1. Laughlin SK, Schroeder JC, Baird DD. New directions in the epidemiology of uterine fibroids. Semin Reprod Med. 2010;28:204-17.

2. Nivethithai P, Nikhat SR, Rajesh BV. Uterine Fibroids: A Review. Indian J Pharm Pract. 2010;3 (1):6-11.The Genetic Bases of Uterine Fibroids; A Review.

3. Medikare V, Kandukuri LR, Ananthapur V, et al. The Genetic Bases of Uterine Fibroids; A Review. J Reprod Infertil. 2011;12(3):181-91.

4. Blake RE. Leiomyomata uteri: hormonal and mo- lecular determinants of growth. J Natl Med Assoc. 2007;99(10):1170-84.

5. Luo X, Chegini N. The expression and potential regulatory function of microRNAs in the patho- genesis of leiomyoma. Semin Reprod Med. 2008;26(6):500-14.

6. Rein MS. Advances in uterine leiomyoma research: the progesterone hypothesis. Environ Health Perspect. 2000;108(5):791-3.

7. Flake GP, Andersen J, Dixon D. Etiology and pathogenesis of uterine leiomyomas: a review. Environ Health Perspect. 2003;111(8):1037-54.

8. Center for Uterine Fibroids [Internet]. Boston: Brigham and Women's Hospital; 2011. What are fibroids?; 2006 Sept 19 [cited 2011 Mar 13]; [about 3 screens]. Available from: http://www. fibroids. net/aboutfibroids.html.

9. Sandberg AA. Updates on the cytogenetics and molecular genetics of bone and soft tissue tumors: leiomyoma. Cancer Genet Cytogenet. 2005;158(1):1-26.

10. Linder D. Glucose-6-phosphate dehydrogenase mosaicism: Utilisation as a cell marker in the study of leiomyomas. Science. 1965:150:(67)

11. Townsend DE, et al. Unicellular histogenesis of uterine leiomyomas as determined by electrophoresis of glucose-6-phosphate dehydrogenase. Am J Obstet Gynecol. 1970;07:1168-73.

12. GLOWM The Global Library of Women's Medi- cine [Internet]. London: The Foundation for The Global Library of Women's Medicine; 2010. Genetics of uterine leiomyomas; 2009 May [cited 2011 Mar 13]. Available from: http://www.glowm.com/?p=glowm.cml/section_view&articleid=363.

13. Faerstein E, Szklo M, Rosenshein NB. Risk factors for uterine leiomyoma: A practice-based case-control study. II. Atherogenic risk factors and potential sources of uterine irritation Am J Epidemiol. 2001;153(1):11-19.

14. Marshall LM, et al. Variation in the incidence of uterine leiomyomata among premenopausal women by age and race. Obstet Gynecol. 1997;90:967-73.

15. Treloar SA, et al. Pathways to hysterectomy: Insights from longitudinal twin research. Am J Obstet Gynecol. 1992;167(1):82-88.

16. Winkler VDH, Hoffmann W. Regarding the question of inheritance of uterine myoma. Deutsche-Medizinische Wochenschrift. 1938;68(8):235-57.

17. Luoto R, et al. Heritability and risk factors of uterine fibroids-the Finnish Twin Cohort study. Maturitas. 2000;37(1):15-26.

18. Sudarshan S, Pinto PA, Neckers L, et al. Mechanisms of disease: hereditary leiomyomatosis and renal cell cancer—a distinct form of hereditary kidney cancer. Nat Clin Pract Urol. 2007;4:104-10.

19. Walker CL, Stewart EA. Uterine fibroids: the elephant in the room. Science. 2005;308:1589-92.

20. Uliana V, Marcocci E, Mucciolo M, et al. Alport syndrome and leiomyomatosis: the first deletion extending beyond COL4A6 intron 2. Pediatr Nephrol. 2011;26:717-24.

21. Levy B, Mukherjee T, Hirschhorn K. Molecular cytogenetic analysis of uterine leiomyoma and leiomyosarcoma by comparative genomic hybridization. Cancer Genet Cytogenet. 2000;121(1):1-8.

22. Packenham JP, du Manoir S, Schrock E, et al. Analysis of genetic alterations in uterine leiomyomas and leiomyo-sarcomas by comparative genomic hybridization. Mol Carcinog. 1997;19(4):273-9.

23. Gross KL, Morton CC. Genetics and the development of fibroids. Clin Obstet Gynecol. 2001;44:335-49.

24. Mäkinen N, Vahteristo P, Kämpjärvi K, et al. MED12 exon 2 mutations in histopathological uterine leiomyoma variants. European Journal of Human Genetics. 2013;21(11):1300-03. doi:10.1038/ejhg.2013.33.

25. Asada H, Yamagata Y, Taketani T, et al. Potential link between estrogen receptor-alpha gene hypomethylation and uterine fibroid formation. Mol Hum Reprod. 2008;14:539-45.

26. Yamagata Y, Maekawa R, Asada H, et al. Aberrant DNA methylation status in human uterine leiomyoma. Mol Hum Reprod. 2009;15:259-67.

27. Fusco A, Fedele M. Roles of HMGA proteins in cancer. Nat Rev Cancer. 2007;7:899-910.

28. Kazmierczak B, Dal Cin P, Wanschura S, et al. HMGIY is the target of 6p21.3 rearrangements in various benign mesen-chymal tumors. Genes Chromosomes Cancer. 1998;23:279-85.

29. Sornberger KS, Weremowicz S, Wil- liams AJ, et al. Expression of HMGIY in three uterine leiomyomata with complex rearrangements of chromosome 6. Cancer Genet Cytogenet. 1999;114:9-16.

30. Thacker J. The RAD51 gene family, genetic instability and cancer. Cancer Lett. 2005;219:125-35.

31. Conaway RC, Conaway JW. Function and regulation of the Mediator complex. Curr Opin Genet Dev 2011;21:225-30.P. Cha, A. Takahashi, N. Hosono et al., "A genome-wide asso-ciation study identi es three loci associated with susceptibility to uterine broids," Nature Genetics, Vol. 43, No. 5, pp. 447-451, 2011.

32. Cha PC, Takahashi A, Hosono N, Low SK, Kamatani N, Kubo M, et al. A genome-wide association study identifies three loci associated with   susceptibility to uterine fibroids. Nat Genet. 2011;43:447–50.

33. Rogers R, Norian J, Malik M, Christman G, Abu-Asab M, Chen F, et al. Mechanical homeostasis is altered in uterine leiomyoma. Am J Obstet Gynecol. 2008;198:474. e1–11.

34. Leppert PC, Catherino WH, Segars JH. A new hypothesis about the origin of uterine fibroids based on gene expression profiling with microarrays. Am J Obstet Gynecol. 2006;195:415-20.

35. Malik M, Norian J, McCarthy-Keith D, et al. Why leiomyomas are called fibroids: the central role of extracel- lular matrix in symptomatic women. Semin Reprod Med. 2010;28:169-79.

36. Joseph DS, Malik M, Nurudeen S, Catherino WH. Myometrial cells undergo fibrotic transformation under the influence of trans-forming growth factor beta-3. Fertil Steril. 2010;93:1500-8.

37. Laping NJ, Everitt JI, Frazier KS, et al. Tumorspecific efficacy of transforming growth factor- beta RI inhibition in Eker rats. Clin Cancer Res. 2007;13:3087-99.

38. Malik M, Webb J, Catherino WH. Retinoic acid treatment of human leiomyoma cells transformed the cell phenotype to one strongly resembling myometrial cells. Clin Endocrinol (Oxf). 2008;69:462-70.

CHAPTER 5

Classification of Fibroids

●Jnaneswari TL

Leiomyomas of uterus are the most common benign neoplasms of the uterus. They are also one of the most common indications for hysterectomy in gynaecology. Uterine fibroids are the most common benign tumour of the female genital tract. However, their true prevalence is probably under estimated, as the incidence at histology is more than double the clinical incidence.

Recent longitudinal studies have estimated that the lifetime risk of fibroids in a woman over the age of 45 years is more than 60%, with incidence higher in blacks than in whites.[1] They are usually asymptomatic, but may cause serious morbidity depending on the location, size and complications in them. A concrete impediment to innovation is the heterogeneity of disease in terms of size, location, growth trajectory and symptomatology of leiomyomas.

Symptomatic leiomyomas range from sizes small enough not to be palpable or visible by ultrasonography to ones large enough to distort a woman's abdominal contour mimicking pregnancy. Having a single therapy such as hysterectomy obviates the complicated decision-making brought on by a disease with many presentations.[2] Classifying myomas based on symptoms, clinical implications and prognosis helps us in taking clinical decisions easily and individualising the treatment approach.

We can classify leiomyomas on the basis of their location (Fig. 5.1), symptoms they cause and the ease of removal/ resection (Table 5.1).

■ CLASSIFICATION OF LEIOMYOMA BASED ON THEIR LOCATION

Table 5.1: Classification of leiomyoma

Uterine	Extra uterine	Unusual variants
Fundus	Cervical	Diffuse leiomyomatosis
Body	Peritoneal	Lipoleiomatosis
Cornual	Broad ligament true pseudo	Leiomyosarcoma
Lower segment	Parasitic fibroid	
Lateral wall		

Relation Between Location and Management

Cornual Fibroid

They are important as they can be a cause of infertility due to their strategic position and their removal, if not careful may lead to damage to the fallopian tubes.

Fundal Fibroid

They can arise from the anterior or the posterior wall. The incision for enucleation must be put in such a way that it does not extend to involve the fallopian tubes.

Lateral Wall

The fibroids located here are difficult to access and there is always a danger of injuring the uterine arteries, while

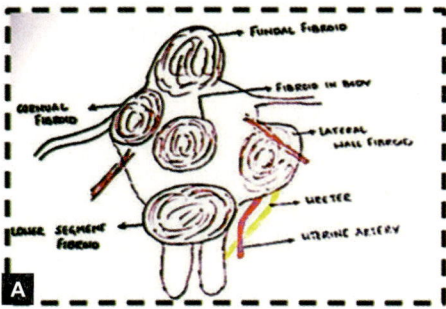

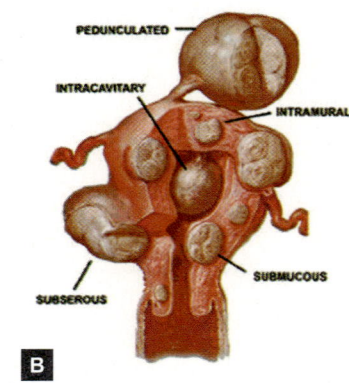

Figs 5.1A and B: Location of fibroid in uterus

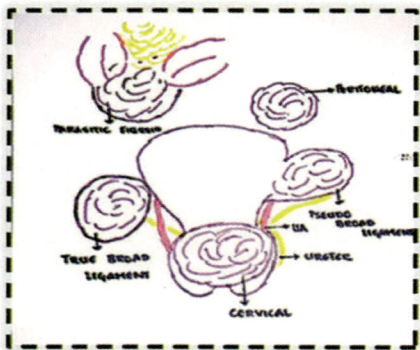

Fig. 5.2: Extra uterine leiomyoma

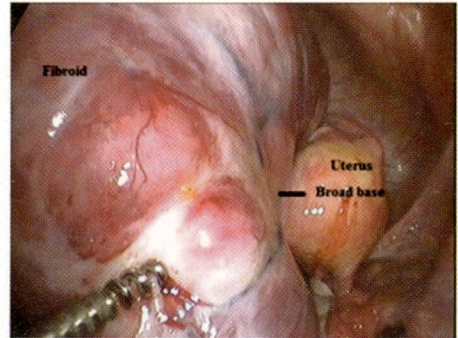

Fig. 5.3: Lateral wall fibroid

Cervix (Figs 5.5A and B) Leiomyomas located in the cervix cause distortion of the pelvic anatomy and push the ureters laterally and can be injured during dissection. The cervical canal usually opens up during enucleation, necessitating repair. They can also cause infertility due to obstruction of cervical canal and cause complications during labour.

Broad Ligament Fibroids

These are further divided into true broad ligament and pseudo broad ligament fibroids. The position of the ureters is medial in true broad ligament fibroids, while laterally pushed in pseudo broad ligament fibroids (Fig. 5.6).

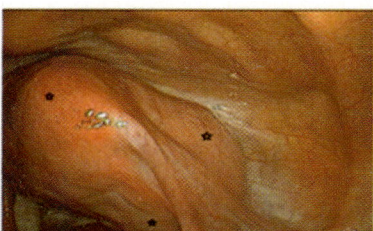

Fig. 5.4: Fibroid in the lower segment.

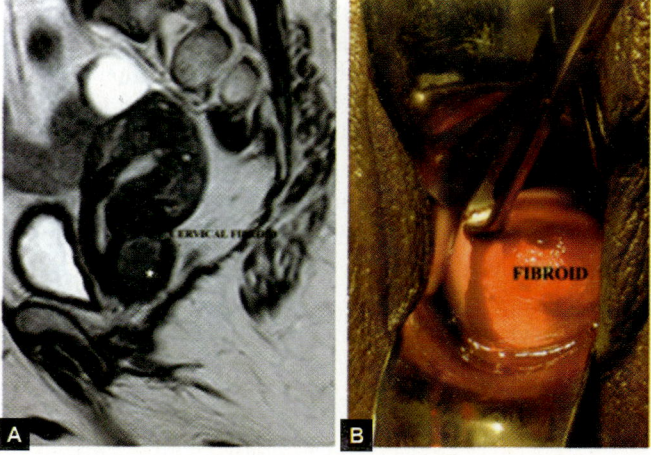

Figs 5.5A and B: Cervical fibroid presenting as mass per vaginum. **A.** Magnetic resonance imaging (MRI) sagittal section; **B.** Same fibroid on clinical examination.

enucleating them. The fibroid may grow into the broad ligament and cause ureteric displacements (Fig. 5.3).

Lower Segment

Fibroids that arise from the lower segment need dissection of the uterovesical fold and dissecting the bladder away. They interfere in labour causing malpresentations and obstructed labour and also interfere during lower segment caesarean section (LSCS). Removal may be considered before the patient gets pregnant (Fig. 5.4).

The leiomyomas in the posterior wall are more difficult to enucleate and suture due to their inaccessibility, except when they are at the fundus.

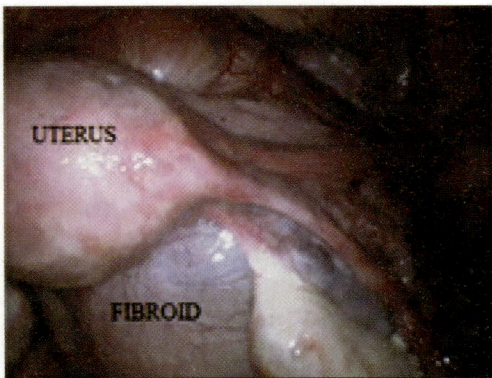

Fig. 5.6: Broad ligament fibroids

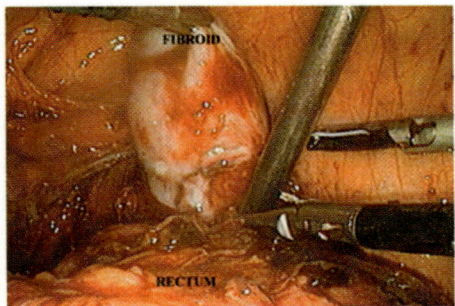

Fig. 5.7: Parasitic fibroids

Parasitic Fibroids

These fibroids pose a difficult challenge as they get their blood supply from a different structure and are usually adherent to the adjacent organs, most probably the bowel (Fig. 5.7).

■ UNUSUAL VARIANTS

Diffuse Leiomyomatosis (Fig. 5.8)

Diffuse leiomyomatosis is a rare condition that consists of diffuse involvement of the myometrium by innumerable small fibroids, which results in symmetrical enlargement of the uterus. Although histologically benign, there may be dissemination through the peritoneal cavity or occasionally metastases to distant organs. Leiomyomatosis peritonealis disseminata is an exceedingly rare benign disorder characterized by multiple vascular leiomyomas growing along the submesothelial tissues of the abdominopelvic peritoneum.[3]

This rare condition is characterized by numerous well-differentiated leiomyomas at sites distant from the uterus. The lesions are histologically identical to their uterine counterparts.[3]

Intravenous Leiomyomatosis

Intravenous leiomyomatosis is a rare disease that is histologically benign, but clinically aggressive—is

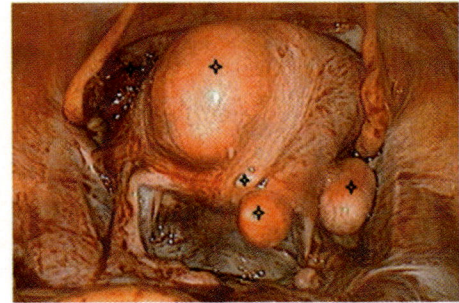

Fig. 5.8: Benign metastasizing leiomyoma

characterized by the intraluminal growth of leiomyomas in intrauterine and systemic veins. These lesions are implants from coexistent or previously resected uterine fibroids. Fewer than 150 cases of intravenous leiomyomatosis are described in the literature. Tumour growth into the venous channels of the myometrium and parametrium occurs in an estimated 80% of cases and cardiac involvement is seen in 10% to 40% of cases.[4,5]

Retroperitoneal Leiomyomatosis

Retroperitoneal growth is yet another unusual growth pattern of leiomyomas. Multiple leiomyomatous masses are usually seen in the pelvic retroperitoneum in women with a concurrent uterine leiomyoma or a history of uterine leiomyoma. Rarely, the extrauterine masses may extend to the upper retroperitoneum, as high as the level of the renal hilum. With regard to their pathologic origin, it is unclear whether these retroperitoneal lesions represent metastatic or synchronous primary lesions and whether they arise from the hormonally sensitive smooth muscle elements[6] or from the embryonal remnants of müllerian or wolffian ducts.[7]

Lipoleiomyosis

Lipoleiomyomas are rare fat-containing fibroids, with a reported prevalence of between 0.005 and 0.2%.[8] They are benign and present with the same symptoms as uterine fibroids. The most likely cause is thought to be fatty metamorphosis of the smooth muscle cells of a leiomyoma.

Leiomyosarcoma

Leiomyosarcomas may occasionally arise in a preexisting fibroid, but are usually known to occur de novo. The patient classically presents with a pelvic mass that has shown a recent or rapid increase in size. They are typically large, heterogeneous masses containing areas of haemorrhage. They usually undergo marked post contrast enhancement and have more ill defined, irregular margins than benign uterine fibroids. The fibroids can occur at unusual sites like vulva, ovary or urethra also.

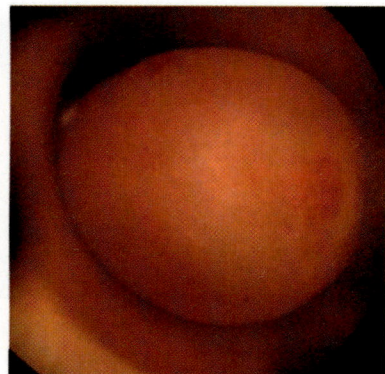

Fig. 5.9: Type 0 submucosal fibroid

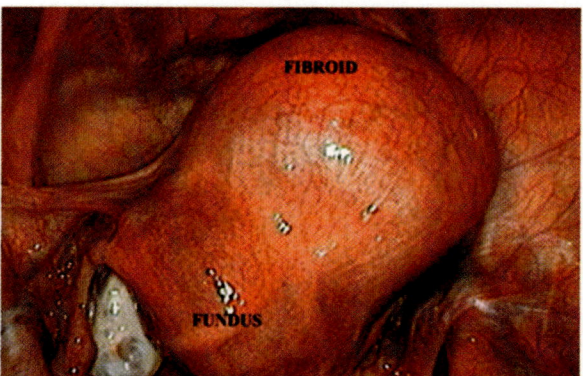

Fig. 5.11: Subserous fibroid

■ CLASSIFICATION OF LEIOMYOMAS BASED ON THEIR LOCATION IN THE UTERINE WALL

The classification of leiomyomas based on their location in the uterine wall are as follows:
1. Submucous fibroids cause menorrhagia, dysmenorrhoea and infertility and need to be treated (Fig. 5.9).
2. Intramural fibroids can be left alone if they are asymptomatic until they are more than 4 to 5 cm (Fig. 5.10A and B).
3. Subserous fibroids are usually asymptomatic and rarely cause any complications (Fig. 5.11).

Classification of submucous fibroids has been proposed on the basis of feasibility of hysteroscopic resection of the same. This scoring system gives a fair idea about the possibility of complete hysteroscopic resection, necessity of multiple

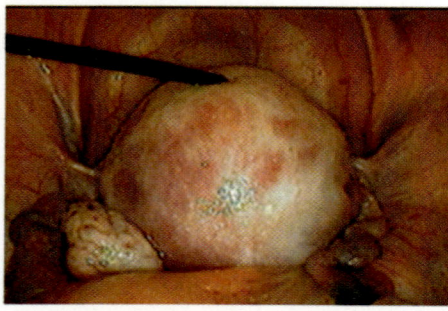

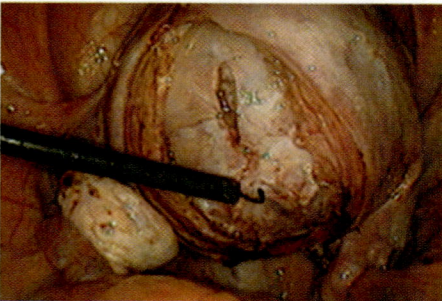

Figs 5.10A and B: Single intramural posterior wall fibroid of size 8 × 10 cm. **A.** Panoramic view; **B.** Enucleation by hysterotomy.

settings, need of laparoscopic assistance and the probability of increased incidence of complications. This enables the operating team to formulate the approach strategy and helps in discussing the various options with the patient and preparing them for the outcome.

■ CLASSIFICATION OF SUBMUCOUS MYOMAS (ESGE)

Based on the European Society of Gynecological Endoscopy (ESGE) the classification of submucous myomas are as follows:
1. Type 0: Entirely within endometrial cavity, no myometrial extension (pedunculated).
2. Type I: < 50% myometrial extension (sessile), < 90 degree angle of myoma surface to uterine wall.
3. Type II: > 50% myometrial extension (sessile), > 90 degree angle of myoma surface to uterine wall.
   (Modified from Wamsteker et al. Obstet Gynecol. 1993;82:736-740).

In addition, this system allows categorisation of the relationship of the leiomyoma outer boundary with the uterine serosa, a relationship that is important when evaluating women for resectoscopic surgery. Thus, a ESGE type 2 leiomyoma that reaches the serosa is considered to be a type 2 to 5 lesion and therefore is not a candidate for resectoscopic surgery.

Consequently, several issues were considered when constructing the classification system, including the relationship of the leiomyoma to the endometrium and the serosa; the uterine location of the leiomyoma (upper segment, lower segment; cervix, anterior, posterior, lateral); the size of the lesions; the number of lesions; and existing leiomyoma classification systems.[11] In addition to the primary classification system, both secondary and tertiary classification systems for leiomyomas are submitted; these latter systems have potential clinical applications, but should also be useful for clinical investigation.

Table 5.2: Presurgical classification of submucous myomas (FIGO classification)

Points	Penetration of myometrium	Largest myoma diameter	Extension of myoma base to endometrial cavity surface	Location along uterine wall (third)	Lateral wall (1+)
0	0	0–2 cm	< 1/3rd	Lower	
1	< 50%	2–5 cm	1/3rd–2/3rd	Middle	
2	> 50%	> 5 cm	> 2/3rd	Upper	
Total score					

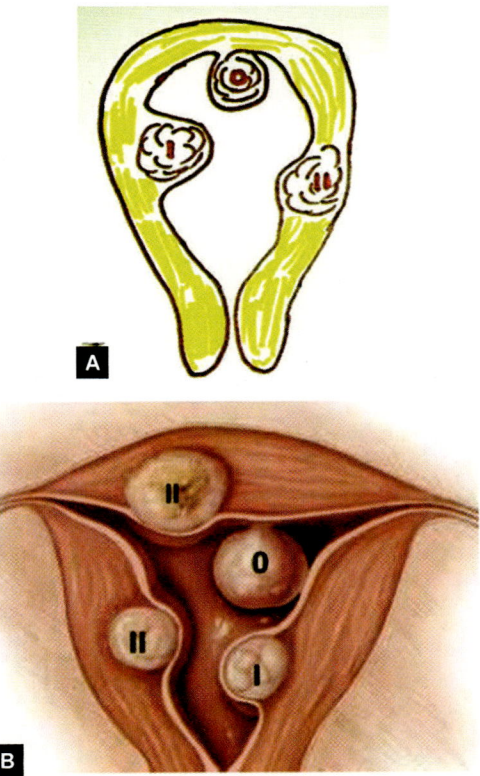

Figs 5.12A and B: Submucous myoma

The primary classification system reflects only the presence or absence of 1 or more leiomyomas, regardless of the location, number and size. It is proposed that the criteria for determining the presence of leiomyomas would require only sonographic examination confirming that 1 or more such lesions are present.

In the secondary system, the clinician is required to distinguish leiomyomas involving the endometrial cavity (submucosal [SM]) from others (O) because it is generally considered that submucosal lesions are the most likely to contribute to the genesis of AUB.

The root of the tertiary classification system is a design for subendometrial or submucosal leiomyomas that was originally submitted by Wamsteker et al.

Inspite of all the detailed classifications available on the submucous fibroids, none of them answer all the questions or the problems caused due to the fibroids. A study was conducted on 108 women using the ESGE system to evaluate infertility and heavy menstrual bleeding outcomes.

For women with type 0 or I submucous leiomyomas 5 cm or less in mean diameter, the decision-making is straightforward. This is the subgroup of leiomyomas in which the evidence is strongest for fertility impairment and hysteroscopic myomectomy has few fertility-inhibiting side effects.[12]

In general, submucous myomas (types 0, 1 and 2) up to 4 to 5 cm diameter can be removed under hysteroscopic direction[14] by experienced surgeons, whereas larger and multiple myomas are best removed abdominally. Type 2 myomas are more likely to require a multi-staged procedure than types 0 and 1.[11,12,14]

Fertility rates after treatment at a mean of 41 months were 49%, 36% and 33% in type 0, 1, and 2 lesions, respectively.[13] Those women with a normal uterine size and not more than two submucous myomas, identified at hysteroscopy were projected to have a risk of needing more surgery within 5 years of 9.7%, whereas those with an enlarged uterus and 3 or more submucous myomas had a risk of further surgery that was greater than 35% at 5 years.

It has been proposed that further research is necessary in using both these classifications in routine practice and reporting the various modalities like operative time, fluid deficit, intraoperative bleeding, feasibility of the approach, number of sittings of the planned hysteroscopic procedure, return of fertility, treatment of heavy menstrual bleeding and long term follow-up.

Table 5.3: Classification of leiomyoma based on complications to the leiomyoma

Uncomplicated	Complicated
	Degeneration
	Torsion
	Haemorrhage
	Malignant transformations

■ CLASSIFICATION OF LEIOMYOMAS BASED ON THE SYMPTOMS

Symptoms

The symptoms are of two types:
1. Symptomatic: Menorrhagia, adjacent organ compression.
2. Asymptomatic.

The number of the leiomyomas, size of the individual myomas and location play an important role in deciding the surgical method for them. Classification of the fibroids should be individualised in each patient according to its size, number, location, symptomatology and prognosis, as the treatment approach is different for each parameter. Clinicians and radiologists, while examining and reporting a case should keep all the aspects in their mind and construct a comprehensive picture for every patient according to the clinical presentation.

■ REFERENCES

1. Okolo S. Incidence, aetiology and epidemiology of uterine fibroids. Best Pract Res Clin Obstet Gynaecol. 2008;22(4):571-88. doi: 10.1016/j.bpobgyn.2008.04.002. Epub 2008 Jun 4.

2. Shannon K, Laughlin MD, MPH and Elizabeth A. et al. Uterine Leiomyomas Individualizing the Approach to a Heterogeneous Condition Obstet Gynecol. 2011;117(2 Pt 1):396-403.

3. N Fasih. Leiomyomas beyond the Uterus: Unusual Locations, Rare pubs.rsna.org/doi/full/10.1148/rg.287085095.

4. Kocia MJ, Vranes MR, Kostic D, et al. Intravenous leiomyomatosis with extension to the heart: rare or underestimated? J Thorac Cardiovasc Surg. 2005;130(6):1724-26.

5. Andrade LA, Torresan RZ, Sales JF Jr, et al. Intravenous leiomyomatosis of the uterus: a report of three cases. Pathol Oncol Res. 1998;4(1):44-47.

6. Billings SD, Folpe AL, Weiss SW. Do leiomyomas of deep soft tissue exist? An analysis of highly differentiated smooth muscle tumors of deep soft tissue supporting two distinct subtypes. Am J Surg Pathol. 2001;25(9):1134-42.

7. Stutterecker D, Umek W, Tunn R, et al. Leiomyoma in the space of Retzius: a report of 2 cases. Am J Obstet Gynecol. 2001;185(1): 248-49.

8. Maebayashi T, Imai K, Takekawa Y, et al. Radiologic features of uterine lipoleiomyoma. J Comput Assist Tomogr. 2003;27:162-5.

9. Walker CL, Stewart EA. Uterine Fibroids: The Elephant in the Room Science. 2005;308:1589–93.

10. Wamsteker K, Emanuel MH, de Kruif JH. Transcervical hysteroscopic resection of submucous fibroids for abnormal uterine bleeding: results regarding the degree of intramural extension. Obstet Gynecol. 1993;82(5):736-40.

11. Alternatives to hysterectomy in the management of leiomyomas. ACOG Practice Bulletin. American College of Obstetricians and Gynecologists. Obstet Gynecol. 2008;112:387-400.

12. Parker WH, Fu YS, Berek JS. Uterine sarcoma in patients operated on for presumed leiomyoma and rapidly growing leiomyoma. Obstet Gynecol. 1994;83:414-8.

13. Vercellini P, Zaina B, Yaylayan L, et al. Hysteroscopic myomectomy: long-term effects on menstrual pattern and fertility. Obstet Gynecol. 1999;94:341-347(II-2).

14. Lasmar RB, Barrozo PR, Dias R, et al. Submucous myomas: a new presurgical classification to evaluate the viability of hysteroscopic surgical treatment—preliminary report. J Minim Invasive Gynecol. 2005;12:308-311(II-2).

SECTION 2

Investigations and Diagnosis

CHAPTER 6

Clinical Features of Fibroids

● Geeta Uttur

Fibromyomas are generally benign neoplasms of the uterus affecting 5% to 20% of women in reproductive age group. Nearly 50% of women with fibroids are asymptomatic. These fibroids are discovered incidentally during a routine pelvic examination or ultrasound done for some unrelated symptoms. But women having symptomatic fibroids bear an enormous disease burden and reduced quality of life.

Clinical symptoms experienced by the women depend on the number, location and size of the myomas present.

■ SYMPTOMS

- Abnormal uterine bleeding
- Chronic pelvic pain/dysmenorrhoea
- Abdominal lump
- Decreased fertility/sterility
- Pressure symptoms (urological or gastroenterological)
- Pregnancy-related complications
- Asymptomatic.

A particular woman may have more than one symptom depending on the size and location of the fibroid. It is quite common to diagnose an untreated fibroid of considerable size to be diagnosed incidentally. Asymptomatic fibroids are more likely to be smaller and probably located in the subserosal and intramural portion of the uterus. Conversely a very small submucous fibroid can cause significant menstrual blood loss and recurrent pregnancy loss. It is estimated that 21% of women with fibroids seek care each year and over 90% of them will be treated with medical or surgical therapy.[1]

Abnormal Uterine Bleeding

Almost one third of women with fibroids will experience abnormal uterine bleeding.[2,3] The most common pattern is cyclical bleeding of increased quantity and/or duration. Excessive bleeding can cause reduction in a woman's quality of life and sometimes be life-threatening, since it can lead to acute blood loss requiring hospitalisation and blood transfusion. Submucous, large intramural and fibroids with intracavitary extension can cause more bleeding.[4] Irregular bleeding is not characteristic of myoma and should be investigated to rule out endometrial disease.[5] However, pedunculated submucous tumours with infection and ulceration can produce acyclical bleeding with/without purulent discharge (Fig. 6.1).

Several theories have been offered as an explanation for the excessive bleeding:
- Increased surface area
- Associated endometrial hyperplasia
- Increased vascularity and congestion
- Interference with normal uterine contractile pattern of the musculature
- Local endocrinological changes within the myoma.

One or more of these mechanisms may contribute to the finding that symptoms of heavy bleeding were equally present in patients regardless of the presence of fibroid in the uterine cavity.[6] Some studies suggest that only 40% of hysterectomy specimens, done for fibroids with menorrhagia have submucous tumours.[7]

Pelvic Pain/Pressure

Pain is not frequent symptom with fibroid. However pelvic pain such as dysmenorrhoea, dyspareunia and non-cyclical pain/discomfort/heaviness in the lower abdomen all are associated with myoma. Dysmenorrhoea can occur in a third of patients. However, there appeared to be no relationship between pelvic pain and the total volume and quantity of fibroids present (Fig. 6.2).[8]

Symptoms secondary to the displacement of surrounding organs or tissues depends on the location of fibroid. Anterior myoma can cause urinary symptoms varying from frequency to difficulty emptying of bladder and in very rare, but extreme situations, urinary obstructions leading to hydronephrosis and chronic kidney disease.[9] Posterior fibroid can cause rectal pressure, backache, tenesmus and even constipation.

Cervical and broad ligament fibroids produce no menstrual disturbances, but only pressure symptoms including ureteric obstruction. Some large tumours may be discovered by the patient herself.

Rarely fibroids produce acute pain due to torsion (subserous pedunculated), red degeneration, infection and sarcomatous degeneration. It should be noted that other degenerative changes such as hyaline, cystic and calcification of fibroids do not cause any type of pain.[10] Attempted expulsion of submucous pedunculated myoma through cervix can cause spasmodic type of pain.

However, it is always important to keep in mind that not all the pelvic pain is due to fibroids and other etiologies must be considered before we consider treating myoma for pelvic pain.

Infertility

Fibroids are present in approximately 5% to 10% of patients with infertility and are the only abnormality seen in 1% to 2.4% of patients with infertility. Fibroids might reduce fertility by the following mechanisms:[11]
- Obstruction of fallopian tubes (Fig. 6.3)
- Impaired gamete transport

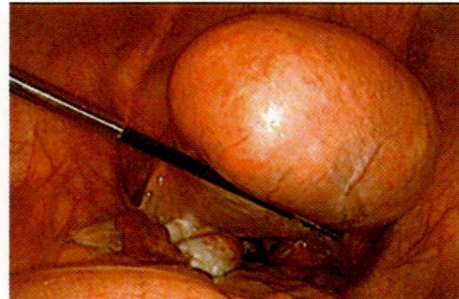

Fig. 6.1: Single intramural fibroid presenting as abnormal uterine bleeding (AUB)

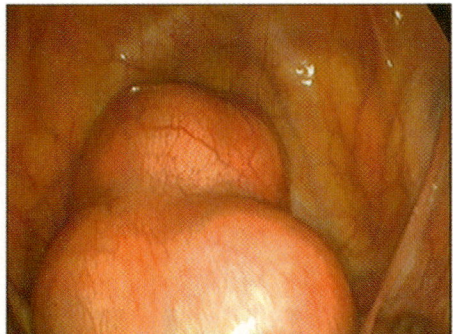

Fig. 6.2: Multiple fibroids in a young lady presenting as dysmenorrhoea

- Abnormal endometrial receptivity
- Distortion of the endometrial cavity
- Impaired uterine contractility
- Impaired blood supply to endometrium
- Abnormal hormonal milieu.

Clinical pregnancy, implantation and live birth rates are significantly impaired in woman with any location of fibroid.[12,13] The effect of fibroids on fertility depends on the location of fibroid with submucous and intracavitary fibroids having the greatest effect. The effect of submucosal fibroids remains unclear, but myomectomy prior to in vitro fertilisation (IVF) in patients with intramural fibroids greater than 50 mm has been shown to be beneficial to pregnancy outcomes.[14] Subserosal fibroids are thought to have little to no effect on fertility but the classification of some fibroids as subserosal is controversial. Myomectomy for subserosal fibroids likely has no effect on pregnancy outcomes (IFigs 6.4A and B).[11]

◼ OBSTETRIC OUTCOMES AND UTERINE FIBROIDS

Incidence of pregnancies affected by presence of fibroid is between 1% and 4%. Majority of these do not change during pregnancy and mostly remain asymptomatic. Only 20% to 30% of the fibroids increase in size and the increase is not more than 25% in volume and occur mostly in first trimester.[15] In about 5% to 10% of pregnant women with fibroids, the fibroids undergo red degeneration. This is a form of coagulative necrosis resulting in a haemorrhagic, meaty cut surface and areas of cystic degeneration causing severe abdominal pain and mild fever often requiring a short hospital stay and conservative management. A similar clinical picture may be often seen after gonadotrophin-releasing hormone (GnRH) agonist treatment or uterine artery embolisation (UAE).

However, regression in the size of the fibroid has been demonstrated in 70% of women following live births. These women have more than 50% reduction in volume of fibroid between early gestation and 3 to 6 months post partum.[16]

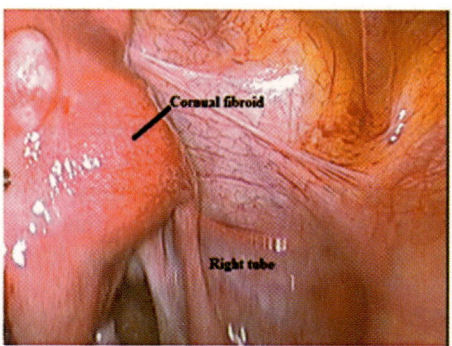

Fig. 6.3: Cornual fibroid in an infertility patient

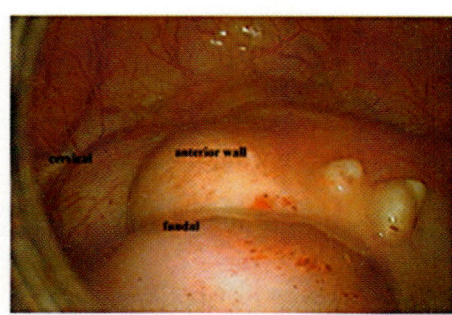

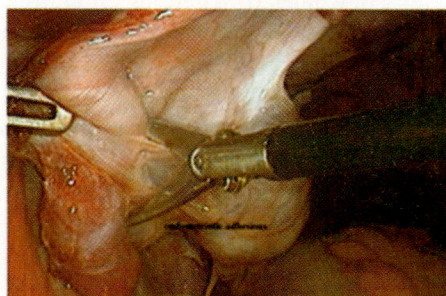

Figs 6.4A and B: A. Multiple intramural and subserosal fibroids (largest being 4 cm) in an infertile female, with previous invitro fertilisation (IVF) failures; B. Same patient with associated endometriosis, distorting tubal anatomy.

Unfavourable outcomes of pregnancy resulting from existence of myoma is quite uncommon. Possible effects of fibroid on pregnancy include:

- Miscarriage(s)
- Preterm labour
- Placental abruption
- Intra uterine growth retardation (IUGR)
- Malpresentations
- Obstructed labour
- Caesarean section and caesarean hysterectomy
- Postpartum haemorrhage (PPH).

Data indicate that fibroids in all locations have an impact on pregnancy outcome and lower live birth rates compared to women without fibroids.[13] Patients with submucous and intramural fibroids have significantly higher spontaneous abortion rate unlike subserosal fibroid with no difference in abortion rates compared to women without fibroids.[13]

Fibroids have been shown to increase risk of preterm delivery particularly, if they are large or multiple. Placental abruption and IUGR can result if the placenta is adjacent to or overlying the fibroid. Large submucous fibroids can distort the uterine cavity and can result in fetal malpresentation. Incidence of malpresentations is significantly higher in women with fibroids compared to women without fibroid,[17] thereby increasing the risk of caesarean section and in turn increasing maternal morbidity.

In coordinate uterine muscle contraction can result in uterine inertia, prolonged labour and post partum haemorrhage after delivery.

SEXUAL PROBLEMS AND FIBROIDS

Patients with uterine fibroids are noted to have significant impairment in sexual function with high rate of dyspareunia.[18] Women with fibroid often feel different, less attractive and inadequate, which adversely affects their sexual function. Fundal and anterior fibroid cause more intense deep dyspareunia than fibroids in other location.[19]

UNCOMMON/UNUSUAL CLINICAL FEATURES OF FIBROIDS

1. Polycythemia is seen occasionally with uterine lieomyomas. This is believed to be the result of autonomous production of erythropoietin by a myoma.[20]
2. Ascites in association with pedunculated or subserous tumours, can result in pseudo Meig syndrome.
3. Disseminated peritoneal myomatous nodules (leiomyoma peritonealis disseminata).
4. Uterine inversion (chronic) with pedunculated submucous fibroids.
5. Very rarely a tumour may get adhered to adjacent viscera, obtain a fresh blood supply from these adhesions and finally be detached completely from the uterus. It is called 'wandering fibroid'/'parasitic fibroid'.

SARCOMATOUS CHANGE IN MYOMA— WHAT IS THE EVIDENCE?

Leiomyosarcoma is the malignant counterpart of benign uterine small leiomyoma accounting for 1% to 2% of all uterine malignancies.

There is no evidence that women with uterine myoma are at increased risk for this malignant neoplasm. Therefore, labeling leiomyosarcoma as a form of 'malignant change' in preexisting myoma is a misnomer. Most leiomyosarcoma occur later in life (fifth/sixth decade) as compared to benign leiomyomas. They may be found concurrently with or rarely may originate from a benign uterine leiomyoma.[21] Because there is no pathognomonic imaging feature that can distinguish leiomyosarcoma from benign leiomyoma, identification of this rare malignancy often occurs after surgery for a presumed benign condition. Abnormal uterine bleeding and rapid growth of the uterus in a postmenopausal women may suggest the possibility.

Because of the rarity of the tumour and lack of evidence, myomectomy/hysterectomy in women with asymptomatic fibroids is not justified for the fear of 'sarcomatom change' in a fibroid.

FIBROIDS AND QUALITY OF LIFE ISSUES

Fibroids can affect many other areas of patient's lives, including activity level, energy, mood and sexual life. To assess the impact of symptomatic fibroids, on patients quality of life and to quantitatively measure symptoms related to fibroid disease the research team led by Spies developed the uterine fibroid symptom and quality of life (UFS-QOL) questionnaire.[22] It revealed that women with fibroids experienced significantly elevated level of symptom distress and lower health related quality of life compared to patients without fibroids. Significant improvement in all parameter of quality of life was observed after treatment of fibroid with UAE, myomectomy and hysterectomy, improvement being greater with hysterectomy.

CLINICAL SIGNS

Progressive anaemia may be noted due to chronic blood loss. An abdominal lump may be felt arising from the pelvis. The mass usually is firm in consistency with well-defined margins and smooth or bossy surface depending on the number and location of the fibroids. The tumour is mobile from side-to-side unless fixed by large size or adhesions or by coexisting conditions like endometriosis. Ascites is rare.

Bimanual examination will reveal an enlarged uterus with regular or bossy surface. The cervix moves with swelling, which is not felt separate from the uterus. Pedunculated fibroid is seen as separate mass. In broad ligament fibroids, uterus is displaced to the opposite side and fibroid is felt as adnexal mass.

In cervical fibroid uterus is found sitting over the mass. In a fibroid polyp, cervical os is felt open and lower pole of the fibroid felt per vaginum. In chronic inversion with fibroid polyp, the fundus of the uterus cannot be felt.

In about 90% of the cases clinical examination is sufficient to make the diagnosis, which can be confirmed by imaging technologies.

CONCLUSION

Uterine fibroids form a significant disease entity affecting 5% to 20% of women of reproductive age group of which 50% of them are symptomatic. Symptoms are varied and include abnormal uterine bleeding, pain, recurrent pregnancy loss, adverse obstetric outcome, infertility, urological and gastrointestinal complications, sexual dysfunction and pelvic pressure. These symptoms affect the quality of life significantly resulting in considerable morbidity and loss of work.

Considering the clinical significance of fibroid uterus more research into aetiology, risk factors and growth of fibroids is needed, so as to better understand the disease process and form strategies to prevent the disease from occurring.

KEY POINTS

- Fibroids or leiomyomas are benign tumours of the uterus affecting 5% to 20% of the reproductive age group of women.
- Majority of the myomas are asymptomatic. 20% to 50% of them may present with varying symptoms depending on the size, number and location of fibroids.
- The one third of women with fibroids suffer from abnormal uterine bleeding, which may result in severe anaemia requiring hospitalisation and blood transfusion.
- Fibroids are responsible for infertility in 5% to 10% of patients—submucous and intramural myomas more responsible than subserous myoma. However removal of intramural myoma of > 4 cm significantly improves assisted reproductive techniques (ART) outcomes.
- 20% to 30% of fibroids increase in size during pregnancy and increase is no more than 25% of the total volume. In 5% to 10 % pregnant women with fibroids, red degeneration can occur resulting in acute pain abdomen.
- Adverse obstetric outcomes resulting from fibroids are uncommon, but include recurrent abortion, preterm labour, placental abruption, IUGR, malpresentations, obstructed labour, caesarean section and postpatrum haemorrhage.
- Fibroids can cause significant impairment in sexual function and quality of life.
- Sarcomatous change in a fibroid is a rare occurence and prophylactic myomectomy or hysterectomy on this basis, in a woman with asymptomatic fibroid is not justified.
- All symptoms due to fibroids are non-specific and all other differential diagnosis are to be considered before treating fibroid for a particular symptom.

REFERENCES

1. Carls GS, Lee DW, Ozminkowlski RJ, et al. What are the total costs of surgical treatment for uterine fibroids? J Women's Health (Larchmt). 2008;17:1119-32.

2. Lumsden MA, Wallace EM: Clinical presentation of uterine fibroids. Bailliere's Clin Obst and Gyne. 1998;12(2):177-95.

3. Gupta S, Jose J, Manyonda I. Clinical presentation of fibroids. Best Pract-Res Clin Obstet Gynaecol 2008;22:615-26.

4. Bukulmez O. Doody KJ. Clinical features of myomas. Obstat Gynaecol Clin North AM. 2006;33:69-84.

5. Stewart-EA Uterine fibroids. Lancet. 2001;357:293-8.

6. Wegienka G, Baird DD, Hertz-Pocciotto I, et al. Self reported heavy bleeding associated with uterine Leiomyoma. Obstet Gynecol. 2003;101:431-7.

7. Lumsden MA. Fibroids and menorrhagia. In Shaw RW, Uterine fibroids: Time for review,UK. Parthenon publishing. 1992;57-68.

8. Lippman SA, Warner M, Samuel S, et al. Uterine fibroids and gynecologic pain symptoms in a population-based study. Fertil Steril. 2003;80:1488-94.

9. Bansal T, Mehrotra P, Jayasena D, et al. Obstructive nephropathy and chronic kidney disease secondary to uterine leiomeyomas. Arch Gynecol Obstet. 2009;279:785-8.

10. Persaud V, Arjoon PD. Uterine leiomyomata; Incidence of degenerative change and correlation of associated symptoms. Obstet Gynecol. 1970;35:432-6.

11. Cook H, Ezzati M, Segars JH. et al. The impact of uterine leiomyomas on reproductive outcomes. Minerva Ginecol. 2010;62:225-36.

12. Somigliana E, Vercellini P, Daguati R, et al. Fibroids and female reproduction; a critical analysis of the evidence. Hum Reprod update. 2007;13:465-76.

13. Pritts EA, Parker WH, Olive DL. Fibroids and infertility; an updated systematic review of the evidence. Fertil Steril. 2009;91:1215-23.

14. Bulletti C. Ziegler D, Levisetti P, Cicinelli E, et al. Myomas, pregnancy outcome and invitro fertilization. Ann N Y Acad Sci. 2004;1034:84-92.

15. Stovall DW. Clinical symptomatology of uterine leiomyomas. Clin Obst and Gyne. 2001;44(2):364-71.

16. Laughter SK, Hartmann KE, Baird DD. Postpartum factors and natural fibroid regression. A M J Obstet Gyneocol. 2011;204:496.

17. Ouyang DW. Economy KE, Norwitz ER :Obstetric complications of fibroids. Obstet Gynecol Clin North AM. 2006;33:153-69.

18. Lippman SA, Warner M, Samuels S, et al. Uterine fibroids and gynecological pain symptoms in a population based study. Fertil steril. 2003;80:1488-94.

19. Ferreros, Abbamonte CH, Giordanom Parisi M, et al. Uterine myomas dyspareunia and sexual dysfunction: Fertil Steril. 2006;86:1504-10.

20. Raj R, et al. Polycythemia associated with lieomyoma of the uterus. Lake Y BR J Obstet Gynecol. 1992;99(911):923-5.

21. D'Angelo E, Prat J. Uterine sarcomas; a review: Gynaecol oncol. 2010;116:131-9.

22. Spies JB, Coyne K, Guaou Guoaou N, et al. The USF-QOL ,a new disease specific symptoms and health related quality of life Questionnaire for Leimyomata. Obstet Gynaecol Clin North AM. 2006;385-95.

CHAPTER 7

Imaging of Uterine Fibroids

● Ramachandra C, Raghunatha Rao

■ INTRODUCTION

Uterine fibroid, also known as leiomyoma, are the commonest uterine neoplasm. Although benign, they can be associated with significant morbidity and are the commonest indication for hysterectomy. Fibroid could be single or multiple and occur at multiple locations in uterus or outside the uterus (Fig. 7.1). The size range from subcentimeter to huge ones, measuring several centimetres, extending beyond pelvis. Histologically, they are benign tumours composed predominantly of smooth muscle cells separated by variable amounts of fibrous connective tissue.[1,2] Although there is no true capsule, these tumours are well circumscribed and surrounded by a pseudo capsule. Several observations suggest that oestrogen and progesterone play an important role in the growth of leiomyomas. Leiomyomas occur in women of reproductive age, often enlarge during pregnancy or during oral contraceptive use, and regress after menopause.[3] They are often discovered incidentally when performing imaging for other reasons. Usually first identified with ultrasonography (USG), they can be further characterized with magnetic resonance imaging (MRI), if there is a clinical need. They are usually easily recognizable, but degenerated fibroids can have unusual appearances. In this chapter, the appearances of typical and atypical uterine fibroids, unusual fibroid variants and fibroid mimics are described on different imaging modalities. Knowledge of the different appearances of fibroids on imaging is essential as it enables prompt diagnosis and guides treatment.

Intravenous leiomyomatosis, metastasizing leiomyoma, diffuse leiomyomatosis, and peritoneal disseminated leiomyomatosis represent unusual growth patterns. Other unusual growth patterns include retroperitoneal and parasitic growth.[4]

Lieomyosarcoma is a very rare entity that should be suspected in postmenopausal women with increasing size of the fibroid.

■ CLASSIFICATION

Three primary or common types of uterine fibroids, classified according to location in the uterus are listed in Tables 7.1. Other systems of classification are described in Table 7.2 and 7.3.

Table 7.1: Common types of uterine fibroids

Types	Features
Submucosal	Least common, nearly 5%. In rare instances, sub mucosal leiomyomas may become pedunculated and protrude into the cervical canal or vagina as a polyp
Intramural	Most common and, are most often asymptomatic
Subserosal	Asymptomatic or presentation may be due pressure effect on the adjoining organs. However, pedunculated subserosal leiomyomas may undergo torsion, which results in infarction accompanied by pain.[5,6]

Uncommon extrauterine fibroids are broad ligament (Figs 7.37 to 7.39), parasitic and cervical fibroids (Figs 7.16, 7.29 and 7.35). Specific types of unusual leiomyomas include lipoleiomyoma and myxoid leiomyoma, which may have MRI features characteristic enough to allow differentiation from other gynaecologic and non-gynaecologic diseases (Figs

7.40 and 7.41). Intravenous leiomyomatosis, metastasizing leiomyoma, diffuse leiomyomatosis and peritoneal disseminated leiomyomatosis represent unusual growth patterns; other unusual growth patterns are retroperitoneal growth and parasitic growth.

Table 7.2: Classification based on MR signal (T2WI)

Type	Appearance on MRI	Fibroid vascularity
Type 1	Low signal intensity as that of skeletal muscle (Fig. 20A.)	Hypovascular
Type 2	Intermediate signal intensity, lower than myometrium, but higher than skeletal muscle (Fig. 20E.)	Intermediate vascularity
Type 3	High signal intensity, same or higher than myometrium (Fig. 20C)	Hypervascular

Funaki K, Sawada K, Maeda F, et al. Subjective effect of magnetic resonance-guided focused ultrasound surgery for uterine fibroids.

Table 7.3: FIGO classification of leiomyomas

Submucosal	0	Pedunculated intracavitory
	1	< 50% Intramural
	2	≥ 50% Intramural
O others	3	Contacts endometrium: 100% intramural
	4	Intramural
	5	Subserosal ≥ 50% intramural
	6	Subserosal < 50% intramural
	7	Subserosal pedunculated
	8	Others (specify, e.g. cervical, parasitic)
Hybrid leiomyomas (impact both endometrium and serosa)	Two numbers are listed separated by a hyphen. By convention first refers to the relationship with the endometrium, while the second refers to the relationship with serosa. One example is below	
	2–5	Submucosal and subserosal, each with less than half of half of the diameter endometrial and peritoneal cavities, respectively

Teaching point: Types 0 and I are hysteroscopically resectable, although significant hysteroscopic expertise may be needed to resect type I masses.

◼ IMAGING TOOLS

Radiography/Contrast Radiography

Conventional radiographs have a limited role in the diagnosis of uterine fibroids. Only calcified fibroids are depicted on the radiographs. Classical appearance of a calcified fibroid is cotton wool appearance, pop corn or amorphous calcifications (Fig. 7.2). Extreme enlargement of the uterus resulting from

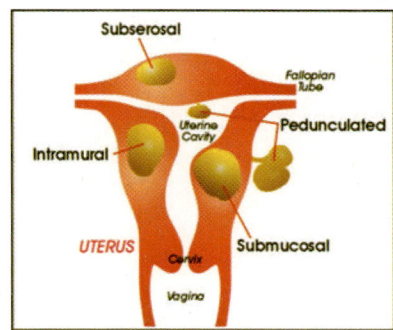

Fig. 7.1: Graphic illustration of different locations of fibroids

fibroids may be seen as a non-specific soft-tissue mass of the pelvis that possibly displaces loops of bowel. In the intravenous urogram (IVU) study, urinary bladder and ureteric compression and consequent hydroureteronephrosis may be seen.

Computed Tomography

Like radiography, computer tomography (CT) scanning also has a limited role in the diagnosis of uterine fibroids. May be incidentally detected when performed for other indications. On CT scans, fibroids are usually indistinguishable from healthy myometrium unless they are calcified or necrotic. Calcifications may be more visible on CT scans than on conventional radiographs because of the superior contrast resolution. The typical finding is a bulky, irregular uterus or a mass in continuity with the uterus (Fig. 7.3). Degenerated fibroids may appear complex and contain areas of fluid attenuation. Calcification is seen in approximately 4% of fibroids4 and is typically dense and amorphous. However, calcification can also be confined to the periphery of the fibroid, when it is thought to be secondary to thrombosed veins from previous red degeneration.

Ultrasonography

Ultrasonography is the imaging modality of choice in the detection and evaluation of uterine fibroids.[7,8,9] While a cost-effective instrument, ultrasound has been criticized for its significant operator dependence, resulting in inferior reproducibility when compared to MRI.[10–13] Ideally, both transabdominal (TA) and transvaginal (TV) scans should be performed. Transvaginal scans are more sensitive for the diagnosis of small fibroids (Figs 7.4A and B); however, when the uterus is bulky, the uterine fundus may lie outside of the field of view. Transabdominal views are often of limited value, if the patient is obese. Ultrasonography is highly operator dependent, but with the present day technical advances and in skilled hands, fibroids as small as 5 mm can be demonstrated on TV USG. Uterine fibroids most often

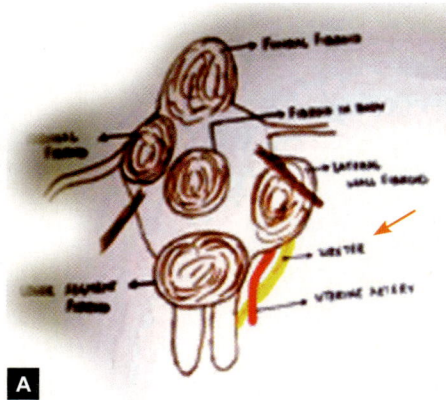

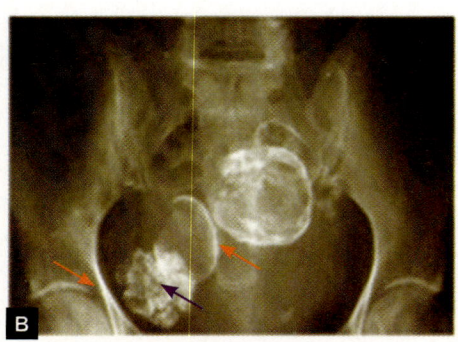

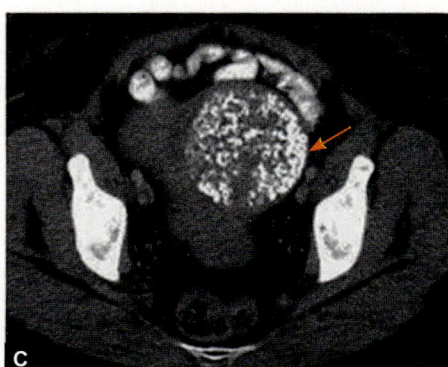

Figs 7.2:A to C: Plain radiograph of pelvis done for unrelated issue in a post-menopausal patient, showing a large dense amorphous calcified fibroid (orange arrow). A. Diagrammatic representation of uterus with multiple fibroid; **B.** Multiple fibroids with peripheral and amorphous dense calcifications and **C.** Axial non-contrast CT of another 42 years. Old female showing amorphous calcifications in a subserous fibroid on left side (orange arrow).

appear on ultrasonograms as concentric, solid, hypoechoic masses (Fig. 7.5). These solid masses absorb sound waves and therefore cause a variable amount of acoustic shadowing. Fibroids may vary in their degree of echogenicity; they can be heterogeneous or hyperechoic, depending on the amount of fibrous tissue and/or calcification. Fibroids may have anechoic components resulting from necrosis or degeneration (Fig. 7.6). The echogenic endometrial stripe may be displaced by a fibroid. Calcifications are hyperechoic, with sharp acoustic shadowing. Diffuse leiomyomatosis appears as an enlarged uterus with abnormal echogenicity (Figs 7.7A and B to 7.11A to C).

Saline Infusion Sonohysterography

Saline infusion sonohysterography[14] based imaging is usually used as a supplementary or adjunct imaging modality for characterization of focal uterine masses bulging into the uterine cavity. It is often difficult on routine scan, to distinguish a leiomyoma from a blood clot or a polyp, and leiomyomas also may obscure the endometrium on imaging or cause an overestimation of endometrial thickness. Fibroids appear as hypoechoic masses in contrast to endometrial polyps, which

are usually hyperechoic with respect to the myometrium. In addition, the echogenic endometrium can be seen draping over the fibroid. Recurrent refractive shadowing is reported to be a particularly useful sign for uterine leiomyomas. The extent to which the fibroid projects into the lumen of the endometrial cavity is of clinical importance. If the fibroid projects into the lumen by more than 50% of its surface, then it can be resected by hysteroscopy, obviating an abdominal surgical procedure. Endometrial polyps, may appear as hyperechoic masses surrounded by a hypoechoic endometrium.

Magnetic Resonance Imaging

Magnetic resonance imaging is considered the most accurate imaging technique for detection and localisation of leiomyomas (Figs 7.12A and B to 7.31). MR imaging has been shown to be more sensitive than US in detection of leiomyomas.[16] Unlike with MR imaging, accurate assessment of an enlarged, myomatous uterus (> 140 cm³) is not consistently possible with US because of the limited field of view.[17] The capability of MR imaging for excellent demonstration of the uterine zonal anatomy enables accurate classification of individual masses as submucosal, intramural or subserosal (Figs 7.32 tp

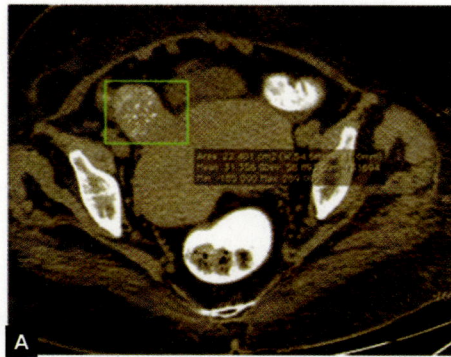

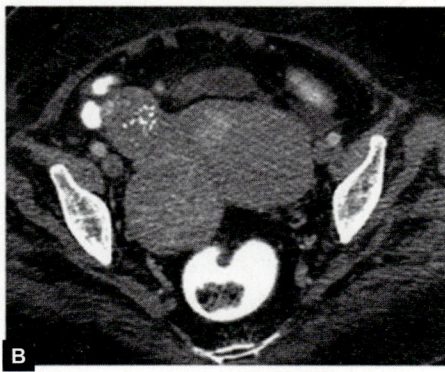

Figs 7.3A and B: Pre- and post-IV contrast axial CT sections through pelvis showing multiple isodense, mildly enhancing intramural and subserous fibroids and a subserous fibroid on right side showing amorphous calcifications (green box).

7.35).[18] MR imaging has been shown to be more accurate than US or hysterosalpingography for determining the location of leiomyomas in infertile women prior to myomectomy.[17]

◼ SUBMUCOSAL LEIOMYOMA

Ultrasonography

1. Hypoechoic subendometrial mass.
2. Stretched, but intact overlying echogenic endometrium.
3. In continuity with myometrium.
4. May attenuate sound or cause edge shadow.
5. Pulsed doppler: Variable resistive indices depending on its vascularity.
6. Colour doppler: Wide range of vascularity depending on cellularity or presence of degeneration. Highly vascular lesion may show central vascularity as well as vessels draped around the mass. If broad based may find multiple vascular pedicles.
7. Sonohysterography: Mass indenting the endometrial cavity, intraluminal mass. Intraluminal projection should be more than 50% of total thickness to be eligible for hysteroscopic removal (Figs 7.13 to 7.19A to C).

Teaching point: Ultrasound appearance of fibroid depends on the amount of fibrosis and muscle components. If muscle component is predominant it will appear as hypoechoic and if fibrosis is more it will be echogenic.

Teaching point: The TVS is for initial imaging and diagnosis. Sonohysterography for surgical planning. MRI scan, in case multiple leiomyomas causing uterine distortion or to differentiate leiomyomas from adenomyoma. MRI has a major role in treatment planning and response assessment.

MRI Findings

Generally well-defined mass arising from myometrium:
1. T1WI: Homogenous, isointense to myometrium or hyper intense, if there is haemorrhagic degeneration.
2. T2WI: Homogenously hypointense to myometrium. Hyperintense if highly cellular or vascular (Figs 7.20A to E).

Contrast Scan

Variable enhancement, enhances less than normal myometrium on delayed scan. Hypervascular fibroids enhances more (Figs 7.21A and B).

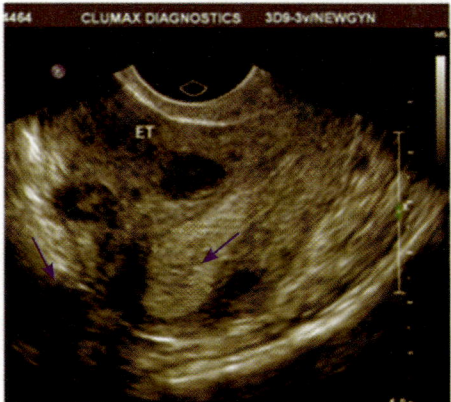

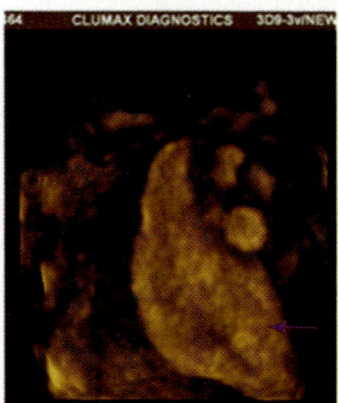

Figs 7.4A and B: A. Sagittal transvaginal sonogram showing multiple intramural hypoechoic fibroids (blue arrows) and **B.** 3D scan showing intramural fibroids (blue arrow).

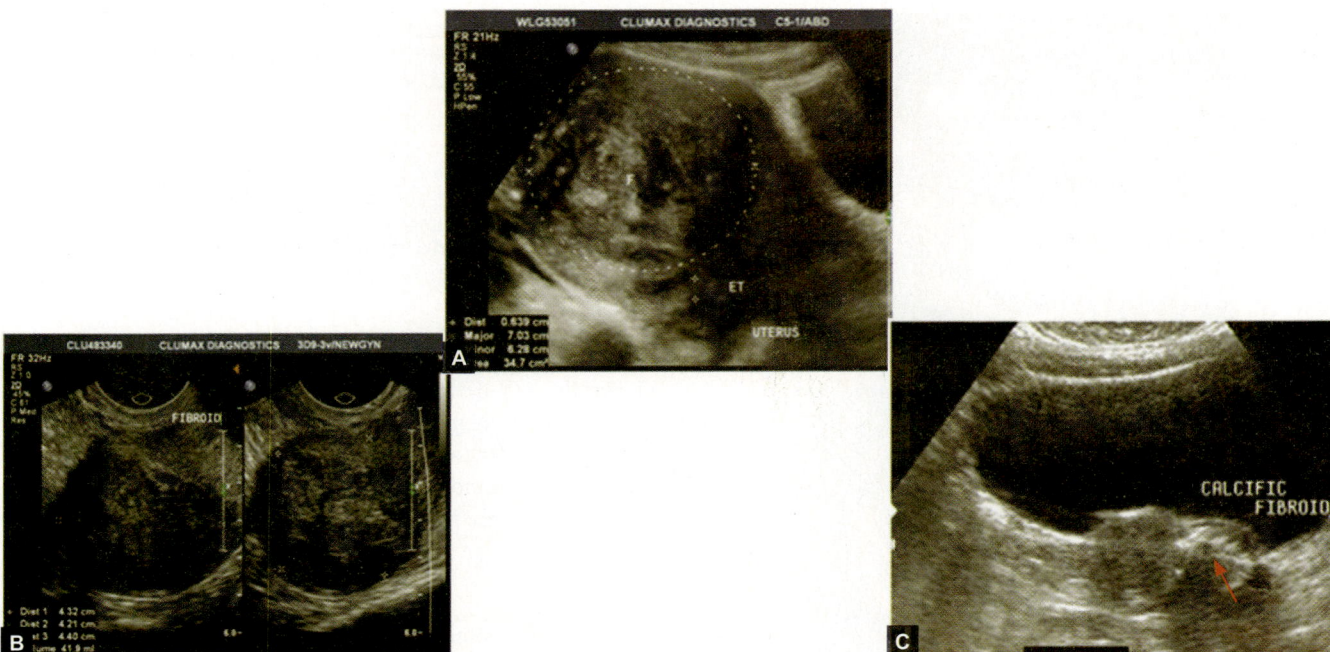

Figs 7.5A to C: A. Sagittal transabdominal sonogram showing large intramural mixed echoic fibroid; **B.** TVS scan showing well-defined hypoechoic subserosal fundal and posterior wall fibroid; **C.** Calcified fibroid in the left lateral wall (red arrow head).

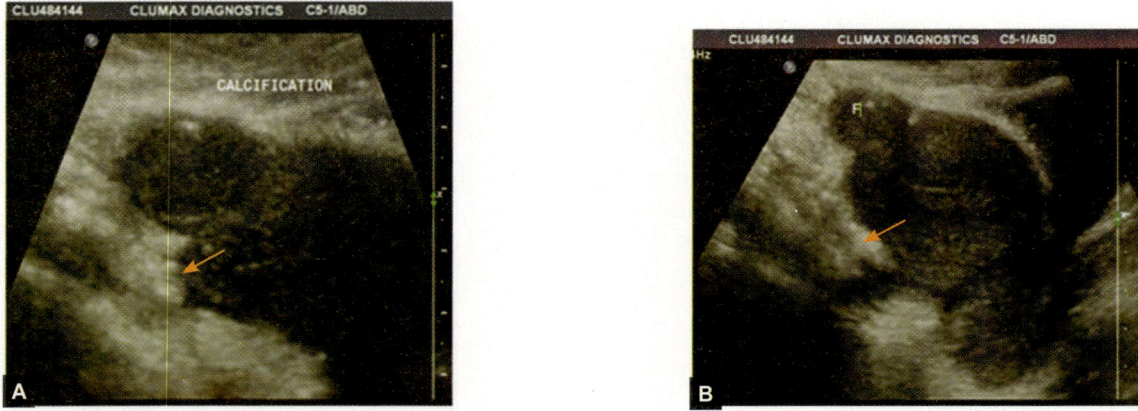

Figs 7.6A and B: Transverse and sagittal transabdominal scan showing small fundal subserosal hypoechoic fibroid with a peripheral calcifications, which are seen as a bright foci (orange arrows).

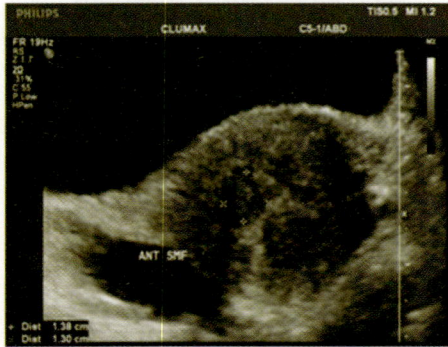

Fig. 7.7: Transabdominal transverse sonogram showing small submucosal fibroid in a 26 years old, presented with menorrhagia

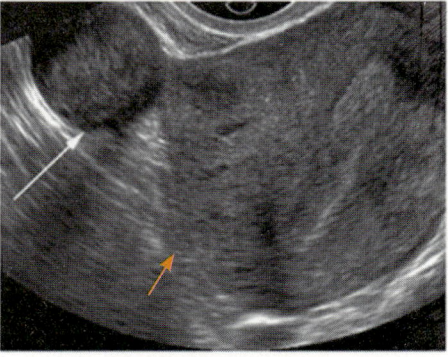

Fig. 7.8: Transvaginal transverse sonogram showing pedunculated (orange arrow) subserosal fibroid (white arrow)

Differential Diagnosis

Endometrial Polyp

TVS

No stretched endometrial lining overlying the mass. No continuity with underlying myometrium single vascular pedicle.

MRI

High signal intensity on T2WI and endometrial origin, enhances with contrast.

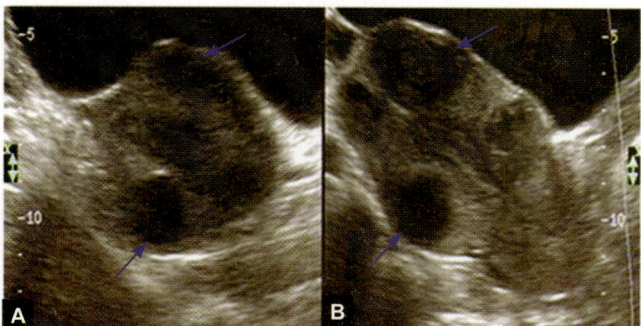

Figs 7.9A and B: Transverse and sagittal transabdominal sonogram showing multiple intramural hypoechoic fibroids (blue arrows)

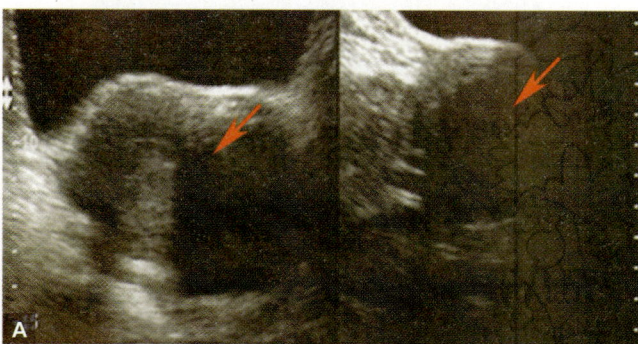

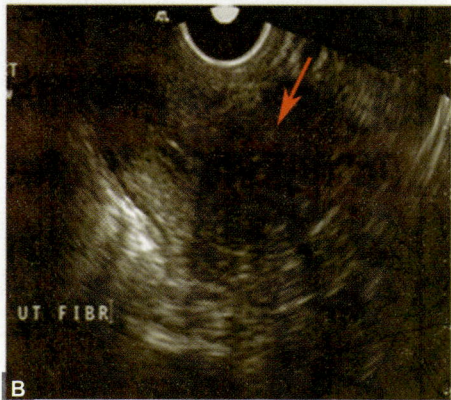

Figs 7.10 A and B: A. Transverse and sagittal transabdominal sonogram of an intramural fibroid showing dense shadowing (red arrows); **B.** Transvaginal scan shows shadowing from an intramural fibroid in another patient.

Adenomyosis

Loss of junctional zone anatomy, poorly defined lesion with cystic foci within. No contour abnormality (Figs 7.22A and B to 7.24A and B).

Endometrial Carcinoma

Usually no endometrial stripe in TVS.

Heterogeneous signal intensity on T2WI and enhances with contrast.

■ INTRAMURAL LEIOMYOMA

Radiograph

Calcifications; common pattern—dense amorphous. Ring-like peripheral rare, represents thrombosed veins from past red degeneration. Displacement of bowel loops if large, as well as compression of ureters and urinary bladder on IVU.

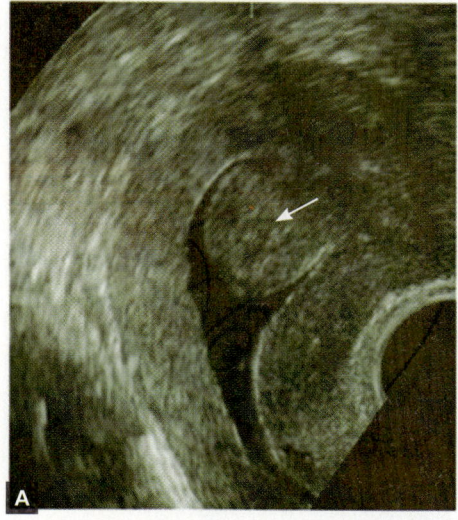

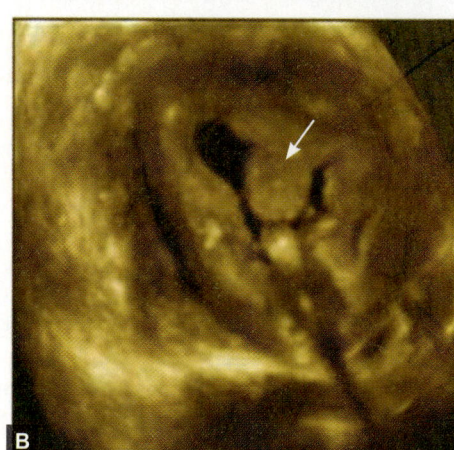

Figs 7.11A and B: A. Saline Sonohysterography showing hypoechoic submucosal fibroid bulging in to the endometrial cavity, which is distended with saline (white arrow); **B.** 3D image in another patient showing similar finding.

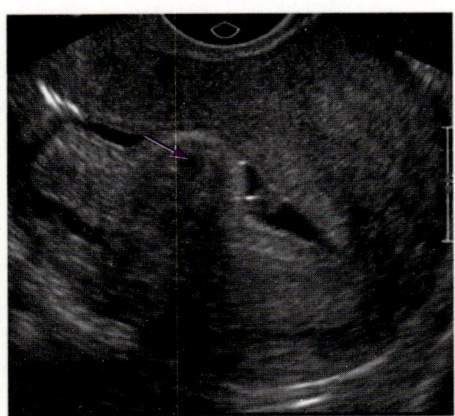

Fig. 7.12: Sagittal transvaginal sonogram showing intramural hypoechoic fibroid (blue arrow) bulging into the endometrial cavity

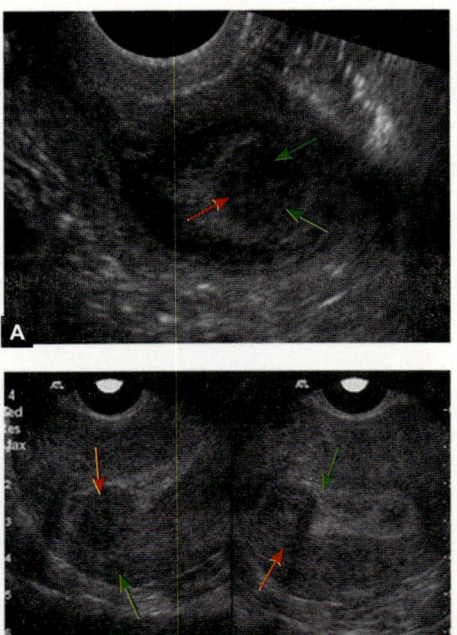

Figs 7.13A and B: Transverse transvaginal sonogram showing hypoechoic submucosal fibroid (green arrows) and hyperechoic compressed endometrium (red arrow)

Ultrasonography

Enlarged lobulated uterus homogenous hypoechoic mass or cystic/heterogeneous (if degenerated). Hyperechoic echogenic foci with posterior shadowing- if calcification.

Areas of sound attenuation, shadowing/obscuration of deeper structures. Colour doppler show peripheral flow with decreased central flow or an avascular core.

Computed Tomography Scan

Homogenous attenuation similar to myometrium-solid mass enlarged uterus with contour deformity calcification/cystic changes, if degenerated. Contrast CT—enhancement less than myometrium, but large degenerated/hyper vascular fibroid may show heterogeneous/increased enhancement.

MRI Findings

TWI

Intermediate/Isointense signal intensity with lobulated outline. If degenerated, high or low signal intensity.

T2WI

Best sequence for leiomyoma, commonly, homogenous, well defined and hypointense to myometrium with a pseudo capsule of compressed myometrium. Hyperintense rim could be due to edema, dilated lymphatics and veins.

Homogenously high signal intensity—if high cellularity and/or vascularity. Heterogeneous signal intensity.

T2*GRE

Foci of dark signal, if calcified.

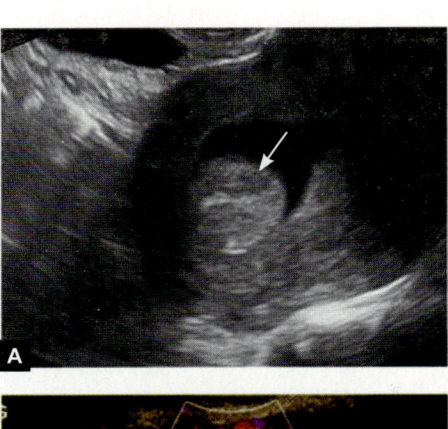

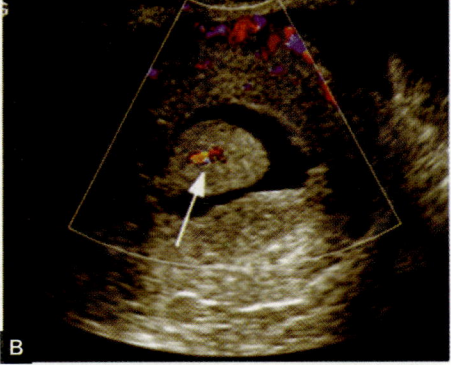

Figs 7.14A and B: Endometrial polyp. **A.** Transvaginal sonogram showing hyperechoic intraluminal lesion with no stretched echogenic endometrium (white arrow) and **B.** Single vascular pedicle on colour Doppler study (white arrow).

Contrast Scan

Generally not indicated well defined with variable enhancement (Fig. 7.21).

Enhancing halo of dilated lymphatics and veins.

Non-enhancing areas—represents haemorrhagic, cystic or necrotic changes.

Fat Sat T1WI

High signal in case of haemorrhagic/carneous degeneration (Figs 7.25A and B to 7.28A to D).

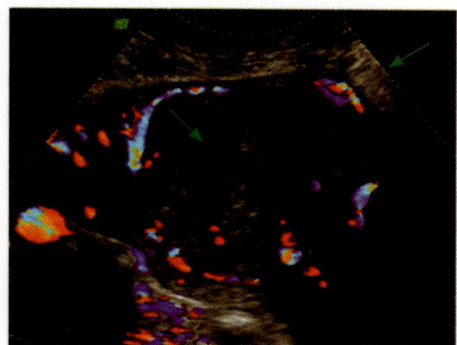

Fig. 7.15: Transverse transabdominal Doppler showing hypoechoic intramural fibroid with peripheral vascularity (green arrows)

Differential Diagnosis

Adenomyosis

No contour abnormalities, poorly marginated, focal or diffuse, minimal mass effect. Adenomyoma may show focal contour bulge.

USG

Poorly defined abnormal myometrial echotexture, may see myometrial cyst and/or echogenic striations into the myometrium (Fig 7.22).

MRI T2WI

Widening of junctional zone, more than 12 mm, ill-defined hypointense lesion with tiny foci of high signal intensity representing cysts (Figs 7.23 and 7.24).

■ SUBSEROSAL LEIOMYOMA

Sessile or pedunculated well-defined rounded masses, arising just deep to and abutting the serosa. Normal myometrium does not surround the entire mass.

Radiography

Displaced bowel loops.

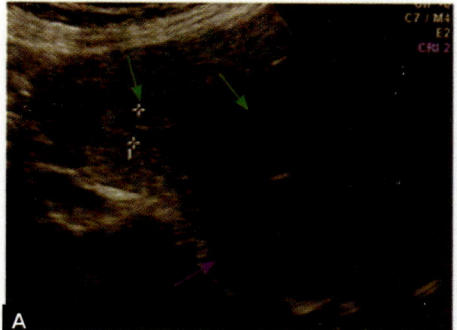

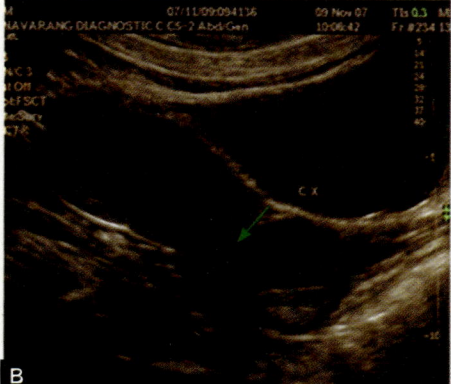

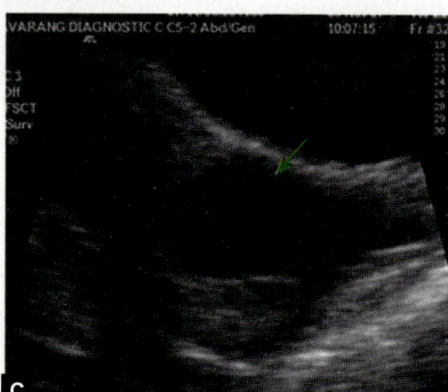

Figs 7.16A to C: Sagittal transabdominal sonogram. **A.** Large hypoechoic cervical fibroid with shadowing (green arrows) and endometrium (blue arrow); **B and C:** Sag and transverse images showing small cervical fibroid (green arrow).

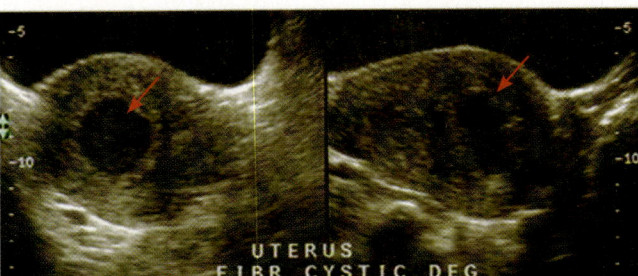

Fig. 7.17: Transverse and sagittal transabdominal sonogram showing intramural fibroid in the right lateral wall showing cystic degeneration (red arrows)

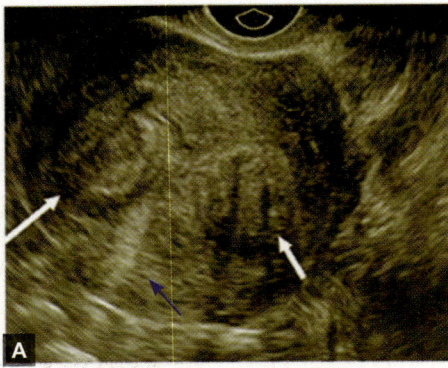

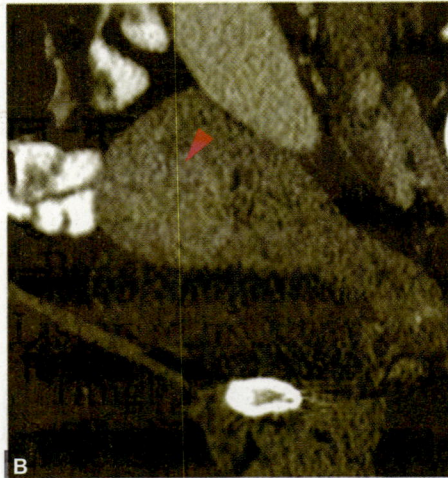

Figs 7.18A and B: A. Transverse transvaginal sonogram showing two intramural fibroids having heterogeneous echotexture (blue arrows). Endometrium –black arrow;[18] **B.** Sag CT reformation of post iv contrast study showing hypervascular intramural fibroid (red arrow head).

IVU

Mass effect on urinary bladder and compression/displacement of ureters.

Ultrasonography

Enlarged lobulated uterus on transabdominal scan.

TVS Scan

Homogenous well defined, hypoechoic mass with poor sound transmission. If degenerated, heterogeneous with or without calcification. Not useful for pedunculated type, since fibroid may not be seen.

Colour Doppler

Show peripheral flow with decreased central flow or an avascular core. Pedunculated fibroid may show vessels in the stalk.

CT scan

Projecting from uterus with similar attenuation to myometrium. In contrast CT most enhance less than myometrium, some may be isodense or enhance more than myometrium. Calcification and/or necrosis if degenerated (Fig 7.2C). Claw of myometrium partially surrounding the tumour.

MRI Findings

T1WI: Hypo to iso intense to myometrium no fat plane separating the mass from uterine surface.

Hyperintense, if carneous/haemorrhagic degeneration.

T2WI: Claw of myometrium partially surrounding tumour.

Generally homogenous low signal intensity mass protruding from uterus (Fig 7.25A). Hyperintense signal indicates high cellularity and/or vascularity (Fig 7.25B).

If pedunculated, the pedicle appear low signal intensity (Fig 7.27B).

Enhancement

Variable depending of the histology and degeneration.

Differential Diagnosis

Ovarian neoplasm: Originates from and inseparable from ovary.

Broad ligament fibroid: No demonstrable connection to the uterus.

Parasitic leiomyoma: Uterine subserosal or pedunculated or freely detached fibroid that recruits blood supply from adjoining structures, which could be lying free in pelvis or attached to uterus by a stalk.

May even recruit blood supply from omentum or intestine. May see large draining veins. If torsed from uterine blood supply, fibroid can be free in peritoneum. Common sites of attachment and/or arterial recruitment are fallopian tubes, broad ligament and omentum. Imaging features are like any other typical uterine leiomyoma.

Contrast enhanced MRI scan with MR angiography: It is the modality of choice since the enhancing vasculature can be traced to the parasitized end organ and may see draining veins.

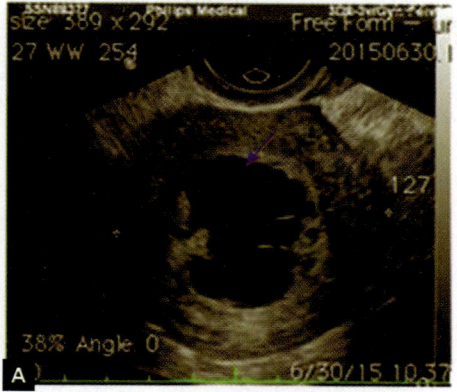
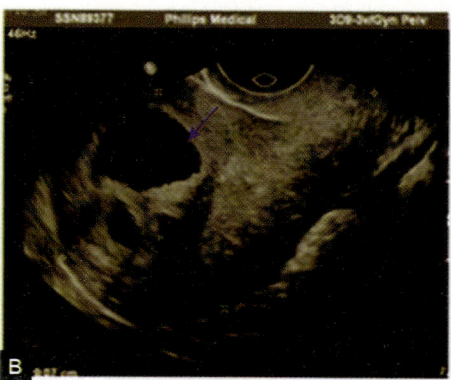
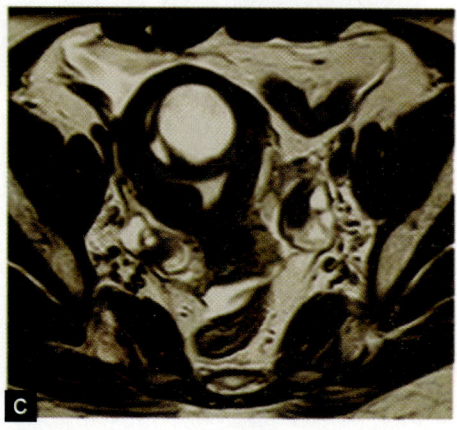
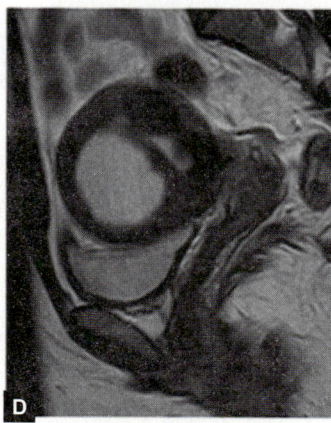

Figs 7.19A to D: **A and B.** Transverse and sagittal transabdominal sonogram showing intramural fibroid in the anterior wall showing cystic degeneration (blue arrows); **C and D.** Same patient's MRI scan T2WI axial and sagittal images showing intra mural fibroid with hyperintense signal changes(was hypointense in T1WI not shown here) consistent cystic degeneration (blue arrows) endometrium (red arrows).

Differential Diagnosis

- Ovarian tumours
- Drop metastasis
- Adnexal masses/lesions
- Lymph nodal masses
- May recur after resection and may
- Show hormone responsive behaviour.

■ DIFFUSE LEIOMYOMATOSIS[19]

Smooth muscle proliferation with unusual growth pattern involving uterus. Smooth muscle nodules range from microscopic to 3 cm in size with diffuse involvement resulting in an enlarged lobulated uterus (Fig 7.28).

Ultrasonography: Enlarged uterus with multiple nodules and heterogeneous echogenicity.

CT features: Multiple enhancing nodules causing diffuse thickening of myometrium.

MRI: Refer figure 7.28 for details.

TWI: Nodules of varying sizes, isointense to muscle.
T2WI: Ill-defined nodules of intermediate signal intensity.
Contrast scan: Diffuse and marked enhancement of nodules.

Differential Diagnosis

Multiple uterine leiomyoma: well circumscribed unlike diffuse leiomyomatosis that are ill defined.

The typical MR imaging feature of leiomyoma, distinct low signal intensity on T2-weighted images-is due to extensive hyalinization.[4,20,21]

Increased contrast enhancement of a fibroid is also presumably indicative of a lesion with increased vascularity and might be expected to be predictive of a better response for uterine artery embolisation.

> **Teaching point:** T2WI sequence in MRI is very important, since it reflects histology of fibroid thus helps to decide treatment options, patient selection and predict treatment response.

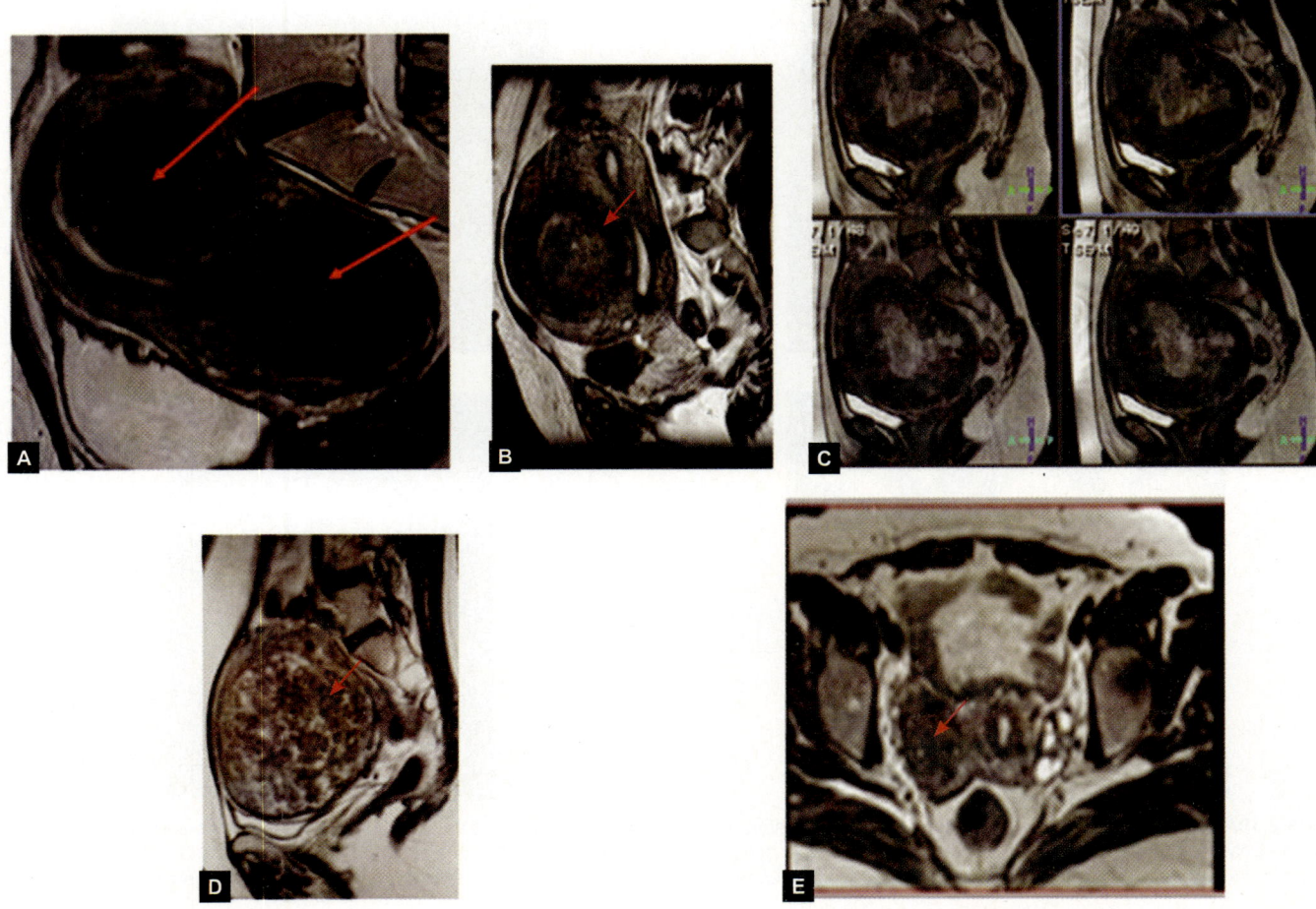

Figs 7.20A to E: A. Sag T2, MR images, showing enlarged uterus with two large hypointense intramural fibroid in the posterior wall compressing the endometrium; **B.** Sag T2, MR image, showing enlarged uterus with anterior wall hyperintense intramural fibroid (white arrow); **C.** Sag T2, MR images, showing large hypointense intramural fibroid with cystic degeneration; **D.** Heterogenous signal intensity intramural fibroid; **E.** Subseroral fibroid on right side, mildly hypointense compared to myometrium.

DISSEMINATED PERITONEAL LEIOMYOMATOSIS[22,23]

Benign condition characterized by multiple smooth muscle nodules arising in pelvic and abdominal cavities. Mostly seen in reproductive age. May range is size from few millimetres to several centimetres. Grossly malignant but histologically benign. Spontaneous regression when exposure to oestrogen is reduced.

Ultrasonography

Solid or complex soft tissue peritoneal masses.

CT Findings

1. Solid and complex masses in the peritoneum, uterus, broad ligaments, ovaries, mesentery, intestines and omentum.

2. Enhancement similar to uterus or heterogeneous.
3. Not associated with infiltration of omentum, ascites or liver metastasis.

MRI Findings

1. T1WI: Masses similar in signal intensity to skeletal muscles or uterine parenchyma.
2. T2WI: Low signal intensity due to smooth muscle.
3. Contrast scan: Variable enhancement.

PET-CT Scan

Peritoneal nodules do not show increased uptake of F-18 FDG as would be seen in lieomyosarcoma. Differential diagnosis mimics peritoneal carcinomatosis. Metastatic malignant neoplasm.

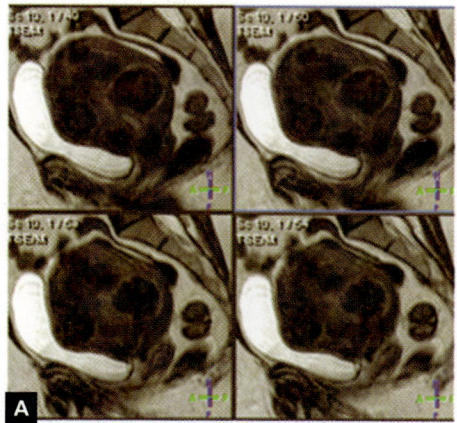

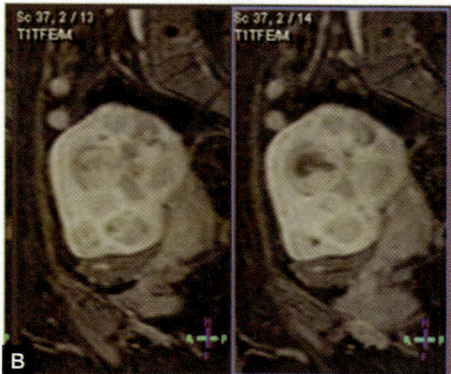

Figs 7.21A and B: Sag T2 and contrast enhanced MR sagittal images of a 24 years old female presented with menorrhagia, showing multiple intramural and submucosal fibroids causing contour deformity and endometrial distortion. All are hypovascular in contrast study and one of the fundal fibroid show cystic degeneration (black arrow head).

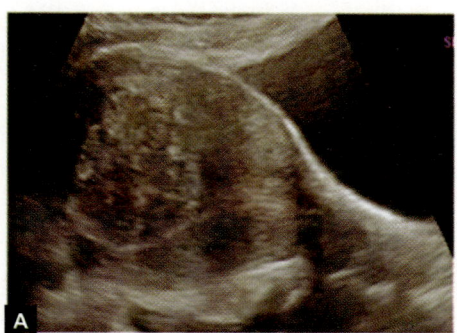

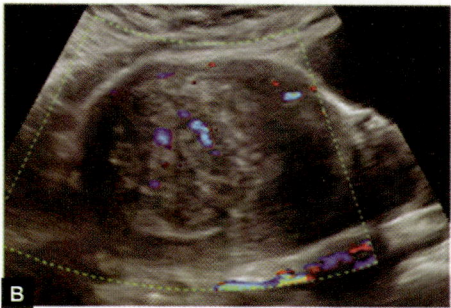

Figs 7.22A and B: Adenomyosis. **A.** Sagittal transabdominal sonogram showing bulky uterus with heterogeneous echogenicity lesion with ill-defined margin and endometrium; **B.** Colour flow mapping shows central scattered vessels.

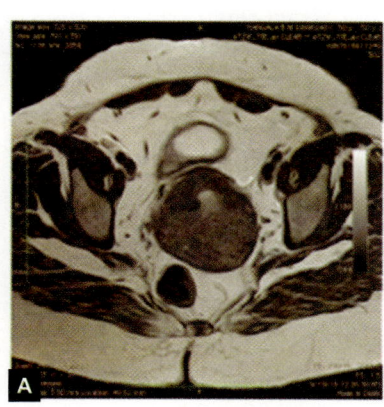

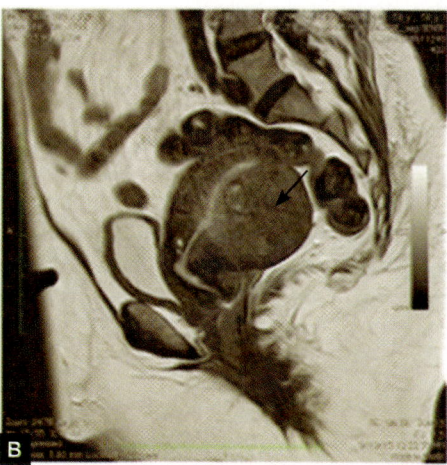

Figs 7.23A and B: Axial and sag T2WI of a 50 years old female showing an intermediate signal intensity posterior wall uterine lesion, causing posterior wall bulge, loss of normal junctional zone and indentation on the endometrium. Note few tiny cystic intensity foci within (black arrow) typical of adenomyoma.

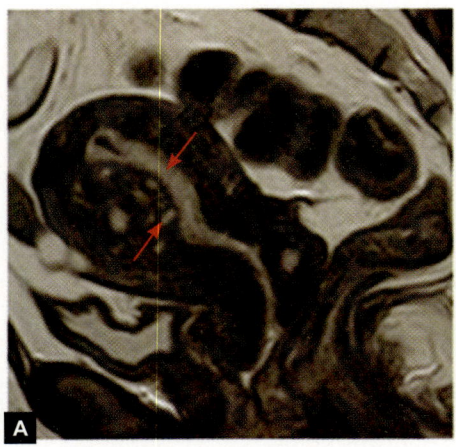

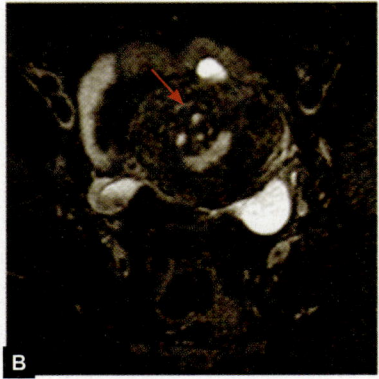

Figs 7.24A and B: Sag T2WI and Coronal FS images of a 32 years old female with severe menorrhagia showing a poorly marginated hypointense signal intensity anterior wall uterine lesion, with loss of normal junctional zone and indentation on the endometrium (red arrow). Note few tiny cystic intensity foci within (white arrow) typical of adenomyoma which may mimic fibroid on ultrasonography.

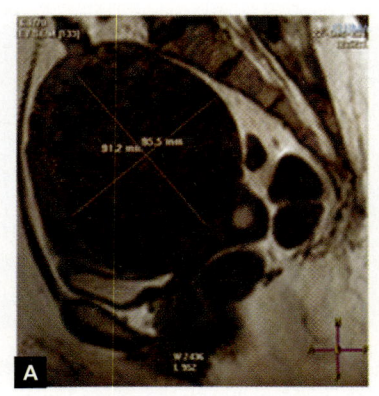

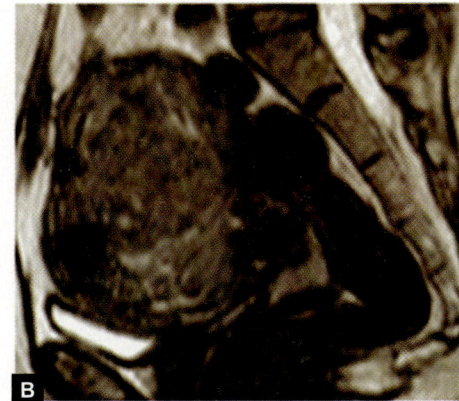

Figs 7.25A and B: A. Sag T2, MR images of a 42 years old female who presented with increased frequency of urination and hardness in lower abdomen, showing large hypointense subserosal fibroid, causing mass effect on urinary bladder and contour deformity; **B.** Hyperintense subserosal fibroid in another patient.

◼ BENIGN METASTASIZING LEIOMYOMA

Asymptomatic extra uterine benign leiomyoma, usually affects women after hysterectomy for leiomyoma. Multiple well-defined nodules ranging from few mms to centimetres affecting multiple extra-uterine sites about 3 months to 20 years post hysterectomy. Most commonly pulmonary, and other sites involved are lymph nodes, peritoneum and retroperitoneum.

Radiograph

Multiple well-defined bilateral lung nodules—common. Less common military pattern, pedunculated pulmonary lesion with large cyst, giant cyst with multiple pulmonary nodules. No pleural effusion, mediastinal lymphadenopathy or calcifications may be associated pneumothorax. Often incidental findings on chest X-ray.

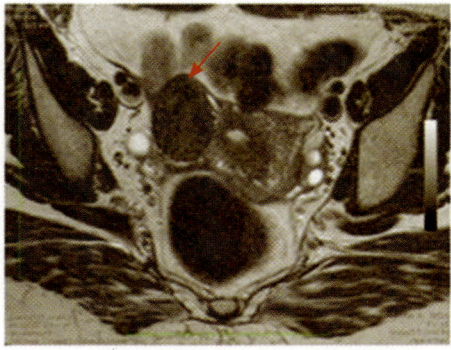

Fig. 7.26: Axial T2WI of show subserosal hypointense fibroid (blue arrow) on right side

CT Scan

1. Multiple bilateral well defined pulmonary nodules.
2. Less commonly cavitary nodules.

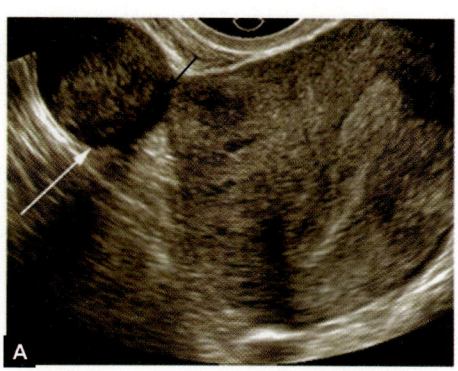

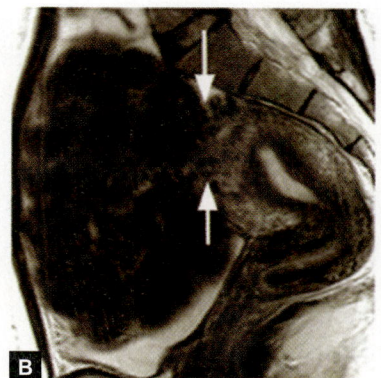

Figs 7.27A and B: A. Transvaginal transverse sonogram showing pedunculated (black arrow) subserosal fibroid (white arrow); **B.** T2W sagittal MR image showing large pedunculated (white arrow) hypointense fibroid anteriorly.

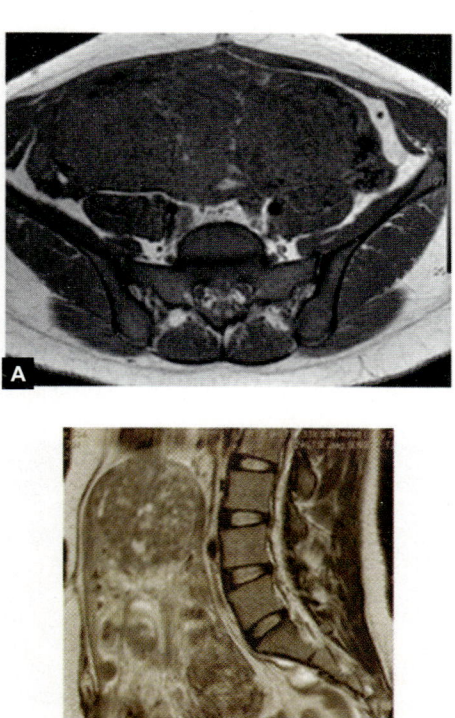

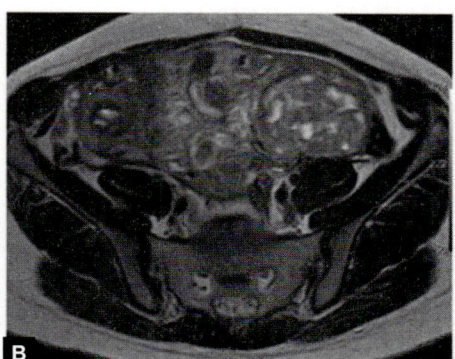

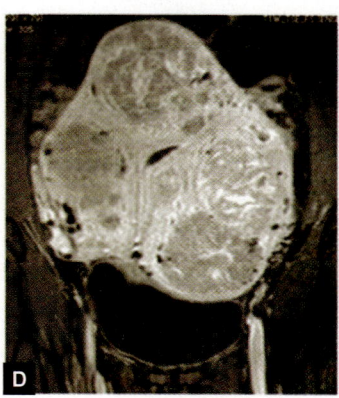

Figs 7.28A to D: Axial T1WI, T2WI, Sag T2 and coronal contrast enhanced MR images of a 28 years old female presented with lower abdominal pain, menorrhagia. Grossly enlarged uterus showing diffuse ill defined T2 heterogeneous signal intensity intramural innumerable fibroids distorting the endometrium, displacing the bowel loops out of pelvis. Varying enhancement pattern noted with contrast.

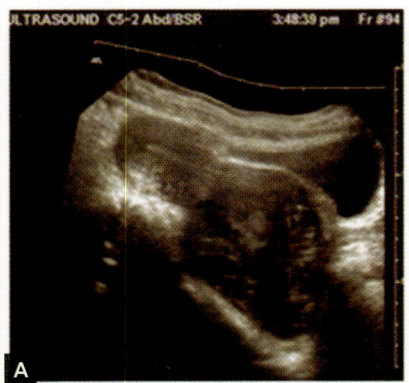
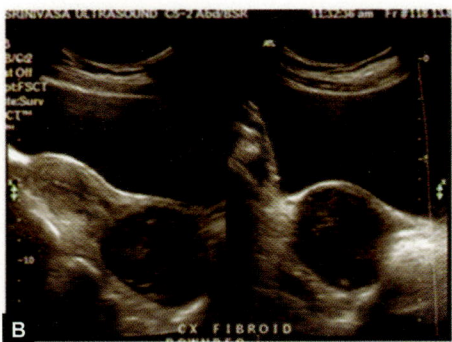

Figs 7.29A and B: A. Sagittal transabdominal sonogram showing large hypoechoic cervical fibroid (blue arrows); **B.** Sagittal and axial sonogram of same patient after down regulation showing shrinkage (star). Patient history of above sonogram 24 years female presented with mass per vagina and bleeding PV.

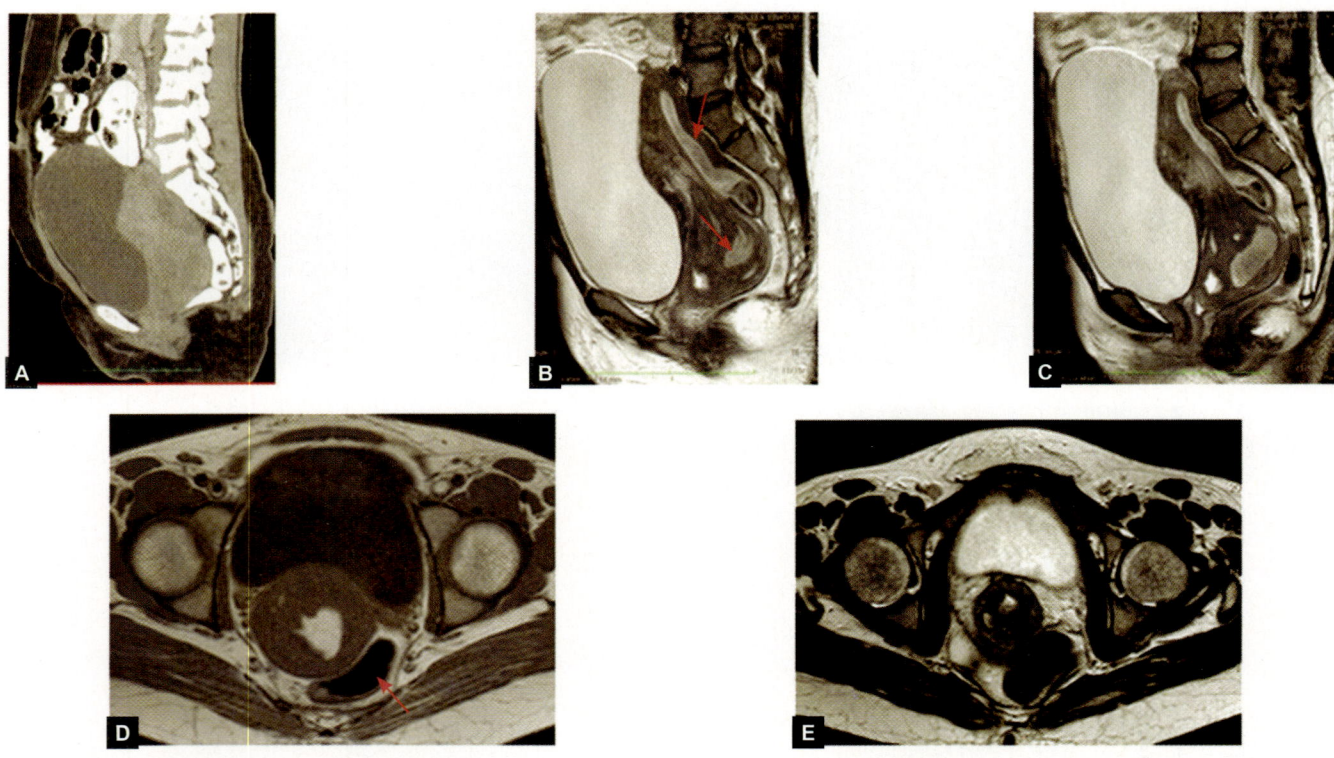

Figs 7.30A to E: A. Sagittal CT reformation showing heterogeneous low density lesion bulging through cervix into the vagina; **B and C.** Sagittal T2WI showing bulky uterus with a large prolapsing submucosal leiomyoma into the vagina, appearing as low to intermediate signal (red arrow) with few haemorrhagic foci. stretched endometrium; **D.** Axial T1WI showing low signal well defined lesion in vagina with bright foci (black notched arrow) representing haemorrhage; **E.** T2WI AXIAL image showing prolapsing submucosal leiomyoma as a well-defined mixed signal intensity intravaginal mass.

3. No significant contrast enhancement.
4. Absence of pleural effusion, lymphadenopathy or calcification.

Differential Diagnosis

1. Leiomyomatosis peritonealis disseminata
2. Proliferation of smooth muscle cells on the peritoneal surface.

3. Affects women during reproductive period and may present during pregnancy.
4. Related to hormonal factor, progresses with oestrogen and regression with progesterone.
5. No extraperitoneal manifestations.
6. Lymphangiomyomatosis.
7. Benign smooth muscle cell proliferation from lymphatic walls in lungs and lymph nodes.

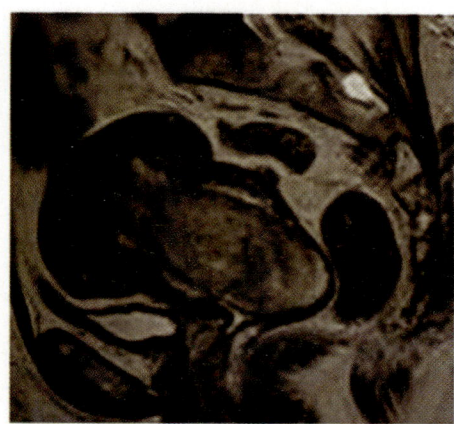

Fig. 7.31: sagittal T2WI showing uterus with a large prolapsing submucosal leiomyoma into the cervix, appearing as heterogeneous (mildly hyperintense) signal (red arrow)

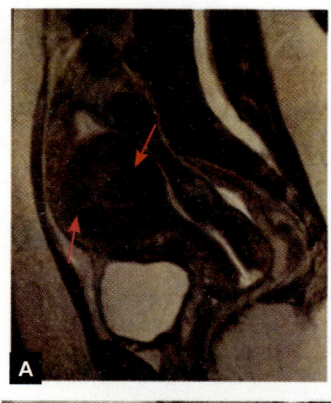

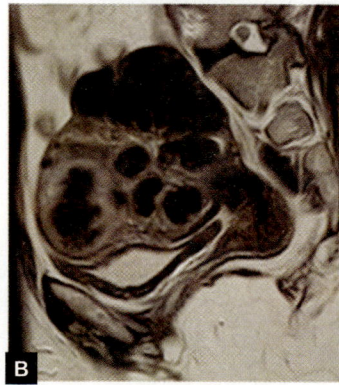

Figs 7.32A and B: A. T2WI SAG MRI image. Shows a hypo to intermediate signal fibroid with submucosal and intramural components (dark arrow). Compressed endometrium, seen as bright line (white arrow); **B.** Sag T2WI showing multiple hypointense fibroids in all locations.

8. Young women; spontaneous pneumothorax, chylous pleural effusion or progressive dyspnoea.
9. No association with uterine leiomyoma.
10. Metastatic leiomyosarcoma.
11. Other metastatic disease.

12. Lipoleiomyoma (Fig 7.40): Lipoleiomyoma is a specific type of leiomyoma that contains a substantial amount of fat. The reported prevalence of lipoleiomyoma is 0.8%.[24] Ultrasonography shows hyperechoic mass. At MR imaging, the fatty tissue demonstrates signal intensity similar to that of subcutaneous fat with all pulse sequences and in CT study, density will be of fat (~ –20 to –120 HU).

■ INTRAVENOUS LEIOMYOMATOSIS

It is a rare condition characterized by growth of smooth muscle cells into the myometrial or pelvic veins. Convoluted, worm-like masses growing within the veins are the hallmark of intravenous leiomyomatosis.[25,26]

Tumour extends from uterus to the extrauterine pelvic veins. Majority of cases, involves unilateral vein, uterine vein more common than ovarian vein. 40% extends into IVC and heart. Best imaging tool, contrast enhanced MR or CT.

Fibroid in Pregnancy (Fig. 7.42)

The prevalence of uterine fibroids in pregnancy varies between 1.6% and 10.7%, depending upon the trimester of assessment and the size threshold.[28–33] In one study, 4% of 12,708 pregnant patients had fibroids with a diameter > 3 cm. In another, 1.6% of 12,600 consecutive pregnant patients had fibroids > 1 cm.[29] A third series in over 15,000 women with non-anomalous singleton pregnancies undergoing routine second trimester ultrasonography reported that 2.7% had fibroids ≥ 1 cm.[30] A fourth series of 4271 first trimester or post-miscarriage ultrasound examinations observed 10.7% of women had a fibroid of ≥ 0.5 cm.[31] The prevalence of fibroids increases with age and is higher in African-American women than in white or Hispanic women.[31] Increasing parity and prolonged duration of breastfeeding are associated with a small, but statistically significant, reduction in prevalence.[33]

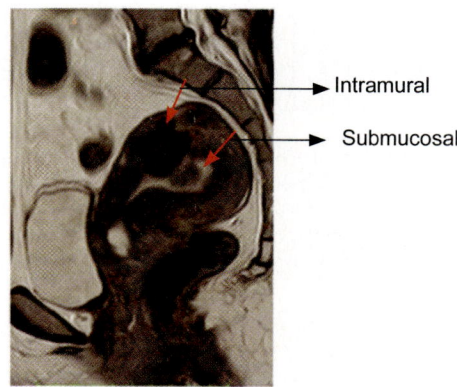

Intramural

Submucosal

Fig. 7.33: Sag T2, MR image, showing retroverted enlarged uterus with intramural (blue arrow) and submucosal fibroid (black arrow)

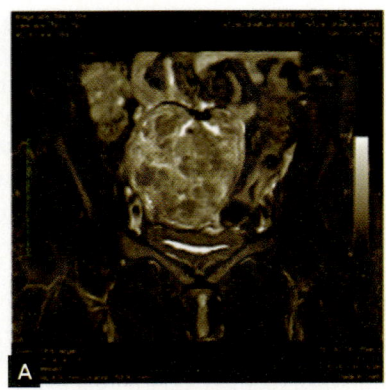

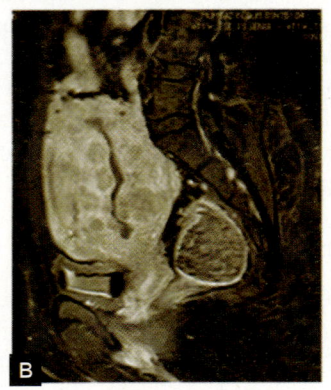

Figs 7.34A and B: A. Coronal T2FS, MR image, showing enlarged uterus with multiple intramural and submucosal hypointense fibroids of varying sizes; **B.** Gadolinium enhanced Sag T1FS image showing them to be less enhancing than normal myometrium-hypovascular.

Table 7.4: Types of fibroid degeneration

Hyaline degeneration	Focal or generalised hyalinization: This is the most common type of degeneration (can occur in 60% of cases)[4]
Cystic degeneration	4%
Myxoid degeneration (Fig 7.41)	Generally considered uncommon although reported as high a 50% by some authors[27]
Red/Carneous degeneration	Due to haemorrhagic infarction, which can occur particularly during pregnancy, and may present with acute abdominal pain

Teaching point: There is no pelvic imaging modality that can reliably differentiate between benign leiomyomas and uterine sarcomas. Leiomyomas and uterine sarcomas appear similar; both are focal masses within the uterus and both often have central necrosis. The diagnosis of uterine sarcoma is based upon histologic examination.

■ LEIOMYOSARCOMA

Uterine lieomyosarcoma is a rare neoplasm with an annual incidence of 0.64 per 100,000 women (Fig. 43).[34] It accounts for < 5% of all uterine malignancies and approximately

30% of all uterine sarcomas. Most lieomyosarcoma occur in women over 40 years of age, with a median age of 60 years. Some data suggest that ill-defined margins are consistent with a sarcoma.[35] Two small studies using different techniques of MRI with gadolinium contrast have reported specificities of 93% to 100% and positive predictive values of 53% to 100%.[36,37] Further study of use of MRI for this purpose

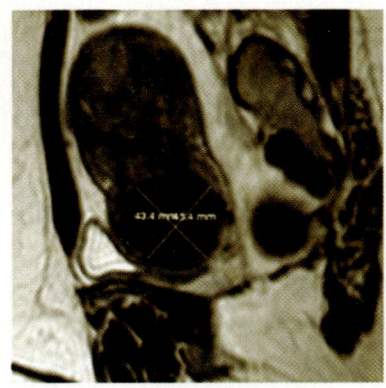

Fig. 7.35: Sag T2, MR image, showing uterus with a hypointense cervical fibroid

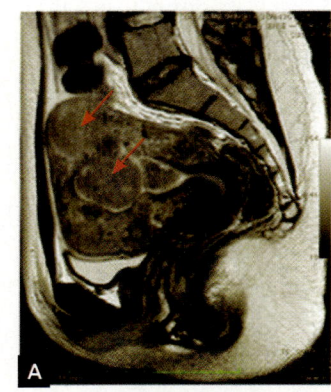

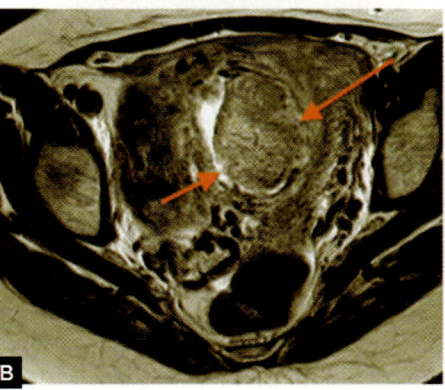

Figs 7.36A and B: A. Sag T2, MR image, showing enlarged uterus with multiple hyperintense intramural and submucosal fibroids; **B.** Axial T2WI image of 26 years old patient with severe menorrhagia showing a hyperintense intra and submucosal fibroid compressing the endometrium.

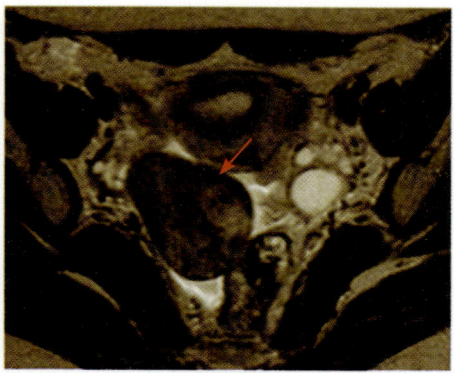

Fig. 7.37: Axial T2WI MRI imaging showing broad ligament fibroid on right side posterior to the uterus seen as T2 hypointense well defined lesion separate from uterus

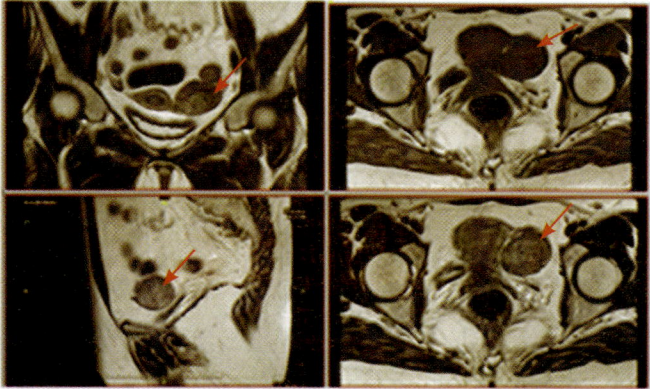

Fig. 7.38: Coronal, axial , Sag T2WI and axial T1WI ,showing broad ligament fibroid on left side seen as T1 Isointense and T2 mildly hyperintense well defined lesion separate from uterus

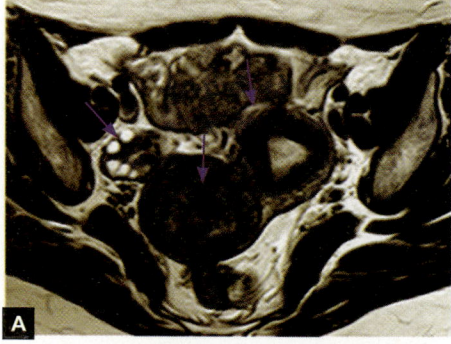

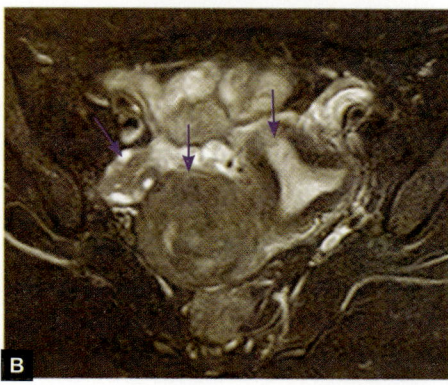

Fig. 7.39A and B: Axial T2WI and axial T2 fat sat images in a 35 years old female, showing broad ligament fibroid on right side seen as hypointense well defined lesion (red arrow) between uterus (displaced to the left-white arrow head) and right ovary (green arrow).

is needed. Positron emission tomography (PET)/CT with fluorodeoxyglucose (FDG) does not appear to be useful to distinguish between leiomyomas and uterine sarcomas. While the FDG uptake is generally high in sarcomas and low in leiomyomas, the uptake varies across individual tumours.[38] A consistent finding in leiomyosarcomas is the absence of calcifications. Occasionally, the presenting manifestations of leiomyosarcoma are related to tumour rupture (haemoperitoneum), extra-uterine extension (one third to one half of cases), or metastases.[39] Most leiomyosarcoma arise de novo, but an apparent minority of leiomyosarcoma may represent leiomyomas that have undergone malignant transformation.[37] A 70 year woman presented with case reference metastasised breast cancer to bone. An evaluation of CT made showed enlarged uterus and tumour. The tumour was a lecomyma in which lecomyosaccuma with osteoclast-like giant cell as well as metastasis of ductal breast carcinoma was present.[40]

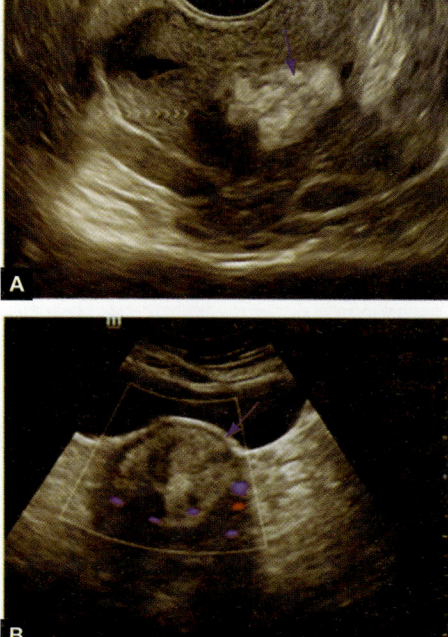

Figs 7.40A and B: A. TVS sagittal section showing echogenic lesion (blue arrow) with peripheral hypoechoic components (blue arrow), in the posterior wall of body of uterus; another patient; **B.** Transabdominal Transverse sonogram showing mixed echoic (hyper- and hypo-echoic components) lesion, indicative of lipoleiomyoma.

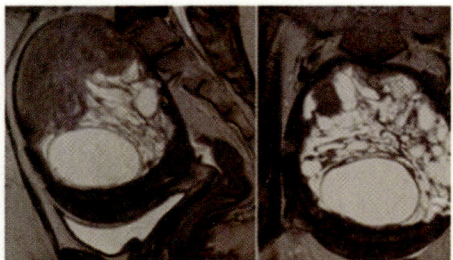

Fig. 7.41: Sag and coronal T2WI show subserosal large intermediate signal intensity fibroid with complex cystic areas—myxoid degeneration in a fibroid

MRI

TWI: Large infiltrating myometrial mass of heterogeneous hypointensity, with regular and ill-defined margins.

T2-weighted images: Usually show intermediate-to-high signal intensity, with central hyperintensity indicative of extensive necrosis (present in > 50% of cases).

Gradient/T1WI: Haemorrhage is common, and foci of calcifications may be present.

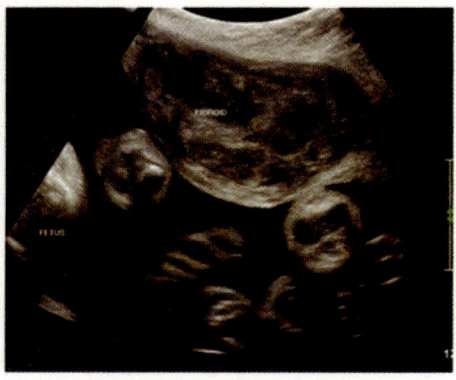

Fig. 7.42: Transabdominal transverse sonogram showing anterior wall intramural fibroid in a pregnant lady. 64 years female known to have fibroid, presented with pain abdomen with sudden increase in size.

Contrast scan: Early heterogeneous enhancement, due to the areas of necrosis and haemorrhage.

Bridging Vascular Sign

MRI feature that is helpful in the evaluation of large pelvic masses, consists of vessels and/or signal voids that extend

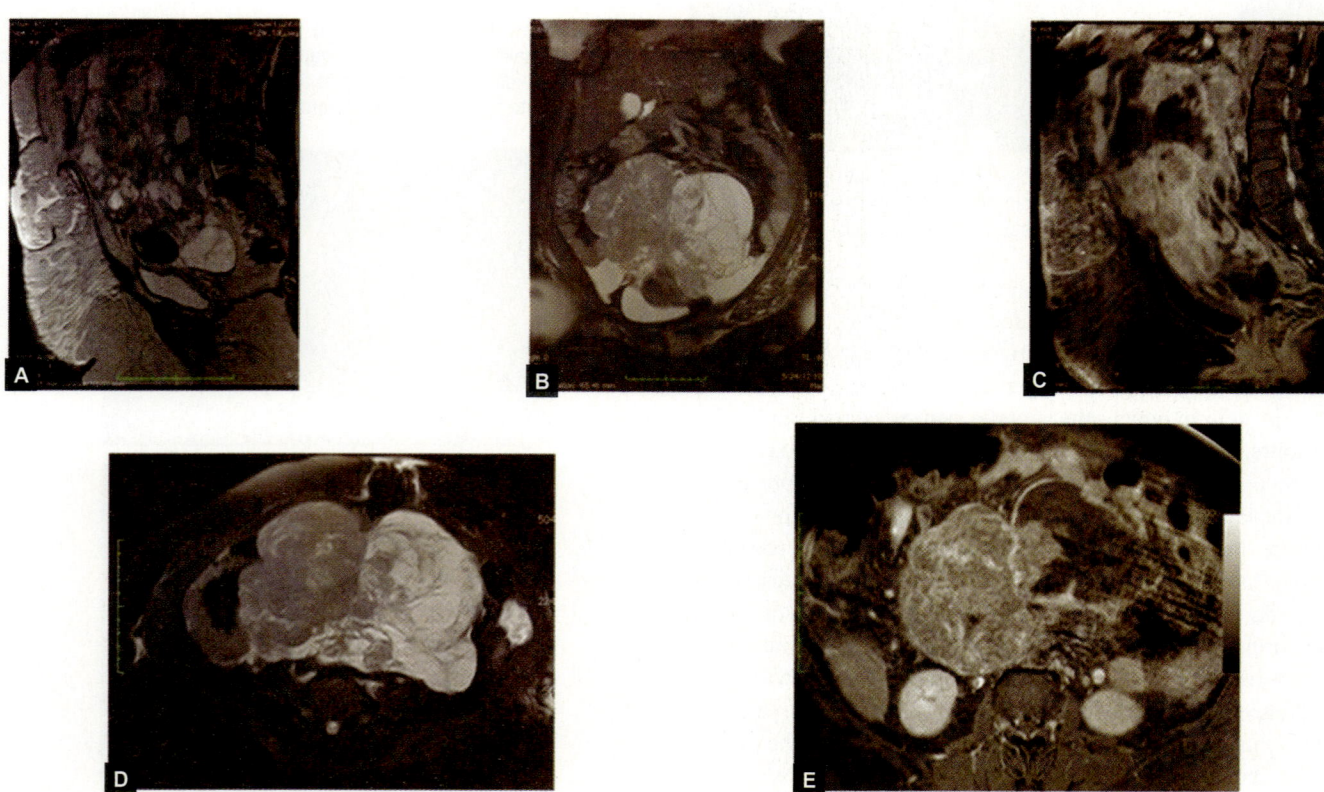

Figs 7.43A to E: A and B. Sagittal T2WI; **C.** Coronal T2 FS; **D and E.** T1 FS with contrast showing huge pelvi abdominal mass from uterus, having irregular lobulated outline, and heterogeneous signal intensity. Ascites and bowel loop adhesion was also demonstrated. Gadolinium enhanced scan show heterogeneous enhancement with large areas of necrosis. Note a component of the mass lesion is herniating through the anterior abdominal wall defect. Surgical excision confirmed to be a lieomyosarcoma.

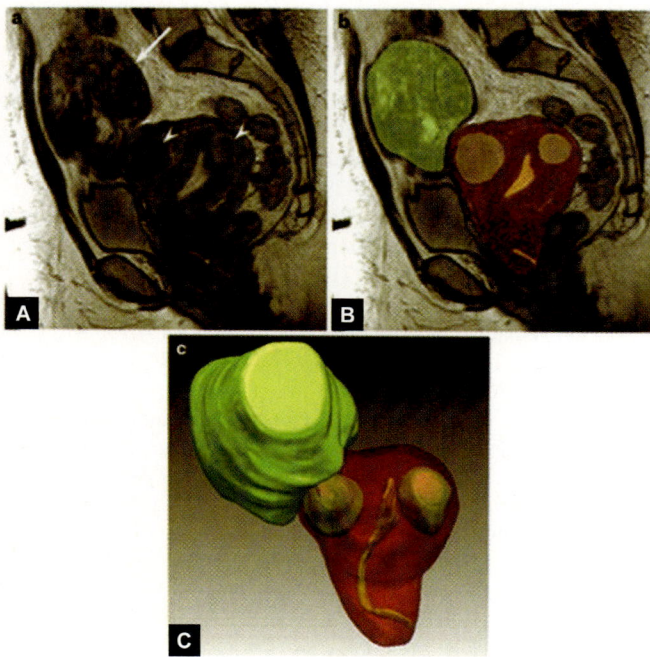

Figs 7.44A to C: A. A Sagittal 3D VISTA image indicates a subserosal fibroid (arrow) and intramural fibroids (arrow heads); **B.** The segmentation results of the target regions indicate the uterine body as a red colour, the endometrium as a yellow colour and fibroids as a green colour; **C.** A 3D SR image precisely indicates the positional relationship of the uterine body (red), endometrium (yellow) and fibroids (green).

from the uterus to supply a pelvic mass. The identification of the bridging vascular sign increases the diagnostic confidence that a large pelvic mass is a uterine leiomyoma.[421] The bridging vessels can be identified as enhancing tubular structures on contrast-enhanced T1W imaging or as flow voids on a T2W fast spin-echo sequence.

Table 7.5: Comparison between leiomyoma and adenomyomas

Leiyomyoma	Adenomyosis
Hypoechoic	Heterogeneous echo pattern, hyper- and hypo-echoic regions
Well-defined margins	Margins ill defined, no capsule
Blotchy shadowing	Streaky shadowing (venetian blinds)
Rim or central calcifications	No calcifications, probe tenderness
Cystic degeneration	Small cystic spaces
Contour bumps and lobularity	No contour abnormalities (exception-adenomyoma)
Commonly multiple	Diffuse often asymmetric myometrial hyperplasia
Peripheral vascularity	Diffuse vascularity
Focal impingement into cavity	Endo/Myometrial interphase ill defined

USEFULNESS OF 3D-SURFACE RENDERED (SR) IMAGES FOR SURGICAL PLANNING

In a study, by Sayed Ahmad Zikri B Sayed Aluwee et al,[43] 10 patients with uterine fibroids underwent 3D volume isotropic turbo spin-echo acquisition (VISTA) sequences in sagittal planes. SR images showing the uterine body, endometrium and fibroids were extracted from the raw MR data. The preoperative assessment for fertility-preserving fibroid enucleation was independently performed by two gynaecologists using 2D sagittal and 3D SR images separately. The required time for the various surgical planning procedures was recorded. Their interpretations were compared with a highly experienced third gynaecologist, whose observations were considered as gold standard. Compared with 2D T2-weighted imaging, advantages offered by 3D T2-weighted imaging include a higher signal-to-noise ratio (SNR), greater tumour conspicuity, fewer artifacts, and the ability to perform multi-planar reformation (Fig. 7.44).

In conclusion, 3D-rendered images could significantly reduce the time required for surgical planning of uterine fibroids without sacrificing the accuracy of the preoperative assessment in comparison with sagittal images. By using 3D-rendered images, spatial recognition becomes stunningly easy, especially for less-experienced gynaecologists. Therefore, 3D-rendered images might be useful for education and may aid in reducing the burden on gynaecologists.

CONCLUSION

Uterine fibroids are common tumours and although benign they can be associated with significant morbidity. They may be encountered incidentally when performing imaging for other reasons and are usually easily recognizable. However, degenerate fibroids can have unusual appearances. Awareness of the various appearances enables a prompt diagnosis and can guide treatment. Ultrasound is the basic imaging modality for diagnosis and follow up. Radiographs, and CT scan play limited role and MRI scan is the modality of choice when diagnosis is in doubt, for accurate localisation, and is of immense help in the evaluation of treatment options.

KEY WORDS

Fibroid, leiomyoma, submucosal, intramural, subserosal, degeneration, hyperintense, hypointense, calcification, lieomyosarcoma, lipoleiomyoma, parasitic leiomyoma, broad ligament leiomyoma, benign metastasizing leiomyoma, adenomyosis, intravenous leiomyomatosis, saline sonohysterography. 3D surface rendered MR images. Myxoid, lipoleiomyoma, Hyaline, Cystic.

■ REFERENCES

1. Prayson RA, Hart WR. Pathologic considerations of uterine smooth muscle tumors. Obstet Gynecol Clin North Am. 1995;22:637-57.
2. Rein MS, Barbieri RL, Friedman AJ. Progesterone: A critical role in the pathogenesis of uterine myomas. Am J Obstet Gynecol. 1995;172:14-8.
3. Andersen J. Growth factors and cytokines in uterine leiomyomas. SeminReprodEndocrinol. 1996;14(3):269-82.
4. Ueda H, Togashi K, Konishi I, et al. Unusual Appearances of Uterine Leiomyomas: MR Imaging Findings and Their Histopathologic Backgrounds Radiographics. 1999;19:S131-S145.
5. Creasman WT. Disorders of the uterine corpus. In: Scott JR, DiSaia PJ, Hammond CB, Spellacy WN (Eds). Danforth's obstetrics and gynecology. Philadelphia, Pa: Lippincott; 1994;925-55.
6. Gompel C, Silverberg SG. The corpus uteri. In: Gompel C, Silverberg SG (Eds). Pathology in gynecology and obstetrics. Philadelphia, Pa: Lippincott; 1994:163-28344.
7. Callen PW. Ultrasonography in Obstetrics and Gynecology, 5th ed. Philadelphia, Pa: Saunders Elsevier; 2007.
8. Kurtz AB, Middleton WD. Ultrasound. St Louis, Mo: Mosby; 1996.
9. Sauerbrel EE, Nguyen KT, Nolan RL. A Practical Guide to Ultrasound in Obstetrics and Gynecology, 2nd ed. Philadelphia, Pa: Lippincott-Raven; 1998. 52-8.
10. Volkers NA, Hehenkamp WJ, Spijkerboer AM, et al. MR reproducibility in the assessment of uterine fibroids for patients scheduled for uterine artery embolization. CardiovascInterventRadiol. 2008;31:260-8.
11. Zawin M, McCarthy S, Scoutt LM, et al. High-field MRI and US evaluation of the pelvis in women with leiomyomas. MagnReson Imaging. 1990;8:371-6.
12. Dueholm M, Lundorf E, Hansen ES, et al. Evaluation of the uterine cavity with magnetic resonance imaging, transvaginal sonography, hysterosonographic examination and diagnostic hysteroscopy. Fertil Steril. 2001;76:350-7.
13. Dueholm M, Lundorf E, Sorensen JS, et al. Reproducibility of evaluation of the uterus by transvaginal sonography, hysterosonographic examination, hysteroscopy and magnetic resonance imaging. Hum Reprod. 2002;17:195-200
14. Omari EA, Varghese T, Kliewer MA. A novel saline infusion sonohysterography-based strain imaging approach for evaluation of uterine abnormalities in vivo: preliminary results. J Ultrasound Med. 2012;31(4):609-15.
15. Davidson KG, Dubinsky TJ. Ultrasonographic evaluation of the endometrium in postmenopausal vaginal bleeding. RadiolClin North Am. 2003;41:769-80.
16. Dudiak CM, Turner DA, Patel SK, et al. Uterine leiomyomas in the infertile patient: preoperative localization with MR imaging versus US and hysterosalpingography. Radiology. 1988;167:627-30.
17. Zawin M, McCarthy S, Scoutt LM, et al. High-field MRI and US evaluation of the pelvis in women with leiomyomas. MagnReson Imaging. 1990;8:371-6

18. Hricak H, Tscholakoff D, Heinrichs L, et al. Uterine leiomyomas: correlation of MR, histopathologic findings, and symptoms. Radiology. 1986;158:385-91.
19. Cohen DT, Oliva E, Hahn PF, et al. Uterine Smooth-Muscle Tumors with Unusual Growth Patterns. AJR 2007;188:246-55.
20. Rosai J. Ackerman's surgical pathology 8th ed. St Louis, Mo: Mosby-Year Book. 1996;1429-33.
21. Aggarwal B K, Panwar S, Rajan S, et al. Varied appearances & signal characteristics of leiomyomas on MR imaging. Indian J Radiol Imaging. 2005;15:271-6.
22. Advincula AP. Images in reproductive medicine. Disseminated Leiomyomatosis peritonei.Fertilsteril. 2005;84(5):1505-7.
23. Diagnostic imaging Gynecology: Edited by HedvigHricak, 1st ed, AMIRSYS Inc. 2007.
24. Dellacha A, Di Marco A, Foglia G, et al. Lipoleiomyoma of the uterus. Pathologica. 1997;89:737-41.
25. Rotter AJ, Lundell CJ. MR of intravenous leiomyomatosis of the uterus extending into the inferior vena cava. J Comput Assist Tomogr. 1991;15:690-3. CrossRef, Medline.
26. Kawakami S, Sagoh T, Kumada H, et al. Intravenous leiomyomatosis of uterus: MR appearance. J Comput Assist Tomogr. 1991;15:686-9.
27. Low G, Rouget AC, Crawley C. Case 188: Intravenous leiomyomatosis with intracaval and intracardiac involvement. Radiology. 2012;265(3):971-5.doi:10.1148/radiol.12111246.
28. Qidwai GI, Caughey AB, Jacoby AF. Obstetric outcomes in women with sonographically identified uterine leiomyomata. ObstetGynecol. 2006;107:376.
29. Exacoustòs C, Rosati P. Ultrasound diagnosis of uterine myomas and complications in pregnancy. ObstetGynecol. 1993;82:97.
30. Strobelt N, Ghidini A, Cavallone M, et al. Natural history of uterine leiomyomas in pregnancy. J Ultrasound Med. 1994;13:399.
31. Laughlin SK, Baird DD, Savitz DA, et al. Prevalence of uterine leiomyomas in the first trimester of pregnancy: an ultrasound-screening study. ObstetGynecol. 2009;113:630.
32. Stout MJ, Odibo AO, Graseck AS, et al. Leiomyomas at routine second-trimester ultrasound examination and adverse obstetric outcomes. ObstetGynecol. 2010;116:1056.
33. Terry KL, De Vivo I, Hankinson SE, et al. Reproductive characteristics and risk of uterine leiomyomata. FertilSteril. 2010;94:2703.
34. Harlow BL, Weiss NS, Lofton S. The epidemiology of sarcomas of the uterus. J Natl Cancer Inst.1986;76(29):399-402.
35. Schwartz LB, Zawin M, Carcangiu ML, et al. Does pelvic magnetic resonance imaging differentiate among the histologic subtypes of uterine leiomyomata?
36. Goto A, Takeuchi S, Sugimura K, et al. Usefulness of Gd-DTPA contrast-enhanced dynamic MRI and serum determination of LDH and its isozymes in the differential diagnosis of leiomyosarcoma from degenerated leiomyoma of the uterus. Int J Gynecol Cancer. 2002;12(4):354.
37. Tanaka YO, Nishida M, Tsunoda H, et al. Smooth muscle tumors of uncertain malignant potential and leiomyosarcom as of the uterus: MR findings.MagnReson Imaging. 2004;20(6):998.

38. Kitajima K, Murakami K, Kaji Y, et al. Spectrum of FDG PET/CT findings of uterine tumors. AJR Am J Roentgenol. 2010;195:737.

39. D'Angelo E, Prat J. Uterine sarcomas: a review. GynecolOncol. 200:116(1)131–139. [PubMed].

40. Van Meurs HS, Dieles JJ, Stel HV. A uterine leiomyoma in which a leiomyosarcoma with osteoclast-like giant cells and a metastasis of a ductal breast carcinoma are present. Ann Diagn Pathol. 2012;16(1):67-70.

41. Kim JC, Kim SS, Park JY. "Bridging vascular sign" in the MR diagnosis of exophytic uterine leiomyoma. J Comput Assist Tomogr. 2000;24:57-60.

42. Magnetic resonance imaging of uterine fibroids: a preliminary investigation into the usefulness of 3D-rendered images for surgical planning. Sayed Ahmad Zikri B Sayed Aluwee, Hiroki Kato, Xiangrong Zhou, Takeshi Hara,Hiroshi Fujita, Masayuki Kanematsu, Tatsuro Furui, Ryuichiro Yano, Nao Miyai and Ken-ichirou Morishige.

CHAPTER 8

Differential Diagnosis of Fibroid Uterus

● M K Pathanjali Prasanna

Uterine fibroids (myomas or leiomyomas) are benign, monoclonal tumours of the smooth muscle cells found in the human uterus. Despite the fact that their cause is still unknown, yet there is considerable evidence that oestrogens and progestogens proliferate tumour growth, as the fibroids rarely appear before menarche and regress after menopause.

Approaches to differentiating benign uterine leiomyomas from other uterine and extrauterine masses are reviewed here.

Defining the correct origin is the first diagnostic step in defining the site of origin the differential diagnoses and treatment options often differ completely.

■ DIFFERENTIAL DIAGNOSIS OF A UTERINE MASS

The challenge of differentiating a leiomyoma from an uterine mass is one part of the diagnostic process for all women with a uterine mass. The differential diagnosis of an enlarged uterus includes both benign and malignant conditions:[1]

- Full bladder
- Pregnancy
- Haematometra
- Endometrial polyp
- Uterine adenomyoma or diffuse adenomyosis
- Solid ovarian tumours
- Transient myometrial contraction
- Uterine malignancies: Uterine sarcoma carcinosarcoma (considered an epithelial neoplasm) endometrial carcinoma metastatic disease (typically from another reproductive tract primary).

Full Bladder

A fibroid apparently may be confused with the full bladder (depending on the size). Hence it is mandatory to examine the patient with the bladder empty. If necessary, following catheterisation. One should not be confused with overflow incontinence in chronic retention as normal urination, as stated by the patient.[1,2]

Pregnancy

In reproductive age group women, any enlarged uterus, pregnancy first to be ruled out.

A pregnancy of 16–18 weeks is very much deceptive and one should be very much careful to exclude pregnancy during child bearing period irrespective of the status of the women.[1]

Diagnosis

Ultrasonogram, if necessary X-ray. The sound policy is to re-examine the patient after 4 weeks when all the features of the pregnancy will be clinically evident.

Haematometra

In this condition, menstrual outflow obstruction at the level of the cervix or higher traps blood and distends the uterus. In this setting, haematocolpos that is trapped blood that distends the vagina is also commonly associated with haematosalpinx. The aetiology could be due to congenital or acquired abnormalities of the outflow of genital tract (Fig. 8.1).

Symptoms classically complain of cyclic, midline pain.

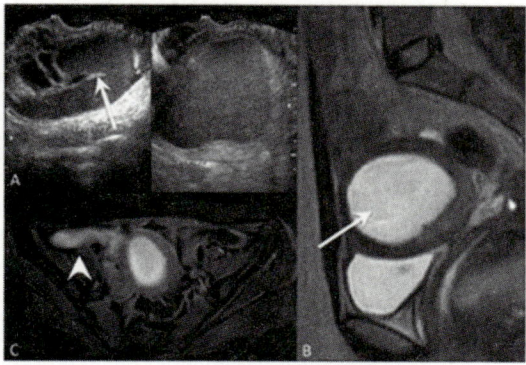

Fig. 8.1: MRI T2W (haematometra)

With total obstruction, there is amenorroea. Partial obstruction causes pain accompanied by scant dark bleeding that may have a foul odour and may not be cyclic.

Clinical findings may mimic early pregnancy, cystic degenerated leiomyoma, leiomyosarcoma and gestational trophoblastic disease1.

Diagnosis

Sonography (Fig. 8.2) is the principal diagnostic tool, which shows a smooth, symmetric hypoechoic enlargement of the uterine cavity. Low level internal echoes may variably be present. A haematosalpinx is seen less commonly and is identified as hypoechoic tubular distensions lateral to a hypoechoic uterus.

Endometrial Polyp

Endometrial polyps are discreet outgrowths of the endometrium that contains a variable amount of gland stroma and blood vessel. They are attached to the endometrium by a pedicle and they may be pedunculated or sessile. It would appear that they are relatively insensitive to cyclical hormonal changes and so are not shed at the time of menstruation. In addition they may contain hyperplastic foci particularly in those that are symptomatic. Histologically, characterised as localised hyperplastic overgrowths of glands and stroma and one of the entities included in a differential of endometrial thickening and fibroid uterus.[3,4] 2%–4% of 'benign' polyps with have a small focus of cancer within them.[5]

Presentation

Unscheduled vaginal bleeding or spotting is the commonest presentation for endometrial polyps. They are frequently found in association with women experiencing abnormal bleeding, while taking hormone replacement theory (HRT) or tamoxifen. In the latter case, the whole endometrial surface may appear polypoid.

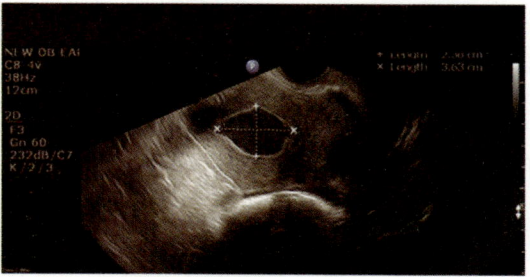

Fig. 8.2: Haematometra (USG)

They can often be suggested on ultrasound or magnetic resonance imaging (MRI) studies, but may require sonohysterography or direct visualisation for confirmation. There are other variants of polyps like adenomyomatous endometrial polyp.

Location: There may be a predilection towards the fundal and cornual regions within the uterus.

Diagnostic Findings

Ultrasound (Fig. 8.3)

Although endometrial polyps may be visualised at transvaginal ultrasound as non-specific endometrial thickening, they may also be identified as focal masses within the endometrial canal:

1. A stalk to the polyp may either be thin or broad based.
2. A feeding vessel may be seen extending to the polyp on colour Doppler imaging.
3. Cystic spaces corresponding to dilated glands filled with proteinaceous fluid may be seen within the polyp and is considered a relatively characteristic feature.[3]
4. May appear as just diffusely thickened endometrium, without visualisation of a discrete mass (mimicking endometrial hyperplasia).
5. Colour doppler: May show flow within the stalk. The 3D ultrasound may be useful to help delineate the borders of a polyp.

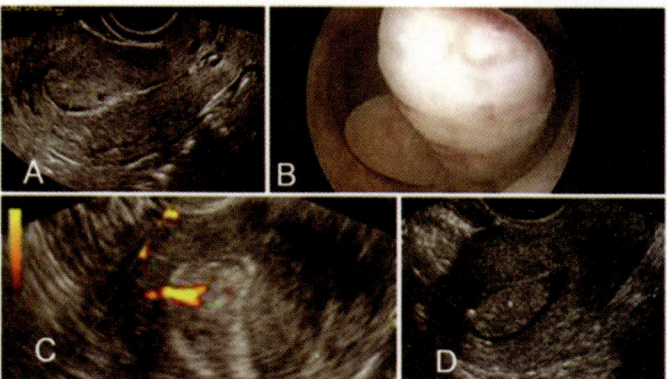

Figs 8.3A to D: A. USG—findings of cervical polyp; **B.** Hysteroscopic cervical polyp; **C.** SIS—endometrial polyp;

Sonohysterography

Although not always necessary for a diagnosis, polyps are well characterised on sonohysterography and appear as echogenic, smooth, intracavitary masses outlined by the fluid. The typical appearance of an endometrial polyp at sonohysterography is as a well defined, homogeneous, polypoid lesion that is isoechoic to the endometrium with preservation of the endometrial-myometrial interface. There is usually a well-defined vascular pedicle within the stalk.

Pelvic MRI

Signal characteristics include in T1W1 image an often isointense signal to endometrium. In T2W1 images they are often seen as hypointense intracavitary masses surrounded by hyperintense fluid and endometrium. In T1 C+ (Gd): can show either homogeneous or heterogeneous enhancement. There are other differential diagnosis for endometrial polyp is foci of endometrial hyperplasia and endometrial carcinoma. For hyperechoic content within the endometrium should also consider the intrauterine blood clot or retained products of conception.

Adenomyoma

Leiomyomas have to be distinguished from all other causes of enlargement of the uterus and, so far as adenomyosis is concerned, this may be impossible (Table 8.1).

Adenomyosis is a common non-neoplastic gynecologic disease characterized by the presence of ectopic endometrium within the myometrium. Adenomyosis typically affects multiparous, premenopausal women over 30 years of age and may cause dysmenorrhoea, menorrhagia, and abnormal uterine bleeding the thickened myometrium composed of haphazardly distributed hypertrophied muscular trabeculae surrounding ectopic endometrial tissue. Brownish old haemorrhagic foci corresponding to haemolysed blood and haemosiderin pigment deposits may be contained within the area of adenomyosis Because the junctional zone is an anatomical land mark in the assessment of adenomyosis, other causes of junctional zone alternatives or a broad and ill-defined junctional zone in the early postpartum period should also be considered in the differential diagnosis of adenomyosis. 20% of cases is associated with coexistent endometriosis.[6]

Clinical Features

The most common symptom is menorrhagia, which is found in approximately 75% of cases. It is gradually progressive over several years and is caused by enlargement of the uterine cavity (bleeding area) and by an increased blood supply. Other theoretical causes for the menorrhagia are impaired contractility of the myometrium and associated endometrial hyperplasia. Dysmenorrhoea is noted by only 30% of patients and, when it occurs, it is mainly intramenstrual. It is more

Table 8.1: Leiomyoma and adenomyosis

	Leiomyoma	Adenomyosis
Location	Typically in uterine corpus/fundus, maybe in cervix (< 8%), rarely parasitic	More often in posterior wall of uterus and fundus, does not involve cervix
Growth pattern	Spherical round lesion with well-defined margins with pseudocapsule	Poorly defined margins blend with surrounding myometrium lacks pseudocapsule
TVUSG	Hypoechoic round lesions sharply demarcated from uterus	Areas of reduced echogenicity or heterogenous appearance Poor definition of endomyometrial junction presence of myometrial cysts
Colour coded duplex usG (CCDU)	Shows central vessel or marginal vascular network	Increased vascularisation
Applicable on T1	Isointense to myometrium peripheral hypointense rim indicates calcification	Mostly isointense, may show hyperintense foci correspondence to small areas of haemorrhage
Applicable on T2	Variable in general hypointense mass related to myometrium Homogenously high SI often seen in cellular myomas High SI rim represents dilated lymphatics in large myoma	Low SI uterine lesion with or without punctuate high SI foci scattered throughout lesion or high SI linear striations extending from endometrium that may lead to pseudowidening of endometrium High SI cysts may be seen (< 5 mm)
Applicable on G enhanced T1	Can appear hypo-iso and hyperintense Hypervascularity often seen in cellular leiomyoma Pseudocapsule more prominent absence of enhancement seen in partially or completely infracted leiomyoma (bridging vascular sign)	Can appear hypo-iso and hyperintense relative to myometrium Perfusion abnormalities may be seen on dynamic contrast enhanced MRI
CT	Calcification is most specific seen upto 10% case may be mottled, streaked or whorled or well defined peripheral rim	Cannot reliably identify adenomyosis enlargement is seen while clear mass lesion or distortion of uterine contour is absent

likely when the myometrium is deeply penetrated and is probably caused by disturbed uterine contractions rather than by tarry cyst formation. The increased size of the uterus can cause diurnal frequency, a sensation of weight in the pelvis, and a noticeable abdominal tumour. The patient may also complain of infertility. The enlargement of the uterus is detected on bimanual examination. The organ is mobile and there is usually no evidence of extrauterine endometriosis. The symptoms and signs are so similar that it may be impossible to distinguish clinically between adenomyosis and leiomyoma.

Pointers in favour of adenomyosis are it tends to occur at a younger age; it rarely enlarges the uterus to more than the size of a 12 to 14 weeks' pregnancy; it causes a regular rather than a nodular uterine enlargement.

A clinical suspicion of adenomyosis can be suggested by imaging studies, including transvaginal ultrasonography (TVUS) and MRI. TVS has several advantages over MRI. It is widely available, relatively inexpensive compared to MRI. It is well tolerated by most patients and generates high quality images not limited by patient size or uterine position. However, it has its limitations. It is operator dependent and may not be reproducible in patients on follow-up. The presence of intramural fibroids can hinder assessment of the adjacent myometrium. MRI, on the other hand, is less operator-dependent.

Diagnostic Findings

Imaging features are variable and in many instances very subtle. Three (some say four) forms can be distinguished.
1. **Diffuse adenomyosis:** Most common.
2. **Focal adenomyosis and adenomyoma:** Some consider these as separate (refer below).
3. **Cystic adenomyosis and adenomyotic cyst:** Rare.

Adenomyosis is usually relatively generalised, affecting large portions of the uterus (typically the posterior wall), but sparing the cervix. Despite often marked enlargement of the uterus, the overall contour is usually preserved.[7]

In some, adenomyosis may be localised, forming a mass. In such cases, the term adenomyoma may be used, although there appears to be some disagreement about whether the terms focal adenomyosis and adenomyoma refer to exactly the same entity. A rare variant is cystic adenomyosis, which is believed to be the result of repeated focal haemorrhages resulting in cystic spaces filled with altered blood products7.

Pelvic Ultrasound

Ultrasound is usually the first and often the only imaging modality employed to investigate menorrhagia and dysmenorrhoea. Unfortunately, the sonographic features of adenomyosis are variable and may be absent. The reported sensitivity and specificity of trans-abdominal ultrasound

are 32% to 63% and 95% to 97% 'respectively.[8,9] There are spectrum of findings which includes:
- Normal appearing uterus
- Focal or diffuse myometrial bulkiness, typically of the posterior wall
- Thickening of the transition zone can sometimes be visualised as a hypoechoic halo surrounding the endometrial layer of ≥ 12 mm thickness
- Subendometrial echogenic linear striations
- Subendometrial echogenic nodules (specific sign)
- Small myometrial cysts/sub endometrial cysts (specific sign)
- Heterogeneous echogenicity (heterogenous myometrial echotexture)
- Hyperechoic: Islands of endometrial glands
- Hypoechoic: Associated muscle hypertrophy
- 'Venetian blind' appearance may be seen due to subendometrial echogenic linear striations and acoustic shadowing where endometrial tissues cause a hyperplastic reaction.

When an adenomyoma is present, then appearances may closely mimic those of a uterine fibroid, which may also coexist.

Hysterosalpingogram (Figs 8.4A to D)

May show diverticula extending into the myometrium.

Computed Tomography

Computed tomography (CT) is unable to diagnose adenomyosis, but may suggest its presence when uterine enlargement is present. Distinguishing between adenomyosis and uterine fibroids on CT is difficult, although the presence of calcifications strongly favours the latter.

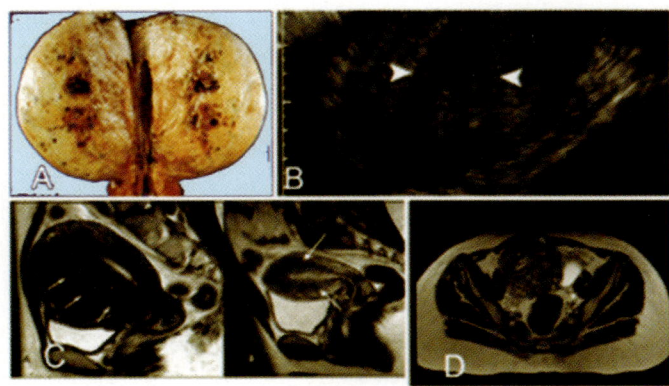

Figs 8.4A to D: A. Adenomyosis (sagittal cut section), ill defined lesion in uterine wall—arrows indicate innumerable hyperintense foci; **B.** Ultrasonography of adenomyosis (venetian bands). Marked enlargement of the junctional zone, arrows indicate MRI appearance of adenomyosis; **C.** T1W1 images (adenomyosis-coronal section); **D.** MRI-T2W.

Pelvic MRI

The MRI is the modality of choice to diagnose and characterise adenomyosis, and T2 weighted images (sagittal and axial) are most useful. MRI has a sensitivity of 78% to 88% and a specificity of 67% to 93%.[10]

The most easily recognised feature is thickening of the junctional zone of the uterus to more than 12 mm, either diffusely or focally (normal junctional zone measures no more than 5 mm). In T2 weighed images, typically a region of adenomyosis appears as an ill-defined ovoid/diffuse region of thickening, often with small high T2 signal regions representing small regions of cystic change, the region may also have a striated appearance. In T1 weighed images, foci of high T1 signal are often seen, indicating menstrual haemorrhage into the ectopic endometrial tissues. Routinely, T1 contrast + (gadiolinium) weighed images , contrast enhanced MR evaluation is usually not indicated for evaluation of adenomyosis, however, if performed, it shows enhancement of the ectopic endometrial glands.[11,12]

Dynamic contrast-enhanced imaging may have greater accuracy than T2-weighted imaging when adenomyosis and endometrial cancer coexist. A specific investigation called Cine MRI, which is cine mode display of serial T2-weighted images obtained at an interval of a few seconds by using an ultrafast sequence, allows visualisation of uterine motion. Cine MR imaging is mainly useful in differentiating a transient myometrial contraction from focal adenomyosis and in determining the origin of exophytic uterine lesions.[13]

A Special Emphasising on the Cystic Lesions in the Female Pelvis

Cystic lesions in female pelvis most often originate in the ovary.[14] Non-ovarian cystic pelvic lesions may include or broad ligament leiomyomas with cystic degeneration, cystic adenomyosis, peritoneal inclusion cysts, paraovarian cysts, mucocele of appendix, hydrosalpinx, subserosal, cystic degeneration of lymph nodes, haematoma, abscess, spinal meningeal cysts and lymphoceles.

The 4% of fibroids undergo cystic degeneration with extensive edema forming cystic, fluid-filled spaces. In such cases, vessels bridging the mass and the myometrial tissue, termed bridging vessel sign is useful in diagnosing the case as leiomyoma.[15]

Solid Ovarian Tumours

Solid ovarian tumour are another differential diagnosis as leiomyomata are common benign tumours of smooth muscle origin and specially when they are subserous origin, or found on the broad ligament.[16] Fibroids may resemble a suspicious ovarian mass on imaging when pedunculating in to the posterior cul-de-sac or degenerated.

Differential Diagnosis for Adnexal Mass

(Courtesy: Nezhat's. Video assisted and robotic assisted laparoscopy and hysteroscopy, 4th edition).

Table 8.2: Differential diagnosis for adnexal mass

Organ	Cystic	Solid
Ovary	Functional cyst	Benign
	Endometrial cyst	Malignant
	Cystic neoplasm Benign Malignant	
Fallopian tube	Tubo-ovarian abscess or hydrosalpinx	Ectopic pregnancy Tubo-ovarian abscess
Uterus	Intrauterine pregnancy	Myoma
Bowel	Distended colon with gas and/or faeces	Appendicitis Diverticulitis Diverticular abscess Colon cancer
Other	Distended bladder	Abdominal wall Haematoma or abscess Pelvic kidney Retroperitoneal neoplasm

Size, architecture and location may appear similar in adnexal, extra-adnexal peritoneal masses and even extraperitoneal lesions. However, special features determining the anatomical relationship of mass and the surrounding pelvic anatomical structures can assist in their differentiation. These parameters include visualisation of ovarian structures, the type of contour deformity at the interface between the ovary and the pelvic mass and the displacement pattern of the vessels, ureters and other pelvic organs.[18]

Defining the ovarian vascular pedicle allows the differentiation from lesions mimicking ovarian tumours such as subserosal uterine leiomyoma. Further more in the majority of leiomyoma cases, a vascular bridging sign at the interface between uterus and leiomyoma can be observed, which is not the case in ovarian lesions.[19] A multivariate analysis reported optimal lesion characterisation when combination of morphologic sonographic and colour Doppler information is used.

The various solid ovarian tumours are neoplasms of stromal origin—fibroma, fibrothecoma, solid teratoma of ovary, dysgerminoma, Brenners tumour, carcinoid tumours and granulosa cell tumours.

Point of Note

If the mass can be definitively separated from the ovaries or is contiguous with the round ligament, then an ovarian aetiology is unlikely.

For instance, the directionality of ureteral displacement can suggest if a mass is intra or extraperitoneal. Then entities such as leiomyomas, nerve sheath tumours, congenital uterine anomalies, and vascular abnormalities (ovarian torsion or iliac vessel aneurysm) in particular are often accurately characterized with sonography and/or MRI.

Diagnosis

Despite advances in technology, gray-scale transvaginal ultrasonography remains the standard for the evaluation of adnexal masses. Ultrasonography should assess size, mass characteristics (cystic, solid or both), complexity (internal septae, excrescences [a disfiguring addition] and papillae), and the presence or absence of abdominal or pelvic fluid (ascites or blood). Ultrasonography characteristics of simple cysts include anechoic mass; smooth, thin walls; no mural nodules or septations and association with acoustic enhancement. The combination of ultrasonography and Doppler flow studies is superior to either alone. In one study, three-dimensional ultrasonography was superior to two-dimensional ultrasonography for the prediction of malignant cases.[20] Ultrasonography and computed tomography have similar sensitivity and specificity for evaluation of adnexal masses, but ultrasonography is generally more cost-effective. In the future, MRI and positron emission tomography may have a role in the evaluation of adnexal masses.

Brief discussion on the few commonest solid ovarian tumours.[21]

Ovarian Fibromas

Ovarian fibromas are a benign ovarian tumour of sex cord/stromal origin. Although fibromas account for approximately 4% of all ovarian neoplasms, they are the most common sex cord ovarian tumour.

Epidemiology

Fibromas occur at all ages, but are most frequently seen in middle-aged women.

Clinical Presentation

Fibromas are generally asymptomatic and are often detected at palpation during routine gynaecologic examination. Tumours can reach a large size at presentation.

Pathology

The tumour belongs to the same histopathologic spectrum as an ovarian thecoma /ovarian fibrothecoma. Fibromas have no (or very few) thecal cells and no (or minimal) oestrogen activity.

It is composed of spindle cells forming variable amounts of collagen. Sectioning of a fibroma typically reveals a chalky-white surface that has a whorled appearance, similar to that of a uterine fibroid. Areas of oedema, occasionally with cyst formation, are also relatively common.

Associations

They are associated with ascites in 40% of cases and with pleural effusions in a small percentage of cases:[22]

Meigs Syndrome

Consists of an ovarian fibroma with ascites and a pleural effusion fibromas are seen in 75% of patients with Nevoid basal cell carcinoma syndrome.[23]

Diagnosis

Ultrasound

On ultrasound, fibromas most commonly manifest as solid, hypoechoic masses with ultrasound beam attenuation. As such, they may appear similar to a pedunculated subserosal uterine fibroid (Fig. 8.5).

However, the sonographic appearance can be variable and some tumours can rarely have cystic components. CT fibromas usually manifest as diffuse, slightly hypoattenuating masses with poor, very slow contrast enhancement. Calcification and bilaterality are both uncommon. In the MRI signal characteristics include in T1: fibromas usually demonstrate homogeneous low signal intensity, in T2 fibromas appear as well-circumscribed masses with low signal intensity may contain scattered hyperintense areas representing oedema cystic degeneration. a band of T2 hypointensity separating the tumour from the uterus on all imaging planes is also considered a characteristic feature T1 C+ (Gd): usually shows heterogenous enhancement (Figs 8.6A and B).

In the differential diagnosis general considerations include:
- Malignant ascites and pleural effusion in the presence of an aggressive ovarian tumour
- Pseudo-Meigs syndrome: Benign reversible pleural effusion in the presence of a primary tumour other than solid ovarian tumours, e.g. broad ligament leiomyoma.

Brenner Tumour

A Brenner tumour is an uncommon surface epithelial tumour of the ovary. It was originally known as a transitional cell

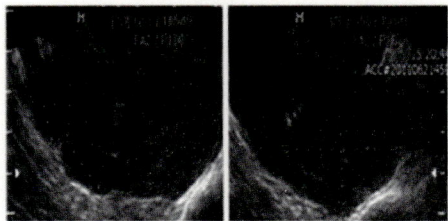

Fig. 8.5: Ultrasonography (ovarian fibroma appearance right ovary)

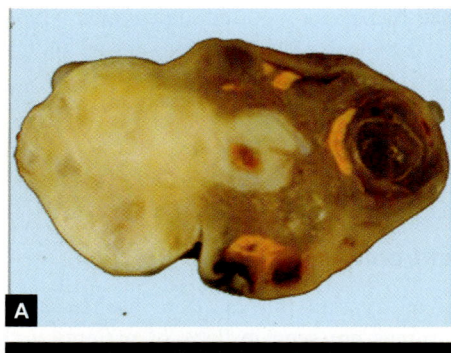

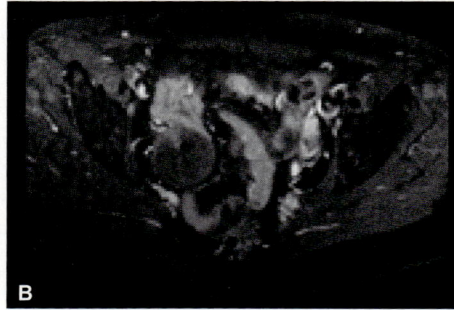

Figs 8.6A and B: A. MRI-T1W1 (image ovarian fibroma);
B. Cut section (ovarian fibroma).

tumour due to its histological similarity to the urothelium. Brenner tumours account for up to 3.2% of ovarian epithelial neoplasms. They can very rarely can occur in other locations, including the testis (Fig. 8.7).

Epidemiology

Most often found incidentally in women between their 5th and 7th decades of life.

Clinical Presentation

They are most frequently found incidentally on pelvic examination or at laparotomy.

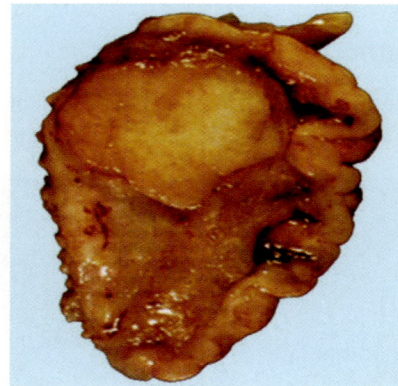

Fig. 8.7: Brenner tumour- cutsection

Pathology

Histological specimens often show transitional cells similar to neoplasms of the urothelium24.

Associations

Brenner tumours are associated with another epithelial ovarian neoplasm of either the ipsilateral or contralateral ovary in 30% of cases.[6] Approximately 6%–7% of Brenner tumours can be bilateral.[25]

Diagnosis

It Often manifest as a multilocular cystic mass with a solid component or as a mostly solid mass. Tumours are usually small (< 2 cm). Even with the occasional large tumour (> 10 cm), there is often a lack of local invasion, lymphadenopathy, ascites, or metastases (i.e. peritoneal metastases and omental caking) which help distinguish it from other malignant ovarian neoplasms.[26] In the Pelvic ultrasound Brenner tumours are similar to other solid ovarian neoplasms, particularly fibromas-thecomas, and can also be confused with pedunculated leiomyomas. They are mainly hypoechoic solid masses. Calcifications have been reported in 50% of Brenner tumours on ultrasound. In CT calcifications have been reported in ~ 83% of Brenner tumours on CT. solid component may show mild to moderate enhancement post contrast. In Pelvic MRI due to its predominantly fibrous content they appear hypointense on T2 weighted sequences.

■ OVARIAN DYSGERMINOMA

Ovarian dysgerminomas are a type of germ cell tumour of the ovary. They are the most common malignant germ cell tumours of the ovary and are thought to account for ~1% of all ovarian neoplasms.[27]

Epidemiologically they are rare ovarian tumours that occur predominantly in young women (majority occurring in the 2nd to 3rd decades[28]). Approximately 10–20 of cases can occur in pregnancy.

Pathology

The tumour is thought to arise from primordial germ cells and is considered an ovarian counterpart of seminoma of the testis. They are usually solid and multi-lobulated. The tumours are usually hormonally inert and in its pure form is not associated with endocrine hormone secretion. However, syncytiotrophoblastic giant cells, which produce HCG, are present in 5% of dysgerminomas and can cause elevation of serum HCG levels.

Approximately 15% of tumours can contain other malignant germ cell variants in which instance they are termed malignant

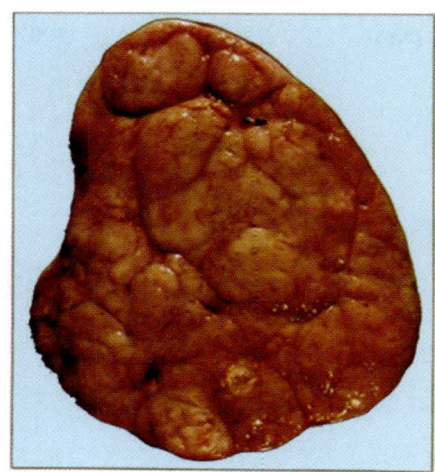

Fig. 8.8: Dysgerminoma cut section.

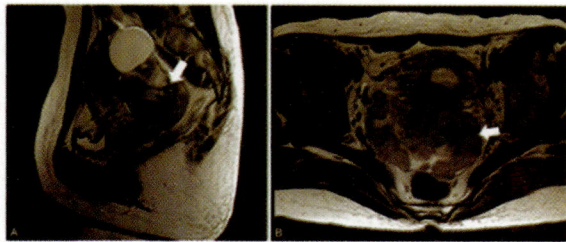

Figs 8.9A and B: MRI dysgerminoma. It measured a 5.8 × 9.8 cm in sized and was a lobulating contoured mass with intermediate signal intensity in T2 images. And a 4.3 × 3.3 cm sized cystic lesion was also observed. **A.** Sagittal view; **B.** Axial view. Arrows: dysgerminoma.

mixed germ cell tumours of the ovary . Approximately 10-17% of tumours can be bilateral.

Diagnosis

In the ultrasound is seen septated ovarian mass with varying echotexture. Colour Doppler interrogation may show prominent flow signal within the fibrovascular septa . In the CT calcification may be present in a speckled pattern. Characteristic imaging findings include multilobulated solid masses with prominent fibrovascular septa. Post contrast imaging can often show enhancement of the septae.[29] In the MRI Tumours are often seen divided into lobules by septa.[30]

Reported signal characteristics including in T2: the septae are often hypointense or isointense 3T1 C+ (Gd)—the septae often show marked enhancement.

Uterine Sarcoma

Rarely, uterine leiomyomas (Fig. 8.10) may undergo malignant degeneration to become a sarcoma. The true incidence of malignant transformation is difficult to determine,

because leiomyomas are common, whereas malignant leiomyosarcomas are rare and can arise de novo (Table 8.3). The incidence of malignant degeneration is less than 1.0% and has been estimated to be as low as 0.2%.[31]

The challenge of differentiating a leiomyoma from a uterine sarcoma is one part of the diagnostic process for all women with a uterine mass. The differential diagnosis of an enlarged uterus includes both benign and malignant conditions.

Rapid growth may occur in either a sarcoma or a benign leiomyoma. In addition, it is theoretically possible for a sarcoma to remain indolent for a long period of time and only come to diagnostic attention when a more aggressive phase of disease is entered. Particularly for postmenopausal women, a new or growing uterine mass warrants further evaluation for uterine sarcoma. The level of suspicion may be lower in women who are on postmenopausal estrgen therapy and have a small increase in the size of a fibroid known to present prior to menopause. In this subgroup, stopping postmenopausal oestrogen therapy is also an option to see, if regression occurs.

Clinical Manifestations

Abnormal uterine bleeding, pelvic pain/pressure, and a pelvic mass are the primary presenting symptoms and signs for both leiomyomas and sarcoma, making it difficult to differentiate between the two on this basis. Some women with sarcoma present with a foul-smelling vaginal discharge, but this is not a reliable indicator of malignancy, since vaginal discharge is a common gynecologic symptom.

Diagnosis

Choice of Imaging Modality

There is no pelvic imaging modality that can reliably differentiate between benign leiomyomas and uterine sarcomas. Leiomyomas and uterine sarcomas appear similar, both are focal masses within the uterus and both often have central necrosis.

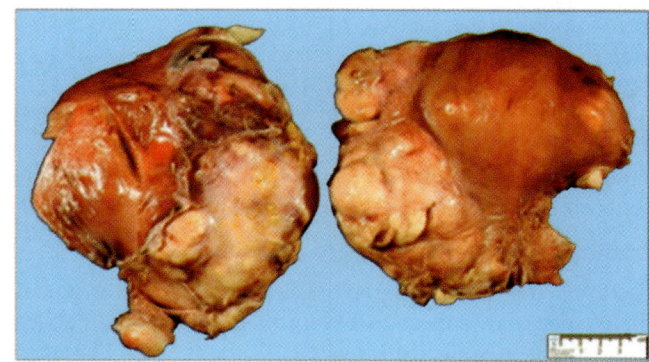

Fig. 8.10: Uterine leiomyosarcoma

Table 8.3: Leiomyoma and leiomyosarcoma

	Leiomyoma	Leiomyosarcoma
Incidence	More frequent	Rare (1:2000) (incidentally discovered)
Peak age	4th decade	6th decade
Growth rate	Slow	Rapid growth especially in postmenopausal women
Characteristics	Benign	Malignant (invasiveness and metastasis seen)
MRI (T1)	Isointense to myometrium peripheral hypointense rim indicates calcification	Haemorrhagic changes with high signal intensity
MRI (T2)	Variable in general hypointense mass related to myometrium Homogenously high SI often seen in cellular myomas High SI rim represents dilated lymphatics in large myoma	Irregular contour, inhomogeneous appearance with pockets of high signal intensity
LDH	Usually normal	Raised LDH levels

Pelvic Ultrasound

It is typically the first-line study to evaluate women for potential uterine pathology. Sonographic evaluation of a uterine mass may identify features suggestive of sarcoma with mixed echogenic and poor echogenic parts, central necrosis, and colour Doppler findings of irregular vessel distribution, low impedance to flow, and high peak systolic velocity. However, many of these characteristics may also be found in benign leiomyomas.

MRI

MRI may be helpful in women in whom there is a suspicion of sarcoma; however, it does not provide a definitive diagnosis. High signal intensity is not a reliable indicator of uterine sarcoma. A consistent finding in leiomyosarcomas is the absence of calcifications. Some data suggest that ill-defined margins are consistent with a sarcoma.[32] Two small studies using different techniques of MRI with gadolinium contrast have reported specificities of 93% to 100% and positive predictive values of 53% to 100%.[33] Further study of use of MRI for this purpose is needed (Figs 8.11A and B).

Computed Tomography

Computed tomography (CT) does not reliably differentiate between leiomyomas and uterine sarcomas.

Positron Emission Tomography/CT

Positron emission tomography/CT with fluorodeoxyglucose (FDG) does not appear to be useful to distinguish between leiomyomas and uterine sarcomas. While the FDG uptake is generally high in sarcomas and low in leiomyomas, the uptake varies across individual tumours.

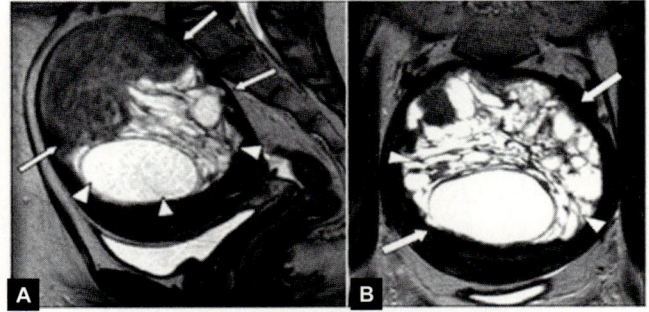

Figs 8.11A and B: MRI T2W images-uterine sarcoma

Transient Myometrial Contraction

Transient myometrial contraction as a physiological phenomenon may simulate a pathological condition such as focal or diffuse adenomyosis. Most common in a non-pregnant woman originate exclusively from the junctional zone and their amplitude frequency and direction depend on the phase of the menstrual cycle. Clinician should be aware of this phenomenon and imaging should be repeated after a suitable interval when the nature of a bulge or a region of low intensity in the myometrium is in doubt.[34]

A transitional zone is an anatomical landmark in the assessment of adenomyosis. Transient uterine contraction that causes a focal area of low signal intensity with an increased in thickness of transitional zone should not be misinterpreted as an organic lesion. Besides depicting many organic lesions. MRI is able to demonstrate the variability in the appearance of the normal uterus.

In women of reproductive age group, three distinct layers can be identified with in the uterine corpus on T2 weighted MR images. A central strip of high signal intensity corresponds in the endometrium and endometrial secretions. A ban of low signal intensity surrounding the endometrium is termed as Transitional zone or inner myometrium. Finally, the peripheral zone of intermediate signal intensity is the outer endometrium. Although there is no obvious histological zonal equivalent on light microscopy morphometric studies have shown that the transitional zone represents the innermost layer of the myometrium. In comparison with the outer myometrium, the transitional zone has an increased nuclear area per unit area, a decreased extracellular matrix per unit volume and a lower water content. The increased nuclear area reflects an increased nuclear cytoplasmic ratio of the myocytes and increased smooth muscle density. This may explain the observed decreased signal intensity on T2 weighted, MR images (Fig. 8.12).

Mark et al first published that the diagnosis of adenomyosis can be made with confidence when the transition zone measures more than 5 mm in the thickness.[34] However the published data do not adequately support this statement. Recently Kang et al reported that taking 8 mm as the upper

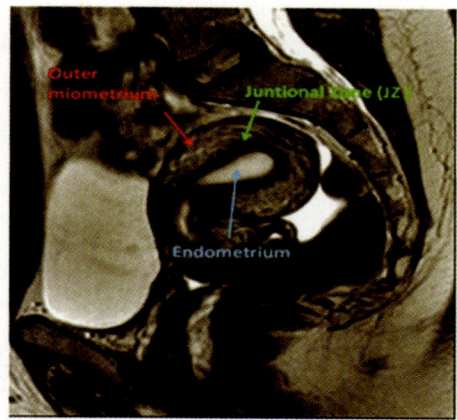

Fig. 8.12: Transient uterine contraction-MRI T2W

limit of normal thickness of the transitional zone may improve the specificity of MRI for diagnosing adenomyosis in the symptomatic patient population up to 100%.[35]

Because the transitional zone is anatomical land mark in the assessment of adenomyosis. Other causes of transitional zone alternations such as diffuse smooth muscle hypertrophy with an increase in the thickness or a broad and ill-defined transition zone in the early post partum period should also be considered in the differential diagnosis of adenomyosis.

Togashi et al have noted this phenomenon in women of reproductive age in the secretary phase of the menstrual cycle.[34]

OTHER RARE DIFFERENTIAL DIAGNOSIS

Disseminated Leiomyomatosis Peritonei

Is a rare benign condition causing multiple smooth muscle, myofibroblastic and fibroblastic nodules in the intraperitoneal cavity.[36] Although the exact aetiology is unknown, it is thought to be caused by smooth muscle metaplasia of the subperitoneal multipotential mesenchymal cells. Due to the diffuse nature of the disease, surgical resection is not potentially curative, but can be used to treat symptomatic lesions or if patients develop intestinal obstruction. However, reduction in lesion .size has been described following chemotherapy in one case.[37,38]

Lymphangioleiomyomatosis (LAM)

Is a rare multi-system disorder that can occur either sporadically or in association with the tuberous sclerosis complex (TSC) and is often considered a forme fruste of TSC.[39] It almost exclusively affects women of child-bearing age39. The estimated incidence is 1:400,000. The disease is characterised by the persistence of dilated lymphatics and interstitial proliferation of abnormal smooth muscle that in turn can obstruct venules, lymphatics, and small airways.

In the chest, there are two phases of proliferation in lymphangioleiomyomatosis. The early phase is characterised by proliferation of immature muscle cells that cover alveolar walls, bronchioles, pleura and vessels, including lymphatic routes. In the late phase, there is a development of cystic spaces and wider proliferation of muscle cells throughout the lung.[40,41]

CONCLUSION

1. Differentiation is clinically very important because of differences in treatment and prognostic implications. MRI in combination with the patient's clinical findings can be invaluable in making this distinction and can avoid unnecessary laparoscopy and/or exploratory surgery. Location is an important distinguishing characteristic.
2. Approach focuses first on the use of anatomic relationships and interactions of various pelvic structures to localize the mass' origin.
3. Extrauterine leiomyomas mimics ovarian tumours on clinical and radiological examination. Broad ligament leiomyoma should be kept important differential diagnosis for such solid adnexal or ovarian mass.
4. Key discriminating imaging features, such as the presence of fat, hypervascularity, or low T2 signal on magnetic resonance imaging (MRI) can be applied to further narrow the list of diagnostic possibilities.
5. Preoperative and intraoperative findings are of limited value in estimating the likelihood that a mass is a uterine sarcoma. Magnetic resonance imaging (MRI) and endometrial sampling are the most potentially useful techniques

REFERENCES

1. Kumar P, Malhotra N. Jeffcoate's Principles of Gynaecology. Tumors of the corpus uteri; 7th ed. New Delhi: Jaypee Brothers; 2008. p. 492.
2. Barek JS. Novack's Gynaecology, 15th ed. New Delhi: Lippincott Williams and Wilkins, Wolters Kluwer (India); 2007. Benign diseases of the female reproductive tract; p. 470.
3. Jorizzo JR, Chen MY, Riccio GJ. Endometrial polyps: sonohysterographic evaluation. AJR Am J Roentgenol. 2001;176 (3): 617-21.
4. Davis PC, O'neill MJ, Yoder IC et-al. Sonohysterographic findings of endometrial and subendometrial conditions. Radiographics. 22(4):803-16.
5. Machtinger R, Korach J, Padoa A, et al. Transvaginal ultrasound and diagnostic hysteroscopy as a predictor of endometrial polyps: risk factors for premalignancy and malignancy. Int. J. Gynecol. Cancer. 15(2):325-8. doi:10.1111/j.1525-1438.2005.15224.x - Pubmed citation.
6. Matalliotakis IM, Kourtis AI, Panidis DK. Adenomyosis. Obstet Gynecol Clin North Am. 2003;30(1):63-82. Cross Ref. Medline.

7. Reinhold C, Tafazoli F, Mehio A, et al.. Uterine adenomyosis: endovaginal US and MR imaging features with histopathologic correlation. RadioGraphics 1999;19 (spec no):S147–S160. Abstract, Medline.

8. Tamai K, Togashi K, Ito T, et al. MR imaging findings of adenomyosis: correlation with histopathologic features and diagnostic pitfalls. RadioGraphics. 2005;25(1):21-40.

9. Takeuchi M, Matsuzaki K, Nishitani H. Susceptibility-weighted MRI of endometrioma: preliminary results. AJR Am J Roentgenol. 2008;191(5):1366-70.

10. Takeuchi M, Matsuzaki K, Nishitani H. Susceptibility-weighted imaging for the evaluation of gynecologic diseases [abstr]. In: Proceedings of the 17th meeting of the International Society for Magnetic Resonance in Medicine. Berkeley, Calif: International Society for Magnetic Resonance in Medicine. 2009;4146.

11. Takeuchi M, Matsuzaki K, Nishitani H. Hyperintense uterine myometrial masses on T2-weighted magnetic resonance imaging: differentiation with diffusion-weighted magnetic resonance imaging. J Comput Assist Tomogr. 2009;33(6):834-7.

12. Fujiwara T, Togashi K, Yamaoka T, et al. Kinematics of the uterus: cine mode MR imaging. RadioGraphics. 2004;24(1):19.

13. Low SC, Chong CL. A case of cystic leiomyoma mimicking an ovarian malignancy. Ann Acad Med Singapore. 2004;33:371-4.

14. Kaushik C, Prasad A, Singh Y, et al. Case series: Cystic degeneration in uterine leiomyomas. Indian J Radiol, imaging. 2008;18:69-72.

15. Fasih N, Prasad Shanbhogue AK, Macdonald DB, et al. Leiomyomas beyond the uterus: Unusuallocations, rare manifestations. Radiographics. 2008;28:1931-48.

16. Camran Nezhat, FarrNezhat. Nezat's Video assisted and Robotic Assisted laparoscopy and hysteroscopy, 4th edition. Management of adnexal masses. p 185.

17. Bohm-Velez M, Fleischer AC, Andreotti RF, et al. Expert Panel on Women's Imaging. Suspected adnexal masses. Reston, Va: American College of Radiology 0(ACR); 2005.http://www.guidelines.gov/summary/summary.aspx?view_id=1&a mp;doc_id=83Point 21. Accessed August 3, 2009.

18. Patel MD. Practical approach to the adnexal mass. Radiol Clin North Am. 2006;44(6):879-99.

19. Adusumilli S, Hussain HK, Caoili EM, et al. MRI of sonographically indeterminate adnexal masses.AJR Am J Roentgenol. 2006;187(3):732-40.

20. Jung SE, Lee JM, Rha SE et al. CT and MR imaging of ovarian tumors with emphasis on differential diagnosis. Radiographics. 22(6):1305- 25. doi:10.1148/rg.226025033.

21. Vijayaraghavan GR, Levine D. Case 109: Meigs syndrome. Radiology. 2007;242(3):940-4. doi:10.1148/radiol.2423040775.

22. Chourmouzi D, Papadopoulou E, Drevelegas A. Magnetic resonance imaging findings in pseudo-Meigs' syndrome associated with a large uterine leiomyoma: a case report. J Med Case Reports. 2010;4:120. doi:10.1186/1752-1947-4-120 -Free text at pubmed - Pubmed citation.

23. Green GE, Mortele KJ, Glickman JN, et al. Brenner tumors of the ovary: sonographic and computed tomographic imaging features. J Ultrasound Med. 2006;25(10):1245-51. J Ultrasound Med (full text)-Pubmed citation.

24. Samanth KK, Black WC. Benign ovarian stromal tumors associated with free peritoneal fluid. Am J Obstet Gynecol. 1970;107(4):538-45.

25. Moon WJ, Koh BH, Kim SK, et al. Brenner tumor of the ovary: CT and MR findings. +*3J Comput Assist Tomogr. 24(1):72-6. J Comput Assist Tomogr (link)-Pubmed citation.

26. Jung SE, Lee JM, Rha SE, et al. CT and MR imaging of ovarian tumors with emphasis on differential diagnosis. Radiographics. 22(6):1305-25. doi:10.1148/rg.226025033.

27. Bierman SM, Reuter KL, Hunter RE. Meigs syndrome and ovarian fibroma: CT findings. J Comput Assist Tomogr. 14(5):833-4.

28. Kim SH, Kang SB. Ovarian dysgerminoma: colour Doppler ultrasonographic findings and comparison with CT and MR imaging findings. J Ultrasound Med. 1995;14(11):843-8. J Ultrasound Med (abstract)-Pubmed citation.

29. Tanaka YO, Kurosaki Y, Nishida M et-al. Ovarian dysgerminoma: MR and CT appearance. J Comput Assist Tomogr. 18 (3): 443-8. - Pubmed citation.

30. Tamai K, Koyama T, Saga T, et al. The utility of diffusion-weighted MR imaging for differentiating uterine sarcomas from benign leiomyomas. Eur Radiol 2008;18(4):723-30. CrossRef, Medline.

31. Oyama T, Togashi K, Konishi I, et al. MR imaging of endometrial stromal sarcoma: correlation with pathologic findings. AJR Am J Roentgenol. 1999;173(3):767-72. CrossRef, Medline.

32. Fujii S, Kaneda S, Tsukamoto K, et al.. Diffusion-weighted imaging of uterine endometrial stromal sarcoma: a report of 2 cases.J Comput Assist Tomogr. 2010;34(3):377-79. CrossRef, Medline.

33. Togashi K, Kawakami S, Kimura I, et al. Uterine contractions: possible diagnostic pitfall at MR imaging. J Magn Reson Imaging. 1993;3(6):889-93. CrossRef, Medline.

34. Ozsarlak O, Schepens E, de Schepper AM, et al. Transient uterine contraction mimicking adenomyosis on MRI. Eur Radiol. 1998;8(1):54-6. CrossRef, Medline.

35. Karaşahin KE, Gezginç K, Ulubay M, et al. Disseminated peritoneal leiomyomatosis. Taiwan J Obstet Gynecol 2008;47:123-5 [PubMed].

36. Lin YC, Wei LH, Shun CT, et al. Disseminated peritoneal leiomyomatosis responds to systemic chemotherapy. Oncology. 2009;76:55-8 [PubMed].

37. Paul PG, Naik S. Disseminated leiomyomatosis peritonei. Incidental finding in laparoscopy: a case report.Surg Laparosc Endosc Percutan Tech. 2010;20:e123–4 [PubMed].

38. Aberle DR, Hansell DM, Brown K, et al. Lymphangiomyomatosis: CT, chest radiographic, and functional correlations. Radiology. 1990;176(2):381-7. Radiology (abstract)-Pubmed citation.

39. Attili AK, Kazerooni EA. Case 116: lymphangioleiomyomatosis. Radiology. 2007;244(1):303-8. doi:10.1148/radiol.2441040790 -Pubmed citation.

40. Avila NA, Kelly JA, Chu SC, et al. Lymphangioleiomyomatosis: abdominopelvic CT and US findings. Radiology. 2000;216(1):147-53. Radiology (full text)-Pubmed citation.

41. Byun JY, Kim SE, Choi BG, et al. Diffuse and focal adenomyosis: MR imaging findings Radiographics. 1999;161-70.

CHAPTER 9

Complications of Fibroid Uterus

● Satwik B Metgud

Fibroid uterus is the most common gynaecological tumours found in women and more than 50% of the patients with fibroids have complications.[1] Although they are mainly a problem in the reproductive years, there are reports of problems from fibroids in postmenopausal women. In this chapter, we focus on special issues highlighting the complications, which are caused by fibroids, the degenerative changes of fibroid and also those which can arise as a result of the treatment. Although often asymptomatic, they may cause menorrhagia, metrorrhagia, infertility, pain, pressure symptoms haemorrhage and repeated abortions. Hence, it is of importance that the clinicians are aware of the complications of fibroids (Table 9.1).

■ SECONDARY CHANGES

The process of leiomyoma degeneration usually begins when the leiomyoma grows so large that the nearby blood vessels can no longer supply it with oxygen and nutrients. Uterine myomas have been identified to undergo several secondary changes and histological variants of uterine smooth muscle tumours. Secondary changes happening in leiomyomas are demonstrable in approximately 65% of cases.[2] These include hyaline change, mucoid, myxoid or myxomatous change, calcification, cystic changes and fatty metamorphosis. Histological variantsinclude cellular leiomyoma, apoplectic leiomyoma, leiomyoma with lymphoid infiltration, atypical (bizarre, symplastic or pleomorphic) leiomyoma, lipoleiomyoma, epithelioid (clear cell) leiomyoma, cotyledonoid dissecting leiomyoma, parasitic leiomyoma, leiomyoma with skeletal muscle differentiation, diffuse leiomyomatosis, intravenous leiomyomatosis, benign metastasizing leiomyoma and mitotically active leiomyoma. In general, hyaline degeneration is the most common (63%) form of degeneration, while the others occur less frequently, such as myxomatous changes (13%), calcification (8%), mucoid changes (6%), cystic degeneration (4%), red degeneration (3%) and fatty changes (3%)2.

Table 9.1: Complications of fibroid uterus

Complications related to pregnancy (antenatal)	Complications not related to pregnancy
Red degeneration	Degeneration (65%)
Preterm labour	AUB/Anaemia
Pain and tenderness	Urinary or bowel obstruction
Spontaneous abortions	Infection
During labour	
	Malignant transformation (< 1%)
Uterine inertia	Infertility
Malpresentation	Torsion of pedunculated subserous fibroid
Obstruction of the birth canal due to cervical or isthmic myoma	Intraperitoneal haemorrhage from rupture of a large vein on the surface of myoma (rare)
	Infection of submucous myoma (rare)
PPH	Polycythemia (rare)
Increased lower segment caesarian section	

Benign Degeneration

Hyaline Degeneration

It is thought to occur in up to 60% of uterine leiomyomas.[3] As with many other types of degeneration, it happens when fibroids outgrow their blood supply.[4] Hyaline degeneration involves the presence of homogeneous eosinophilic bands or plaques in the extracellular space, which represent accumulation of proteinaceous tissue.[5] It produces a hyperechoic appearance on ultrasound and loss of the usual myomatous architecture. On MRI there is a low SI on T2WI, without contrast enhancement.[5] The tumour is soft, gelatinous in consistency and pale on cut section. The hyalinized areas interspersed among the whorls are translucent and may be either small and localised or extensive. On histologic examination, typical hyaline changes are characterized by a diffuse, amorphous reddish-pink pattern and marked cellularity.[6]

Red Degeneration

Red degeneration is a haemorrhagic infarction of the uterine leiomyoma, which is a well-known complication, especially during pregnancy. Red degeneration occurs in 8% of tumours complicating pregnancy, although the prevalence is about 3% of all uterine leiomyoma.[7] The mechanism of red degeneration is suggested to begin with venous obstruction at the periphery of the lesion, which induces haemorrhagic infarction and extensive necrosis that involves the entire lesion. Grossly, the tumour presents a mottled, dark red appearance, not unlike that of uncooked beef. On histologic examination, there is patchy necrosis and haemorrhage in the muscle fibres. Red degenerations are painful, but often self-limiting (Box 9.1).

Box 9.1: Mechanism of severe pain associated with red degeneration

Rapid fibroid growth results in the tissue outgrowing its blood supply leading to tissue anoxia, necrosis and infarction[21]
The growing uterus results in a change in the architecture (kinking) of the blood supply to the fibroid leading to ischemia and necrosis[21]
Release of prostaglandins from cellular damage within the fibroid[23]

Cystic Degeneration

Cystic degeneration occurs in approximately 4% of leiomyomas. It typically occurs after hyaline degeneration8. There is a tendency for hyalinization to undergo liquefaction with the formation of cystic spaces of varying sizes (Fig. 9.1), but without an epithelial lining. The greater part of the tumour may be cystic, the cysts containing colourless or blood-stained fluid. The cystic areas are not well demarcated from the rest of the tumour (Figs 9.2 and 9.3A and B), and irregular strands of tissue lining the cavities may traverse them. Myomatous and mucoid degenerations may also result in cystic change.

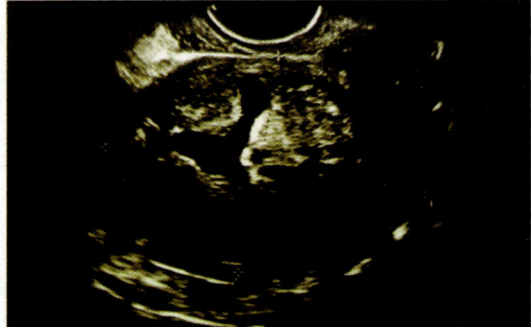

Fig. 9.1: Ultrasound image of cystic degeneration of fibroid

Calcification

This dystrophic change is seen in 8% of leiomyoma9. The circulatory deprivation which leads to precipitation of calcium carbonate and phosphate, may be focal or diffuse, and may be seen on preoperative X-ray films. The finding of a calcified leiomyoma (Fig. 9.4) is more common in postmenopausal woman. The calcareous material is recognized histologically by the purplish amorphous lake produced with hematoxylin.

Myxomatous Degeneration

While this type of degeneration is generally considered rare. The higher end of prevalence for this type of degeneration has been reported up to 50% of all degenerations10. Fibroids that have undergone myxoid degeneration are filled with a gelatinous material and can be difficult to differentiate from fibroids that have undergone cystic degeneration , however, they typically appear as more complex cystic masses.This is characterized grossly by a pasty gelatinous appearance. Usually the change is mild and patchy. On histologic examination, the myxomatous tissue appears pale when stained with haematoxylin and eosin. Smooth muscle cells are sparse and are seen as thin wavy fibrils in a clear background.

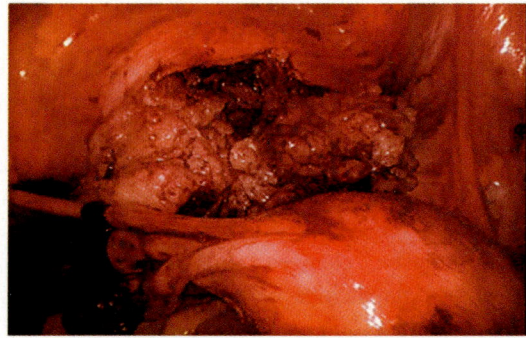

Fig. 9.2: Laparoscopic image of myomectomy in a degenerated fibroid

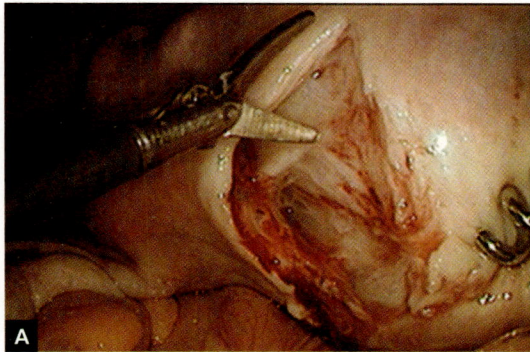

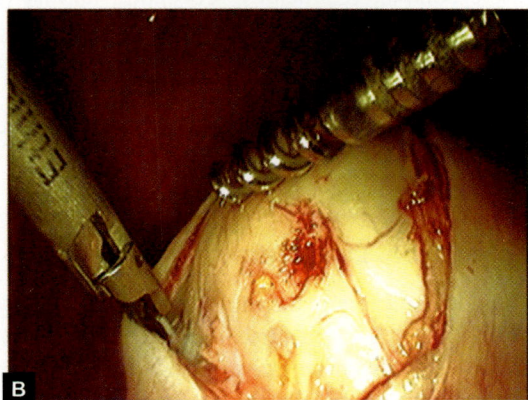

Figs 9.3A and B: A. Cystic degeneration of fibroid, with difficulty in getting the correct plane, proceeded with excision of fibroid as it was a subserous fibroid; **B.** A nondegenerated fibroid with pseudocapsule, connective tissue being separated to obtain correct plane for enucleation.

Mucoid Degeneration

The gross charecteristics do not differ significantly from those seen in the myxomatous type. The differences are mainly microscopic, the mucoid areas appear bluish and amorphous. They are usually circumscribed and may form cysts.

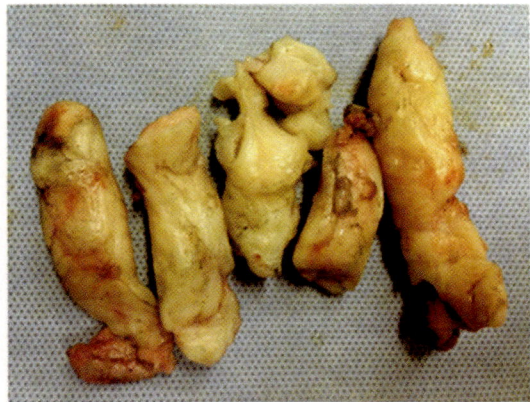

Fig. 9.4: Subserosal calcified fibroid, difficult to morcellate-specimen

Fatty Degeneration

This type of degeneration is usually associated with hyaline change. It has to be differentiated from uterine lipoma. On histologic examination, fatty degeneration is characterized by small vacuolated cells containing fat, which is identified in frozen sections stained for lipid.

■ INFECTION AND NECROSIS

Uterine fibroid necrosis and infection changes are rare but potentially serious event. It usually accompanies a degenerating or dying fibroid and can cause painful infection to the surrounding uterine tissue. Surgical removal is usually a preferred option. There is an association of increased incidence of fibroids in patients with history of PID, chlamydia, trichomonas, or herpes, but lacks conclusive evidence from larger studies.[11,12]

Necrosis may result from torsion or twisting of a pedunculated leiomyoma and is often associated with pregnancy or the use of contraceptive drugs.[13,14] Unlike other types of degeneration, it produces clinical symptoms of abdominal pain and tenderness.[15]

The triad of bacteremia or sepsis, leiomyoma uteri and no other apparent source of infection should suggest the diagnosis of pyomyoma.[16]

■ SARCOMATOUS CHANGE

Uterine sarcoma is rare (3–7 per 100,000) with a poor prognosis.[17] Malignant transformation in leiomyomas can be extremely difficult to recognize by gross appearance at operation. Changes in colour and consistency of the tumour are important since the sarcomatous tissue produces variegation and a soft consistency. A similar picture, however, can be seen in non-malignant degenerative changes. All fibroids showing these features should therefore be subjected to careful microscopic examination.

Sarcomatous change in leiomyomas must be differentiated microscopically from both leiomyosarcoma arising from the myometrium and cellular leiomyoma. When there has been malignant change, the most useful microscopic criterion is the demonstration is areas in the malignant tumour where there are features of a benign growth. In the cellular leiomyoma, there is an increase in the number of nuclei, but these are regular and not pleomorphic. Mitotic figures are found in both the cellular leiomyoma and the sarcoma.

In studies and systematic reviews of women undergoing hysterectomy or myomectomy for a myometrial mass, the prevalence of sarcoma is approximately 0.20% (1 in 500) in most studies.[18–20]

■ COMPLICATIONS IN PREGNANCY

Pain is the most common complication of fibroids in pregnancy and is seen most often in women with large fibroids (> 5 cm) during the second and third trimesters of pregnancy.[21,22] Three main theories have been proposed to explain the severe pain associated with red degeneration.

Leiomyomas during pregnancy may also initiate preterm labour. Most cases can be managed conservatively with adequate rest, analgesics and tocolytics if indicated. The complications of fibroids in pregnancy and its management is covered in detail in the section Fibroids in fertility and pregnancy.

In early pregnancy, spontaneous miscarriage rates are greatly increased in pregnant women with fibroids compared with those without fibroids and bleeding is significantly more common, if the placenta implants close to the fibroid. In late pregnancy, such complications include preterm labour, placental abruption, placenta previa and fetal anomalies.

Prior to pregnancy, myomectomy can be considered in women with unexplained infertility or recurrent pregnancy loss, although whether this intervention improves fertility rates and perinatal outcome remains unclear.[24]

During Labour

1. Malpresentation, labour dystocia, and caesarean delivery. Large fibroids, multiple fibroids and fibroids in the lower uterine segment have all been reported as independent risk factors for malpresentation.[25] Numerous studies have shown that uterine fibroids are a risk factor for caesarean delivery.[26] This is due in part to an increase in labour dystocia, which is increased two-fold in pregnant women with fibroids.
2. Retained placenta: One study reported that retained placenta was more common in women with fibroids, but only if the fibroid was located in the lower uterine segment.
3. PPH: Reports on the association between fibroids and postpartum haemorrhage are conflicting. Pooled cumulative data suggest that postpartum haemorrhage is significantly more likely in women with fibroids compared with control subjects.[27] Fibroids may distort the uterine architecture and interfere with myometrial contractions leading to uterine atony and postpartum haemorrhage.[28]

■ COMPLICATIONS IN NON-PREGNANT WOMEN

Leiomyoma causing heavy bleeding with anaemia is the most common complication and problems like urinary or bowel obstruction is least common complication. The risk of malignant transformation is less than 2%.

Abnormal Uterine Bleeding

Abnormal uterine bleeding is seen in 30% of the patients with myoma and plays a significant role is causing iron deficiency anaemia. Submucous myoma produces the most pronounced symptoms of menorrhagia, premenstrual and post menstrual spotting. The mechanism by which fibroids cause menorrhagia is not well understood, the possible explanations are:[29]

1. Interruption of blood supply to the endometrium or distortion and congestion of the surrounding vessels.
2. Fibroids located within the uterine wall may inhibit muscle contracture, thereby preventing normal uterine attempts at haemostasis.
3. Fibroids increase the size and volume of the uterus and there by uterine lining, hence increased bleeding.
4. Pedunculated submucous myomas can lead to areas of venous thrombosis and necrosis on the surface, which cause intermenstrual bleeding

Haematological Disorders

Iron deficiency anaemia is the most common haematological disorder secondary to uterine haemorrhage. However women with fibroids can also have polycythemia[30] due to increased production of erythropoietin and also thrombocytosis in response to excess bleeding.[31] These two haematological complications are known to be associated with venous thromboembolism.

Pain

Pain is the commonest complication in women with fibroid uterus and typically have spasmodic dysmenorrhoea.[32] The uterus goes into spasms as it tries to expel the large clots and excess blood. The pain typically starts with the bleeding and ends abruptly with the end of the bleeding. The main factor for pain is the vascular occlusion, which leads to necrosis and infection. The other causes are:

- Torsion of a pedunculated fibroid
- Myometrial contractions to expel the myoma
- Red degeneration
- Heaviness fullness in the pelvic area
- Feeling a mass
- Myoma impacted in the pelvis causes back pain radiating to the lower extremities
- Dyspareunea if it is protruding to vagina.

Pressure Effects

A large myoma may distort or obstruct other organs like ureters, bladder or rectum and cause urinary symptoms, hydroureter, constipation, pelvic venous congestion and lower limb edema. Rarely a posterior fundal tumour can cause

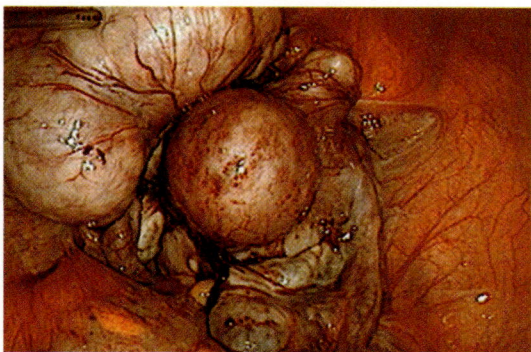

Fig. 9.5: Moderate endometriosis coexisting with fibroid

retention of urine in case of extreme retroflexion of the uterus distorting the bladder base. Parasitic tumour may cause bowel obstruction. Cervical tumours can cause serosanguineous vaginal discharge, bleeding, dyspareunia or infertility. These problems are more likely with large fibroids. Renal and venous obstruction are potentially life-threatening and need to have the fibroids removed to prevent permanent damage.

Infertility

Approximately 5% to 10% of infertile women have fibroids.[33] Their size and location determines whether fibroids affect fertility. The current data suggest that only those fibroids with a submucosal or an intracavitary component are associated with decreased reproductive outcome.[34] Surgical removal of these type of fibroids may be of benefit. The association of uterine fibroids with infertility is an important concern to the clinicians and is dealt in detail in the section Fibroids in fertility and pregnancy.

Box 9.2: Pelvic pathologies commonly coexistent with fibroid uterus

Endometrial hyperplasia and endometrial polyps[35]
Endometriosis[36] (Fig. 9.5)
Anovulation and dysfunctional uterine bleeding
Pelvic inflammatory disease[37]
Tubal pregnancy

■ REFERENCES

1. Horace Fletcher, 1 Celia Burrell, et al Complications of Uterine Fibroids and Their Management. Obstetrics and Gynecology International Volume 2012, Article ID 932436, 2 pages doi:10.1155/2012/932436.
2. Persaud V, Arjoon PD. Uterine leiomyoma. Incidence of degenerative change and a correlation of associated symptoms. Obstet Gynecol. 1970;35:432-6.
3. Ueda H, Togashi K, Konishi I, et al. Unusual appearances of uterine leiomyomas: MR imaging findings and their histopathologic backgrounds. Radiographics. 1999;19:S131-45.
4. Hamm B, Baert AL, Beinder E, et al. MRI and CT of the Female Pelvis. Springer Verlag. 2010.
5. Okizuka H, Sugimura K, Takemori M, et al. MR detection of degenerating uterine leiomyomas. J Comput Assist Tomogr. 1993;17:760-6.
6. In: Nucci MR, Oliva E (Eds). Gynecologic Pathology. A Volume in the Series Foundations in Diagnostic Pathology. Elsevier Churchill Livingstone: 2009. pp. 261-89.
7. Kawakami S, Togashi K, Konishi I, et al. Red degeneration of uterine leiomyoma: MR appearance. J Comput Assist Tomogr. 1994;18:925-8.
8. Manjula K, Kadam SR, Chandrasekhar HR. Variants of Leiomyoma: Histomorphological Study of Tumors of Myometrium. JSAFOG. 2011;3:89-92.
9. Danforth DN, Scott JR. Benign lesions of corpus uteri. In: Danforth DN, Scott JR, (Eds). Obstetrics and Gynecology, 5th ed. Philadelphia: Lippincott; 1986;1073-9.
10. Dähnert W. Radiology Review Manual. Lippincott Williams & Wilkins. 2011.
11. Sterling L, Boutet M, Colak E, et al. Fibroid infected with Escherichia coli requiring surgical removal following uterine artery embolization. J Obstet Gynaecol Can. 2013;35(9):823-6.
12. Moore Kristen R, Cole Stephen R, Dittmer Dirk P, et al. Self-Reported Reproductive Tract Infections and Ultrasound Diagnosed Uterine Fibroids in African-American Women. Journal of Women's Health. 2015;24(6):489-95. doi:10.1089/jwh.2014.5051.
13. Laughlin SK, Schroeder JC, Baird DD. New directions in the epidemiology of uterine fibroids. Semin Reprod Med. 2010;28:204-17.
14. Faerstein E, Szklo M, Rosenshein NB. Risk factors for uterine leiomyoma: A practice-based case-control study II. Atherogenic risk factors and potential sources of uterine irritation. Am J Epidemiol. 2001;153:11-9.
15. Merrill JA & Creasman WT. Disorders of the uterine corpus. In: JR Scott, PJ DiSaia, B Hammond and WN Spellacy: Danforth's obstetrics and gynecology, p.1027. Edited by JB Lippincott Company, Philadelphia. 1990.
16. JS Greenspoon, M Ault, BA James, "Pyomyoma associated with polymicrobial bacteremia and fatal septic shock: case report and review of the literature," Obstetrical and Gynecological Survey. 1990;45(9):563-9.
17. Brooks SE, Zhan M, Cote T, et al. Surveillance, epidemiology, and end results analysis of 2677 cases of uterine sarcoma 1989-1999. Gynecol Oncol 2004;93:204.
18. http://www.fda.gov/downloads/AdvisoryCommittees/CommitteesMeetingMaterials/MedicalDevices/MedicalDevicesAdvisoryCommittee/ObstetricsandGynecologyDevices/UCM404148.pdf (Accessed on November 24, 2014).
19. Parker WH, Fu YS, Berek JS. Uterine sarcoma in patients operated on for presumed leiomyoma and rapidly growing leiomyoma. Obstet Gynecol. 1994;83:414.
20. Leung F, Terzibachian JJ, Gay C, et al. Hysterectomies performed for presumed leiomyomas: should the fear of leiomyosarcoma make us apprehend non laparotomic surgical routes? Gynecol Obstet Fertil. 2009;37:109.

21. Lee HJ, Norwitz ER, Shaw J. Contemporary Management of Fibroids in Pregnancy. Reviews in Obstetrics and Gynecology. 2010;3(1):20-27.

22. Burton CA, Grimes DA, March CM. Surgical management of leiomyomata during pregnancy. Obstet Gynecol. 1989;74(5):707-9.

23. Katz VL, Dotters DJ, Droegemueller W. Complications of uterine leiomyomas in pregnancy. Obstet Gynecol. 1989;73:593-6.

24. De Carolis S, Fatigante G, Ferrazzani S, et al. Uterine myomectomy in pregnant women. Fetal Diagn Ther. 2001;16:116-9.

25. Lev-Toaff AS, Coleman BG, Arger PH, et al. Leiomyomas in pregnancy: sonographic study. Radiology. 1987;164:375-80.

26. Vergani P, Locatelli A, Ghidini A, et al. Large uterine leiomyomata and risk of cesarean delivery. Obstet Gynecol. 2007;109:410-4.

27. Klatsky PC, Tran ND, Caughey AB, et al. Fibroids and reproductive outcomes: a systematic literature review from conception to delivery. Am J Obstet Gynecol. 2008;198:357-66.

28. Szamatowicz J, Laudanski T, Bulkszas B, et al. Fibromyomas and uterine contractions. Acta Obstet Gynecol Scand. 1997;76:973-76.

29. CP West and MA Lumsden. 'Fibroids and menorrhagia,' Bailliere's Clinical Obstetrics and Gynaecology. 1989;3(2): 357-74.

30. NA Abdul Ghaffar, MP Ismail, NMZ Nik Mahmood, et al. "Huge uterine fibroid in a postmenopausal woman associated with polycythaemia: a case report," Maturitas. 2008;60(2):177-9.

31. JH Witt, MI Marks, and E. I. Smith, "Leiomyoma presenting as prolonged fever, anemia, and thrombocytosis," Cancer. 1983;52(12):2359-62.

32. MY Dawood, 'Dysmenorrhea', Journal of Reproductive Medicine for the Obstetrician and Gynecologist. 1985;30(3):154-67.

33. Pritts, Elizabeth A. MD. Fibroids and Infertility: A Systematic Review of the Evidence Obstetrical & Gynecological Survey. 2001;56(8):483-91

34. Kristin Van Heertum Larry Barmat. Uterine fibroids associated with infertility Summary Women's Health. 10(6):645-53. DOI 10.2217/whe.14.27(doi:10.2217/whe.14.27).

35. American Journal of obstetrics and Gynecology. 1940;41:694-7.

36. Huang JQ, Lathi RB, Lernyre M, et al. Coexistence of endometriosis in woman with symphomatic leconyomas fectal sterl. 2010;94:720-3.

37. Fairsteen E, Myoses S, Rosenshen NB. Risk factors for uterine lecomyoma: a practice based csx-control study II Atecogenis risk factors and potential sources of uterine irritation American journal of Epidenuology. 153(1):11-19.

SECTION 3

Management of Fibroids

CHAPTER 10

Medical Management of Fibroids

● K Jayakrishnan, Niranjana Jayakrishnan

Uterine leiomyomas are the most common gynecological tumours and are present in 30% of women in the reproductive age group. Treatment of leiomyomas must be individualised, based on symptoms, size and rate of growth of the uterus, and the woman's desire for fertility. The majority of uterine leiomyomas are asymptomatic and will not require therapy.

Medical management (Table 10.1) should be tailored to the needs of the woman presenting with uterine fibroids and geared to alleviating the symptoms. Cost and side effects of medical therapies may limit their long-term use (SOGC 111-C).

■ ORAL CONTRACEPTIVE PILLS

The influence of oral contraceptive pill (OCP) on myomata is poorly understood and data on its effect on the size of myomata are conflicting.

Mechanism of Action

By inhibiting ovulation, both OCPs and pregnancy may have a protective effect against the recurrence of fibroids after myomectomy.

Review of Literature

The OCP appear to improve short-term menstrual irregularities through their effects on the endometrium, but they do not reduce the size of myomata.[1] In a meta-analysis, the authors reported a 17% reduction in morbidity among women who had used OCP for 5 years or more.[2]

Side Effects

Early side effects of oral contraceptives (OCs) include bloating, nausea, and breast tenderness. Although they may be bothersome enough to lead to discontinuation of the OC, these side effects usually subside in several months. Abnormal bleeding is a common problem that often resolves. Weight gain is not a consistent finding with low-dose pills

■ TRANEXAMIC ACID (TA)

Mechanism of Action

This antifibrinolytic lysine derivative reduces the amount of bleeding by preventing fibrin degradation.

Dosage

The dose is usually 1–1.5 g 4 times daily; however, patients are advised to use TA sporadically only during acute episodes of heavy bleeding.

Review of Literature

Food drug administration (FDA)-approved for treatment of menorrhagia in 2009, tranexamic acid (TA) decreases menstrual bleeding within 2–3 hours of administration. Low-quality evidence suggests that the drug reduces intraoperative blood loss during myomectomy.[3]

Table 10.1: Various modalities of medical management of fibroids

Treatment	Contraceptive effect	Effect on pain	Effect on bleeding	Fibroid volume	Special Consideration
NSAID	No fertility preserved	Helpful	Reduction shown in HMB	Not evaluated	• Gastric irritation • Patients with asthma • Start at onset of bleeding • Mefenamic acid is the only NSAID with a licence for HMB but other NSAIDs may have a class effect
Tranexamic acid	No fertility preserved	No effect	Reduction shown in HMB	Not evaluated	• (Max daily dose of 4 g best as 1 g four times daily) • Start at onset of bleeding and use for up to 4 days • Available over the counter • Thromboembolic events are rare
LNG-IUS	Yes, reserved on removal	Usually helpful	Significant reduction but may take 6 months	No conclusive evidence	• Not contraindicated in Nulliparous women • Clinicians who fit intrauterine devices should be appropriately trained and attend regular updates to maintain their competence • Progestogenic side-effects tend to be minimal and usually settle after 6 months
CHC	Yes, reserved on stopping	Usually helpful	Reduction shown in HMB Helped by extended use (tricycling or continuous)	Not evaluated	• Commonly used in clinical practice, although oestradiol valerate/dienogest combination is only product licensed in women with HMB, with evidence of 88% reduction in menstrual blood loss • Assess risk of ATE and VTE • Refer to UKMEC
High-dose oral progestogen	No, but not recommended of trying to conceive.	Usually helpful	Reduction shown in HMB ifused on day 5–26 of each cycle (15 mg norethisterone or 20–30 mg/day medroxyprogesterone acetate).	Not evaluated	• Progestogenic side-effects significant and limit long-term continuation • Maybe useful at menopause • Avoid norethisterone if BMI > 30 k/m^2 due to risk of VTE • Use in luteral phase only (i.e. day 19–26) is not efffective
High-dose injected progestogen	Yes, will take up to a year before fertility returns after last injection	Usually helpful	Reduction, with high incidence of amenorrhoea with continuous use	Not evaluated	• Variable weight gain • Caution in women with high risk of osetoporosis or cardiovascular disease due to hypoestrogenic effects
Ulipristal acetate (5mg)	No, additional non-hormonal, contraception, required in women at risk of pregnancy	Yes, effective within first cycle	Rapid reduction in bleeding, with many achieving amenorrhoea within 7–10 days	Significant reduction of 36%–42% by 3 months	• Licensed for women with fibroids suitable for surgery to relieve symptoms • 3-month course can be repeated once; second 3-month course is licensed • Benefit on fibroid volume when stopping may persist for 3–6 months
GnRH analogues	No, additional non-hormonal contraception required in all women at risk of pregnancy	Yes, gradual reduction	Gradual reduction upto 30 days to achieve amenorrhoea.	Significant reduction of 53% by 3 months	• Specialist initiated; for shared care, see local guidelines • Menopausal symptoms usual • Consider add-back HRT (continuous combined or tibolone), if young (< 45 years), high osteoporotic risk, or intractable menopausal symptoms develop • Limited use because of osteroporosis risk

Treatment	Contraceptive effect	Effect on pain	Effect on bleeding	Fibroid volume	Special Consideration

ATE = Arterial thromboembolism, CHC = Combined horomonal contraception, GnRH = Gonadotrophin-releasing hormone; HMB = Heavy menstrual bleeding; HRT = Hormone replacement therapy; LNG-IUS = Levonorgestrel intrauterine system; NSAID = Non-steroidal anti-inflammatory drug; VTE = Venous thromboembolism. See : www.guidelines.co.uk/wpg_uterine_fibroids_2014.

Side Effects

Include dizziness, gastrointestinal symptoms and possible intralesional thrombosis leading to necrosis.

Long-term Disadvantages

Although the evidence for risk of thromboembolic event with TA is controversial, caution should be exercised with its use in combination with hormonal treatment such as OCP.

■ MEDICAL MANAGEMENT

All medications currently available for fibroid treatment including gonadotropin-releasing hormone (GnRH)-agonist and sex steroids are unsuitable for long-term use because of their significant side effects. In recent years, new medications have been introduced that offer the promise of practical, long-term medical therapy for symptomatic fibroids. To date, the most encouraging results in terms of fibroid volume reduction, symptom relief, and compliance with long-term administration have been obtained with mifepristone, a progesterone receptor antagonist and asoprisnil, a selective progesterone receptor modulator.

Progesterone Receptor Agonists and Modulators

Mifepristone

Mechanism of action: Mifepristone has been the first available active antiprogestin. It has been shown to decrease fibroid size and blood flow to the fibroids.

Dosage: Early studies of women with symptomatic fibroids reported that daily administration of mifepristone at doses ranging from 5 to 50 mg for 3 to 6 months resulted in a 26% to 74% reduction in fibroid volume and a decrease in the prevalence and severity of fibroid-related symptoms, including menorrhagia, dysmenorrhoea and pelvic pressure (Steinauer et al, 2004).[4]

Review of literature: More recently, in a randomized, double blinded, placebo-controlled trial including 42 women with symptomatic fibroids, treatment with mifepristone 5 mg/day for 26 weeks led to a 47% reduction in fibroid size and a significant improvement in fibroid-related symptoms (Fiscella et al., 2006). By 12 months, 9 (41%) of 22 women randomized to mifepristone had become amenorrheic (Fiscella et al., 2006).

The drug was well tolerated, and no endometrial hyperplasia was noted in any participant (Fiscella et al, 2006).[5]

Side effects: High incidence (28%) of endometrial hyperplasia was observed in patients screened with endometrial biopsies (Steinauer et al, 2004).[4]

Long-term benefits: Although these data are very encouraging, further studies in larger samples with longer periods of treatment are needed to reliably assess the long-term safety and efficacy of this drug.[6,7]

Asoprisnil

Another promising medication for fibroid treatment is asoprisnil, a selective progesterone receptor modulator with mixed agonist/antagonist activity.

Mechanism of action: This drug has been shown to inhibit proliferation and induce apoptosis in uterine fibroid cells (Chen et al, 2006; Wang et al, 2006). In addition, it has an inhibitory effect on the endometrium as a result of suppressed endometrial angiogenesis and/or function of the spiral arteries (Chwalisz et al, 2004, 2005).[8]

Dosage: Small observational studies of women with symptomatic fibroids showed that daily treatment with asoprisnil at doses ranging from 5 to 25 mg for 3 months reduced fibroid volume in a dose-dependent manner and suppressed both abnormal and normal uterine bleeding, with no effects on circulating oestrogen levels and no breakthrough bleeding (Chwalisz et al, 2005).[8]

Review of literature: In a recent randomized, double blind, placebo-controlled trial involving 129 women, a 3-month treatment with asoprisnil doses of 5, 10 and 25 mg daily suppressed uterine bleeding in 28, 64 and 83% of women, respectively, and reduced fibroid volume and fibroid-related pressure symptoms (Chwalisz et al, 2007).[9]

Side effects: Asoprisnil treatment was associated with follicular-phase oestrogen concentration and minimal hypooestrogenic symptoms (Chwalisz et al, 2007).[9]

Long-term benefits: These promising findings warrant replication through larger controlled trials over extended treatment intervals.

Ulipristal Acetate

The newest SPRM that has both agonist and antagonist selective tissue effect is ulipristal acetate.

Mechanism of action: Induces apoptosis by suppressing neovascularization and cell proliferation without proliferating healthy uterine tissue.

Dosage: At a daily dose of 5–10 mg, ulipristal acetate induced amenorrhea in 50% to 70% of women in 10 days, and resulted in suppression of uterine bleeding in all patients at the end of a 13-week course.

Review of literature: A comparison of monthly injection of leuprolide acetate (3.75 mg) and daily administration 5–10 mg ulipristal for 3 months by Donnez et al found that both drugs had the same effect on myomata. Myomata maintained a size reduction 6 months after discontinuation of ulipristal, eliminating the need for further surgical interventions.

If treatment for more than 3 months is anticipated, a patient must wait for two menstrual periods before restarting ulipristal. In the first study of long-term medical management with ulipristal, four 3-month courses led to a significant reduction in fibroid volume in 80% of cases. The volume of the largest fibroid was decreased by 72%.

Side effects: Headache, nausea, abdominal pain, dizziness, fatigue, dysmennorhea, acne, menstrual irregularity, functional ovarian cysts and hot flushes.

Long-term usage: Clinicians detecting endometrial thickening in women treated with UA need to be aware that administration of UA for longer than 3 months may lead to endometrial thickening. This is related to cystic glandular dilation, not endometrial hyperplasia. However, in absence of robust safety data for a period longer than 3 months or on repeat courses of treatment, treatment duration should not exceed 3 months. Clinicians should be aware of the need to investigate, as per usual clinical practice, persistence of endometrial thickening following treatment discontinuation and return of menstruation to exclude any underlying pathological conditions.

Telepristone

Mostly has progesterone antagonist activity and low antiglucorticoid activity. It was specifically developed for use as an antiprogestin in the treatment of uterine fibroids and endometriosis. It has been shown to reduce fibroid size by up to 40% and significantly decreases vaginal bleeding. While one study reported that telepristone-induced apoptosis in fibroid cells another studies did not confirm this fact. The US FDA placed a full clinical hold on telepristone in August 2009 because of elevated liver enzymes associated with drug treatment.[10]

Progestogen-releasing Intrauterine System

The LNG-IUS was introduced as a contraceptive device, but it was recognized as an effective treatment for non-organic AUB, decreasing its intensity and improving anaemia. Its use for treating related bleeding, therefore, was soon investigated. A prospective study comparing the efficacy of the LNG-IUS in improving AUB in two groups of women, with and without fibroids, has demonstrated an 86% decrease in bleeding intensity in both groups. After 4 years, there was a 99.5% decrease in both groups and also a reduction in uterine volume in the group with fibroids.

Another study, an RCT comparing LNG-IUS with a low-dose COC in women with fibroids, demonstrated that the former was more effective in reducing UF-related bleeding than the latter, although the trial suffered with high attrition rates and assessed uterine bleeding in only 22 patients. In the LNG-IUS group, there was a significant decrease in menstrual blood loss and uterine volume, while haematocrit increased. Both studies excluded women with submucous fibroids that caused distortion of the uterine cavity. Therefore, LNG-IUS is probably an effective option in selected symptomatic women with no endometrial distortion.

Gonadotropin-releasing Hormone Agonist

Mechanism of action: GnRHa works by desensitizing GnRH pituitary receptors. As a result, it is associated with an initial flare effect followed by a hypoestrogenic state after 2 weeks. It has been used to treat uterine myomas for more than 3 decades. The most common GnRHa used for uterine myoma is leuprolide acetate.

Dosage: Intramuscular injection of 3.75 mg monthly—or a single dose of 11.25 mg every 3 months—reduces the mean uterine volume by 36% at 12 weeks and 45% at 24 weeks. However, the effects are temporary.[11]

Review of literature: GnRHa is useful for premenopausal women who opt for medical treatment and for preoperative treatment. It reduces the size of myomata, facilitating surgery with a minimally invasive technique and improving the patient's haematologic status. However, it may lead to degeneration of myomata, making them soft and difficult to manipulate. Occasionally, the cleavage plane between a myoma and the pseudocapsule obliterates, making myoma enucleation challenging. Whether obliteration of the surgical plane is related to the presence of adenomyosis is not entirely clear.

Side effects: GnRHa adverse effects, such as menopausal symptoms, are related to the hypoestrogenic state. When given alone, it is associated with up to 5.5% reduction in bone mass within the first 6 months of use. Due to its adverse effects, GnRHa use should be limited to 3 to 6 months. In order to counter adverse effects and to maintain patient compliance, add-back treatment with low-dose oestrogen and progestin therapy is advisable.

Practice guidelines (Ulipristal versus GnRHa): In women with excessive uterine bleeding, the authors use ulipristal acetate 5 mg daily for 3 months. It is associated with a rapid decrease in uterine bleeding. During the first few days of treatment, when the bleeding is still excessive, supportive treatment with tranexamic acid can be given. A second course of ulipristal is administered after 2 menstrual cycles.

Alternatively, a single course of GnRHa for 3 months can be given. However, it may be associated with increased uterine bleeding in the first week of treatment due to initial stimulation of the endometrium. Because of GnRHA's pronounced menopausal adverse effects, add-back treatment should be considered.

Ulipristal or GnRHa can be given for 3 months preoperatively to reduce fibroid volume before myomectomy by laparoscopy or laparotomy.

For patients undergoing hysteroscopic myomectomy, the authors use GnRHa preoperatively a month before the procedure. It produces a thin endometrium, which facilitates the procedure and decreases fluid absorption. Ulipristal is associated with endometrial changes but not thin endometrium.[11,12]

Side effetcs: Adverse effects are similar to those of GnRHa and disappear after drug discontinuation, with rapid return to the original leiomyoma size. Release of histamine by mast cells is a known adverse effect. Recent preparations are associated with less histamine release and thus better tolerated.

Long-term Benefits: Long-term therapeutic efficacy is yet to be determined.

Gonadotropin-releasing Hormone Antagonist

Mechanism of action: GnRH antagonists exert their action through the direct competitive inhibition of GnRH by occupying the pituitary GnRH receptors, and therefore blocking the access of the endogenous GnRH and exogenously administered agonists to their receptor sites. These agents may induce a deep suppression of gonadotropins and the sex steroids, while avoiding any 'flare up' phenomena, which may lead to a reduction in uterine fibroids size of up to 50%. The compound has been used preoperatively to decrease myomata size before surgery. The drawbacks are absence of a long-acting preparation and cost. Daily administration may decrease patient compliance.

Review of literature: Some of the GnRH antagonists approved for clinical use by the US FDA include cetrorelix (Cetrotide; Serono) and ganirelix (Antagon; Organon International). These agents are usually used as injectables. One of the major limitations to the wide use of the GnRH antagonists in leiomyoma treatment is the short half-life of these agents and the non-availability of the depot formulation, thus require repetitive dosing (daily for most of the antagonists).

Promising GnRH Antagonist (Elagolix)

Elagolix is a second-generation new non-peptide (GnRH) antagonist, highly potent antagonist orally active and rapidly bioavailable after administration that is being developed by Abbott Laboratories (Abbott) in collaboration with Neurocrine Biosciences. It is finalizing the phase III for endometriosis and finalizing phase II for uterine leiomyoma with opportunity to be its first and only approved oral treatment for uterine leiomyoma.

This promising compound inhibits GnRH receptors in the pituitary gland leading to a dose-dependent suppression of LH, FSH and estradiol. Consequently, suppression of E2 is more prolonged at higher doses. Pituitary suppression is maintained for only a portion of the day, and baseline gonadotropin levels return by 24 hours. To date, Elagolix has been studied in 18 clinical trials totaling more than 1,000 subjects.

Dosage: Elagolix seems to be well tolerated for multiple doses up to 200; rapidly absorbed after oral administration, with median time of maximum plasma concentration values ranging from 0.5 to 1 h.

The therapeutic window of E2 levels for suppression of endometriosis is attainable at a dose of 100–150 mg/day with serum estradiol remained between 20 and 50 pg/mL. The Elagolix therapeutic dose for management of uterine fibroid is yet to be determined.

Somatostatin Analogues

Increasing evidence has demonstrated a role for growth factors, such as insulin growth factor-I (IGF-I) and IGF-II, in the initiation and progression of uterine fibroids. Leiomyoma tissue expresses higher levels of IGF-I/IGF-II receptors compared to normal adjacent myometrium. Additionally, these tissues secrete their own IGF-1, probably for autocrine and paracrine use. From a clinical perspective, it has been recently reported that patients with high levels of growth hormone (acromegalic patients) have a higher prevalence of uterine fibroids than the general population.

Lanreotide, which is a long-acting somatostatin analogue that has been shown to reduce growth hormone secretion, has also recently been evaluated in seven women with uterine fibroids in Italy. Interestingly, lanreotide induced a 42% mean myoma volume reduction within a 3-month period. These results show that somatostatin analogues may potentially be a new therapy for uterine fibroids.

The treatment with somatostatin analogues for diseases other than leiomyoma appears to be safe and is usually well tolerated with some reports of gallstone formation. However, the lacking of clinical trials, which test the long-term use of somatostatin analogues along with the severe and adverse health implications such as decreased life expectancy due to accelerated heart disease observed in adults with growth hormone deficiency may hinder its future use for leiomyoma treatment.

Aromatase Inhibitors

Aromatase inhibitors work by directly blocking the conversion of androgen to oestrogen, leading to a decrease in circulating oestrogen levels without causing systemic adverse effects.

Letrozole

This drug is associated with a reduction in fibroid size, thinning of endometrium and cessation of bleeding. Mild side effects of hot flashes, vaginal dryness and musculoskeletal pain are reported. The LEAP (letrozole, exemestane, and anastrozole pharmacodynamics) trial was a phase I pharmacodynamic study comparing the effects of these three AIs on safety parameters such as serum markers of bone formation and resorption, in healthy postmenopausal women with normal bone mineral density. The results demonstrated that all three inhibitors administered for 24 weeks caused incremental increases in bone resorption markers such as C-telopeptide crosslinks.[13]

Anastrozole

This third-generation non-steroidal medication does not alter cortisol or aldosterone levels. It is also not associated with androgenic, progestogenic, or oestrogenic effects. At a dose of 1 mg/day for 12 weeks, anastrozole results in reduction in myoma volume of up to 32% and improves menstrual symptoms.[14]

Fadrozole

Shozu et al reported a case of rapid regression of myoma symptoms and a 71% reduction in their size after the use of fadrozole for 8 weeks. Today, there is still a paucity of information of the use of fadrozole for uterine myomata.[15]

Selective Oestrogen Receptor Modulators

The SERMs, like oestrogen, are agents that elicit tissue-specific responses by intensely interacting with two kinds of oestrogen receptors (ERs), ERα and ERβ, inhomogenously distributed throughout the body. SERMs have complex pharmacokinetics properties due to their vaguely understood physicochemical properties and low solubility in blood (1–200 ng/mL). In addition to analytical detection limitations at such low concentrations, several of the compounds have sufficiently long half lives that impede protocol development. Since SERM are not administered to humans intravenously, the exact bioavailability of any of these drugs has not been evaluated properly. Frequently, differences in SERM activity depend upon the target gene promoter, as well as the background of a desired cell or tissue. SERMs are characterized by their diverse range of agonist/antagonist actions on ER-mediated processes. SERMs belong to several different chemical classes such as benzopyran, benzothiophenes, chromane, indoles, naphtalenes, and triphenylethylenes compounds all of which are not steroidal compounds. Many are available for clinical usage including raloxifene and tamoxifen discussed below. Novel SERMs are currently being tested in clinical trials such as LY353381 (arzoxifene), EM-652 and CP 336,156 and their structures are very similar to known SERMs.

Raloxifene and Tamoxifen

Two of the best characterized SERMs are tamoxifen and raloxifene, which are both considered to act predominantly as oestrogen antagonists, blocking the effects of oestrogens.

Raloxifene is a more complete uterine antagonist than tamoxifen, significantly reducing fibroid size in postmenopausal women yet is less efficacious at reducing tumour volume in premenopausal women. Clinical outcomes in premenopausal women treated with raloxifene suggest that this compound, like tamoxifen, can affect the ovaries via the HPO axis. Tamoxifen is associated with insidious side effects, such as thromboembolic events, vasomotor symptoms and an increased risk of developing endometrial cancer and cataracts.

Non-hormonal Agents

Vitamin D, green tea, heparin and its nonanticoagulant analogs, pioglitazone and pirfenidone have been used to treat myomata. However, their clinical efficacy has not been proven in randomized trials.

Gestrinone

This synthetic steroid is commonly used in endometriosis and suppresses the growth of myomata by regulating the activity of multiple genes without inducing apoptosis. This drug is not available in India.

Cabergoline

Small studies reported a reduction in myomata size with cabergoline, a dopamine agonist used to treat hyperprolactinemia.

Potential of Novel Therapies Enabled by Smart Nanocarriers. The development of nanocarriers designed to deliver and protect drug therapeutics (e.g. anti fibrotic, aromatase inhibitors, progestins, etc.) is an emerging field. Advances in guided-ultrasound technology (e.g. human in vitro fertilisation where oocytes as small as 3–5 mm are manipulated) make it feasible to envision utilizing nanocarriers to create a drug depot inside the fibroid by local injection. Thus, skilled physicians could inject the therapy into the uterine fibroid under guided ultrasound in an outpatient setting. This approach would impede diffusion and distribution of the drug away from the injected fibroid, prolong release, delay inactivation, and therefore reduce the need for repeat injections. Examples of the most promising thermoresponsive delivery systems are given below.[16]

Atrigel

Atrigel comprises a water-insoluble biodegradable polymer. A drug is added, forming a solution or suspension. Leuprolide acetate was incorporated into Atrigel. Clinical studies demonstrated a 22.5 mg leuprolide depot maintained an effective suppression of serum testosterone (50 ng/dL) for more than 3 months.

ReGel

ReGel is a ~4,000 Da triblock copolymer formed from PLGA and polyethylene glycol (PEG, 1000 Da or 1450 Da) in repetitions of PLGA-PEG-PLGA or PEG-PLGA-PEG. ReGel is formulated as a 23 wt% copolymer solution in aqueous media. A drug is added to the solution and upon temperature elevation to 37°C the whole system gels. Degradation of ReGel to final products of lactic acid, glycolic acid and PEG occurs over 1–6 weeks depending on copolymer molar composition. Chemically distinct drugs like porcine growth hormone and glucagon-like peptide-1 (GLP-1) may be incorporated, one at a time, and released from ReGel.

LiquoGel

Works by independent drug delivery routes—entrapment and covalent linkage This later feature distinguishes LiquoGel from other thermoresponsive injectables, as in theory, two or more drugs can be delivered to the tumour site. LiquoGel is a tetrameric copolymer of thermogelling N-isopropylacrylamide; biodegrading macromer of poly (lactic acid) and 2-hydroxyethyl methacrylate; hydrophilic acrylic acid (to maintain solubility of decomposition products); and multifunctional hyperbranched polyglycerol to covalently attach drugs. LiquoGel is formulated as a 16.9 wt% copolymer solution in aqueous media. The solution gels at physiological conditions and degrades to release drug contents within 1–6 days.

Antifibrotics

Fibroids are characterized by altered collagen fibrils, fibrosis and tissue stiffness, as well as increased amounts of type I and V collagen.

Selective elimination of collagen producing cells or reducing their state of activation is currently limited to experimental trials. Medical strategies that interfere with collagen formation (e.g. antifibrotic drugs) should be efficacious in fibroid treatment.

A high throughput screening assay has been developed to indentify drug candidates that show antifibroitc activity.

Two promising antifibrotic candidates are highlighted below, but in general this class of pharmaceuticals presents undesirable side effects when systemically administered.

Pirfenidone

Pirfenidone is an orally bioavailable antifibrotic agent that has been shown to regulate fibrosis. Pirfenidone inhibits fibroblast proliferation, diminishes the messenger ribonucleic acid (RNA) levels of collagen types I and III in a dose-dependent manner, and effectively inhibits myometrial and fibroid cell proliferation in vitro. The drug is currently in phase III clinical trials for the treatment of pulmonary fibrosis.[17] Oral administration of pirfenidone in clinical trials is associated with undesirable side effects including vomiting, fever, abnormality of hepatic function, dizziness, facial paralysis, hepatoma, and skin photosensitivity.

Halofuginone

As an extract from hydrangeas, halofuginone is a small organic molecule exhibiting coccidiostat benefits in birds and more recently antifibrotic activity against fibroid cells. Halofuginone inhibits both fibroid and myometrial smooth muscle cell proliferation by rapidly inhibiting DNA synthesis and later inducing apoptosis. In addition, halofuginone significantly suppressed TGFβI mRNA production.[18,19]

At 3.5 mg/day, nausea, vomiting and fatigue were reported. Several patients experienced bleeding complications on treatment with halofuginone in which a causal relationship could not be excluded. This medication is not currently used in humans and its toxicity is unknown.

Reported side effects of halofuginone when taken in patients with advanced solid tumours were nausea, vomiting and fatigue.

Purified Collagenase

Collagenase clostridium histolyticum is a FDA approved drug targeting Dupuytren's contracture in adults with a palpable cord. This drug comprises a fixed ratio mixture of two classes of purified collagenases; type I and type II collagenase. Both are metalloproteinases requiring zinc and calcium for full activity and have selective activity against collagen. These two classes of enzymes are not immunologically cross-reactive and differ from each other in domain structure substrate affinity and catalytic efficiency. When combined, they demonstrate synergistic collagenolytic activity.

In vivo, clostridial histolyticum collagenase is not effective in degrading type IV collagen. Thus in clinical studies, purified clostridial histolyticum collagenase did not degrade large blood vessel membranes or nerves.

The dose used for treatment of a Dupuytren's contracted joint is 0.58 mg per direct injection into the cord. Up to three injections may be given per affected joint. This drug is approved by FDA for the treatment of Dupuytren's contracture of the adult hand with a palpable cord present and has not yet been used in clinical trials for fibroids.

■ CONCLUSION

About 30% percent of women have uterine fibroids and the majority of them will not require intervention. For those women who present with symptoms, the menu of options for the treatment of uterine leiomyomas is expanding. These technologies are relatively new and although many are promising, they often lack long-term data, which interferes with our ability to present all risks and benefits with assurance. Ongoing research and data collection will help us assess the relative merit of newer options as the technology continues to expand.

■ REFERENCES

1. Rackow BW, Arici A. Options for medical treatment of myomas. Obstet Gynecol Clin North Am. 2006;33(1):97-113.
2. Qin J, Yang T, Kong F, et al. Oral contraceptive use and uterine leiomyoma risk: a meta-analysis based on cohort and case-control studies. Arch Gynecol Obstet. 2013;288(1):139-48.
3. Kongnyuy EJ, Wiysonge CS. Interventions to reduce haemorrhage during myomectomy for fibroids. Cochrane Database Syst Rev. 2009;(3):CD005355.
4. Machado RB, de Souza IM, Beltrame A, et al. The levonorgestrel-releasing intrauterine system: its effect on the number of hysterectomies performed in perimenopausal women with uterine fibroids. Gynecol Endocrinol. 2013;29(5):492-5.
5. Fedele L, Bianchi S, Marchini M, et al. Histological impact of medical therapy–clinical implications. J Obstet Gynaecol. 1995;102(12):8-11.
6. Friedman AJ , Hoffman DI , Comite F, et al. Treatment of leiomyomata uteri with leuprolide acetate depot: a double-blind, placebo-controlled, multicenter study. The Leuprolide Study Group. Obstet Gynecol. 1991;77(5):720-5.
7. Koechling W, Hjortkjaer R, Tankó LB. Degarelix, a novel GnRH antagonist, causes minimal histamine release compared with cetrorelix, abarelix and ganirelix in an ex vivo model of human skin samples. Br J Clin Pharmacol. 2010;70(4):580-7.
8. Chwalisz K, DeManno D, Garg R, et al. Therapeutic potential for the selective progesterone receptor modulator asoprisnil in the treatment of leiomyomata. Semin Reprod Med. 2004;22(2):113-9.
9. Chwalisz K, Larsen L, Mattia-Goldberg C, et al. A randomized, controlled trial of asoprisnil, a novel selective progesterone receptor modulator, in women with uterine leiomyomata. Fertil Steril. 2007;87(6):1399-412.
10. Luo X, et al. The selective progesterone receptor modulator cdb4124 inhibits proliferation and induces apoptosis in uterine leiomyoma cells. Fertility and Sterility. 2010;93(8):2668–2673. [PMC free article] [PubMed].
11. Donnez J, Tatarchuk TF, Bouchard P, et al; PEARL I Study Group. Ulipristal acetate versus placebo for fibroid treatment before surgery. N Engl J Med. 2012;366(5):409-20.
12. Donnez J, Vázquez F, Tomaszewski J, et al; PEARL III and PEARL III Extension Study Group. Long-term treatment of uterine fibroids with ulipristal acetate. Fertil Steril. 2014;101(6):1565-73. e1–18.
13. Darlene K, Taylor and Phyllis C, Leppert .Treatment for Uterine Fibroids: Searching for Effective Drug Therapies.
14. Donnez J, Vázquez F, Tomaszewski J, et al. PEARL III and PEARL III Extension Study Group. Long-term treatment of uterine fibroids with ulipristal acetate. Fertil Steril. 2014;101(6):1565-73. e1–18.
15. Hilário SG, Bozzini N, Borsari R, et al. Action of aromatase inhibitor for treatment of uterine leiomyoma in perimenopausal patients. Fertil Steril. 2009;91(1):240-3.
16. Wikland M, et al. A randomized controlled study comparing pain experience between a newly designed needle with a thin tip and a standard needle for oocyte aspiration. Hum. Reprod. 2011;26(6):1377-83. [PMC free article] [PubMed].
17. Macias-Barragan J, et al. The multifaceted role of pirfenidone and its novel targets. Fibrogenesis & Tissue Repair. 2010;3(1):16. [PubMed].
18. Grudzien MM, et al. The antifibrotic drug halofuginone inhibits proliferation and collagen production by human leiomyoma and myometrial smooth muscle cells. Fertility and Sterility. 2010;93(4):1290-8. [PMC free article] [PubMed].
19. Tantibhedhyangkul JA, Behera M. Non-surgical treatment options for symptomatic uterine leiomyomas. Current Women's Health Reviews. 2010;6(2):146-60.

CHAPTER 11

Surgical Management of Fibroids

● Chandana Anantha Rama Reddy

■ INTRODUCTION

Uterine myomas are the most common benign neoplasms of the female reproductive tract, originating from the uterine smooth muscle. They occur in 25% to 30% of women of reproductive age, as many as 50% of women over the age of 35 years and approximately 70% of women over the age of 50 years; the prevalence of uterine leiomyomas increases during reproductive age and decreases after menopause.[1,2]

Leiomyomas vary in size from small to large masses that can distort and enlarge the uterus. Hysterectomy has been a very common therapy in patients who have completed reproduction. Interest in uterine preservation and organ preserving surgery through techniques of minimally invasive surgery has increased, since the first reports of laparoscopic myomectomy in 1980.

Compared with the laparotomic approach, laparoscopic myomectomy has some advantages including less pain and reduced blood loss, faster recovery, less morbidity, and fewer complications. However, some gynecologic surgeons consider laparoscopic myomectomy a challenge because of the skill in suturing, risk of recurrence, cost, risk of conversion to an open procedure and limits in terms of number and size of myomas.

Laparoscopic myomectomy has evolved into a safe, efficient, and cost effective approach for the treatment of intramural, subserosal and pedunculated fibroids. At first the surgical approach was limited by the technology available for myoma morcellation and uterine repair. Now with the availability of the electro-mechanical morcellator, the harmonic scalpel and the development of instrumentation for suturing, linear stapling, and combined bipolar coagulation with knife blade cutting the laparoscopic myomectomy is a procedure, which can readily become part of the armamentarium for all advanced laparoendoscopic surgeons.

■ INDICATIONS

The decision to perform surgery for uterine leiomyomata is complex and varies from patient-to-patient based on their medical comorbidities, surgical history, clinical scenario and patient preference.

This procedure is considered when patient either has a desire for future fertility or feels strongly about retaining her uterus. The criteria are directed at relieving symptoms or improving quality of life by decreasing the patient's concerns. No indications exist for removing asymptomatic fibroids.

Excessive Uterine Bleeding

1. Profuse bleeding causing lifestyle derangements that is refractory to medical management.
2. Uterine bleeding that results in anaemia.
3. Pelvic discomfort caused by myomata.
4. Acute and severe chronic lower abdominal pain or low back or pelvic pressure with evidence of sizeable leiomyoma on imaging studies.

Leiomyomata that are palpable abdominally.

A definite risk exists for myoma recurrence after myomectomy and, with it, the need for a repeat surgical procedure in the future. If the patient no longer desires to retain her fertility or her uterus, hysterectomy is the usual procedure of choice

■ CONTRAINDICATIONS FOR LAPAROSCOPIC MYOMECTOMY

The surgical techniques involved present a challenge to gynecologists. Location, size and number of fibroids should be taken into consideration when choosing patients as surgical candidates. A relative contraindication to myomectomy is the strong possibility that a functional uterus could not be reconstructed after excision of the myomas. For myomectomy to be considered successful, reconstructing the uterus must be possible. The following conditions should be regarded as relative contraindications for laparoscopic myomectomy (LM):

1. Diffuse leiomyomata.
2. Existence of more than three fibroids > 7 cm.
3. Uterine size greater than 20 weeks' gestation.
4. One fibroid > 15 cm.
5. Women who have completed childbearing and who desire hysterectomy.
6. Any medical condition that is not suitable for anaesthesia or prolonged laparoscopic surgery.

It should not be performed, if the possibility of endometrial cancer or uterine sarcoma have not been excluded.

■ PREOPERATIVE EVALUATION AND TREATMENT

For all the listed indications, other possible causes should be thoroughly excluded. When no other correctable findings are identified, the patient must decide if her symptoms are sufficiently severe to require surgery.[3] In women who complain of menorrhagia, the haematocrit is used to assess the degree of anaemia. For anaemic patients, preoperative gonadotrophin releasing hormone agonists (GnRHa) treatment may enable restoration of a normal haematocrit, decrease the size of myoma and reduce the need for transfusion. While some studies show a decrease in intraoperative blood loss after a course of GnRHa therapy.[4] Some surgeons have also found that pretreatment with GnRHa is associated with loss of cleavage planes as there is hydropic degeneration of myoma. This may make dissection difficult in some patients.[5]

Ultrasonography provides information about the site, size and number of fibroids. Fluid contrast ultrasonography determines endometrial distortion by submucous fibroids. Periodic pelvic ultrasound examinations help monitor the growth rate of asymptomatic myomas. Submucous tumours can be detected by pelvic ultrasound, a hysterogram or hysteroscopy. The presence of large broad ligament myoma emphasizes the need for an intravenous urography to look for ureteral obstruction. Since small interstitial myomas palpated during laparotomy can be missed at laparoscopy, a vaginal ultrasound should be done preoperatively, and can also be performed intraoperatively to aid in myoma identification and localisation. Patients are counseled regarding the potential for intra- and post-operative bleeding and the possible need for a laparotomy as well as blood transfusion. Although myomectomy may rarely result in hysterectomy, patients should be informed of this possibility.

■ TYPES OF MYOMECTOMY

1. Total laparoscopic myomectomy
2. Laparoscopically assisted myomectomy: Laparoscopically assisted myomectomy (LAM) is a safe alternative to LM. It is less difficult and requires less time to complete The decision to perform LAM usually is made in the operating room after diagnostic laparoscopy and treatment of other pelvic abnormalities are completed. Cases for which LAM may be superior to LM include a myoma greater than 8 cm, many myomas requiring extensive morcellation, and a deep, large, intramural myoma that requires uterine repair in multiple layers.

   Three major objectives of LAM are reduction of blood loss, prevention of postoperative adhesions and maintenance of myometrial integrity. LAM, with 'open' morcellation and conventional suturing, reduces the duration of the operation and the need for more extensive laparoscopic experience. This approach may enable more gynecologists to apply a minimally invasive technique.
3. SILS (myomectomy).
4. Robotic myomectomy and robotically assisted myomectomy: Advances in robotic surgery have increased the popularity of this method of minimally invasive surgery for various reasons. Shorter learning curves, a three-dimensional vision system, wristed instrumentation, and ergonomic positioning are all advantages to straight laparoscopy.[6] Because of the intricate steps required during laparoscopic myomectomy including myoma enucleation and multilayer myometrial closure, straight laparoscopy can be difficult even in the hands of experienced surgeons. Because of its inherent advantages and principles similar to open surgery, robotic technology has the potential to facilitate utilisation of a less invasive approach to the surgical management of myomas, thereby increasing this option for patients.
5. Myolysis: Laparoscopic myolysis or leiomyoma coagulation can be used as an alternative to laparoscopic myomectomy for the treatment of small intramural or subserosal leiomyomas. The procedure was developed in Germany in 1986 and was first performed in the United States by Goldfarb in 1990.[7,8] Myolysis is designed to destroy the blood supply and subsequently cause stromal death of symptomatic myomas in order to achieve a decrease in their size. A neodymium:yttrium-aluminum-garnet (ND:YAG) laser bare fiber was initially used to

perform the procedure, although additional modalities such as the monopolar coagulation needle, bipolar coagulation needle, or the hyperthermia electrode (diathermy) can also be utilised.

6. High-intensity focused ultrasound (HIFU).
7. Uterine artery embolisation: It involves the catheterisation of both uterine arteries and the instillation of microparticles to cause occlusion thereby disrupting the blood supply to the myomas and subsequently leading to devascularisation and infarction. Embolisation did result in significant improvements in patient symptomatology.

◼ REFERENCES

1. Mettler L, Schollmeyer T, Tinelli A, et al. Complications of uterine fibroids and their management, surgical management of fibroids, laparoscopy and hysteroscopy versus hysterectomy, haemorrhage,adhesions, and complications. Obstet Gynecol Int. 2012;2012:791248.

2. Zimmermann A, Bernuit D, Gerlinger C, et al. Prevalence, symptoms and management of uterine fibroids: an international internetbased survey of 21,746 women. BMC Womens Health. 2012;12:6.

3. Bradley S Hurst. Laparoscopic myomectomy. In Ricardo Azziz, Anna Alvarez. Murphy (Eds). Practical manual of operative Laparoscopy and Hysteroscopy, 2nd ed. New York: Springer; 1997:163-72.

4. Zullo F, Pellicano M, Dicarlo C, et al. Ultrasonographic prediction of the efficacy of GnRH agonist therapy before laparoscopic myomectomy. J Am Assoc Gynecol Laparosc. 1998;5(4):361-6.

5. Takahashi K, Kawamura N, Ishiko O, et al. Shrinkage effect of gonadotropin releasing hormone agonist treatment on uterine leiomyomas and t(12;14). Int J Oncol. 2002;20(2):279-83.

6. Visco AG, Advincula AP. Robotic gynecologic surgery. Obstet Gynecol. 2008;112(6):1369-84.

7. Gallinat A, Leuken RP. Current trends in the therapy of myomata. In: Leuken RP, Gallinat A (Eds). Endoscopic Surgery in Gynecology. Berlin, Demeter Verlag. 1993:69-71.

8. Goldfarb HA. Nd:YAG laser laparoscopic coagulation of symptomatic myomas. J Reprod Med. 1992;36:636-38.

CHAPTER 12

Laparoscopic Myomectomy Techniques: Incision, Enucleation, Suturing and Morcellation

● Vivek Salunke

■ INTRODUCTION

Laparoscopic myomectomy was described for the first time as early as 1970s when it was exclusively restricted for subserosal myomas. Surgical science has seen a tremendous shift from open to minimal access surgery and with the recent advances in video endoscopic imaging technology and energy devices coupled with improved skill acquisition of the surgeons, laparoscopic myomectomy is being now preferred at most good centres worldwide. It is not any longer restricted to moderate < 9 cm myoma or less than 5 to 7 myomas. Size, number and location are no longer a restriction in experienced hands, although the technique has its learning curve.

Debatable issues about excessive blood loss, long time involved in surgery and the strength of the obstetric scar are of lesser concern with the evolving trends showing results equal to if not better than the open approach.

However, the recent evolving concern is of morcellation and the upcoming contained bag morcellation is being advocated to combat this debate.

■ TECHNIQUES

Under general anaesthesia (GA) patient is placed supine in Trendelenberg position with her arms by sides. Foleys is put in the bladder.

Role of Hysteroscopy Before Proceeding to Laparoscopy

The author generally likes to take hysteroscopic assessment many times to actually assess the enlargement of the uterine cavity, as this in addition to a transvaginal ultrasound gives a good guide on how deep the myoma is. If the cavity on hysteroscopy is stretched and large it generally indicates that the myoma is a deep intramural one and hysteroscopy will also give a good indication as to its location in laparoscopy (Figs 12.1 to 12.3).

Also the location of the grade 2 bulge seen on hysteroscopy in deep intramural myomas gives a good guidance sometimes as to where exactly we should be placing our incision in cases where the laparoscopic bulge or projection is diffuse (Figs 12.4 to 12.6).

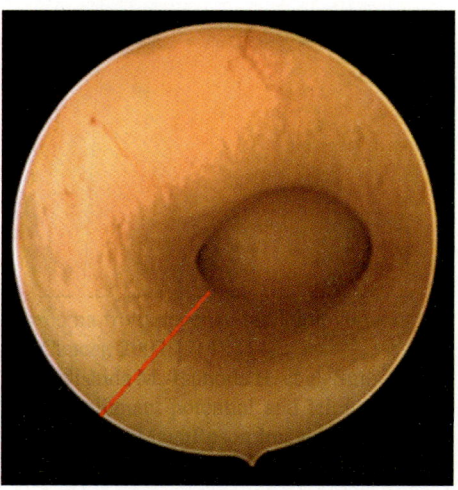

Fig. 12.1: Elongated lower uterine

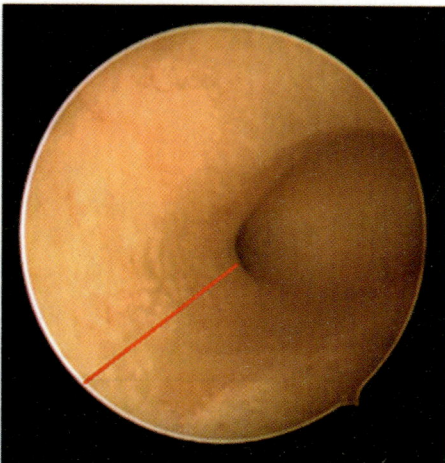

Fig. 12.2: Lower uterine segment appears stretched segment seen on hysteroscopy

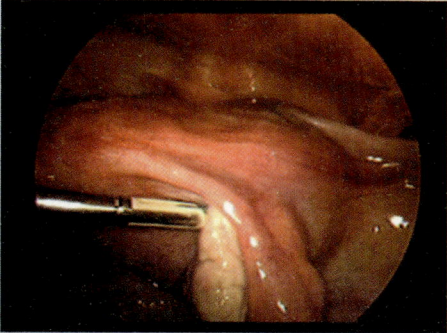

Fig. 12.3: Same fibroid on laparoscopy notice the lower position as predicted by hysteroscopy

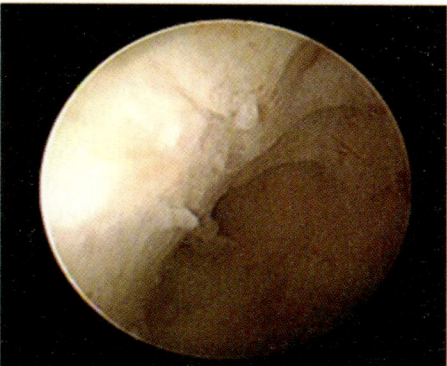

Fig. 12.4: Another case where the grade 2 bulge on hysteroscopy is seen on right fundolateral region

Manipulation of Uterus

Any routine manipulator may be used, but the author personally does not favour the use of manipulators as these make the uterus rigid and may actually make the suturing

of posterior and inferiorly placed fibroids more difficult. On the contrary, the use of assistant's contralateral port for manipulation of uterus serves the best as this port can be used to actually topple and deflect the uterus in any direction (Fig. 12.7). This may be achieved by holding the incision line or suture material by a grasper from the assistant port.

Abdominal Entry and Port Placement Protocol

Each surgeon has his own entry protocol. We generally use the Veress needle through Palmer's point or umbilicus and insufflate to a pneumoperitoneum of about 18 mm Hg. If myoma or pathology is small (size < 8–10 cm), an umbilical trocar (11 mm) is put or else a primary trocar (5 mm) is taken at left upper quadrant which actually visualises the fibroid and

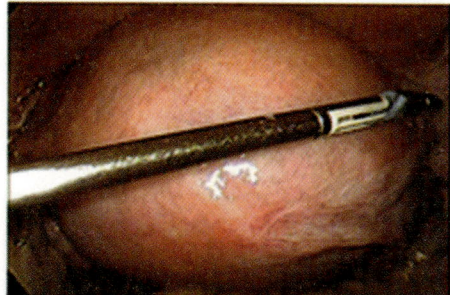

Fig. 12.5: Same fibroid on laparoscopy—difficult to decide the incision

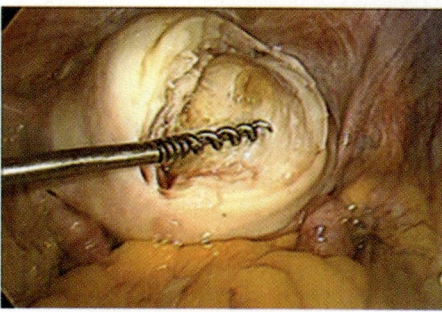

Fig 12.6: Using hysteroscopic guidance incision was correctly taken and identified the myoma on right fundolateral region

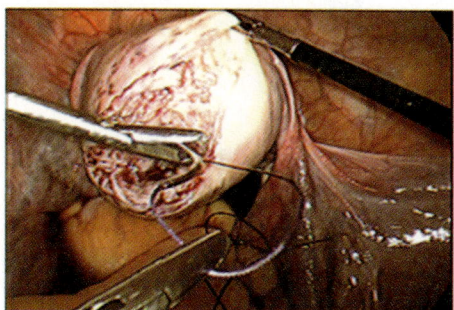

Fig. 12.7: Notice that the assistant side (right) port grasper is used to topple the uterus anteriorly and keeps the uterus stabilised, while the surgeon sutures

overall size of uterus and then accordingly a supra-umbilical entry above the umbilicus is chosen and an 11 mm trocar is introduced under direct vision of 5 mm optical trocar (Fig. 12.8).

A total of three 5 mm working ports are taken, which may be chosen as per the style of suturing preferred by the surgeon. We generally choose two left ports lateral to inferior epigastric vessels and one lower right port for assistant. Many surgeons use a third suprapubic port (Figs 12.9 and 12.10).

Transcervical chromopertubation must be performed prior to procedure because later the methylene blue dye will preferentially draw out of the mucosa.

Some Special Tips to Decrease the Blood Loss

The main aim of surgery is to achieve a clean bloodless dissection with minimal or no use of energy sources and consequent necrosis of myometrium. Suturing should be compact allowing for minimal or no dead space with a consequent strong scar.

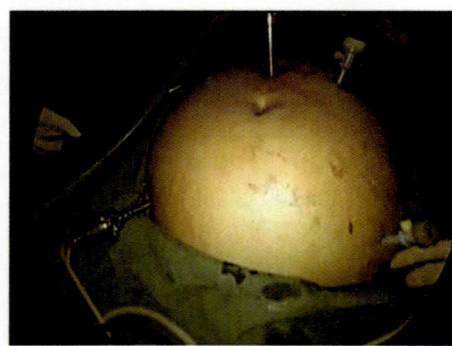

Fig. 12.8: Supraumbilical primary trocar and port placement in a very large 20 cm myoma

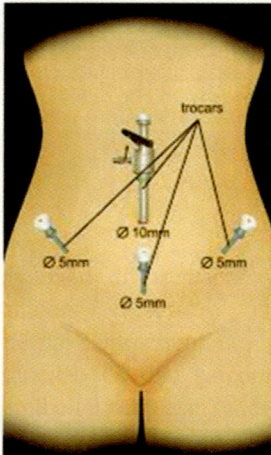

Fig. 12.9: Contralateral port placement

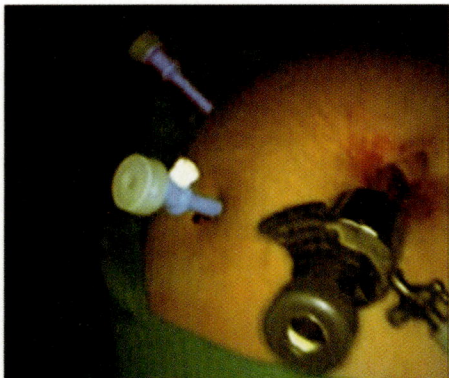

Fig. 12.10: Ipsilateral ports taken for routine 7–8 cm myoma

Use of Vasopressin

8-arginine vasopressin, a synthetic derivative of vasopressin is widely used up to 20 units. Period of action is about 20 to 30 minutes. Dilutions of 20 units in 20 mL normal saline are mentioned.

The author uses vasopressin in a dilute concentration of about 20 units in 300 to 400 mL of normal saline for myomectomy (Figs 12.11 and 12.12). This, in addition to its vasoconstrictive action may also facilitate dissection (hydrodissection) by the fluid entering the plane between the pseudocapsule and the myoma.

Use must be under strict control and monitoring by anaesthetist. Side effects like bronchoconstriction, urticaria, anaphylaxis and myocardial infarction have been reported. Use of Bupivacaine HCl (0.25%) with 0.5 mL of epinephrine (half ampoule of 1 mg/mL) has been reported, but long-term effects are not known.[2]

Role of Uterine Artery Ligation

This method has been adopted by some surgeons to reduce blood loss and in the author's opinion is of use specially when dealing with multiple and large myomas. Transitory ligation at level of internal os after reflecting the uterovesical fold is possible (Figs 12.13 and 12.14). The uterine artery can be

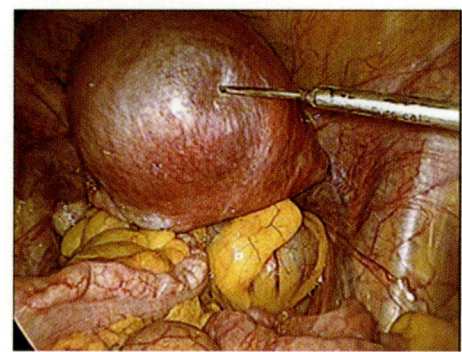

Fig. 12.11: Vasopressin injection into myoma

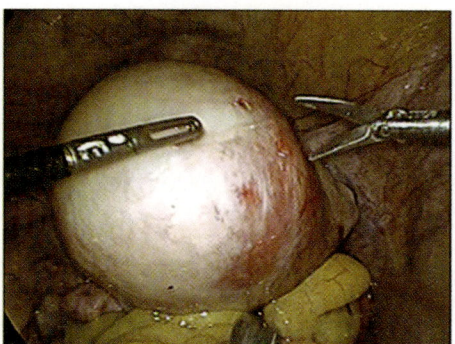

Fig. 12.12: Notice blanching after vasopressin action

ligated at the origin to (Fig. 12.15). The option to permanently leave the suture behind or release the suture remains open.

In a study, which compared uterine artery ligation with a control group with no ligation it was found that although, the mean operative time was larger (107 min vs 93 min; p = 0.03), but there was less blood loss. (84 mL vs 137 mL; p < 0.001) in uterine artery ligation group.[3]

Another study in which temporary clipping of uterine artery was done, documented a statistically effective less haemoglobin drop in clipped group versus control group.[4]

Transitory clipping of uterine arteries at the origin has been described to decrease intraoperative blood loss. At the end of surgery, the declipping is performed, if fertility is desired or may be left occluded if there is no desire for fertility. Also selectively unilateral ligation may be done if largest myoma

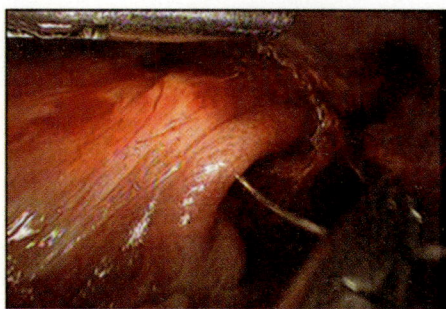

Fig. 12.13: Round body needle seen passing for uterine artery ligation at the internal os

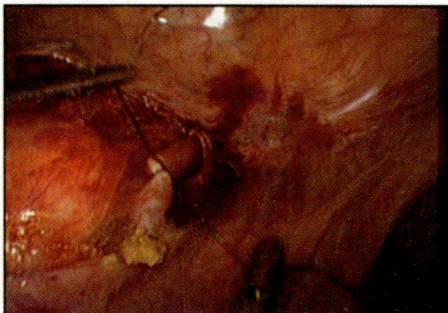

Fig. 12.14: Uterine artery ligated at internal os level on right side

is lateral, e.g. right artery in right lateral myoma. Bilateral occlusion is done if myoma is vascularised by both arteries.[5]

Also observational comparative studies on uterine artery ligation and its effect have found an improvement in the effectiveness of treatment both on the clinical symptoms and recurrence of the leiomyomas.

Other Adjuncts

Several other intraoperative adjuncts to decrease bleeding have been discussed, but none of them are intensively studied.

These include use of misoprostol. A placebo controlled trial showed that misoprostol 400 mcg per vaginally 1 hour prior or per rectally 30 minutes prior to abdominal myomectomy resulted in significant reduction in operative time, operative blood loss, postoperative haemoglobin drop and need for postoperative blood transfusion.[6,7]

Recent evidences suggest the presence of oxytocin receptors also in myomas, but the use of oxytocin as an intraoperative adjunct to decrease bleeding needs to be properly studied and validated.

Use of antifibrinolytics like tranexaemic acid not been studied exclusively for myomas but there is one trial where in 10 mg/kg of the drug was given intravenously to a maximum of 1 g, 15 minutes before skin incision. This trial did show a decreased blood loss of 243 mL but did not reach significant levels.[8]

A gelatin thrombin matrix is also now available which when applied to wet tissue causes rapid haemostasis and may be useful in gynaecological surgeries.[9]

■ OPERATIVE TECHNIQUE

The use of minimally invasive approach raises some peculiar concerns of which the main are:
- Bloodless enucleation
- Compact suturing to get a good quality scar.
- To avoid many incisions: Generally with laparoscopic technique, each myoma needs its own hysterotomy. The traditional approach of Bonney (1931)[10] and Buttram

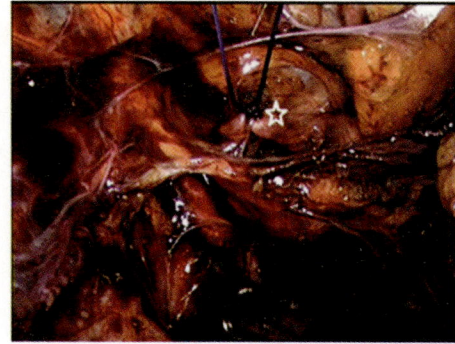

Fig. 12.15: Uterine artery ligation at origin

and Reiter in 1981[11] of removing myomas through a single surgical anterior hysterotomy is not possible with laparoscopic approach.

Incision or Hysterotomy (Length, Depth and Direction)

In laparoscopic approach, the rule of thumb is to create incision taking care that:

1. Length is adequate to allow easy enucleation without excessive extensions of angles at a later stage (Fig. 12.16).
2. Depth is adequate and easily reveals the pseudo-capsule (compressed myometrium) and myoma interphase (Fig. 12.17). This allows healthy adjacent myometrium to be preserved and damage avoided to perimyomatous vessels which are often distended due to compression of myoma.
3. Direction of incision: Vertical or horizontal or even oblique in certain instances is decided depending on proximity to fallopian tubes, utero-ovarian ligament and other vital structures and also whether the surgeon is an ipsilateral or contralateral suturer.
4. Generally ipsilateral suturers prefer horizontal incisions, while contralateral people prefer vertical incisions.
5. Incision may be made with cold scissors (author's preference) or using pure high power cutting current monopolar or even a harmonic scalpel.

6. Myomas are largely recognised by its smooth and bosselated appearance and pearly white colour in contrast to myometrium.
7. Use of cautery should be limited as many reports of rupture after myoma coagulation have been documented. Haemostasis must be achieved by sutures and vasoconstrictive agents.

Enucleation

Dissection of myoma is performed by first identifying the avascular plane of fine interlacing tissue between pseudocapsule and myoma itself. The magnification provided by the laparoscopy makes this very precise and accurate.

Myoma is grasped with a myoma spiral/strong grasping forceps and traction is given. At same time counter traction is applied by surgeon or assistant in opposite direction by pushing the edge of the incision (Fig. 12.18). Plane is identified and fibres transected from superficial to deeper areas, thus slowly enucleating the fibroid out (Fig. 12.19).

In cases of very deep intramural myomas which are indenting the cavity, care and caution should be exercised when enucleating the deeper part of the myoma. The cavity is seen bulging as boggy area and special care should be taken if possible not to breach this (Fig. 12.20). In the event of an inadvertent breach care is taken only to properly exclude it

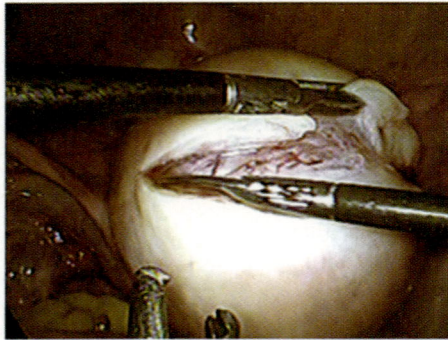

Fig. 12.16: Incision with cold scissors

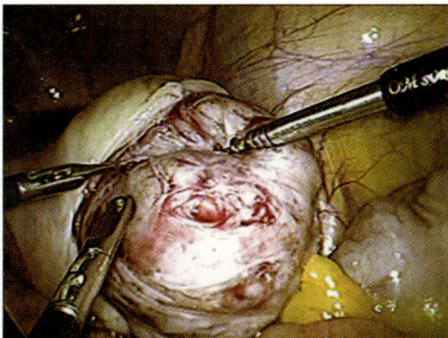

Fig. 12.18: Traction and counter traction being given to enucleate the myoma out

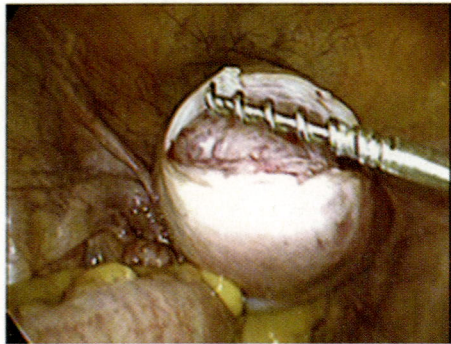

Fig. 12.17: Deciding depth of incision with scissors

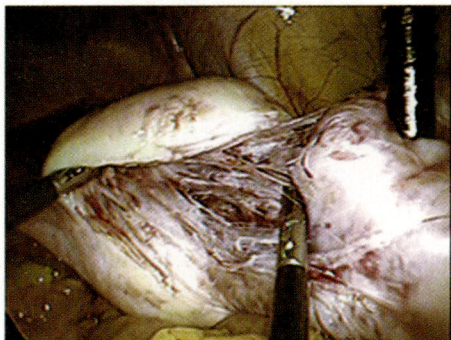

Fig. 12.19: Last phase of enucleation with the interlacing fibres visible

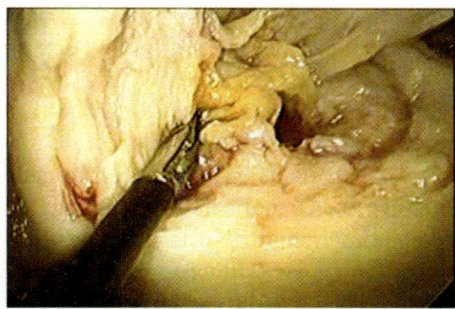

Fig. 12.20: Cavity exposed during enucleation of a deep intramural myoma

while suturing, so that it does not get trapped in the suture as this theoretically may cause iatrogenic adenomyosis or synechiae. The author does not recommend suturing the endometrium separately as is done by some surgeons.

Closure/Suturing the Hysterotomy

This is an important aspect of the surgery as any technical difficulty in carrying out this step may result in a weak scar and uterine rupture in pregnancy. Suture material of choice is (Vicryl-polyglactin 910- Ethicon) mounted on a curved needle 40 mm or a 50 mm needle in case of very large myomas. Needle tip is generally atraumatic, but at times for negotiating

through very large and deep myomas, the author uses an OS needle or cutting needle.

When the myoma is very deeply situated, then we suture in three layers and the first layer is taken deep in the myometrium, so as to get the base compressed and bringing the edges together. This deepest layer stitches go through whole thickness at the level of the base although excluding the cavity carefully and effectively compresses the base.

The needle is passed at the level of the base and first the posterior edge is taken full thickness (Fig. 12.21). There after the anterior edge is taken at same deep level (Fig. 12.22). Now the needle is reversed and passes through anterior edge again at the deep level, but a few centimetres away from the previous site (Fig. 12.23). At the end the needle is now taken out through the posterior edge (Fig 12.24). The two ends are pulled and tied (Figs 12.25 and 12.26).

Another intermediate layer through the myometrium of both anterior and posterior edges (excluding the serosa) using interrupted or figure of '8' sutures can be taken to obliterate the dead space (Fig. 12.27).

Finally the third layer of superficial plane causing end-to-end approximation can be taken as a continuous running sutures or interrupted figure of '8' sutures or even a baseball sutures (Figs 12.28 and 12.29). This leads to a compact closure (Figs 12.30 and 12.31) and adhesion barriers like Interceed

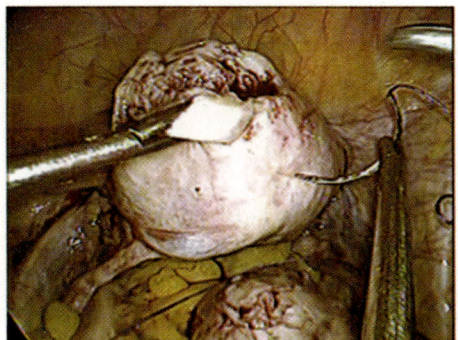

Fig. 12.21: Starting the base closure with the needle taking the posterior flap at the base

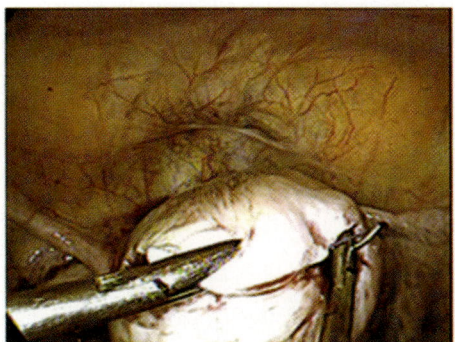

Fig. 12.22: The same needle now passes through anterior flap at the same deep level

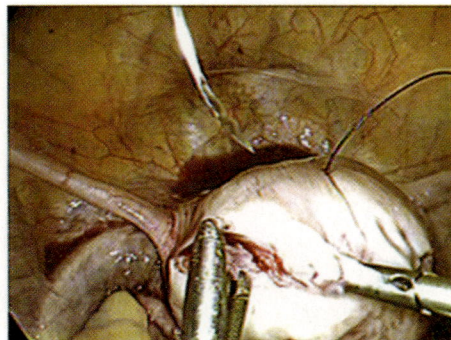

Fig. 12.23: Notice the curve of the needle reversed to pass-through anterior flap in opposite direction

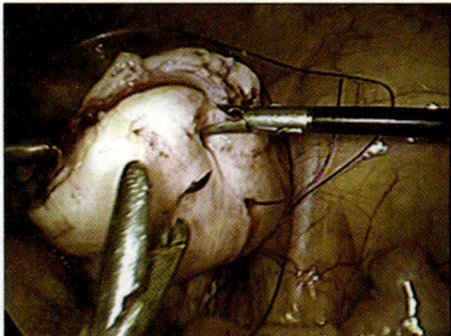

Fig. 12.24: Needle now comes out through the posterior layer

(Fig. 12.33) may be placed over this.

Sometimes in very posteriorly or very anteriorly placed myomas, the angulation of the needle is such that its passage through the incision is difficult to achieve. In such instances, removing the manipulator and asking the assistant to topple and depress the incision line may help. Dr Charles Koh in his concept of suturing in the vertical zone has described myomectomy suturing in 3 layers. First layer is of continuous closure using 2-0 PDS with a CT-1 needle. At the end the first layer is kept tight by holding on traction with a laprotie. Second layer is sutured by using the same suture and moving back towards the first knot. The last layer on the top is subserous type with 4-0 PDS and no suture is visible on the top.

Suture Materials

The author generally either uses standard vicryl polyglactin No 1 or 1-0 on a cutting needle (40 mm size) or (50 mm size) in large myomas for standard suturing. The author also finds the use of barbed suture useful.

Barbed Suture

An Innovation in Suture Design

The bidirectional barb sutures (Fig. 12.34) were first introduced in 2007 in United States (Angiotech Pharmaceuticals). The material is poly-dioxanone, nylon or poly-propylene, but it is the suture design that makes it revolutionary. This suture

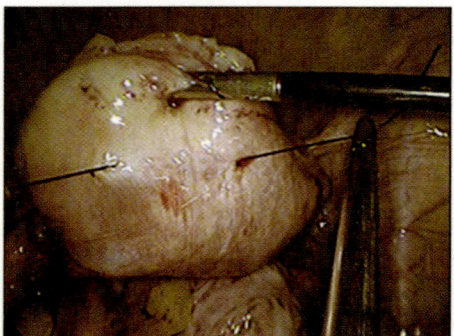

Fig. 12.25: Surgeon now pulls the thread in traction thus compressing the two edges together

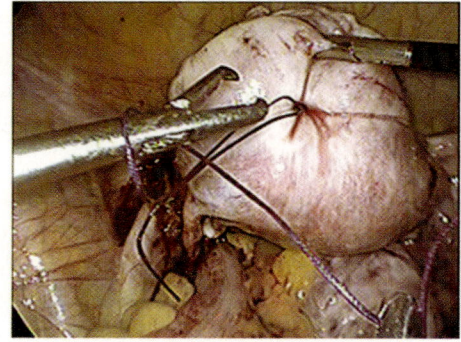

Fig. 12.26: Tying the base knot

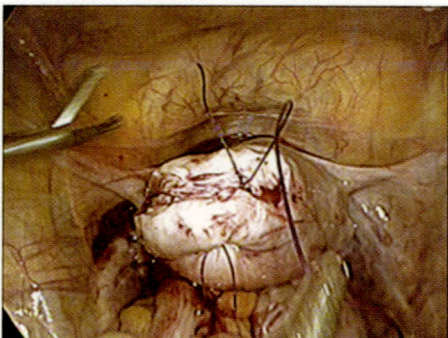

Fig. 12.27: Second layer taken to approximate the inner myometrium

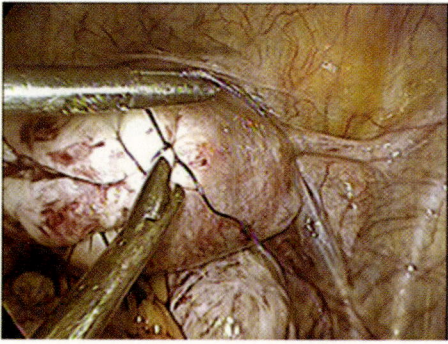

Fig 12.28: Third layer of interrupted figure of 8 sutures

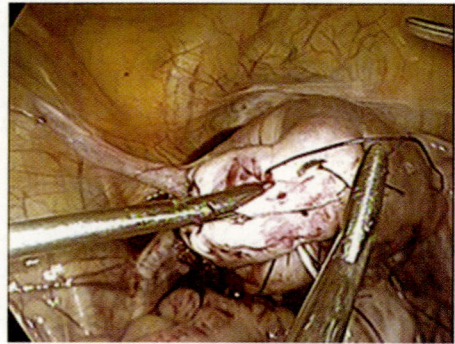

Fig. 12.29: Top layer being continued

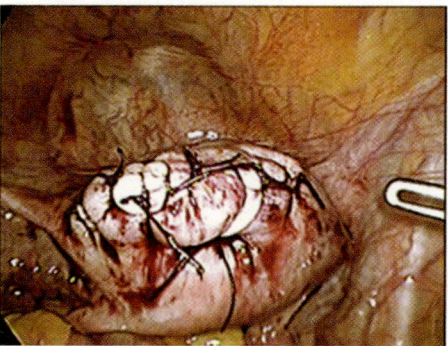

Fig. 12.30: Final look after a compact suturing

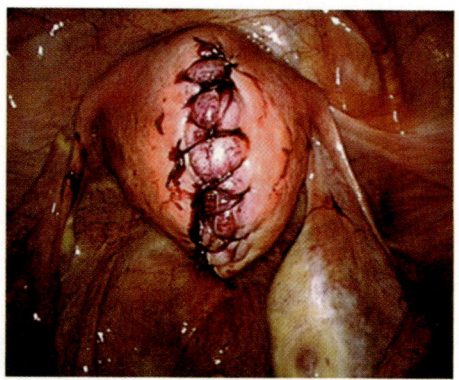

Fig. 12.31: Example of vertical hysterotomy

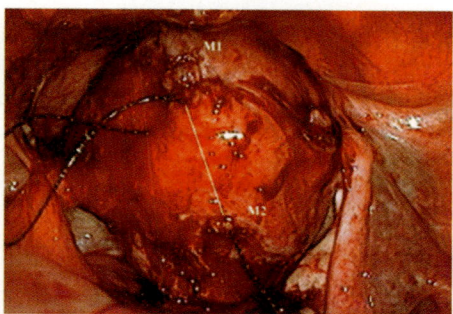

Fig. 12.32: Myoma bed suturing in multiple myomas, figure demonstrates that after closing myoma bed 1 (M1) needle is buried into myometrium and brought out at myoma bed 2 (M2) minimising suture exposure there by avoiding adhesions

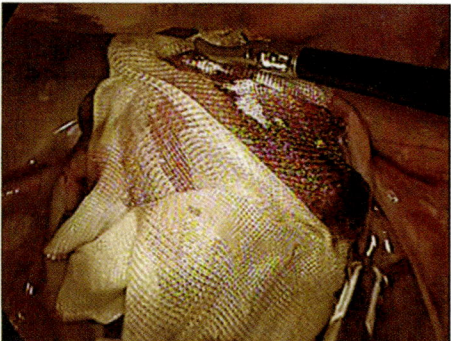

Fig. 12.33: 10 interceed placement

properly is a challenge. In cases where knot tying is difficult, the use of barbed suture can approximate the tissues compactly with less time and with even distribution of tension.[12]

In the author's own experience, the use of barbed suture is very valuable especially when dealing with large myomas, where the suturing time is crucial. Also haemostasis obtained is much better than traditional sutures.[13,14]

The V-LOC suture by Covidien, introduced in 2009, is a unidirectional barbed suture with a loop at one end for

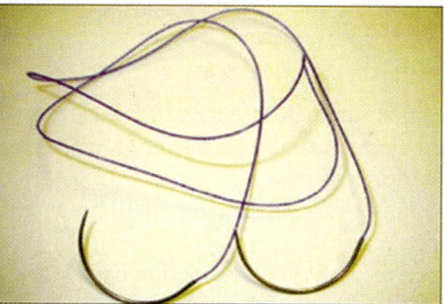

Fig. 12.34: The bidirectional barb suture

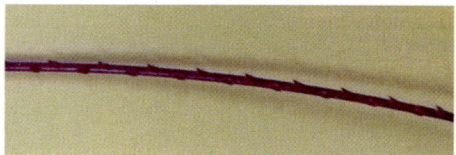

Fig. 12.35: Magnified view of the barbs in the suture[13]

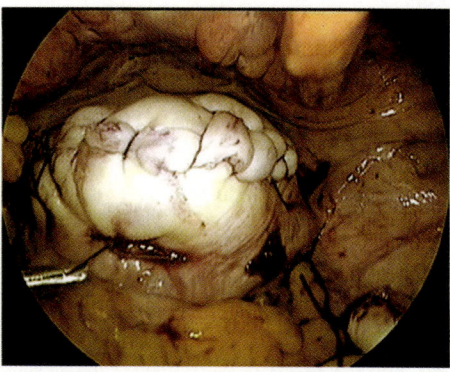

Fig. 12.36: Barbed suture closure—notice the absence of knotting and good haemostasis

consists of standard suture material with tiny barbs cut into the length of filament (Fig. 12.35) in a helical array set facing in opposite directions from mid-point with a needle at each end (Fig. 12.35). This allows tissues to be re-approximated without need of tying a surgical knot (Fig. 12.36). It has had a profound impact on laparoscopic suturing, especially in laparoscopic myomectomies. The tension on the suture material is evenly distributed across the length of suture rather than only on the ends at the knot. Unidirectional barbed sutures are also available.

In minimally invasive surgery, especially laparoscopic myomectomy, the ability to perform suturing quickly and

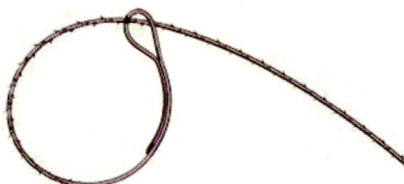

Fig. 12.37: Unidirectional barb suture loaded on a single needle

facilitated fixation (Fig. 12.37). This suture also makes suturing easy and fast.

The Stratafix by ethicon-endosurgery is also available.

The adhesion formation with barbed suture in animal studies has not been found to be different in comparison to standard suture materials.[15]

Significantly faster closure time in myomectomy with barbed suture has been seen in several in vivo studies now.[16] Pregnancy outcomes are also comparable following suturing with barbed suture when compared with standard suture.[17]

Extraction

Various methods are possible for extraction of myomas:
- Standard electromechanical power morcellation
- Via posterior colpotomy
- Via endoknife—appropriate for small myoma < 2–4 cm in diameter
- Contained morcellation in isolation bags
- Via minilaparotomy.

Standard Electromechanical Power Morcellation

This was first introduced in 1993 to improve speed and ease of tissue extraction without the need of laparotomy. Standard morcellation involves extension of the port size to 12–15 mm and guiding the morcellator under vision (Fig. 12.38). It is recommended to activate the blade of the morcellator inside a trocar with an oblique end, so that simple traction on the myoma peels it like an 'orange' without small fragments. 'Swiss cheese' effect should be avoided as this leads to fragmentation.

The technique has potential for vascular and visceral injury and has to be performed under strict visual guidance and control. Concern regarding the power morcellation is further discussed in the upcoming sections.

Posterior Colpotomy

Allows for the large myomata to be extracted.[18] Some people have suggested that this approach may cause postoperative

adhesions in colpotomy site).[19–21] A monopolar hook may be used or even a harmonic scalpel (Fig. 12.39) to create an incision in the posterior vagina (Fig. 12.40) over a colpotomizer through which the fibroid is extracted. This incision may be closed laparoscopically or vaginally (Figs 12.41A and B). Some authors have also described the opening of the posterior fornix under direct vision by a 10–12 mm trocar introduced vaginally in the posterior fornix under laparoscopic vision (Fig. 12.42).

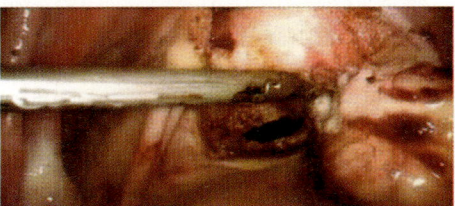

Fig. 12.39: Incision of colpotomy in laparoscopy

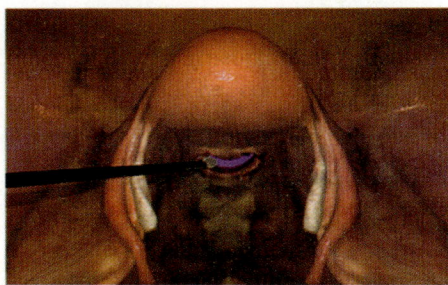

Fig. 12.40: The site of incision between the uterosacral ligaments

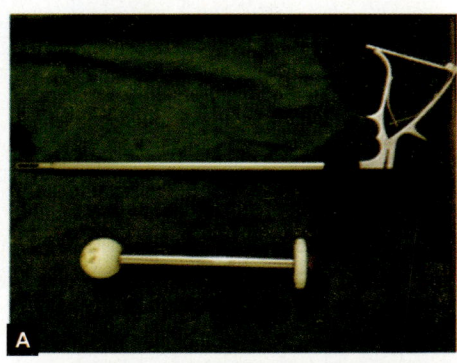

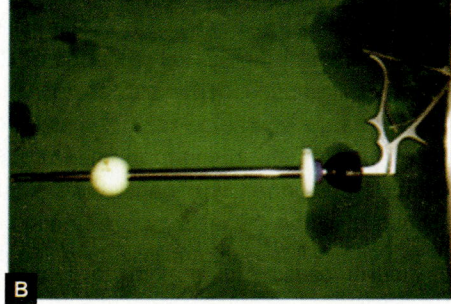

Figs 12.41A and B: Vaginal colpotomizer with a claw forceps to catch the fibroid in vivo

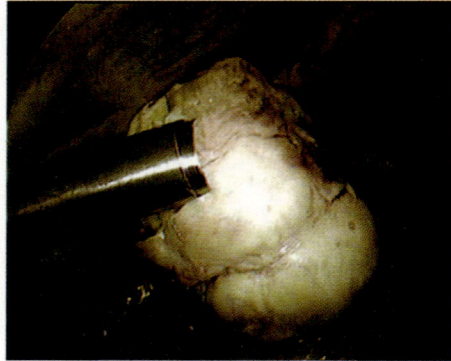

Fig. 12.38: Standard technique of electromechanical morcellation

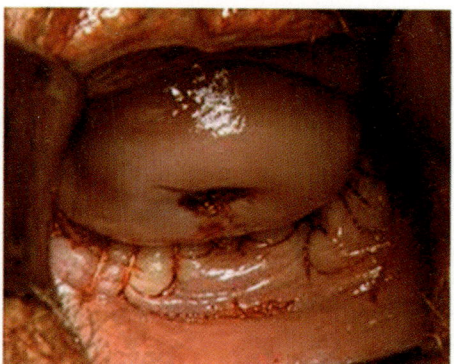

Fig. 12.42: Closure of colpotomy seen from vaginal view

Endoknife

This involves using a classic lancet with an interchangeable blade (Fig. 12.43) which is transformed into an endoscopic instrument, which can be inserted easily through 10 mm trocar. The blade has an automatic retraction system and can be set in standby position for security. Mass is held between the two grasping forceps and held with traction, under vision the knife then cuts the specimen (Figs 12.44 and 12.45). This is simple, safe, reusable and inexpensive method but has limitations when the size of specimen is big.[22]

Contained Morcellation

About 1 in 400 females undergoing surgery of myomas are at risk of having a leiomyosarcoma (American Cancer Society). The 5 year survival for leiomyosarcoma is poor as seen from the data:
– Stage I: 60%
– Stage II: 35%
– Stage III: 22%
– Stage IV: 15%.

Several studies have reported an increase in recurrence rate and decrease in rate of survival following morcellation, which results in upstaging of disease. So, the methods of bag morcellation, minilaparotomy and colpotomy are proposed to overcome this problem. For larger specimens a minilaparotomy with or without use of self-retaining retractors is advised.

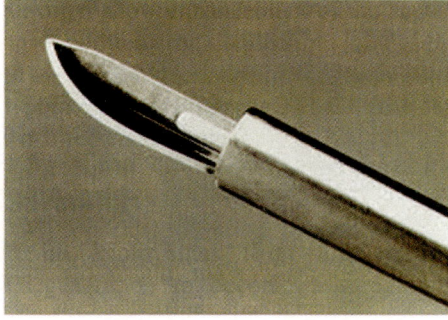

Fig. 12.43: The endoknife mounted with blade

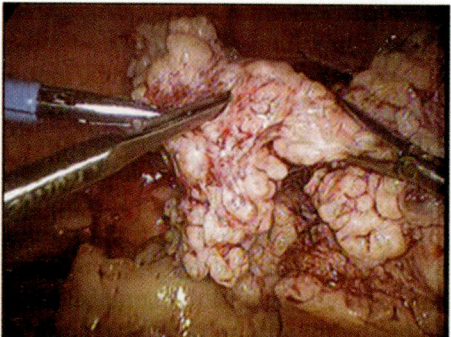

Fig. 12.44: Use of endoknife for morcellation

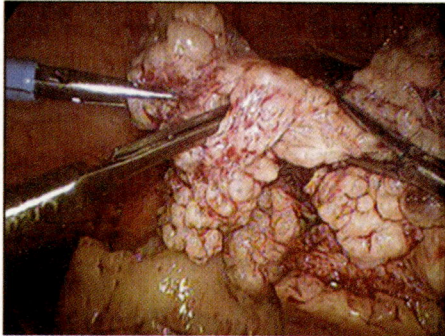

Fig. 12.45: Two graspers stabilizing the myoma

In April 2014, FDA issued a warning about power morcellation, concerning morcellation of unsuspected leiomyosarcomas. AAGL—most females with uterine cancer can be diagnosed prior to surgery. 1 in 400 to 1 in 1,000, females undergoing myomectomy will have uterine leiomyosarcoma, prognosis of these females is unusually poor and may be worsened in setting of power morcellation.

Inbag morcellation seems to be a viable alternative to open power morcellation and offers the advantage of no spillage of tissues or fluids during morcellation.[23]

This technique involves the placement of the specimen into a large plastic bag within abdomen, exteriorising the opening of the bag, insufflating the bag within the peritoneal cavity and then using the power morcellator within the bag to remove the specimen in a contained manner.

A recent study from January 2013 to April 2014 which included 73 patients, concluded this as a feasible technique. Methods of morcellating uterine tissue in a contained manner may provide an option to minimize the risks of open power morcellation, while preserving the benefits of minimally invasive surgery (Level of evidence II).[24]

In the author's own personal experience, this method once a couple of cases are performed is fairly easy to perform and the author has morcellated specimens up to 2.3 kg with relative ease and without spill.

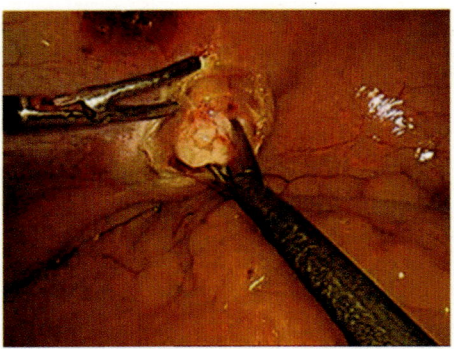

Fig. 12.46: 22 parasitic myoma in the left previous myomectomy port

In addition to the risk involved to viscera and vessels, there has been concern for tissue dissemination. Retrospective studies show that disseminated parasitic myomas occur in 0.1%–1% of cases with power morcellation.[25,26] The use of contained morcellation is likely to substantially reduce this particular complication (Fig. 12.46).

Description of Technique

The isolation bag (Figs 12.47 to 12.50) is available in various sizes. The average size of large bag may be as big as 50 × 50 cm. The basic steps are:

1. First step involves folding the bag in an accordion style and the air is compressed out of it (Fig. 12.51).

2. This folded bag is then placed inside the plastic trocar sleeve (Fig. 12.52), which holds the folded bag completely along its length and this trocar is now introduced through the side port being used for the morcellation (Fig. 12.53).

3. After being completely pushed in the peritoneal cavity the plastic sleeve is withdrawn (Fig. 12.54) and the bag is spread inside in such manner that it gets unfolded by a coordinated action of the surgeon and his assistant (Fig. 12.55).

4. The closed base of the bag is placed snugly at the POD and the bag opened wide with the instruments of the surgeon and assistant ports.

5. Next, the parked specimen (usually right upper quadrant) is grasped and placed into the bag (Figs 12.56 and 12.57).

6. Next the rim of the bag is railroaded out through morcellator port, then the morcellator port and the base is resealed so that gas does not leak out (Fig 12.58).

7. The bag has other additional sleeve which is used for passing the optical trocar with the gas connection. This sleeve is now railroaded out through the optical (11 mm) port (Fig 12.59).

8. Abdomen is now deflated.

9. The sleeve is opened with a small nick and the optical trocar with the scope is introduced inside the bag and the pneumoperitoneum created within the bag (Fig. 12.60).

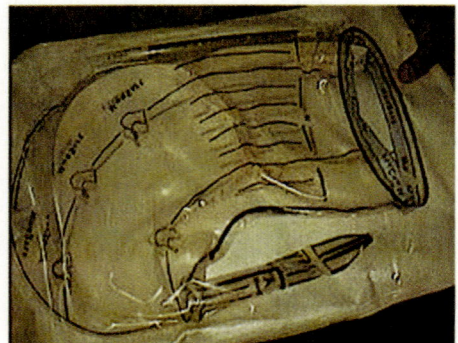

Fig. 12.47: Isolation bag Morsafe

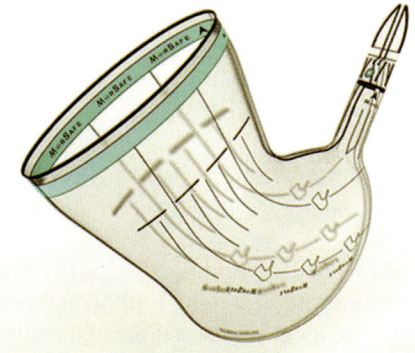

Fig. 12.48: The diagrammatic representation of an isolation bag

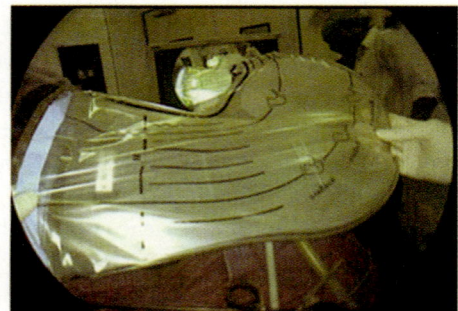

Fig. 12.49: The isolation bag opened up for a full view

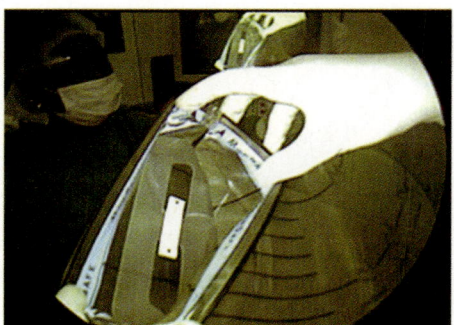

Fig. 12.50: Open rim of bag

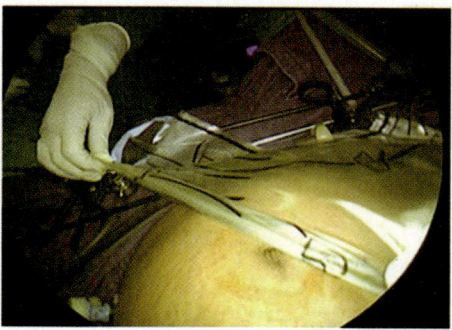

Fig. 12.51: Rolling bag in accordian style

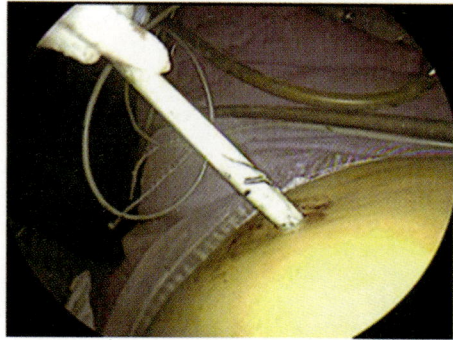

Fig. 12.52: Rolled bag placed inside sleeve

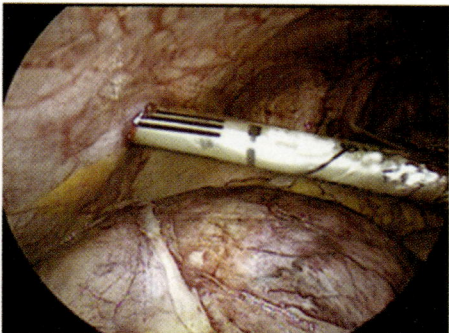

Fig. 12.53: Inside view of bag in the sleeve

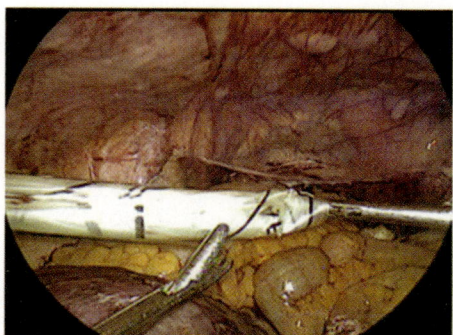

Fig. 12.54: Sleeve is withdrawn and bag retained in

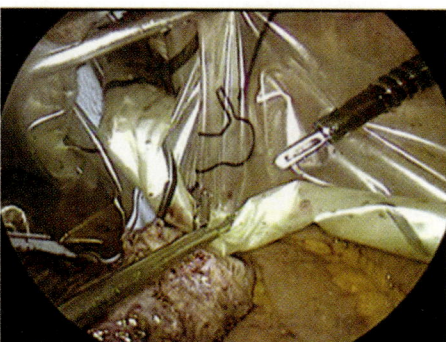

Fig. 12.55: Unrolling the bag

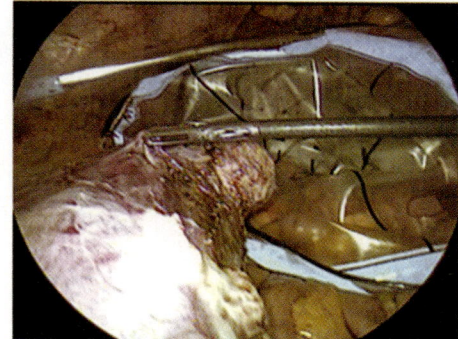

Fig. 12.56: Specimen being placed in bag

10. Once the bag pneumoperitoneum is established, the morcellator is introduced under the vision and entire specimen is morcellated within bag and railroaded out ensuring no spill and also safety to neighbouring viscera and vessels (Figs 12.61 to 12.63).

11. The defect of the morcellator site is closed in standard manner with port closure needle.

Various methods of using these isolation bags in multiport laparoscopic myomectomy, in single port surgery and even in robot-assisted laparoscopic myomectomy have been described. In multiport laparoscopic myomectomy, an alternative technique is also discussed in which the bag is introduced at umbilical port instead of side port with the camera being placed at the lateral port.

Minilaparotomy

This is a safe and effective minimally invasive alternative to laparoscopic myomectomy. Further advantages are that it allows for the freedom to additionally palpate the uterus and also effectively close it in three layers. This makes the technique very important for those surgeons with limited suturing skills.

Minilaparotomy incision (Fig 12.64A and B) may vary from a 3 to 6 cm suprapubic transverse incision. This is adequately small and also cosmetic. The incision is taken 2 to 3 finger breadths above the symphysis pubis. The skin and subcutaneous tissue are incised horizontally till the level of fascia. Next the finger is used to dissect bluntly in the vertical direction, working up towards the umbilicus and down towards the pubis.

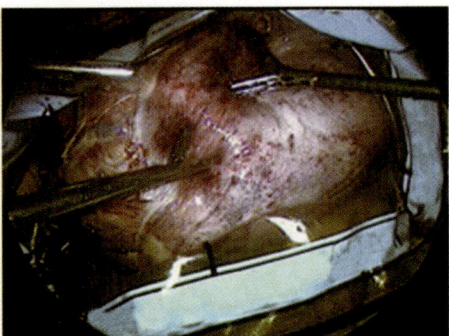

Fig. 12.57: Specimen placed in bag

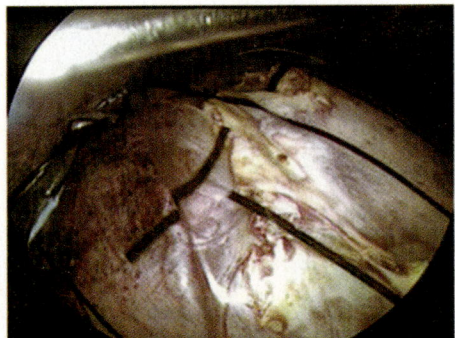

Fig. 12.58: The bag's edges being taken out of morcellator port (with the specimen inside)

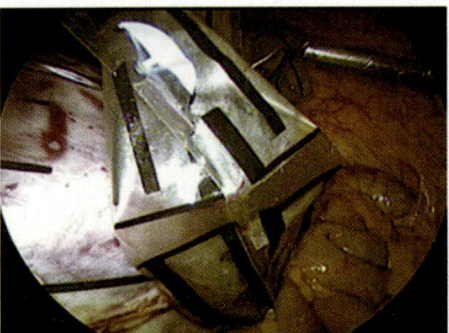

Fig. 12.59: Identifying tail end and railroading it out of primary port

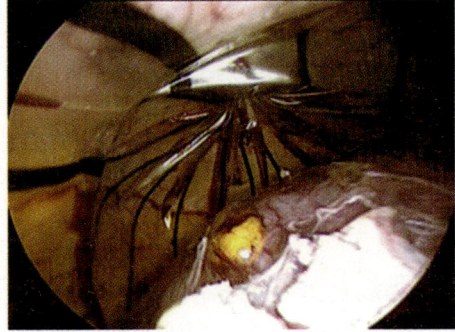

Fig. 12.60: Establishment of pneumoperitoneum in the bag via the extension end

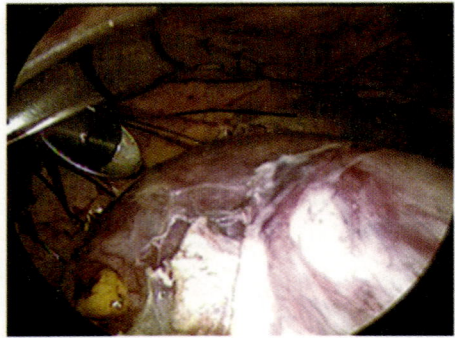

Fig. 12.61: Morcellator being introduced

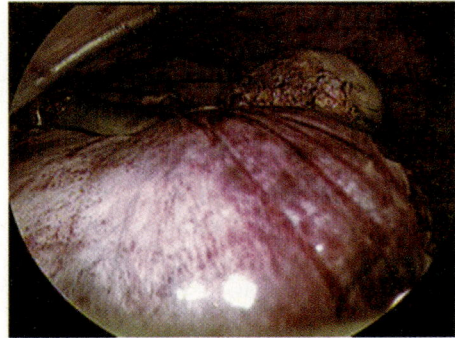

Fig. 12.62: Morcellation being carried out

The fascia is then opened in midline for about 6 cm. The rectus muscle is then separated at midline and peritoneum grasped and nicked vertically taking care not to injure the urinary bladder. Elastic abdominal retractors are now available which are then introduced (Figs 12.65 and 12.66) (e.g. Mobius retractors). The surgeon and assistant both work in coordinated manner to adjust the top and bottom rings so that they adjust firmly and snugly. Usually 2–3 twists of the retractor will give a round opening of ring size and keep the subcutaneous fat, muscle, peritoneum out of the way. This provides the room for removal by morcellation and also for repair of the hysterotomy. If the situation is found to be more complicated as in broad ligament myoma or inaccessible low posterior wall or cervical myoma, then the retractor is removed and incision is extended to conventional laparotomy.

The rules of myomectomy after this manner are same. The only difference is that contrary to laparoscopic myomectomy where in multiple incisions are generally required for enucleating different myomas, here we may attempt the removal of multiple myomas through a single strategic incision and proceed as in the open method.

The myomas are morcellated using number 10/11 blade (Fig 12.67). Thereafter the entire uterus defect can be exteriorised for easy and compact suturing.[27]

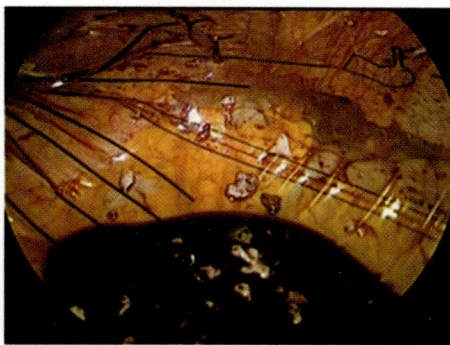

Fig. 12.63: The entire blood and small fragments of myoma collect at the base of bag

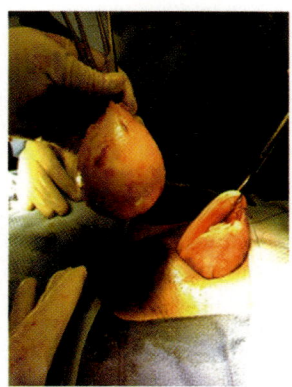

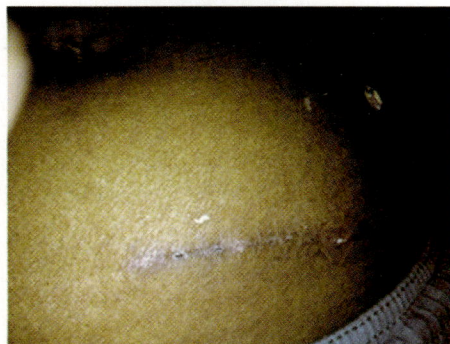

Figs 12.64A and B: Myoma enucleated through minilaparotomy

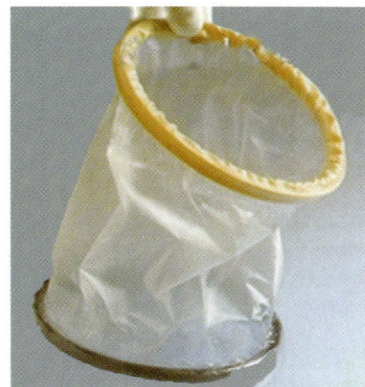

Fig. 12.65: The Mobius retractor for minilap method

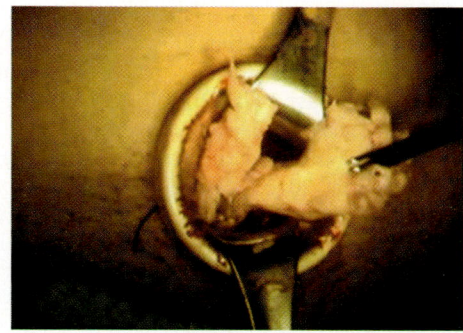

Fig. 12.66: Extraction of the myoma strips via minilap

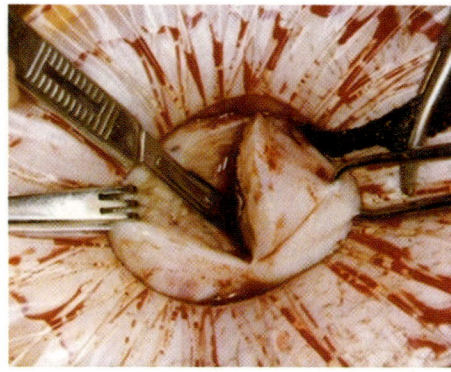

Fig. 12.67: Myoma morcellation in progress through minilap with ring retractor in place

CONCLUSION

Over the last two decades, surgical science has seen a paradigm shift from simple procedures performed through laparoscopy to the present era of laparoscopy permeating the domains of highly complex surgical procedures, including myomectomy. This has raised the certain issues, like morcellation related concerns, but at same time, led to technological advances and solutions in the form of contained morcellation.

Technological advances allow us to perform complex surgical procedures and at the same time, this very need to perform surgical procedures with safety and efficiency, prompts the development of newer technological advances. Symbiosis between the two is undeniable.

Laparoscopic myomectomy is thus a very protocol based surgery of which endosuturing is an integral part. With proper implementation of principles of surgery and technology, the minimal access route is the best in terms of patient outcome.

REFERENCES

1. Malzoni M, Rotond M, Pecone C, et al. Fertility after laparoscopic myomectomy of large uterine myomas. European Journal of Gynaecological Oncology. 2003,24(1):79-82.
2. Zullo F, Palomuba S, Corea D, et al. Bupivacaine plus epinephrine for Laparoscopic Myomectomy: a randomized placebo controlled trial. Obstet Gynecol. 2004;104(2):243-9.

3. Chang WC, Huang PS, Wang PH, et al. Comparison of laparoscopic myomectomy using in situ morcellator with and without Uterine Artery ligation for treatment of symptomatic myomas. J Minim Invasive Gynecol. 2012;19:715-21.

4. Vercellino G, Erdemoglu E, Joe A, et al. Laparoscopic temporary clipping of uterine artery during laparoscopic myomectomy. Arch Gynecol Obstet. 2012;286(5):1181-6.

5. Dubuisson J, Ramyend L, Streuli I. The role of preventive uterine artery occlusion during laparoscopic myomectomy: A review of literature. Arch Gynecol Obstet. 2015;291(4):737-43.

6. Celik H, Sapmaz E. Use of a single preoperative dose of Misoprostol is efficacious for patients who undergo abdominal myomectomy. Fertil Steril. 2003;79:1207-10.

7. Fredrick S, Fredrick J, Fletcher H, et al. A trial comparing the use of rectal misoprostol plus perivascular vasopressin alone to decrease myometrial bleeding at the time of abdominal myomectomy. Fertil Steril 2013;100:1044-9.

8. Caglar GS, Tasci Y, Kayikcioglu F, et al. Intravenous Tranexaemic acid use in myomectomy: a prospective randomized double-blind placebo controlled study. Eur J Obstet Gynecol Reprod Biol. 2008;137:227-31.

9. Kongnyuej EJ, Wiysonge CS. Interventions to reduce haemorrhage during myomectomy for fibroids. Cochrane Database Syst Rev. 2011;(11):CD.

10. Bonney V. The technique and results of myomectomy. Lancet. 1931;220:171-3.

11. Buttram VC, Reiter R. Uterine leiomyomata: etiology, symptomatology and management. Fertil Steril. 1981;36:433-45.

12. James A Greenberg, Rand H Goldman. Barbed suture: A Review of Technology and Clinical Uses in Obstetrics and Gynaecology. Rev Obstet Gynecol. 2013;6(3-4):107-15.

13. Nett M, Avelar R, Sheehan M, et al. Watertight knee arthotomy closure: Comparison of novel single bi-directional barbed self-retaining suture versus conventional interrupted sutures. J Knee Surg. 2011;24:55-9.

14. Gozen AS, Avslan M, Schulze M, et al. Comparison of laparoscopic closure of the bladder with barbed polyglyconate versus polyglactin suture material in the pig bladder model: An experimental in vivo study. J Endourol. 2012;26:732-6.

15. Einarrson II, Vonnahme KA, Sandberg EM, et al. Barbed compared with standard suture: Effects on cellular composition and proliferation of the healthy wound in the ovine uterus. Acta Obstet Gynecol Scand. 2012;91:613-9.

16. Huang MC, Hseih CH, Su TH, et al. Safety and efficacy of unidirectional barbed sutures in minilaparotomy myomectomy. Taiwan J Obstet Gynecol. 2013;52:53-6.

17. Sandberg EM, Cohen SL, Hill Lydecker, et al. Pregnancy outcomes after laparoscopic myomectomy closure with bidirectional barbed suture. J Minimal Invasive Gynecol. 2013;20:492-8.

18. Mangeshikar PR. New instrumentation and technique for laparoscopic myomectomy. J Am. Assoc. Gynecol Laprosc. 1995;2:S29.

19. Milles CE, Johnston M, Rundell M. Laparoscopic myomectomy in the infertile women. J Am Assoc Gynecol Laparosc.1996;3:525-32.

20. Hasson HM, Rotman C, Rana N, et al. Laparoscopic myomectomy. Obstet Gynecol. 1992;80:884-8.

21. Linsday E Clark, Gulden Menderal, et al. A simple approach to specimen retrieval via posterior colpotomy incision. JSLS. 2015;19(2).

22. De Grandi P, Chardonnens E, Gerber S. The morcellator knife: a new laparoscopic instrument for supracervical hysterectomy and morcellation.Obstet Gynecol. 2000;95(5):777-8.

23. Jon I, Einarsson, Sarahl Cohen, et al. In Bag Morcellation Journal of Minimally Invasive Gynaecology. 2014;21(5):951-3.

24. Cohen Sarah L, Einarrson Jon, et al. Contained Power Morcellation with an insufflated isolation bag Obstetrics and Gynaecology. 2014;124(3):491-7.

25. Ciecaella G, Granese R, Calagna G, et al. Parasitic myomas after endoscopic surgery: an emerging complication in the use of morcellator? Description of four cases. Fertile Steril. 2011;96:90-6.

26. Leren V, Langbrekke A, Quigstad E. Parasitic leiomyomas after Laparoscopic surgery with morcellator. Acta Obstet Gynecol Scand. 2012;9:1233-6.

27. Malle H Glasser. Minilaparotomy myomectomy: A minimally invasive alternative for the large fibroid uterus. Journal of Minimally Invasive Gynaecology. 2005;12:275-83.

CHAPTER 13

Hysteroscopic Myomectomy Techniques

● Vidya V Bhat

■ INTRODUCTION

Uterine fibroids (myomas or leiomyomas) are benign growths of uterine muscle that occur commonly in women of reproductive age.[1] Symptoms often attributed to uterine fibroids are heavy menstrual bleeding and pressure symptoms.

On routine histological examinations of hysterectomy specimens of premenopausal age group fibroid were seen in 40% of cases.[2,3] Hysteroscopic series have reported finding submucous fibroids in 6% to 34% of women investigated for abnormal uterine bleeding and 2% to 7% of women investigated for infertility.[4,5]

■ CLASSIFICATION OF FIROIDS

Preoperative classification of leiomyomas makes it possible to determine the best route for surgery.

ESGE Classification

The most commonly used classification system was developed by the European Society of Gynaecological Endoscopy (ESGE),[6] which considers the extent of intramural extension (Table 13.1). Each fibroid under that system is classified as (Fig. 13.1):

1. Type 0: No intramural extension.
2. Type I: Less than 50% extension.
3. Type II: More than 50% extension.

Advantages

1. Useful when considering therapeutic options, including the surgical approach.

2. It provides relationship of the outer boundary of leiomyoma with the uterine serosa, a relationship that is important when evaluating women for resectoscopic surgery.

Table 13.1: European Society of Gynaecological Endoscopy

Score	Size	Topography	Extension	Penetration	Lateral wall
0	2 cm	Lower	1/3	0	
1	2–5 cm	Middle	1/3–2/3	50%	+1
2	> 5 cm	Upper	> 2/3	> 50%	

Disadvantages

Does not give information regarding completeness of surgery, duration of surgery and fluid deficit.

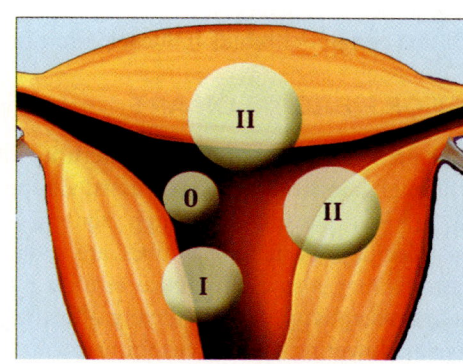

Fig. 13.1: Types of submucus myoma

STEP-W Classification

A second classification system is lasmar's STEP-W classification,[7] which was recently devised to take into account additional features of the fibroid. It considers size, topography, extension, penetration and the lateral wall. There are as follows:

1. Group I: 0 to 4 non complex.
2. Group II: 5 to 7 complex.
3. Group III: 7 to 9 non hysteroscopic.

Advantages

Better correlation with:
- Completeness of myomectomy
- Duration of surgery
- Fluid deficit.

Disadvantages

It does not specify the classification in multiple myomas.

■ BLOOD SUPPLY OF FIBROIDS

1. Arteries are less dense in fibroid than myometrium and do not have a regular pattern of distribution.
2. 1 to 2 major vessels are found at the base or pedicle.
3. Numerous thin walled sinusoidal vessels are found coursing on surface of fibroids.

■ FIBROIDS AND INFERTILITY

Fibroids are present in 5% to 10% of infertile patients, and may be the sole cause of infertility in 1% to 2.4%.[8,9] Fibroids may cause infertility by:

1. Obstruction of the fallopian tubes and impairing gamete transport.
2. It may cause distortion of the endometrial cavity, causing abnormal endometrial receptivity, hormonal milieu and altered endometrial development.[10,11]

However, the issue of whether fibroids can be the sole cause of infertility has been poorly understood.[8] But studies show removing the fibroids increases the pregnancy rate from 25% to 42% and certainly fibroids influence infertility.[12]

■ EFFECT OF FIBROIDS ON ART

The relationship between fibroids and infertility has been elucidated through numerous studies on assisted reproductive technologies (ART) patients. Although abnormal gamete transfer and blockage of fallopian tubes are circumvented by ART, fibroids may also compromise fertility by altering the endometrial receptivity thus negatively affecting embryo implantation and lowering the chances for pregnancy.[10,11]

■ FIBROIDS AND PREGNANCY

The reported incidence of fibroids in pregnancy ranges from 0.1%–10.7% of all pregnancy.[13–15] A study by De Vivo et al[16] reported that 71.4% of fibroids grew during the first and second trimesters, while 66.6% grew between the second and third trimesters. Although most pregnancies with fibroids are uneventful, fibroids increase the risk of pregnancy complications.

■ FIBROIDS AND OBSTETRICAL OUTCOMES

Complications occur in approximately 10% to 40% of pregnancies in the presence of fibroids.[17,18] Fibroids may contribute to recurrent miscarriages.

■ SURGICAL MANAGEMENT

Well-designed surgical intervention trials for myomectomy and infertility are sparse, with a single randomised controlled trail (RCT) published to date. This study demonstrated an improvement in spontaneous conception rates after the surgical removal of submucosal fibroids.[19]

Preoperative Evaluation

A complete history related to symptoms and how they affect quality of life. Preoperative imaging also is imperative—using either 2D or 3D saline infusion sonography or a combination of diagnostic hysteroscopy and transvaginal ultrasound.

Any woman who has abnormal uterine bleeding (AUB) and a risk for endometrial hyperplasia or cancer should undergo endometrial biopsy as well.

Magnetic resonance imaging (MRI), computed tomography (CT) and hysterosalpingography are either prohibitively expensive or of limited value in the initial preoperative assessment of uterine fibroids.

Preoperative Medications

1. Gonadotropin-releasing hormone (GnRH) agonists:[20]
   - Advantages—reduces the size of large fibroids.
   - Disadvantages—the drug complicates dissection of the fibroid from the surrounding capsule.

   Further there is lack of data demonstrating that GnRH agonists decrease blood loss and limit absorption of distension media.
2. Vasopressin: 0.5 mg in 20 cc of saline or 20 U in 100 cc, injecting 5 cc of the solution at 3, 6, 9 and 12 O'clock positions.
   - Advantages: Reduce blood loss during hysteroscopic myomectomy when it is injected into the cervical stroma preoperatively, reduces absorption of distension fluid and facilitates cervical dilation.

3. Misoprostol: To facilitate cervical dilatation specially in nulliparous lady, 200 μg atleast 2 hours before procedure.

HYSTEROSCOPIC MYOMECTOMY

Hysteroscopic myomectomy is the least invasive surgical approach to fibroid removal.[21] It is most effective for patients with submucosal fibroids completely within the uterine cavity (type 0) or with at least 50% of the fibroid volume within the uterine cavity (type I).[22] Fibroids with less than 50% of the fibroid volume in the cavity (type II) are much more difficult to resect completely and are more often associated with the need for repeated procedures. Additionally, it has generally been recommended that hysteroscopic myomectomy can be done for fibroids under 5 cm; however fibroids greater than 5 cm and type II fibroids have been resected hysteroscopically in 2 to 3 settings (Figs 13.2 and 13.3).

Surgical Techniques

1. Office hysteroscopic myomectomy.
2. Excision of intracavitary component.
3. Complete fibroid excision—one step and two step procedure.
4. Resectoscopic excision by slicing.
5. Cutting and excision of base of fibroid.
6. Morcellation by intrauterine morcellator (IUM).
7. Vaporisation of fibroid.
8. Ablation neodymium-doped yttrium aluminum garnet (Nd:YAG) laser (Fig. 13.4).

Instrumentation

Among the options are monopolar and bipolar resectoscopy and the mechanical approach using the Truclear system, which includes a morcellator.[23] Monopolar instrumentation (Fig. 13.5), in particular, carries a risk of energy discharge to healthy tissue (Fig. 13.6). The monopolar resectoscope also has a longer learning curve, compared with the mechanical approach. In order for the current to flow, a non-conductive media must be used, such as sorbitol or glycine.

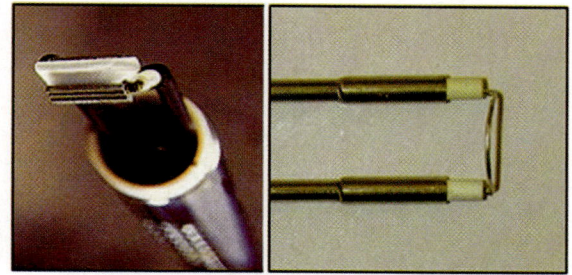

Fig. 13.3: Hysteroscopic morcellator

The bipolar is much safer as the current only passes through that tissue with which the electrode comes into contact. In this setting, conducting distention media can be used safely. The disadvantages are due to small loop, it takes longer time and vision is obscure (Fig. 13.7).

In contrast, the Truclear system requires fewer insertions, has a short learning curve, and omits the need for capture of individual chips, as the mechanical morcellator suctions and captures them throughout the procedure. In addition, because resection is performed mechanically, there is no risk of energy discharge to healthy tissue.

Size of Truclear System

1. The Truclear system also is associated with a significantly shorter operative time, compared with resectoscope.
2. Advantageous for residents, fellows and other physicians learning the procedure.
3. Shorter operative time also may result in lower fluid deficits.
4. In addition, saline distension may reduce the risk of fluid absorption and hyponatremia.
5. The tissue-capture feature allows evaluation of the entire pathologic specimen.
6. Besides hysteroscopic myomectomy, the Truclear system is appropriate for visual dilatation and curettage (D & C), adhesiolysis, polypectomy, and evacuation of retained products of conception.

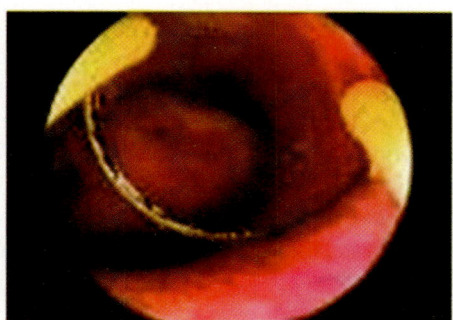

Fig. 13.2: Hysteroscopic resection of polyp

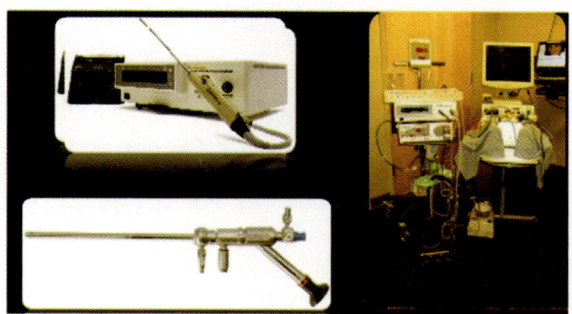

Fig. 13.4: YAG laser

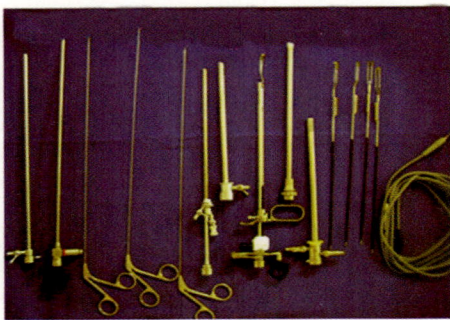

Fig.13.5: Instrumentation

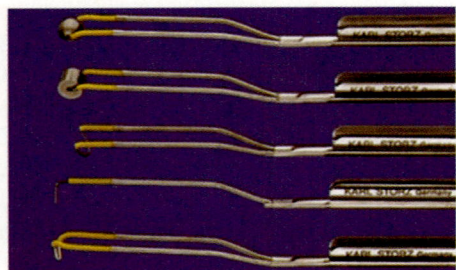

Fig. 13.6: Monopolar instrumentation

Media of Distension[24]

The uterine cavity is a potential space and hence requires some type of medium to distend it so that surgery can be performed.

Ideally the Media

1. Should be isotonic and have little impact on fluid volumes in the body.
2. Should not cause electrolyte abnormalities.
3. Should allow good visualisation.
4. Should not cause haemolysis.
5. Should not conduct electricity.

This perfect medium does not exist; however, one must weigh the risks and benefits of available media when choosing, which one to use for each procedure.

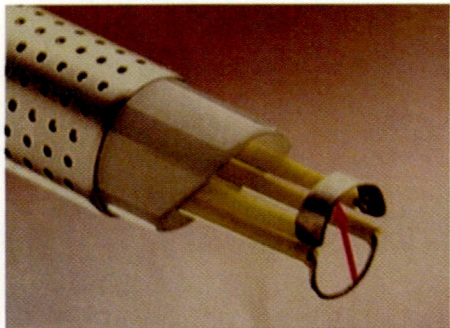

Fig. 13.7: Bipolar electrode

The following media have been used for uterine distention, i.e. carbon dioxide, Hyskon, Ringer's lactate (RL), normal saline (NS), half normal saline, glycine, sorbitol, mannitol, Cytal (sorbitol and mannitol), and dextrose 5% in water (DW).

Carbon Dioxide

Not suitable for operative procedure since concomitant blood and endometrial debris collected and obscure the vision. It can absorb systemically and cause life-threating cardiopulmonary arrest, so not in use nowadays.

Normal Saline

Advantages

1. Isotonic electrolyte rich solution—does not cause electrolyte imbalance.
2. Suitable for morcellator.

Disadvantages

1. Contain electrolytes and are conductive, so the current diffuses in every direction, away from the electrodes, and no cutting effect is found.
2. Not suitable for monopolar resectoscope.
3. Visualisation may be impaired due to bubble formation.

Glycine

Glycine is the fluid most commonly used in resectoscopic surgery today. The fluid is 1.5% of the amino acid in water. It is a hypotonic fluid, having an osmolality of 200 mOSM/L.

Advantage

1. It can be used, while using monopolar and bipolar resectoscope.
2. Due to its osmolality causes minimal haemolysis.
3. It provides excellent visualisation of the uterine cavity.

Disadvantage

It may cause significant hyponatremia and fluid overload.

Technique

Technique of hysteroscopic myomectomy are (Figs 13.8 to 13.11):

1. Effective for Rx of fibroid type 0 and type I.
2. Faster than conventional resectoscopy.
3. Insert the hysteroscope under direct visualisation. Preoperative cervical ripening facilitates the insertion.
4. Distend the uterus with saline and inspect the uterine cavity noting the number, size, location of fibroid and whether they are sessile or pedunculated.
5. Place the morcellator window against the fibroid to begin cutting. Elevate the fibroid with tip of morcellator for easy cutting.

6. Enucleation is largely accompanied by varying intrauterine pressure, which permit uterine decompression and myometrial contraction and render fibroid capsule more visible.

7. If necessary hysteroscopy can be withdrawn to stimulate myometrial contraction, which also help to delineate fibroid capsule.

8. Reinspect the uterus to rule out perforation and to remove any other pathology.

9. Once all the designated fibroid have been removed, withdraw the morcellator and hysteroscope from uterus.

Mechanism of Action

1. Rotary blade: 1,500 rpm—5 mm.
2. Reciprocating blade: 2,500 rpm—7 mm.

Post Operative Care and Follow-up

1. Nonsteroidal anti-inflammatory drugs (NSAIDs) is sufficient to relieve post operative pain and discomfort.
2. Patient can return to normal activity within 24 to 48 hours.
3. Sexual activity is permissible 1 week after the surgery.

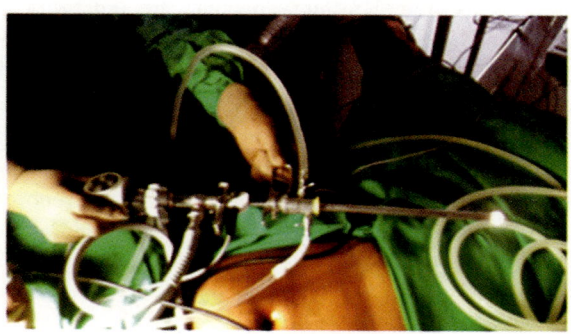

Fig. 13.8: Resectoscope set up

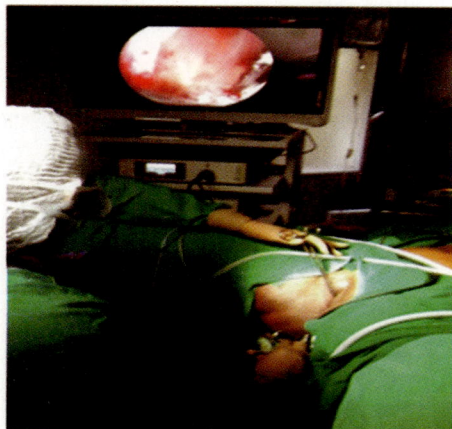

Fig. 13.9: Patient setup for hysteroscopic myomectomy

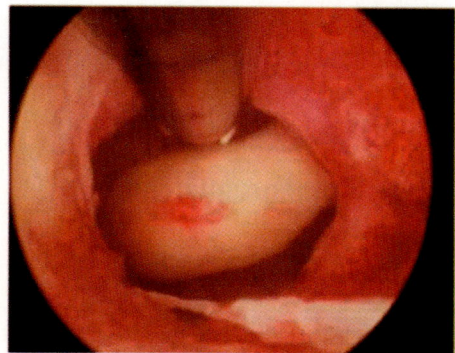

Fig. 13.10: Hysteroscopic morcellation

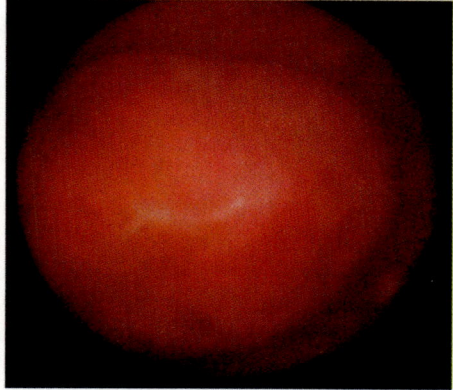

Fig. 13.11: Hysteroscopic view of submucous fibroid

4. Follow-up visit after 4 to 6 weeks of surgery or immediately, if she developed increasing pain, foul-smelling discharge or fever.

Procedure Advantages[25]

Safe

1. Simple, mechanical design eliminates the risk of energy discharge-induced scarring and reduces the risk of air or gas emboli.
2. Localised treatment reduces endometrial damage, which may help preserve the chances of pregnancy.
3. Proprietary suction control technology minimizes fluid use.

Efficient

1. Continuous cutting and tissue removal means only single insertion is necessary.
2. Single insertion means fewer procedural steps than resectoscopy.

Effective

1. Targeted pathology removal under continuous visualisation ensures efficient cut and capture.
2. Tissue capture allows evaluation of entire pathology.

Clear

1. Continuous hysteroscopic outflow and suction helps maintain clear operative field.
2. No tissue floating within the uterine cavity.

Disadvantages of Morcellator

1. Type I and type II.
2. Cannot control haemorrhage.
3. Fibroids more than 4 cm difficult to morcellate.
4. Zero degree telescope, so limited vision.

Complications

Surgical Technique Related: Early Complications

Perforation

Uterine perforation (Fig. 13.12) can happen at any stage during the procedure and is estimated to occur in 0.4% to 1.6% of operative hysteroscopies. It is the most common complication of hysteroscopic surgery. If a surgeon suspects that uterine perforation has occurred, laparoscopy should be performed to assess for intraperitoneal bleeding and damage to other intraperitoneal structures such as the bowel. Small tears measuring less than 5 mm can usually be left to heal themselves unless they are actively bleeding. In some cases of uterine perforation, there will be damage to the bowel, although it is quite rare. Studies have not shown any change in outcome with primary closure of the bowel injury vs colostomy. The use of a drain has not been shown to improve outcomes. Overall, young healthy patients with bowel injury from hysteroscopy tend to do very well (Fig. 13.13).

Haemorrhage

The most common cause of haemorrhage in the setting of hysteroscopy is uterine perforation, which was discussed above. Haemorrhage can be controlled with uterine artery ligation. This can be performed vaginally, if the surgeon has adequate skill. A Bakri intrauterine balloon can also be placed for tamponade, but this is not recommended if the patient has a perforation. Once the balloon is placed, it is left for 24 to 48 hours and then slowly decompressed. In cases of severe, life-threatening haemorrhage, uterine artery ligation, internal iliac artery ligation, UAE may be performed. Lastly hysterectomy may be performed if other techniques failed. As with any surgical haemorrhage, it is important to communicate with the anesthesiologist about ongoing blood loss and transfuse blood components as necessary.

Cervical Lacerations

Bleeding occurring from the tenaculum site on the cervix can usually be controlled with pressure applied with a sponge holder. Haemostatic agents such as silver nitrate sticks and Monsel's solution can also be used. Tears often require suturing (Fig. 13.14).

Prevention

Use two instruments (Tenaculum/Allis forceps) for equal and broad surface distribution of pressure.

Late Complications

Infection: Infection after transcervical myomectomy remains low and it is not currently recommended to give prophylactic antibiotics. Rare infectious complications including toxic shock syndrome, broad ligament abscess and pyometra have also been reported.

Uterine synechiae: Uterine synechiae are emerging as an important complication in operative hysteroscopy, especially when it is performed for the purpose of fertility. A study from France looked at 53 patients who underwent hysteroscopic myomectomy for infertility attributed to submucous myomas. 2 months postoperatively, patients underwent a diagnostic hysteroscopy to assess for synechiae. They reported a synechiae rate of 7.5%, which was lower than previous studies. They attributed their low rate of synechiae to the use of bipolar rather than monopolar cautery.

Media Related

1. Embolism.
2. Anaphylaxis reaction.
3. Pulmonary edema.

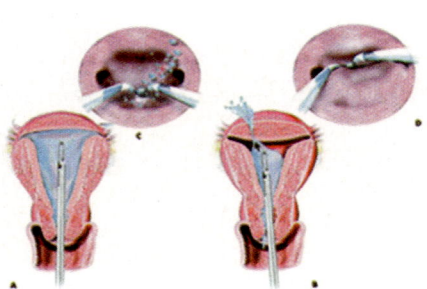

Fig. 13.12: Perforation during hysteroscopy

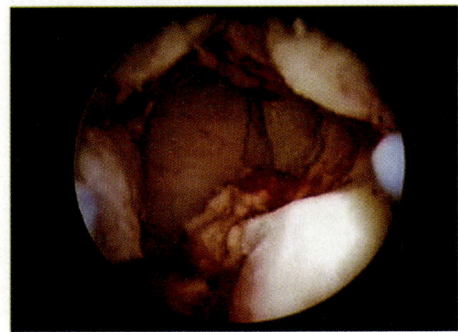

Fig. 13.13: Complex perforation

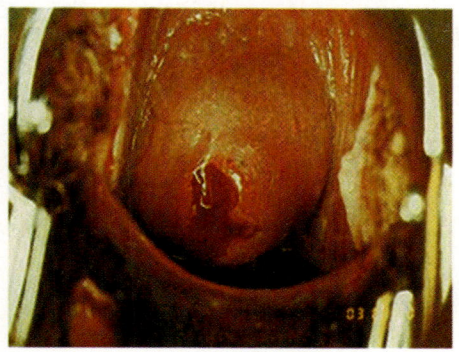

Fig. 13.14: Cervical trauma

4. Renal failure.
5. Bleeding diathesis.
6. Acute hyponatremia and hypoosmolality.

Energy Source Related

1. Electrical shock or low frequency leaks.
2. Burn or high frequency leaks.
3. Neutral electrode site injury.

■ CONCLUSION

Although epidemiological studies have been inconclusive in establishing a relationship between fibroids and infertility, clinical evidence supports the view that submucosal fibroid have a negative impact on pregnancy, ART and pregnancy outcome. Hysteroscopic myomectomy is the least invasive and safe approach for submucosal myoma (type 0 and type I). Hysteroscopic morcellation offers good alternative to conventional resectoscopy in terms of reduced operating time, less visual field obstruction and reduced fluid deficits but the surgical outcome remains similar in both techniques.

■ REFERENCES

1. Grant JM, Hussein IY. An audit of abdominal hysterectomy over decade in district hospital. Br J Gynaecol. 1984;91:73-7.
2. Clarke A, Black N, Rowe P, et al. Indications for and outcome of total abdominal hysterectomy for benign disease: a prospective cohort study. Br J obstet Gynaecol. 1995;120:611-20.
3. Farquhar CM, Sadler L, Harvey S, et al. A longitudinal case control study of premenopausal women undergoing hysterectomy. 2000.
4. Parker WH. Etiology, symptomatology and diagnosis of uterine myomas. Fertil Steril. 2007;87:725-36.
5. Wamsteker K, Emanuel MH, de Kruif JH. Transcervical hysteroscopic resection of submucous fibroids for AUB, results regarding the degree of intramural extension. Obset Gynecol. 1993;82:736-40.
6. Lasmar RB, Barrozo PR, Dias R, et al. Submucous fibroids: a ne presurgerical classification to evaluate the viability of hysteroscopic surgerical treatment- preliminary report. J Minim Invasive Gynecol. 2005;12:308-11.
7. Cook H, Ezzati M, Segars J, et al. The impact of uterine leiomyomas on reproductive outcomes. Minerva Ginecol. 2010;62:225-36.
8. Donnez J, Jadoul P. What are the implication of myomas on fertility? A need for debate? Hum. Reprod. 2002;17:1424-30.
9. Rackow B, Taylor H. Submucosal uterine leiomyomas have a global effect on molecular determinants of endometrial receptivity. Fertil Steril. 2010;93:2027.
10. Sinclair D, Mastroyannis A, Taylor H. Leiomyoma simultaneously impair Endometrial BMP-2- Mediated decidualization an Anticoagulant Expression through secretion of TFG- B3. J clin Endocrinol Metab. 2011;96:412-21.
11. Bulletti C, De Ziegler D, Polli V, et al. The role of leiomyomas in infertility. J Am Asso Gynecol Laparosc. 1999;6:441-5.
12. Coronado G, Marshall L, Schwartz S. Complications in pregnancy, labour and delivery with uterine leiomyomas: A population- based study. Obst Gynaecol. 2000;95:764-9.
13. Qidwai G, Caughey A, Jacoby A. Obstetrics outcomes in women with sonographically identified uterine leiomyomata. Obstet Gynaecol. 2006;107:376-82.
14. Laughlin S, Baird D, Savitz D, et al. Prevalance of uterine leiomyoma in first trimester of pregnancy: An ultrasound screening study. Obstet Gynaecol. 2009;113:630-5.
15. De Vivo A, Mancuso A, Giacobbe A, et al. Uterine myomas during pregnancy: a longitudinal sonographic study: Ultrasound obstet Gynaecol. 2011;37:361-5.
16. Ouyang DW, Economy KE, Norwitz ER. Obstetrics complication of fibroids. Obstet Gynecol Clin North Am. 2006;33:153-69.
17. Exacoustos C, Rosati P. Ultrasound Diagnosis of uterine myomas and complications in pregnancy. Obstet Gynecol. 1993;82:97-101.
18. Goldberg J, Pereira L. Pregnancy outcomes following treatment of fibroids; uterine fibroid embolization versus laproscopic myomectomy. Curr Opin Gynecol. 2006;18:402-6.
19. Surrey ES, Leitz AK, Schoolcraft WB. Impact of intramural leiomyomata in patients with a normal endometrial cavity on in vitro fertilization embryo transfer cycle outcome. Fertil Steril. 2001;75:405-10.
20. Mencaglia L, Tantini C. GnRH agonist analogs and hysteroscopic resection of myomas. Int J Gynecol Obstet. 1993;43(3):285-8.
21. Farhi J, Ashkenazi J, Feldberg D, et al. Effect of uterine leiomyomata on the results of in vitro fertilization treatment. Hum Reprod. 1995;10:2576-8.
22. Van Dongen H, Emanuel MH, wolterbeek R, et al. Hysteroscopic morcellator for removal of intrauterine polyps and myomas: a ramdomized controlled pilot study among residents in training. J Minm invasive Gynecol. 2008;15(4):466-71.
23. Emanual MH Hart A, Wamsteker K, Lammes F. An analysis of fluid loss during transcervical resection of submucous myomas. Fertil Steril. 1997;68(5):881-6.
24. AAGL Practical Report: Practice Guidelines for management of Hysteroscopic Distending Media: J Min Invasiv Gynecol. 2013;20:137-48.
25 Bhat VV, Chandel NP, AS Dinesh, et al. Retrospective analysis of outcomes of hysteroscopic morcellation and conventional resectoscopy of uterine submucous myomas in Indian subcontinent- A multicentre comparative study: Ind Obstet Gynecol. 2015;5(2):25-8.

Laparoendoscopic Single Site Myomectomy

● Madhuri Vidyashankar

Uterine myomas are the most common benign tumours of the female genital tract. More than 20% of all women will develop myomas during their lifetime, and 20% of them will undergo hysterectomy during the reproductive age because of such tumours.[1,2]

Most of the uterine myomas are asymptomatic and can be managed expectantly. However, they can cause abnormal uterine bleeding, pelvic pain and infertility. Women with large myomas may be predisposed to pelvic pressure, dyspareunia, bowel dysfunction, and bladder symptoms such as urinary frequency and urgency.[3]

For women in whom preservation of uterus is desired, minimally invasive methods such as laparoscopic myomectomy, minilaparotomy myomectomy, or laparoscopically assisted myomectomy have been described.[4–6] With the improvement in technical skills and instrumentation, the surgeons have been trying to reduce the number of ports thereby reducing morbidity and improving cosmesis. LESS myomectomy is a step in that direction, which provides these benefits without compromising the result of surgery.

■ INDICATIONS FOR SINGLE-PORT LAPAROSCOPIC MYOMECTOMY

Selection of Myoma

It depends on the size of fibroid, location of the fibroids the surgeon's capabilities and experience. To begin with, fundal, upper body, anterior wall or posterior wall fibroids facilitate easier myoma enucleation and suturing of the myoma bed.

In the initial part of learning curve, smaller myomas may be operated, proceeding to larger myomas with experience.

Relative Contraindications

1. Previous umbilical hernia mesh repair.
2. It may be challenging to apply single-port surgery to more complex disorder such as very large myomas and severe pelvic adhesive disease,[7] large broad ligament fibroids and multiple large fibroids.

Preoperative Patient Counselling

1. The patient is counselled that surgery will be attempted through single-port, however multiple laparoscopic ports may be required to safely and successfully perform the procedure in case of difficult situations.
2. The patient is counselled about potential benefits of improved cosmetic outcome and decreased postoperative pain; with caution that these benefits have not been evaluated thoroughly in randomised trials.
3. The requirement of regular visits to hospital for post operative wound care.[8]

Preoperative Assessment and Planning

1. Selection of patient as discussed in inclusion and exclusion criteria.
2. Deciding the operative technique.
3. Selection of access port.
4. Specialised instruments to be used to overcome the technical challenges unique to single-incision surgery.
5. Preparation of the umbilicus.

Selection of Access Port for LESS Myomectomy

1. Curcillo and King: Greater degrees of triangulation, reduced clashing of hands outside the abdomen reduces instrument collsion inside abdominal cavity
2. SILS port (Covidien): Flexibility with increased instrument manipulation
3. Gelpoint (applied medical system): Better triangulation due to wider platform.

Optics for Single-port Laparoscopic Myomectomy

The extra long laparoscope moves the camera head away from the other instruments at the umbilicus, thereby increasing instrument mobility and reducing hand collisions. The 52 cm long telescope from Karl Storz with 0° and 30° are used. The 30° scope offers the advantage of better vision for deep structures. If available, a flexible tip endoscope (ENDOEYE) may provide better visibility and easier manipulation.

Instruments for Suturing

The difficulties associated with single-incision surgery include limited working space outside of the abdomen for the surgeon and the assistant resulting in hand collisions at

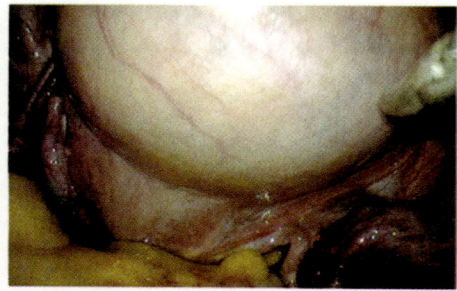

Fig. 14.1: Fundoanterior fibroid around 10 cm

or above the umbilicus. Additionally, within the abdomen, there is limited ability for triangulation or confinement to a single-axis workspace for instruments leading to collision of instruments. These difficulties are specially compounded in suturing. Specialised equipment for single-incision procedures can be used to help overcome these technical challenges including the use of specialised access ports and articulating instruments. These specialised instruments, while increasing the ease and efficiency of surgery also increase the costs as compared to conventional multiport laparoscopy. Use of articulating instruments facilitates triangulation and myoma bed suturing. We believe a combination of straight and articulating instruments is ideal in suturing of myoma in single-port myomectomies.

Operative Procedure

Access to abdominal cavity is gained through a 2 to 3 cm vertical or curvilinear horizontal incision in the umbilicus using one of the access ports as described earlier. A laparoscope, extra long length, with a 30° angle of view or flexible tip endoscope (ENDOEYE), is used. The use of instruments of varying length moves the camera head away from the two operating instruments, allowing for more freedom of movement outside the abdomen. After the trocars are inserted, inspection of the abdominal cavity is done. The number, size and location of fibroid is assessed (Fig. 14.1). The subserosa of the largest myomas is injected with dilute vasopressin, 10 units in 200 mL of saline solution, using only 10 ml with each injection (Figs 14.2A and B). The blanching of the myoma is appreciated after injection (Fig. 14.3). The infiltration of dilute vasopressin creates a plane of dissection between the pseudocapsule of myoma and myometrium and reduces intraoperative bleeding.

The type of incision on the myoma is decided by the location and size of the myoma. A vertical/horizontal/oblique incision is made over the myoma using the Harmonic Ace (Ethicon,

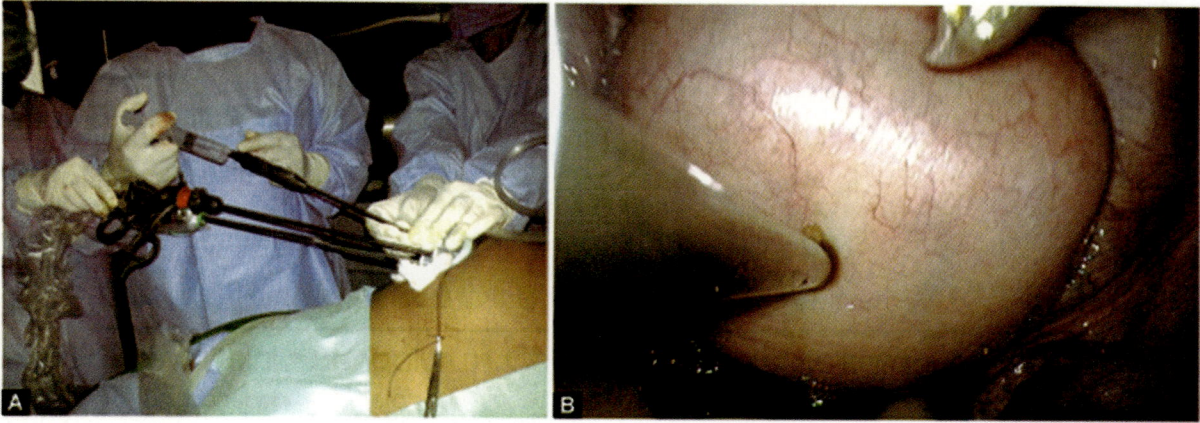

Figs 14.2A and B: Vasopressin infilteration. **A.** Outside view; **B.** Laparoscopic view.

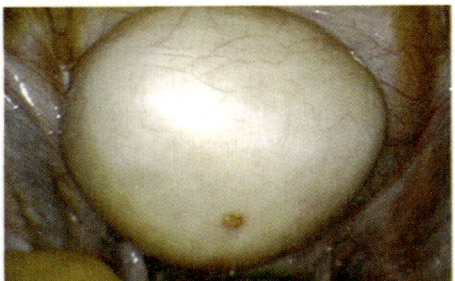

Fig. 14.3: Blanching of the fibroid after vasopressin infiltration

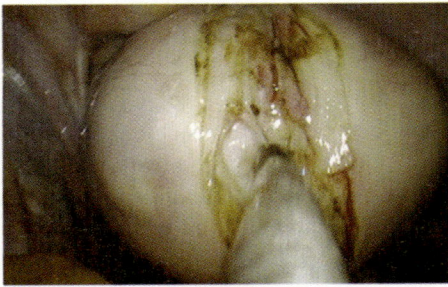

Fig. 14.4: Incision given over the myoma with monopolar hook

Cincinnati, OH) or a monopolar hook (Fig. 14.4) and the myoma is grasped with a single-toothed tenaculum or a myoma spiral (Fig. 14.5A to D). Monopolar hook is avoided in single-port laparoscopic surgery when alternatives are available to avoid electrosurgical injuries.

Traction is placed on the myoma spiral and the myoma is enucleated from the uterus using blunt dissection and counter traction (refer Figs 14.5B to D). The myoma is placed in the posterior cul-de-sac. Then attention is directed towards closing the myometrium (Fig. 14.6). The 14 × 14 cm 0-polydioxanone bidirectional barbed Quill suture (Angiotech, Vancouver, BC) is placed through a 5 mm port by straightening the needles on

each end. Alternatively, the suture is inserted by inserting a 10 mm trocar (Figs 14.7A and B). Once inside the abdomen, the needles are curved back again using a grasper and needle driver. One needle is placed in the peritoneum of the abdominal wall, while the other needle is used for suturing. If a longer length of barbed suture is required, the thread can be cut in the centre and used.

A two layer closure of the uterus is then performed for larger myomas and a single layer closure for smaller myomas. For double layer closure, the deepest layer of myometrium is closed with the first needle; the needle is cut off, straightened and removed from the abdomen. A more superficial layer is

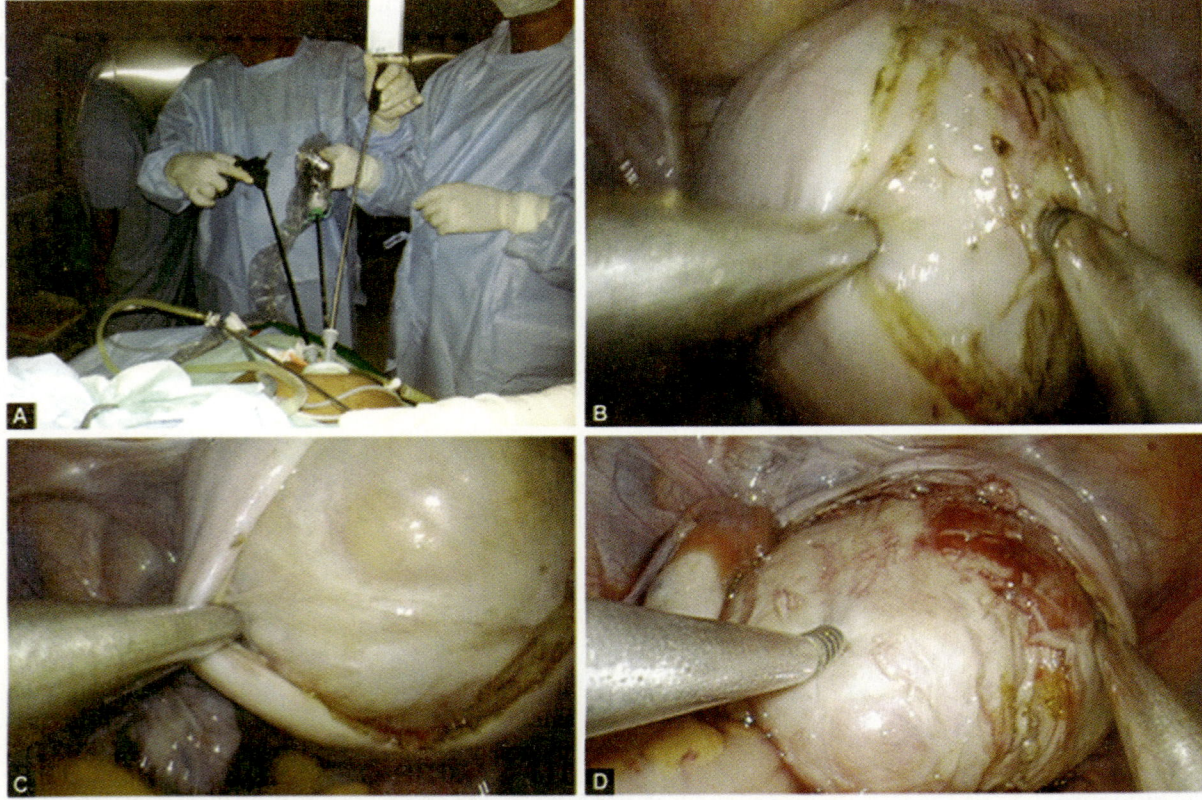

Figs 14.5A to D: A. Myoma screw inserted through 5 mm trocar. ENDOEYE and dissecting instrument is inserted through the other 2 trocars (outside view); **B to D:** Enucleation done by inserting a myoma spiral in the fibroid and using another instrument such as a suction irrigation cannula or scissors. The principle of traction and counter traction is used to separate fibroid's pseudocapsule from the myometrium.

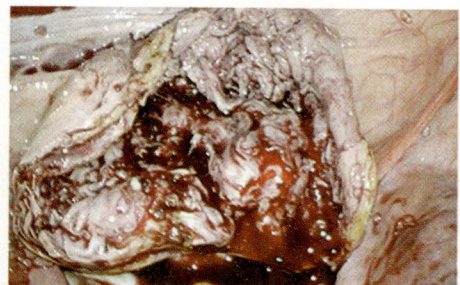

Fig. 14.6: Myoma bed after enucleation

closed with the second needle and likewise the needle is cut off, straightened and removed from the abdomen (Figs 14.8A to D and 14.9). Single layer closure may be adequate for smaller incisions. No knot tying is required if barbed suture is used, but it can be performed. Alternatively suturing devices like Endostitch may be used (Figs 14.10A and B). In selected cases, Interceed (Ethicon, West Somerville, NJ) adhesion barrier is cut in half and introduced through the trocar and may be placed over the hysterotomy scar to prevent postoperative adhesions.

Myoma Morcellation Techniques

1. Transumbilical mechanical.
2. Transumbilical electromechanical.
3. Transvaginal electromechanical.

Transumbilical Mechanical

The myoma is brought up to the incision using the tenaculum after removing the port. Then the myoma is pulled further in the incision and carefully morcellated at the level of the incision using a knife. The fascia is closed with No 1-0 vicryl suture.

Transumbilical Electromechanical (Figs 14.11A to C)

Retrieval of myoma may also be done by electromechanical morcellation through umbilicus or alternatively through the

pouch of Douglas. In umbilical morcellation, 10 or 15 mm morcellator is inserted through one opening in the port and a toothed grasper through another. The toothed grasper is used to feed the myoma, which is held in claw forceps introduced through the morcellator. The claw forceps is then drawn into the morcellator and morcellation is done. The main disadvantage of transumbilical morcellation is that panoramic view of morcellation is not seen and the view of blade is very limited.

Transvaginal Electromechanical

The surgeon inspects the vaginal side. The posterior lip of the cervix is held by an Allis forceps and retracted anteriorly and the vaginal surface is visualised. A sponge on holder is used to push the posterior vaginal fornix and the location is visualised laparoscopically to ensure the correct position between the two uterosacral ligaments and away from rectum. A 1.5 cm transverse superficial incision is made vaginally to facilitate the introduction of the morcellator under continuous laparoscopic vision. The morcellators with long blade like SAWALHE (Karl Storz GmbH & co. KG, Tuttligen Germany) or GYNECARE X TRACT (Ethicon Inc, Somerville, NJ) are preferred for vaginal morcellation. During morcellation, pneumoperitoneum is increased to 20 mm Hg to ensure good visualisation. A 10 mm claw forceps was used to guide the myoma into the morcellator and morcellation was done carefully. The morcellator was removed under vision and the adjacent structures were carefully inspected. The vaginal incision is left unsutured.

The morcellated myoma bits are sent for histopathologic examination. The skin is closed with interrupted 3-0 monocryl suture. 10 mL of 0.5% bupivacaine is injected into the incision site and Dermabond (Ethicon, West Somerville, NJ) adhesive is applied over the incision. The uterine manipulator is removed and Foley's catheter is also removed at the conclusion of the procedure. This surgeon completes a single-incision laparoscopic myomectomy as described in approximately 1 to 2 hours.

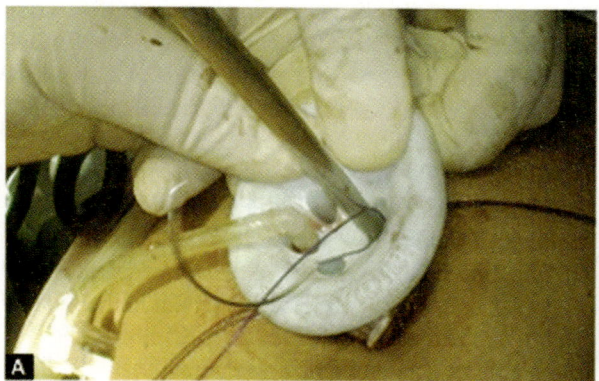
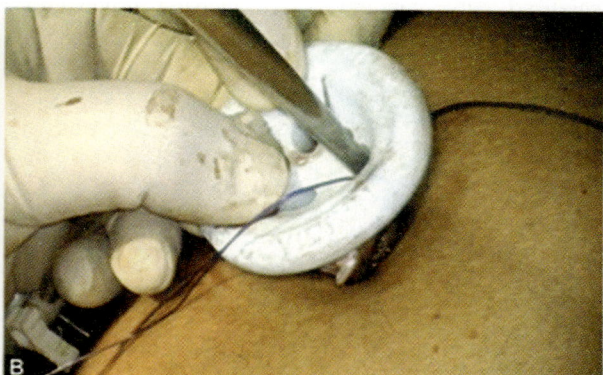

Figs 14.7A and B: Insertion of needle through the access port. Trocar is removed and needle is straightened slightly before insertion.

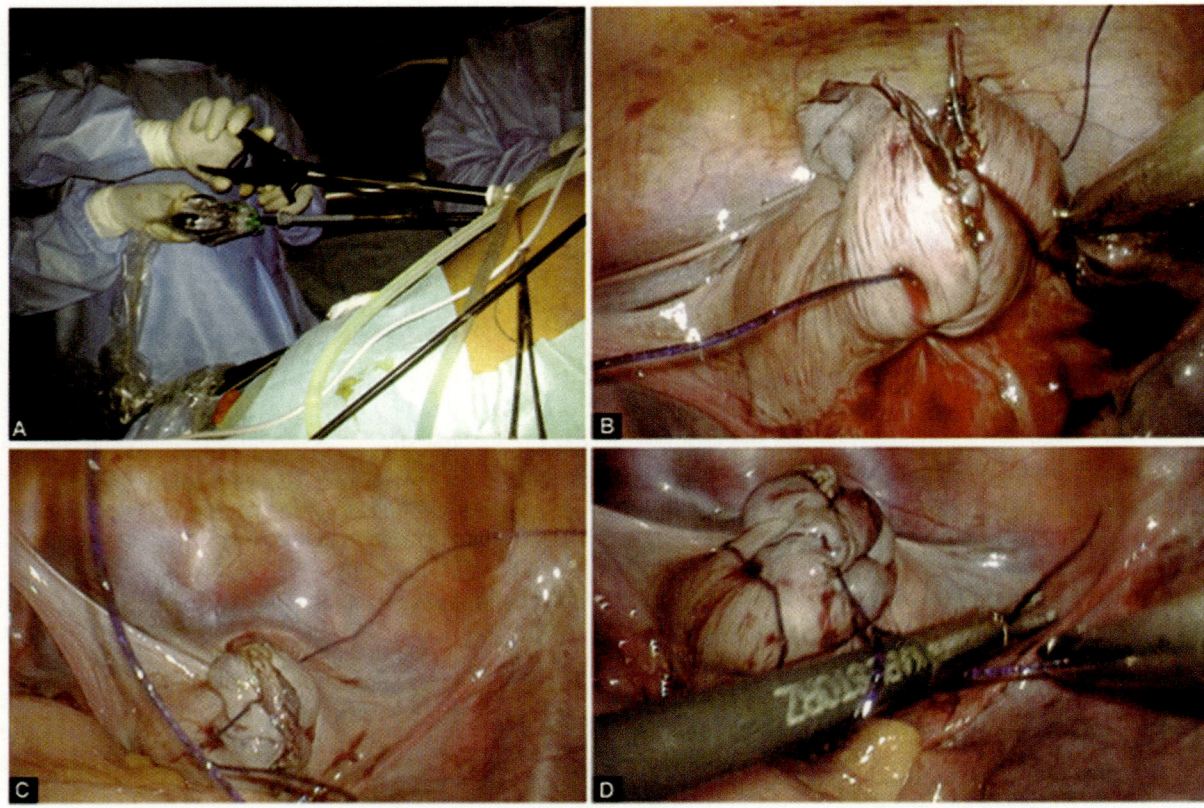

Figs 14.8A to D: Myoma suturing. **A.** A self-righting needle driver inserted through 5 mm port. We use one curved and one straight instrument; **B.** Taking bite through myoma bed; **C and D.** Thread is pulled and knot is being tied.

■ DIFFICULTIES ASSOCIATED WITH SINGLE INCISION LAPAROSCOPIC MYOMECTOMY

Difficulties with Limitation of Triangulation

1. The difficulties associated with single-incision surgery include limited working space outside the abdomen for the surgeon and the assistant resulting in hand collisions at or above the umbilicus.
2. Intraperitoneally, there is lack of triangulation or confinement to a single-axis workspace for instruments. Specialised equipment for single-incision procedures can be used to help overcome these technical challenges including the use of specialised access ports, articulating instruments, a flexible laparoscope or a 30° laparoscope, and instruments of varying lengths.
3. To avoid collision, only the main operating instrument should be kept in the target zone. The instrument handles should be kept apart extra corporeally by dividing the space above into various heights or planes and keeping handles separately. Also, only one instrument should be moved at a time to avoid collisions.[9]

Difficulties with Suturing for Myoma

The most difficult aspect of laparoscopic myomectomies is intracorporeal suturing for uterine closure. The single-incision technique adds an extra dimension of difficulty to this step. After enucleation of myomas, the repair of uterine wall defects may be challenging for surgeons with limited experience in endoscopic suturing. Intracorporeal knots are much more difficult to perform than extracorporeal knots in single-port laparoscopic surgery. Conventional rigid straight instruments can often provide more tension than flexible instruments. Since the conventional rigid straight instruments remain parallel in single-port surgery, it is difficult to roll thread around an instrument with the other instrument. In addition,

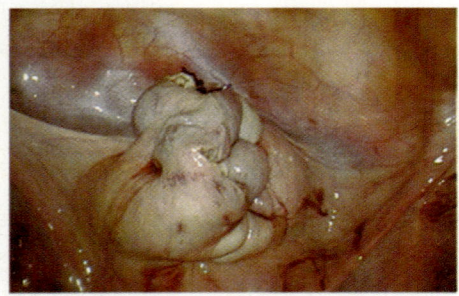

Fig. 14.9: Myoma bed after completion of suturing

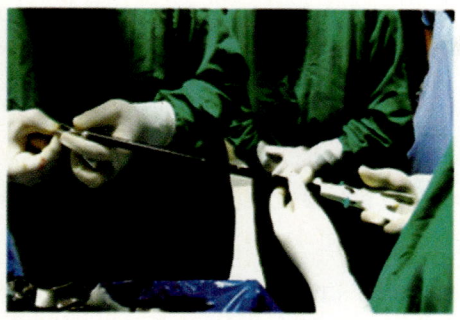 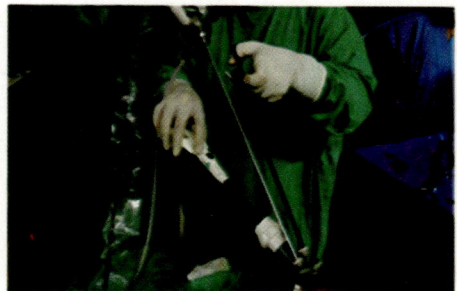

Figs 14.10A and B: Suturing in SILS myomectomy: Outside view. **A.** Loading the needle using the disposable needle loader provided with the suture material; **B.** Suturing with Endostitch.

some surgeons may experience difficulties in maintaining adequate tension of the suture line during suturing, thereby increasing the intraoperative bleeding and facilitating the formation of haematoma.[10]

The various steps that can be used to ease the suturing in LESS myomectomy are:

1. The myometrium can be closed with barbed suture, which has been shown to be feasible and faster for myomectomies.[11] The use of bidirectional barbed suture is safe for uterine closure and facilitates closure through preventing back sliding of the suture and eliminating the need for knot tying.[12] Barbed suture enables continuous, wound closure with even distribution of tensile strength throughout the repair. These benefits of barbed suture are especially valuable in single-incision surgery because intracorporeal knot tying can be more challenging than with the multiport approach.[7] The evaluation of barbed suture showed that it can facilitate closure of the myometrial defect and enable more surgeons to perform laparoscopic myomectomy.[13] One of these novel sutures, the V-Loc TM 180 (Covidien, Mansfield, MA) consists of a barbed absorbable thread, armed with a surgical needle at one end and a loop at the other end, which is used to secure the suture. The barb and loop end allow approximating the tissues without the need to tie surgical knots.[14]

2. Use of one articulating and one straight instrument. If one articulating and one straight instrument are used, the rolling over of instrument over the other to form a knot is simplified.

3. Use of self-righting needle driver. Use of self-righting needle holder makes it easy for surgeon to hold the needle faster and with ease also facilitating single handed suturing.

4. Use of Endostich to facilitate myoma bed suturing (refer Figs 14.10A and B).

5. Extra corporeal suturing of myoma bed using a Clarke's suture driver.

6. Single hand suturing technique.

7. The barrier of intracorporeal suturing has been facilitated for some surgeons by the use of Da Vinci (Intuitive Surgical, Sunnyvale, CA) robot-assisted laparoscopic myomectomies. Although single-incision robot-assisted laparoscopic myomectomies have not been described, the use of robot assistance for other single-incision gynecological laparoscopic surgery is feasible.[15]

Barbed Suture (Figs 14.12A to C)

Barbed suture is a relatively new concept in gynecologic surgery. The Quill bidirectional barbed suture (Angiotech Pharmaceuticals, Inc., Vancouver, BC, Canada) was approved by the US Food and Drug Administration (FDA) for soft tissue approximation in 2004.

Bidirectional barbed sutures are created by cutting barbs into the suture with the barbs facing in a direction opposite

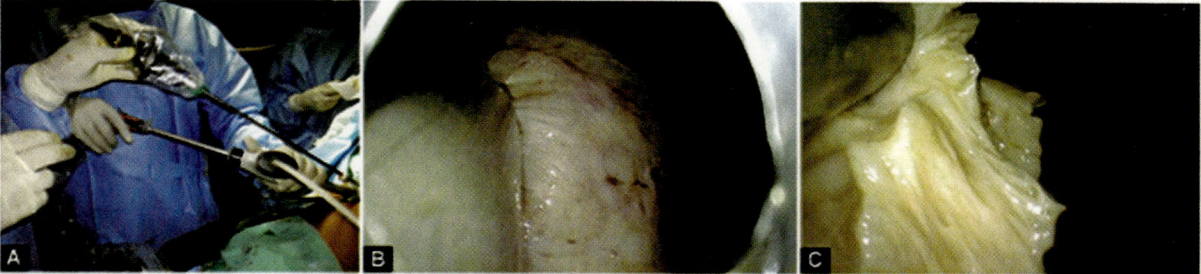

Figs 14.11A to C: Transumbilical electromechanical morcellation. **A.** Outside view: 10 mm claw forceps is inserted through trocar sleeve; **B and C.** Morcellation of fibroid: laparoscopic view. Note the compromised view in transumbilical morcellation.

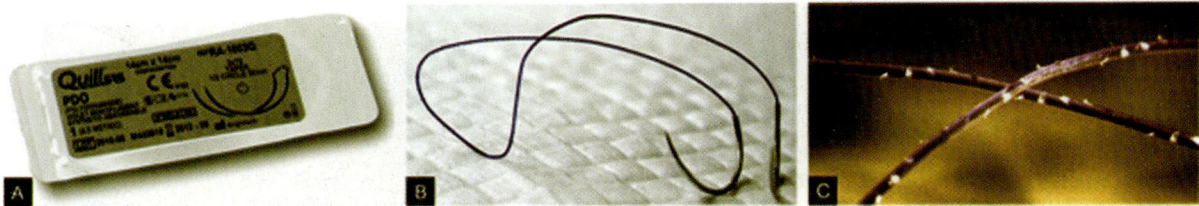

Figs 14.12A to C: Various suture material used for myometrial closure

that of the needle. The barbs change direction at the midpoint of the suture[16] and needles are swaged onto both ends of the suture. Once the bidirectional barbed suture is anchored to the tissue, it resists migration.[17,18] Because bidirectional barbed sutures self-anchor and are balanced by the countervailing barbs, no knots are required. Furthermore, barbed suture self-anchors at every 1 mm of tissue, yielding more consistent wound apposition. Knotless barbed suture can securely reapproximate tissues with less time, cost and aggravation.[19,20] The 14 × 14 cm polydioxanone suture is used for closure of smaller hysterotomy wounds. Larger hysterotomy wounds after removal of deep-seated myoma or large myomas may be sutured using 24 × 24 cm suture either in a single or double layer with the serosa closed in continuous suturing or baseball sutures. The deepest layer is closed with one needle and the subsequent layers including serosa is closed with the other needle. The colpotomy wound after hysterectomy can be safely closed with a 7 × 7 cm suture. Use of bidirectional-barbed suture for hysterotomy closure significantly shortens total operating time during laparoscopic myomectomy and greatly facilitates laparoscopic closure of the hysterotomy site.[13]

Advantages

1. Barbed suture resists migration and aids in maintaining adequate tension of the suture line during suturing.
2. It allows faster closure of the uterine wall defects contributing to the reduction in intraoperative blood loss.

Disadvantages

A potential limitation of the barbed suture may be that it is more expensive than a traditional suture. There have also been concerns about increased chance of inflammation and adhesion formation. A randomized study was done to compare barbed suture with traditional suture with regards to ease of use and adhesion formation. The adhesion rate after myometrial closure with barbed suture was found not to be different from that with standard suture like Vicryl.[21]

■ COMPLICATIONS OF LESS MYOMECTOMY

1. **Haemorrhage:** It a common complication of myomectomy performed by any approach. It can be reduced by using vasopressin, proper planning of uterine incision and suturing in multiple layers.

2. **Requirement of extraport:** Any difficulty during enucleation, suturing or morcellation due to improper visualisation, lack of triangulation or instrument collision may require placement of extra side port. It is important that the surgeon must not hesitate to put an extra port, if the situation demands.

3. **Difficulties with suturing:** Have already been described above.

4. Difficulties with specimen retrieval: Specimen retrieval by mechanical morcellation or by using electromechanical morcellator is difficult due to reduced visualisation, especially in case of larger fibroids. Utmost care must be taken in morcellation more so in LESS myomectomy. The morcellator blade should be visualised at all times and adequate pnemoperitoneum must be maintained. When using electromechanical vaginal morcellation through the pouch of Douglas, a longer blade morcellator should be used.

5. **Postoperative myometrial collection:** It may be caused due to improper closure of the myometrial defect. In a deep defect, multilayered closure is mandatory. Any collection or haematoma may lead further to infection increasing postoperative morbidity. Also, it may weaken the myomectomy scar later and predispose to uterine rupture during pregnancy.

6. **Scar integrity and rupture uterus during pregnancy:** Uterine rupture is a rare event in pregnant patients with a previous laparoscopic myomectomy.[22] Excessive tissue coagulation, use of unsuitable suture size (3–0, 4–0), and development of myometrial haematomas may increase the risk of uterine rupture during pregnancy. The risk of uterine rupture has been described as 1.0% to 3.6% in various studies.[22,23] This risk may be decreased by using proper size suture material, multilayered closure depending on the size of the defect, avoiding unnecessary coagulation and proper haemostasis.[24]

■ CONCLUSION

Laparoscopic myomectomy is currently being used widely as procedure of choice for surgical management of uterine myomas by gynecologic endoscopic surgeons. Prospective, randomized studies comparing abdominal and laparoscopic myomectomy in selected patients show that laparoscopic procedure is associated with less postoperative pain, shorter hospital stay, and shorter recovery than abdominal surgery.[25] The wide application of this approach though, is limited by the size and number of myomas reasonably removed, the technical difficulty of the procedure and of laparoscopic suturing.[26] In single-port surgery, larger and multiple myomas may pose increased technical difficulty, operative time and bleeding. Better and suitable instrumentation, skilled surgeon and improved technique may offset these difficulties. As more and more LESS myomectomies are performed, it may become a safe, feasible and effective alternative to multiport laparoscopic myomectomy in simpler cases without compromising on the principles of surgery.

■ REFERENCES

1. Cramer DW. Epidemiology of myomas. Semin Reprod Endocrinol. 1992;10:320-4.
2. Cramer SF, Patel A. The frequency of uterine leiomyoma. Am J Clin Pathol. 1990;94:435-8.
3. Guarnaccia M, Rein M. Traditional surgical approaches to uterine fibroids: abdominal myomectomy and hysterectomy. Clin Obstet Gynecol. 2001;44:385-400.
4. Alessandri F, Lijoi D, Mistrangelo E, et al. Randomized study of laparoscopy versus minilaparotomic myomectomy for uterine myomas. J Minim Invasive Gynecol. 2006;13:92-7.
5. Palomba S, Zupi E, Falbo A, et al. A multicenter randomized, controlled study comparing laparoscopic versus minilaparotomic myomectomy: short-term outcomes. Fertil Steril. 2007;88:942-51.
6. Prapas Y, Kalogiannidis I, Prapas N. Laparoscopy vs. laparoscopically assisted myomectomy in the management of uterine myomas: a prospective study. Am J Obstet Gynecol. 2009;200:144-6.
7. Jon I. Einarsson Single-Incision Laparoscopic Myomectomy, Journal of Minimally Invasive Gynecology. 2010;17:371-3.
8. Yong-Wook Kim, Byung-Joon Park, Duck-Yeong Ro, et al. Single-Port Laparoscopic Myomectomy Using a New Single-Port Transumbilical Morcellation System: Initial Clinical Study, Journal of Minimally Invasive Gynecology. 2010;17:587-92.
9. Craig Sobolewski, Patrick P Yeung Jr, Stuart Hart. Laparoendoscopic single-site surgery in gynecology. Obstet Gynecol Clin N Am. 2011; 38:741-5.
10. Yuen LT, Hsu LJ, Lee CL, et al. A modified suture technique for laparoscopic myomectomy. J Minim Invasive Gynecol. 2007;14:318-23.
11. Alessandri F, Remorgida V, Venturini PL, et al. Unidirectional barbed suture versus continuous suture with intracorporeal knots in laparoscopic myomectomy: A randomized study. J Minim Invasive Gynecol. 2010.
12. Greenberg JA, Einarsson JI. The use of bidirectional barbed suture in laparoscopic myomectomy and total laparoscopic hysterectomy. J Minim Invasive Gynecol. 2008;15:621-3.
13. JI Einarsson, NR Chavan, Y Suzuki, et al. Use of Bidirectional Barbed Suture in Laparoscopic Myomectomy: Evaluation of Perioperative Outcomes, Safety, and Efficacy, Journal of Minimally Invasive Gynecology. 2011;18:92-5. 2010 AAGL.
14. Franco Alessandri, Valentino Remorgida, Pier Luigi Venturini, et al. Unidirectional Barbed Suture versus Continuous Suture with Intracorporeal Knots in Laparoscopic Myomectomy: A Randomized Study, Journal of Minimally Invasive Gynecology. 2010;17:725-9.
15. Escobar PF, Fader AN, Paraiso MF, et al. Robotic-assisted laparoendoscopic single-site surgery in gynecology: initial report and technique. J Minim Invasive Gynecol. 2009;16(5):589-91.
16. Leung JC. Barbed suture technology: recent advances. MedicalTextiles: Proceedings of the 149th International Conference and Exhibition. Pittsburgh, PA: October 26-27;62-80.
17. Rashid RM, Sartori M, White LE, et al. Breaking strength of barbed polypropylene sutures: rater-blinded, controlled comparison with nonbarbed sutures of various calibers. Arch Dermatol. 2007;143:869-72.
18. Rodeheaver GT, Pineros-Fernandez A, et al. Barbed sutures for wound closure: in vivo wound security, tissue compatibility and cosmesis measurements. Society for Biomaterials 30th Annual Meeting Transactions. 2004;229:232.
19. Greenberg JA, Einarsson JI. The use of bidirectional barbed suture in laparoscopic myomectomy and total laparoscopic hysterectomy. J Minim Invasive Gynecol. 2008;15:621-3.
20. Moran ME, Marsh C, Perrotti M. Bidirectional-barbed sutured knotless running anastomosis v classic Van Velthoven suturing in a model system. J Endourol. 2007;21:1175-8.
21. Jon I Einarsson, Anna T Grazul-Bilska, Kimberly A. Vonnahme, Barbed vs. Standard Suture: Randomized Single-Blinded Comparison of Adhesion Formation and Ease of Use in an Animal Model, Journal of Minimally Invasive Gynecology. 2011;18:716-9.
22. Dubuisson JB, Chapron C. Laparoscopic myomectomy today. A good technique when correctly indicated. Hum Reprod. 1996;11:934-5.
23. Dubuisson JB, Fauconnier A, Deffarges JV, et al. Pregnancy outcome and deliveries following laparoscopic myomectomy. Hum Reprod. 2000;15:869-73.
24. Parker WH, Einarsson J, Istre O, et al. Risk factors for uterine rupture after laparoscopic myomectomy. J Minim Invasive Gynecol. 2010;17:551-4.
25. Mais V, Ajossa S, Guerriero S, et al. Laparoscopic versus abdominal myomectomy: a prospective, randomized trial to evaluate benefits in early outcome. Am J Obstet Gynecol. 1996;174:654-8.
26. Parker WH, Rodi IA. Patient selection for laparoscopic myomectomy. J Am Assoc Gynecol Laparosc. 1994;2:23-6.

CHAPTER 15

Total Laparoscopic Hysterectomy (TLH) in Fibroid Uterus

● Sanjay Patel

Today, laparoscopic hysterectomy is a safe and feasible technique to manage fibroids as it offers minimal postoperative discomfort, shorter hospital stay , rapid convalescence and early return to the activities of daily living. The rationale for total laparoscopic hysterectomy (TLH) is to convert abdominal hysterectomy into a laparoscopic procedure and thereby reduce trauma and morbidity.

■ TYPES OF FIBROID ENCOUNTERED DURING TLH (Figs 15.1 to 15.5)

The difficulties with enlarged uterus are limited access to uterine pedicle, injury to ureter and bowel during dissection depending on size and location of myoma and high risk complication such as bleeding.

Operative theatre (OT) table should be in Trendelenburg position with 30° of angulation. The legs are kept in Lloyd-Davies position (Fig. 15.6), so that the thighs are almost in a straight line with the abdomen.

The patient's buttocks should protrude over the edge of the table to allow good uterine manipulation.

The table should be lowered to the minimum possible height, so that operator's elbows touch his hip to give better control of finer movements.

Veress needle is placed through umbilicus or Palmer's point, after assessing size of uterus. After insufflation with carbondioxide, 10mm trocar may inserted supraumbilically (Fig. 15.7) or at the Palmer point (a point 3 cm below the left costal margin in the midclavicular line).

Entry under vision avoids injury to vessels. This also help to place port at variable site depending on size and site of fibroid.

The pelvis and abdomen are inspected. The size, site and number of myomas are assessed. Sometimes, injection

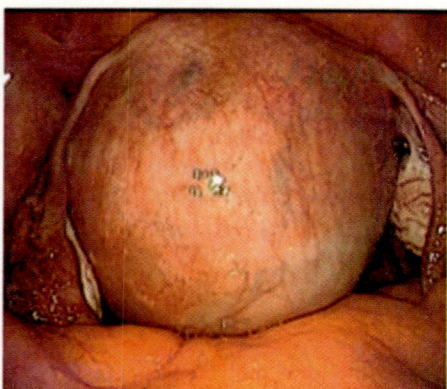

Fig. 15.1: Fibroid uterus

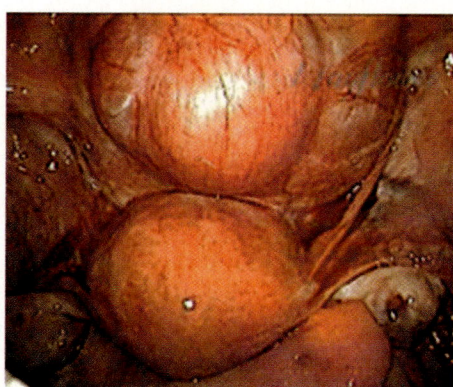

Fig. 15.2: Cervical fibroid uterus

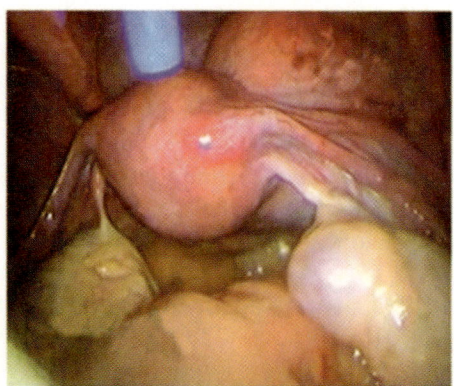

Fig. 15.3: Broad ligament fibroid uterus

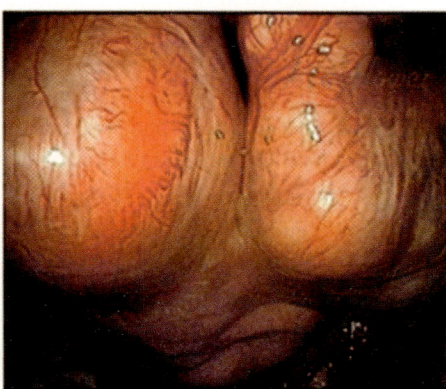

Fig. 15.4: Multiple fibroid uterus

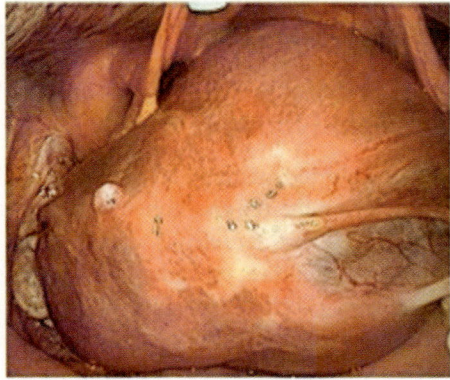

Fig. 15.5: Huge fibroid uterus

Laparoscopic use of tenaculum or myoma screw are also helpful.

The ascending branch of the uterine artery is identified close to the isthmus. Posterior fold of broad ligament is dissected up to uterosacral ligament. A reevaluation of the route of dissection is advised if fat is encountered because the fat belongs to the bladder (Fig. 15.11).

Next, the vesicouterine peritoneal fold is identified (Fig. 15.12) and the dissection is continued anteriorly, thereby

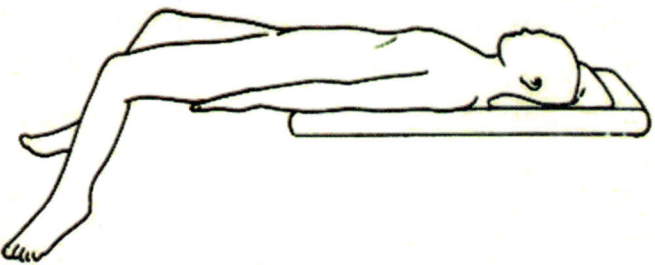

Fig. 15.6: Patient positioning for total laparoscopic hysterectomy

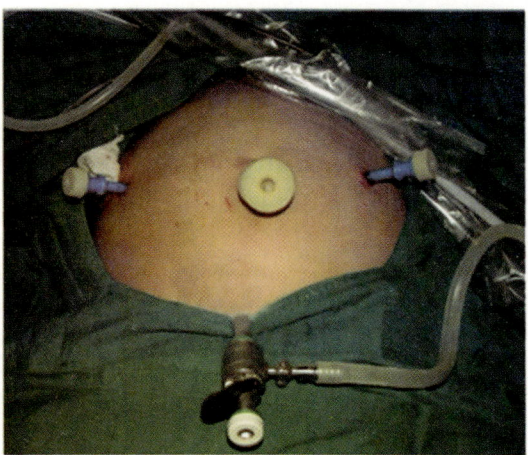

Fig. 15.7: Port placement for total laparoscopic hysterectomy

vasopressin is helpful to control bleeding during debulking procedure. However it is to be avoided in hypertension and heart disease.

Bilateral salpingectomy (Fig. 15.8) done with special care taken to avoid damage to subtubal vessels. Bilateral upper pedicles are dessicated (Fig. 15.9) and cut using Harmonic scalpel. Broad ligament is opened and anterior and posterior folds are dissected. During this step of the procedure, the uterine manipulator (Fig. 15.10) is being pushed upwards and to the contralateral side to provide maximal visualisation.

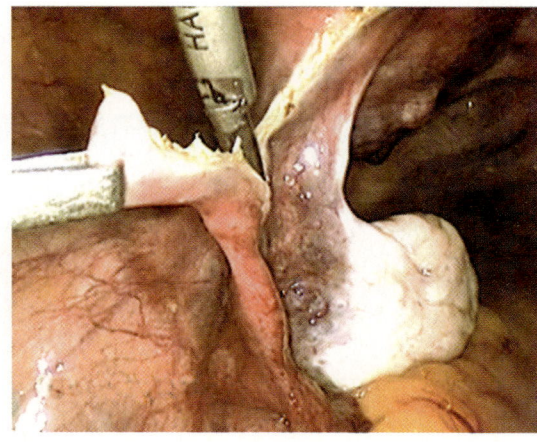

Fig. 15.8: Bilateral salpingectomy

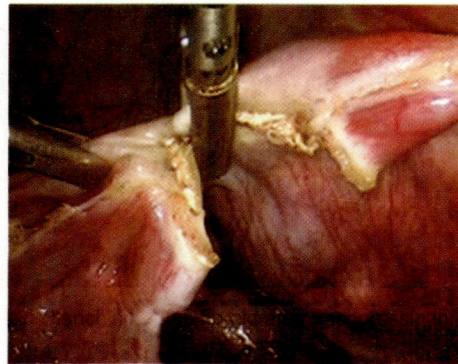

Fig. 15.9: Dessication of upper pedicles

mobilizing the bladder off the lower uterine segment. It is important to stay in the loose areolar tissue as much as possible.

Uterine artery is coagulated and dissected through Ligasure (Fig. 15.13). It is important to take the uterine vessels high and then dissect medially to the uterine vessels down to the cervix. This averts ureteral injury and provides a healthy vascular pedicle that can be safely desiccated further in the event of bleeding. The uterosacral ligaments are then coagulated and sectioned (Fig. 15.14), thus favouring lateralisation of the ureter from the uterus.

Cardinal ligaments are dessicated and cut. The harmonic scalpel is then used to cut circumferentially around the cervix and vaginal vault is opened (Fig. 15.15). The specimen is detached completely.

Specimen is retrived vaginally. In case of uterus more than normal size, vaginal morcellation is useful. The vaginal vault is then sutured with No.1 Vicryl or V-LOC (Fig. 15.16). The pelvis is irrigated and haemostasis attained perfectly. We modify our techniques in different cases as described further.

◼ TLH APPROACH IN DIFFERENT CASES

Multiple Uterine Fibroids (Figs 15.17A to K)

1. Injecting dilute vasopressin (1:200 normal saline) subserosally prior to applying traction to the uterus. This

can reduce bleeding associated with pulling and tearing of the uterine serosa (refer Fig. 15.17 B).
2. In multiple and pedunculated fibroids, myomectomy improves exposure for hysterectomy (refer Figs 15.17 C and D).
3. To minimise bleeding, uterine artery ligation at its origin in pararactal space is helpful prior to hysterectomy (refer Figs 15.17F to K).

Fibroid with Lower Segment Caesarian Section (Figs 15.18A to I)

1. Adhesiolysis for omental adhesion to anterior abdominal wall is best done by using harmonic scalpel (refer Fig. 15.18A) but in cases of bowel adhesions sharp scissors (Figs 15.18B and C) is the best tool.
2. Lateral window technique: Dense adhesions and fibrosis are usually observed in the midline anteriorly at the level of the uterovesical fold and any attempt to push the bladder down on the midline can cause unintentional bladder injuries. A safer approach is from the lateral portion of the cervix. In this area, adhesions are less dense and firm, and the bladder is not in direct contact with the cervix. This plane is always above the level of the uterine vessels. The lateral approach creates a surgical window that enables safe and sharp dissection laparoscopically (refer Figs 15.18D to H).
3. Intra-operative cystoscopic (refer Fig. 15.18I) examination was performed to rule out bladder injuries. Fill the bladder retrograde to check for leaks and bladder margins.

Broad Ligament Fibroid (Figs 15.19A to K)

1. In severely distorted anatomy (refer Figs 15.19A and B) consider entering the retroperitoneum sooner rather than later. The course of the ureter is traced at the beginning and at the end of the procedure. Make a peritoneal incision at pelvic brim between ureter and infudibulo-pelvic ligament. Extend peritoneal incision. Develop the

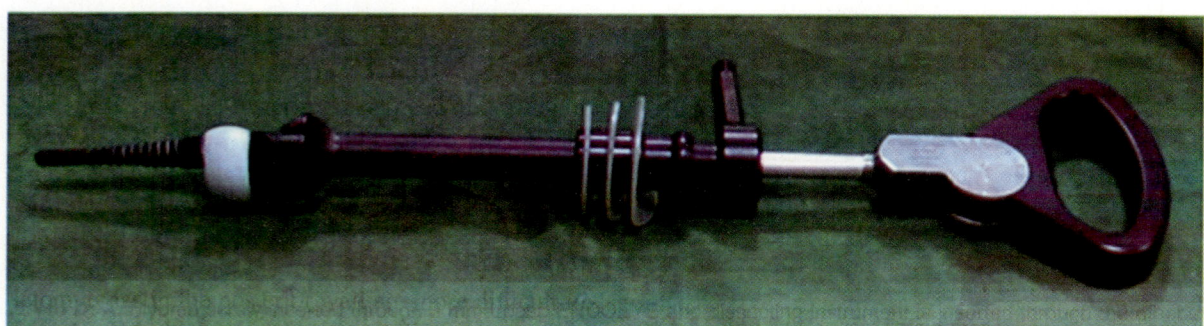

Fig. 15.10: Uterine manipulator

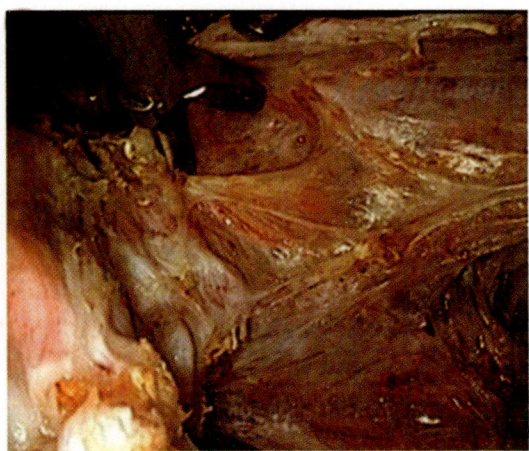

Fig. 15.11: Careful dissection of fat planes during bladder dissection

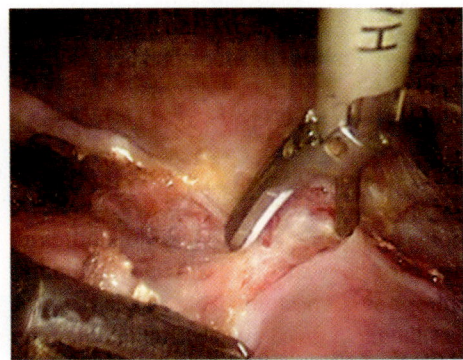

Fig. 15.12: Identification of uterovesical fold

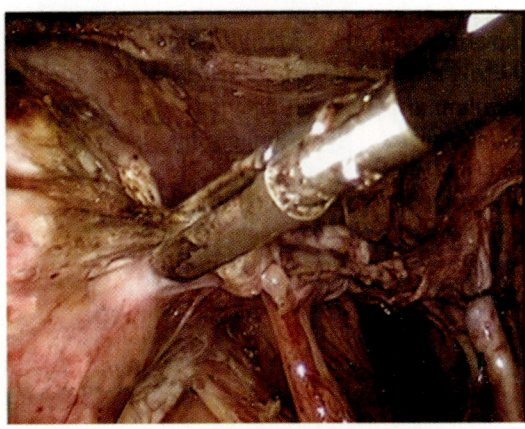

Fig. 15.13: Uterine artery coagulation

Cervical Fibroid (Figs 15.20A to L)

1. The course of the ureter is confirmed with special attention given to the uterosacral ligament attachments, to determine the displacement in the relative position of the uterine arteries or ureter. At times when the myoma is large and boundaries difficult to confirm, the broad ligament is opened with an anterior approach to delineate the myoma (refer Fig. 15.20D)

2. In case of an anterior wall type, a transverse incision is made in the uterovesical pouch and peritoneum, to

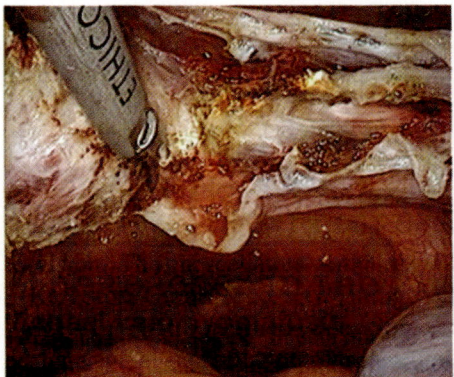

Fig. 15.14: Coagulation of uterosacral ligaments

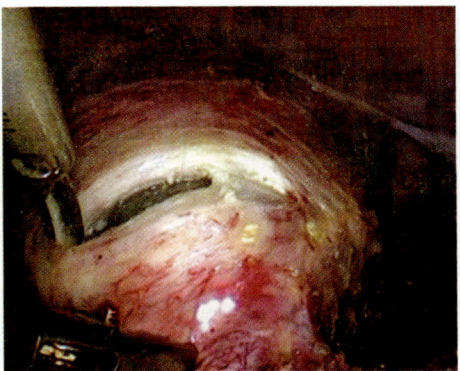

Fig. 15.15: Opening of vault using harmonic

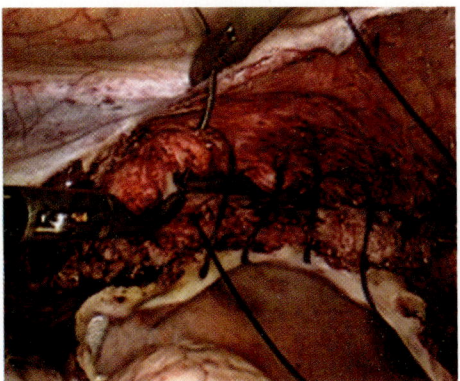

Fig. 15.16: Vault suturing

pararectal space. Identify all borders of pararectal and prevesical space (refer Figs 15.19C to I).

2. Uterine artery always crosses above the ureter (water under the bridge).

3. Internal iliac artery ligation is also helpful to minimize bleeding as pulse pressure is reduced up to 85% allowing haemostasis and clot formation (refer Figs 15.19J and K).

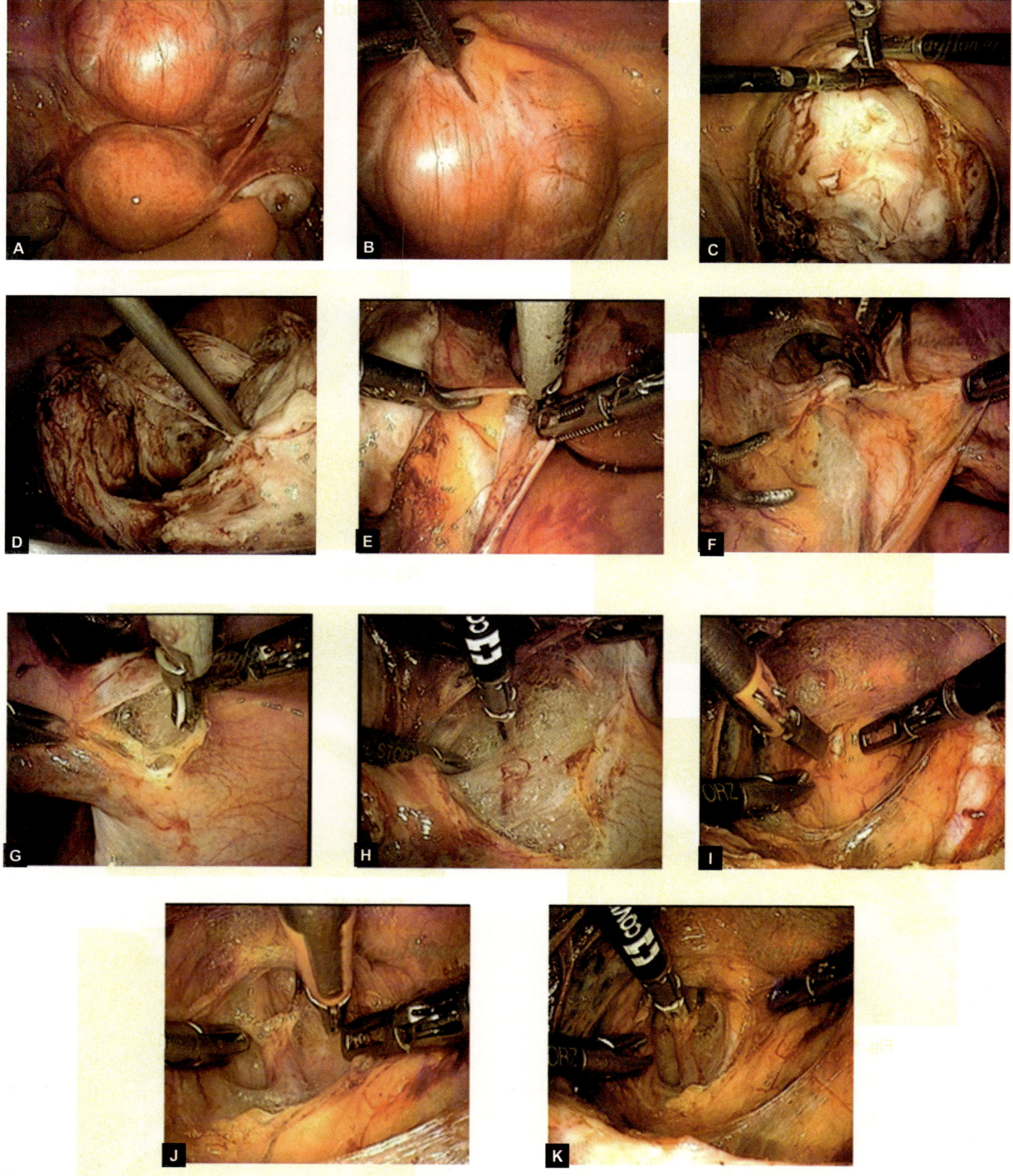

Figs 15.17A to K: Step by step total laparoscopic hysterectomy of uterus with multiple fibroids

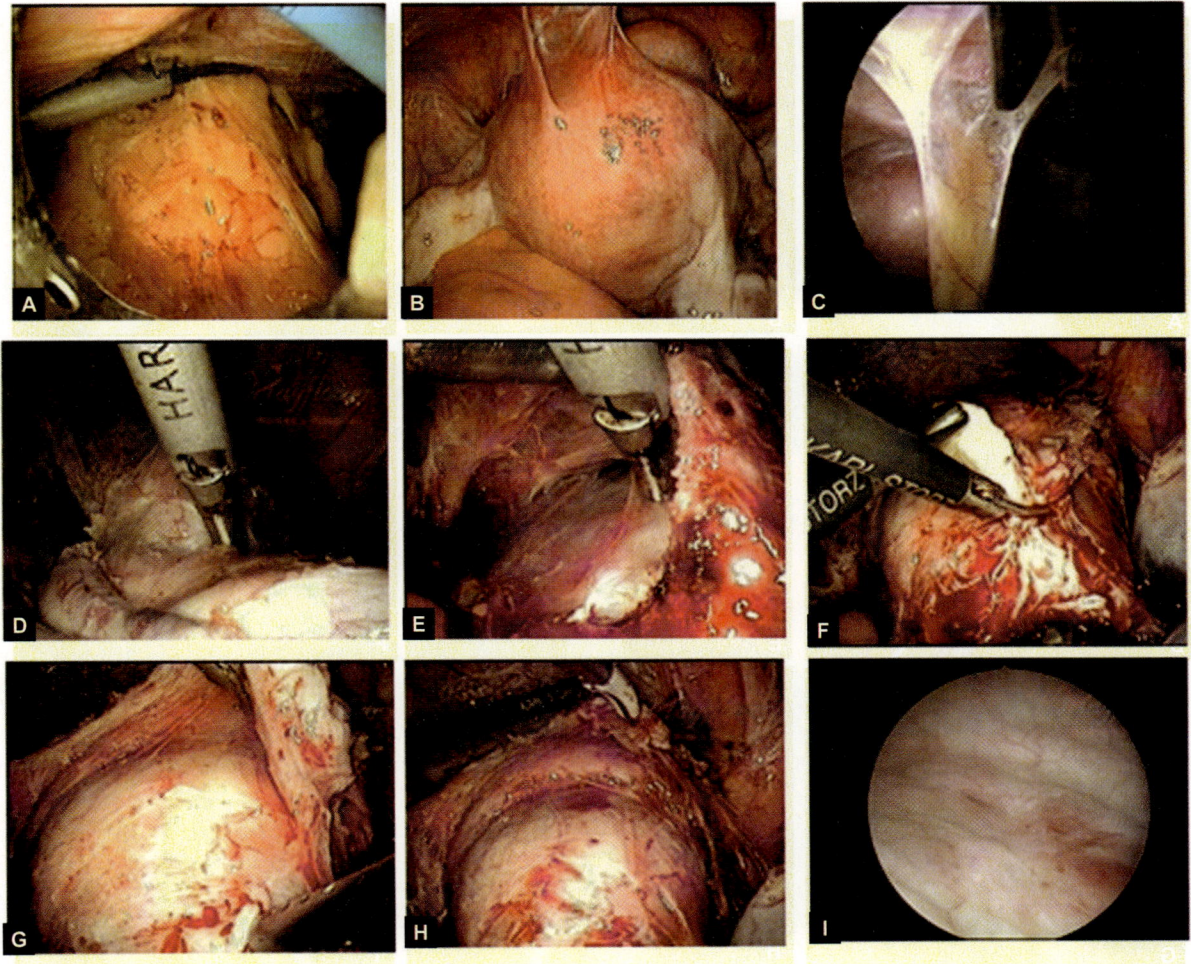

Figs 15.18A to I: Fibroid with LSCS

perform a blunt dissection of the bladder. In case of posterior myomas we prefer a midline vertical incision to avoid injuring the vessels and to stay at a safe distance from the ureter.

3. Prior identification of the ureters with either retroperitoneal dissection or preprocedure cystoscopic ureteric stenting or fibreoptic catheterisation (refer Fig. 15.20L) may be of help in selected cases of very large cervical myomas with lateral projection.

Fibroid with Endometriosis (Figs 15.21A to O)

1. Bowel preparation: Failing to prepare the bowel preoperatively may result in increased risk and limit the surgeons ability to perform a satisfactory resection.

2. It is important to do adhesiolysis (Figs 15.21C to F) first, restore the anatomy to normal as much as it is possible. In difficult cases it is usually easier to start the dissection from lateral aspect and then proceed medially rather than other way round.

3. Medial displacement of the ureter and its prominence may cause misidentification as a uterosacral ligament. This puts the ureter at increased risk if it is not identified. The ureter can be tracked (refer Fig. 15.21M) down from pelvic brim till the uterosacral ligament. If an apparent uterosacral ligament goes over the pelvic brim, it is the ureter and not the uterosacral.

4. Colorectal nodule: It is caused by infiltration of the uterosacral ligaments and rectovaginal septum by endometriotic nodules (refer Figs 15.21I to K).

Huge Fibroid (Figs 15.22A to G)

1. Lateral ports are placed at higher position. Low port placement is for better instrument control. The uterus is released from side walls (Figs 15.22A to C). Vertically grown uterus up to 32 to 34 weeks size having space laterally and pedunculated fibroid can be operated laparoscopically.

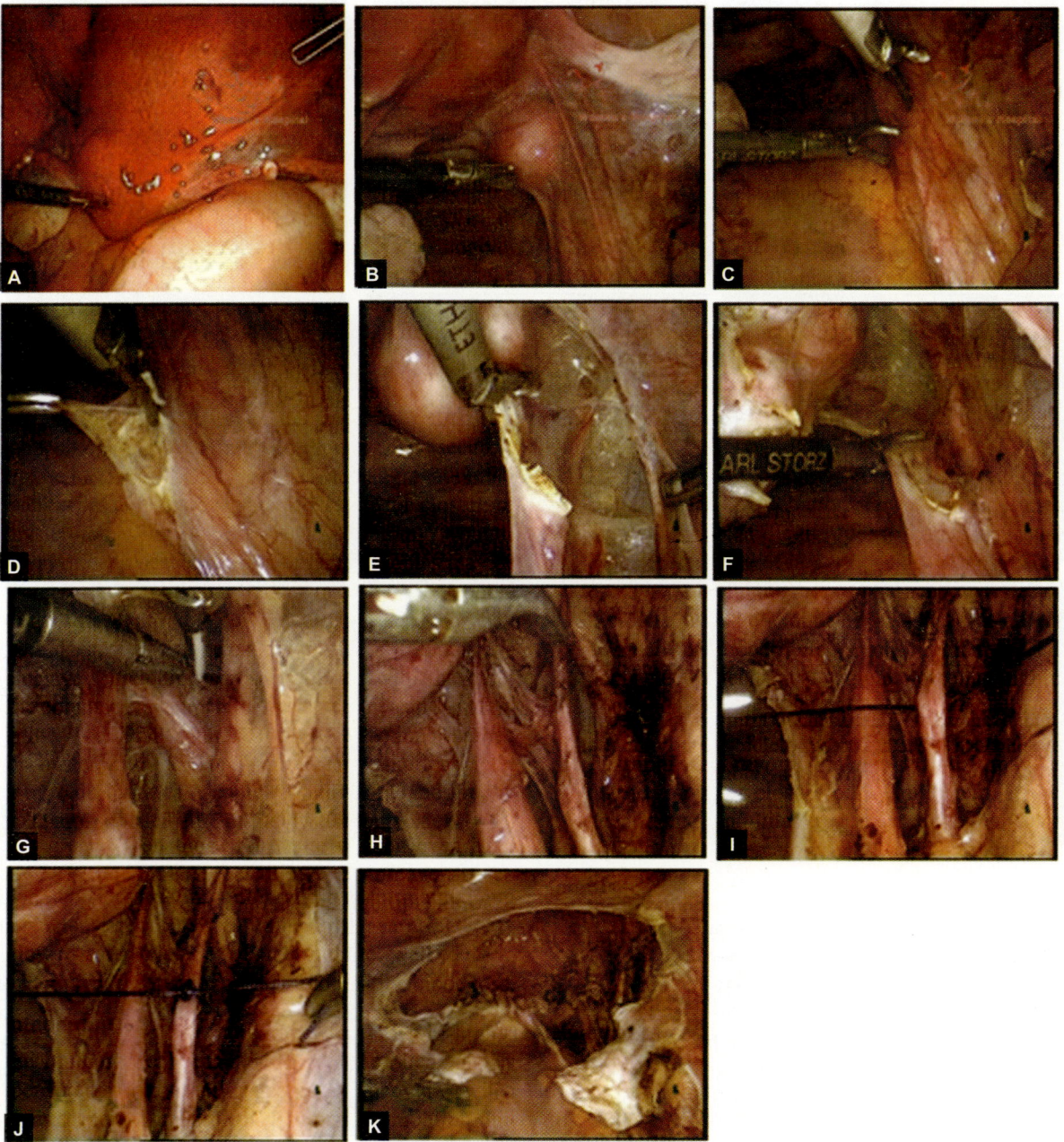

Figs 15.19A to K: Broad ligament fibroid

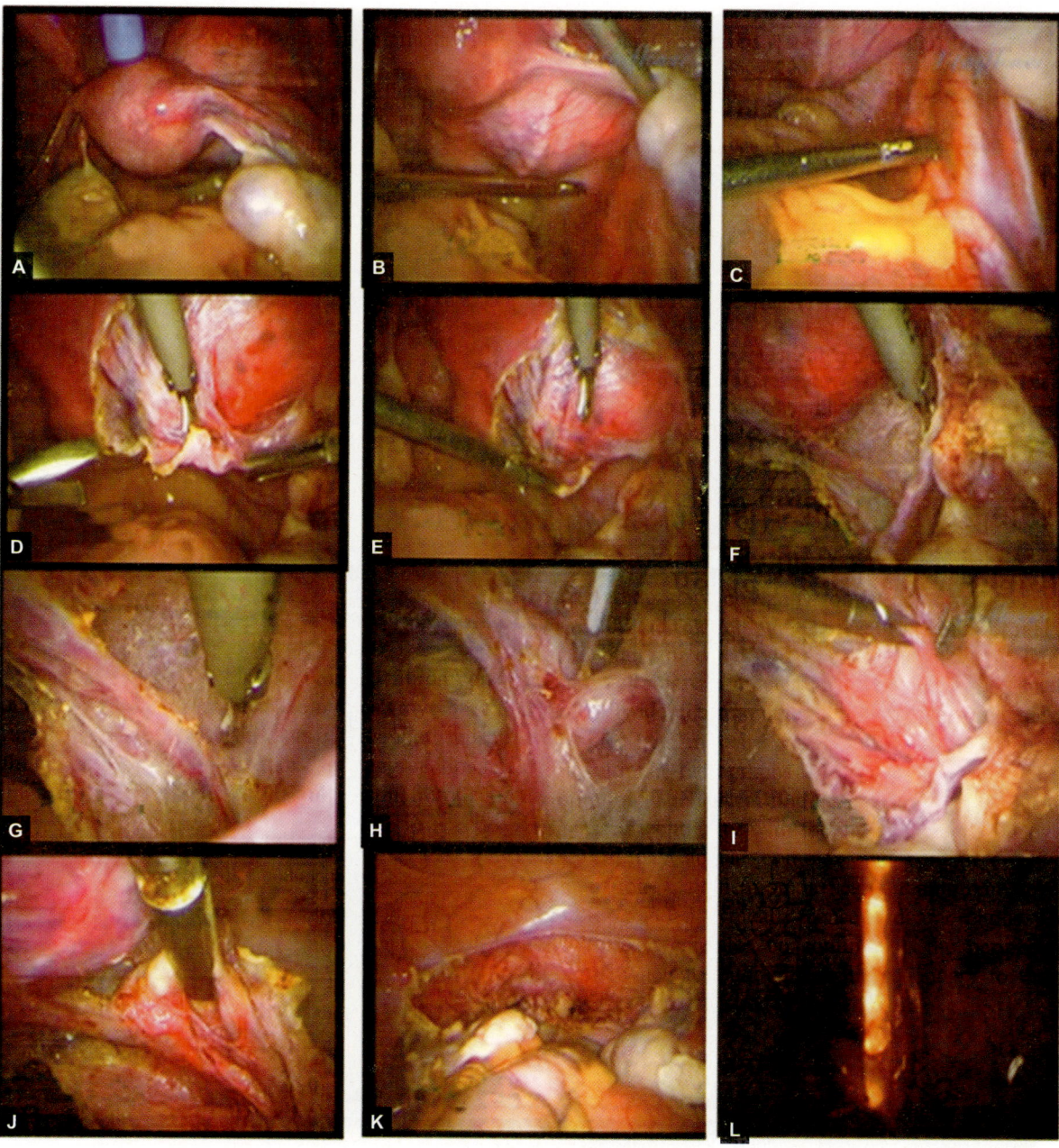

Figs 15.20A to L: Cervical fibroid

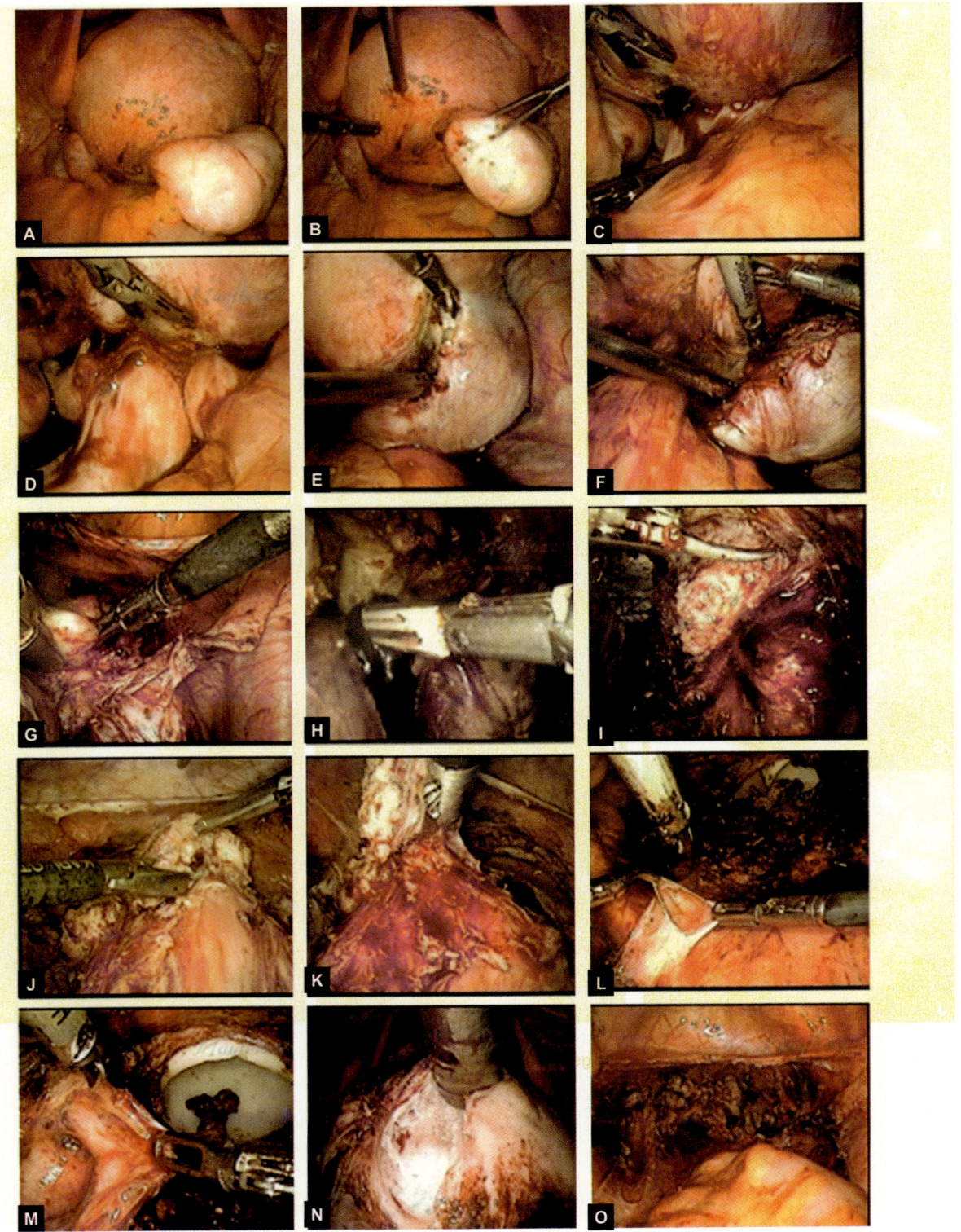

Figs 15.21A to O: Fibroid with endometriosis

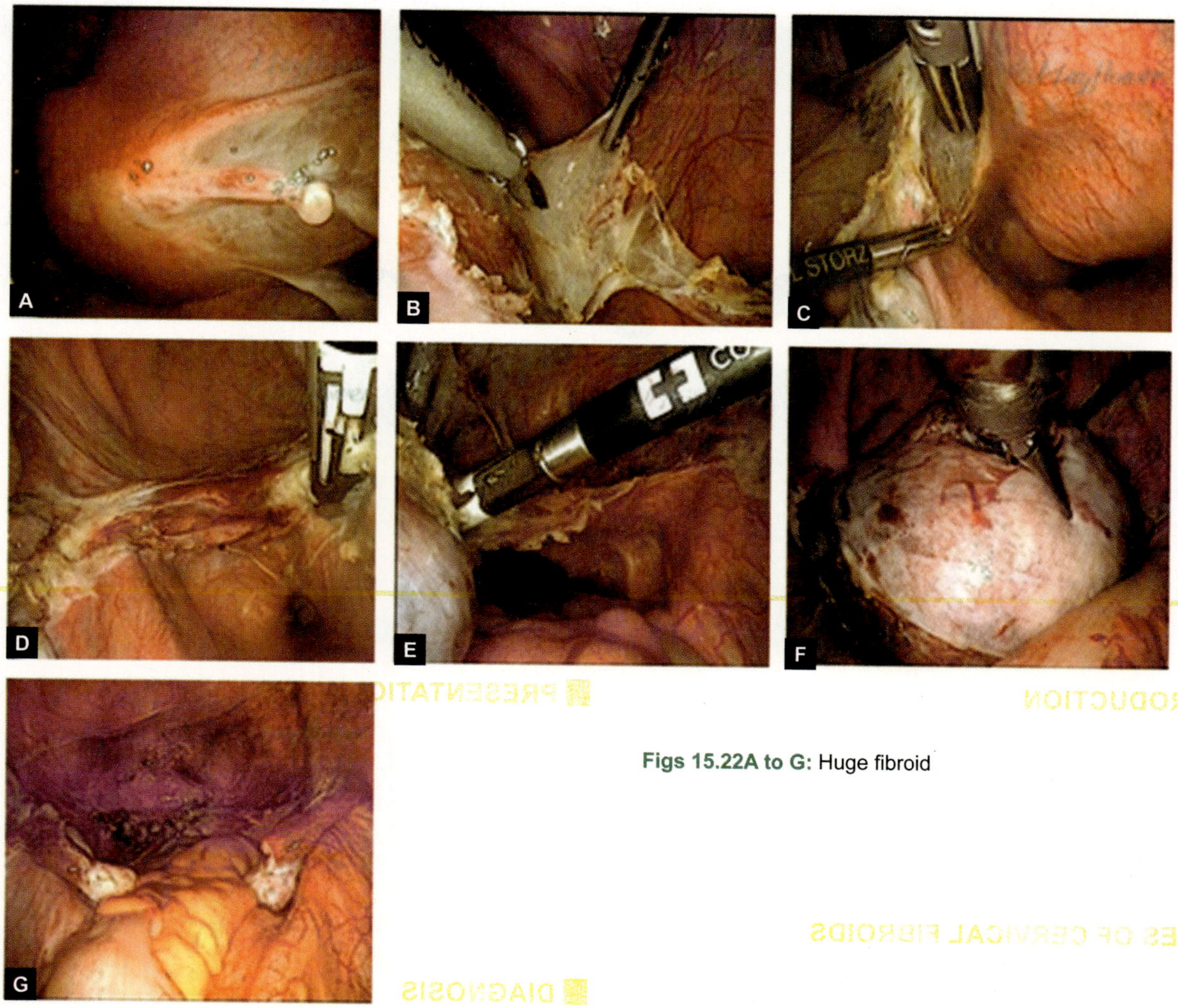

Figs 15.22A to G: Huge fibroid

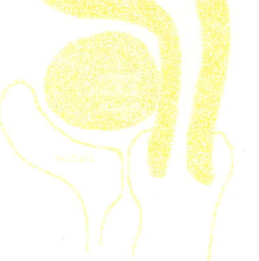

2. Both uterine arteries are sealed before transection (refer Figs 15.22D and E)
3. Debulking specimen in-situ with morcellator (refer Fig. 15.22F) with endobag is also helpful in huge fibroid.

■ CONCLUSION

Total laparoscopic hysterectomy is a technically feasible procedure. It can be performed by experienced surgeons for large uteri regardless of the size , number or location of the myomas. The mean blood loss was significantly less for the laparoscopic hysterectomy.

A major concern is that such distortions as well as the poor exposure may increase the risk of bladder, ureteric and bowel injury. We encountered ureteric injury in two cases of endometriosis and colonic injury in one case of endometriosis. In skilled hands, these patients could benefit all the advantages related to minimally invasive approach such as minimal blood loss, short hospital stay, prompt recovery, obtaining a satisfactory result.

CHAPTER 16

Management of Cervical Fibroid

● Shanthala Thuppanna

■ INTRODUCTION

Uterine leiomyomas are the commonest smooth muscle tumour of the uterus, they are clinically evident in 20%–30% of women over 30 years of age, and are found in about 70% of women by the age of 50 years. After menopause they usually decrease in size.[1]

■ TYPES OF CERVICAL FIBROIDS

About 95% of myomas occur in the uterine corpus, and cervical myomas account for less than 5% of uterine myoma. Cervical myoma are mainly classified into those that occur on the subserosa (extracervical type) and those that occur within the cervix (intracervical type)[2] (Fig. 16.1). They can grow anteriorly (Fig. 16.2), posteriorly, (Fig. 16.3) laterally or central.

■ PRESENTATION

Cervical fibroids can be asymptomatic or can cause symptoms like bleeding, pelvic pain and infertility.

In case of anterior cervical fibroid retention of urine or frequency of urine, rectal symptom like constipation in case of posterior cervical fibroids. In case of intravaginal cervical fibroid, woman may suffer with foul-smelling vaginal discharge with feeling of something coming out.

■ DIAGNOSIS

Occasionally, on speculum examination infravaginal intracervical fibroids can be seen, if it is protruding from external os.

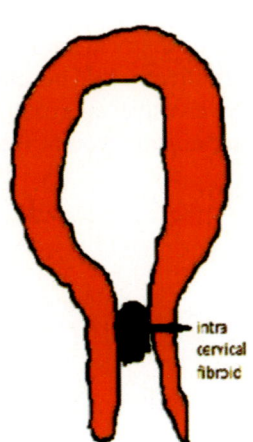

Fig. 16.1: Intracervical fibroid

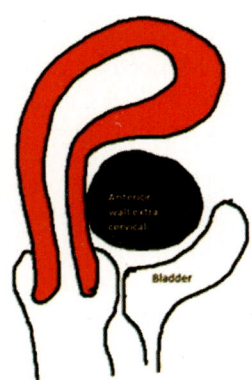

Fig. 16.2: Anterior wall extracervical

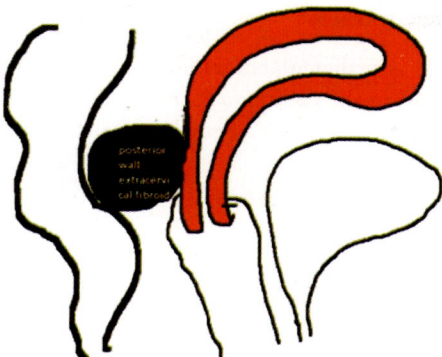

Fig. 16.3: Posterior wall extracervical fibroid

Ultrasonography

Transvaginal scans are more sensitive for the diagnosis, cervical fibroids are usually clearly visible under transvaginal ultrasound, but can be difficult to differentiate from polyps.

Magnetic Resonance Imaging

Magnetic resonance imaging (MRI) (Figs 16.4 and 16.5) is not generally required for diagnosis, except for complex cases. It is however the most accurate modality for detecting, localizing and characterizing fibroids.

■ PREOPERATIVE WORK UP

As a routine all blood investigations should be done. Various methods are followed to reduce the blood supply to the uterus during surgery. This helps in correcting anaemia also.

The reported reduction of uterine volume with the use of a pre-operative gonadotropin-releasing hormone (GnRH) agonist for 3 to 4 month ranges between 35% and 65%, though larger myomas appear to experience a greater reduction in size than smaller ones. It shortens the duration of surgery and blood loss.[3]

Use of GnRh agonist is also restricted by its adverse effects like, delay in definitive surgery, loss of surgical planes, missing of small fibroids and menopausal symptoms.[4]

Diagnostic hysteroscopy performed before planning corrective surgery especially helps to take decision to go ahead with hysteroscopic or laparoscopic approach in case of intracervical fibroid.

■ SURGICAL MANAGEMENT

Either myomectomy or hysterectomy for cervical fibroids is more challenging compared to myomas at the corpus. Cervical fibroids will distort the normal anatomy of the bladder, ureter, blood vessels and rectum making it more complicated for dissection and for suturing.

There are very few reported studies regarding cervical fibroid management, the largest study reported to have 28 cases.[5,6]

Methods to Minimize the Bleeding

Uterine Artery Ligation

Uterine artery ligation has been done routinely by many surgeons. Uterine artery ligation (Fig. 16.6) is done by dissecting the triangle enclosed by the round ligament, external iliac artery, and infundibulopelvic ligament. The ligation is done at the origin of the uterine artery, after identifying the internal iliac vessels, ureter and its relation to the uterine artery to prevent inadvertent ligation.[7,8]

Endovascular Balloon Occlusion

In one study temporary endovascular balloon occlusion of the bilateral internal iliac arteries for control of haemorrhage was done in order to avoid negative effect of permanent uterine artery ligation on ovary and uterus. This is done in a radiology suite by radiologist under fluoroscopic guidance. The bilateral internal iliac arteries were temporally occluded by inflation

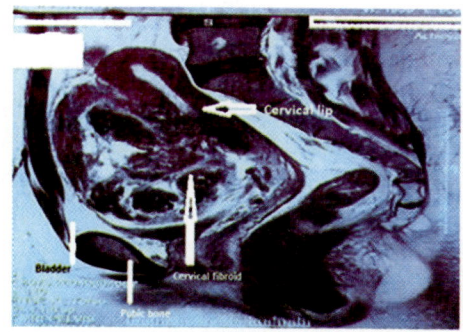

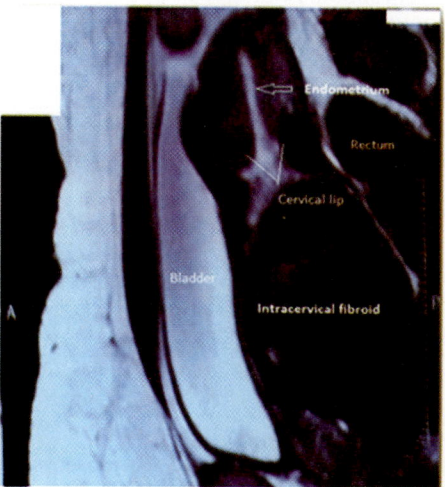

Figs 16.4A and B: A. MRI showing cervical fibroid; **B.** MRI showing cervical fibroid

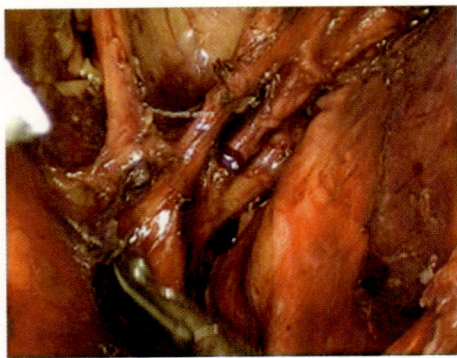

Fig. 16.5: Uterine artery ligation

of the occlusion balloons. The sheaths and deflated balloon catheter were left in place.

Clipping of the Uterine Artery

Clipping of the uterine artery is done after identifying the uterine artery at the origin, blood flow can be reopened so the restoration of blood supply is good for the ovary and uterus. Clipping is therefore effective in controlling the amount of blood loss in patients with myoma who desire to have children.[9]

Vasopressin

Vasopressin has a dual role in normal homeostasis. Its largest role involves regulation of extracellular fluid osmolality. Through a completely different mechanism, it also affects volume and pressure regulation.[10]

Activation of receptor by vasopressin results in vasoconstriction of the vessels and contraction of smooth muscle.[11–14]

Vasopressin should be diluted before use. Tissue infiltration will aid in dissection, higher dilutions should be used to increase the amount of fluid administered (e.g. 20 U in 100 mL saline solution). Almost universally, a total dose of no more than 4 to 6 U was used.[15] The biggest concern about the use of vasopressin is its effects on cardiovascular system.

■ OPERATIVE PROCEDURE

Surgery for cervical fibroids (Fig. 16.6) is removal of uterus or removal of the fibroid to preserve the fertility. In case of extracervical fibroids, abdominal route is chosen, only dilemma is in case of intracervical fibroids when we want to preserve the uterus. There is no defined strategy for removal of intracervical fibroids, various techniques followed are vaginal twisting of fibroid pedicle, hysteroscopic resection of fibroid and even uterine artery embolisation. In this chapter, we are concentrating on the laparoscopic approach.

Vaginal Approach

If the fibroid is pedunculated and its base is seen clearly we may try avulsing the pedicle or can ligate with No. 1 or 1-0 delayed absorbable suture and can take it out vaginally.

Hysteroscopic Approach

Hyteroscopic removal is a good option, if we have good vision. If the fibroid is huge, getting the distension and vision may be difficult. Hysteroscopic resection is done with monopolar resectoscope with electrolyte free media or with bipolar resectoscope with normal saline. It is very difficult to mention up to what size intracervical fibroid can be removed hysteroscopically, as it depends on surgeon's expertise.

Abdominal Approach

Depending on the size, visibility and surgeons expertise, we can decide about hysteroscopic or laparoscopic approach.

Surgery is performed under general anaesthesia with endotracheal intubation with modified lithotomy position. Pneumoperitoneum is created by closed method intraumbilically in case of no previous surgeries and normal size uterus. Palmers point is chosen in case there are any previous scars suspecting adhesions and when uterus is huge.[16–19]

If palmer point is used for the pneumoperitoneum, then the 5 mm trocar is inserted blindly and 5 mm scope is inserted and after inspecting the pelvis, the upper abdomen and the entry point, remaining ports are inserted under direct visualisation in adhesion-free safe entry site to avoid complications. The 10 mm port is inserted in umbilical or supraumbilical area depending on the size of the fibroid and adhesions.[20]

After primary and secondary port insertion, inspection of the uterus, adnexa and relation of fibroid to the other important structures like ureter, bladder and the uterine vessels are noted. Cervix is dilated and the manipulator/Hegar's dilator can be used for uterine manipulation. Type of the incision and dissection depends on the site of the fibroid.

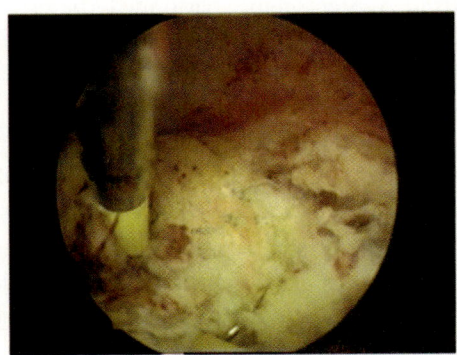

Fig. 16.6: Cervical fibroid

Intracervical Fibroids

Intracervical fibroids, which are huge and cannot be resected hysteroscopically are approached laparoscopically. The anterior incision is preferred because its very difficult to extend incision posteriorly, uterovesical fold of peritoneum is identified and separated from the lower uterine segment, (Fig. 16.7). Usually in cervical fibroids uterovesical fold of peritoneum is loose and it is dissected very easily.

Vasopressin is injected in the cervix where maximum fibroid bulge is seen. We prefer to go for transverse incision with 5 mm harmonic scalpel, alternatively we can use monopolar hook with blended mode for incision. Incision can be decided intraoperatively depending on how far we are from important structures, which will be decided by the fibroid size and position. Once we reach fibroid, 5 mm myoma spiral is used for traction, pedicle is detached, with harmonic scalpel (Fig. 16.8). in case of broad pedicle, we can ligate to avoid bleeding and fibroid is detached.

If the anatomy is difficult and if expecting severe bleeding, uterine artery can be ligated/clipped by opening the broad ligament. We routinely do not ligate uterine artery. Cervix is closed with no. 1 delayed absorbable suture with figure of 8 after excluding the cervical mucosa. After achieving haemostasis, myoma is removed by morcellation.

Extracervical Fibroids

Extracervical fibroid can be on anterior or posterior wall. In case of anterior wall fibroids, uterovesical fold of peritoneum is separated and fibroid is localised. (Figs 16.9 to 13) Vasopressin is injected, incision is given over the maximum bulge with Harmonic scalpel, after enucleating the myoma, bed is obliterated by figure of 8 no-1 delayed absorbable suture. After achieving haemostasis, fibroid is retrieved by morcellation.

In case of posterior wall cervical fibroid we must pay attention to the rectum and ureter. The preferred incision is transverse between the uterosacral ligaments. After enucleating the fibroid, myoma bed is closed with the no. 1 delayed absorbable suture with figure of 8 with one or two layer depending on the depth of base.

Hysterectomy

The difficulties which are commonly encountered are distorted anatomy of uterine artery, ureters. Also introduction of vaginal manipulators for laparoscopic hysterectomy is difficult, we use routinely myoma spiral for uterine manipulation.

In case of severely distorted anatomy, tracing the ureter and ligating the uterine artery at the origin will help to prevent unwanted complication. In extracervical fibroids we may encounter difficulty in approaching vault. in these

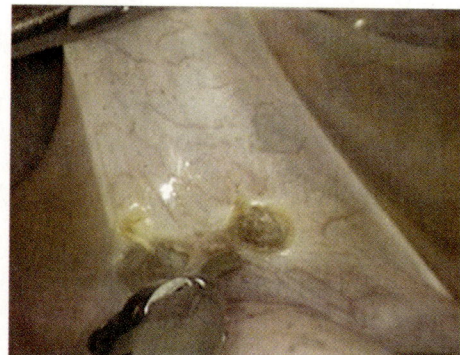

Fig. 16.7: Bladder dissection before approaching cervical fibroid

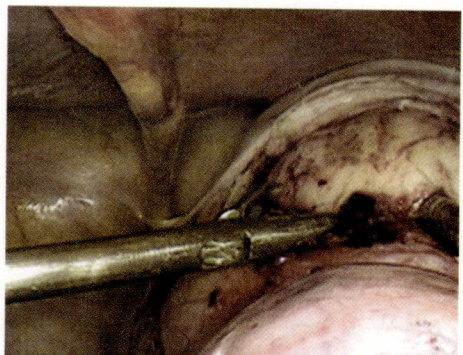

Fig 16.8: Enucleation of Intracervical Fibroid.

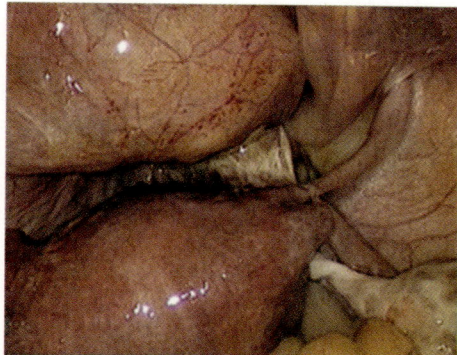

Fig. 16.9: Anterior wall cervical fibroid covered by the bladder

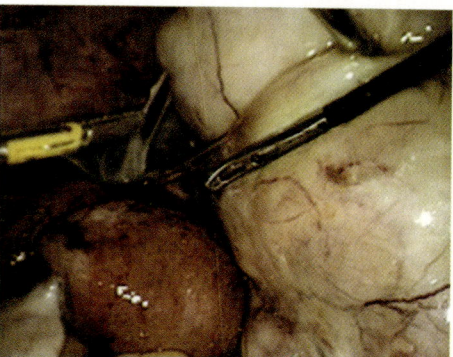

Fig. 16.10: Approaching the cervical fibroid by separation of uterocervical fold of peritoneum

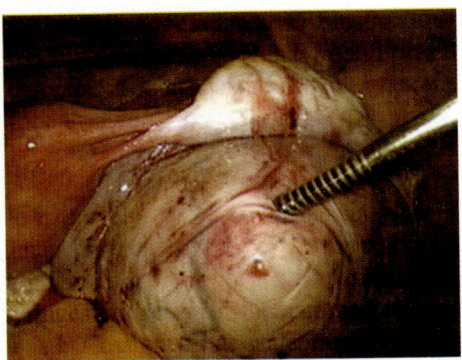

Fig. 16.11: Pseudobroad ligament fibroid

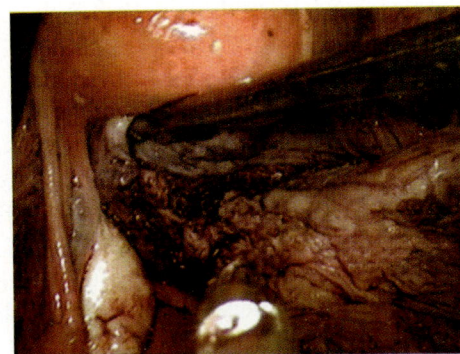

Fig. 16.12: Pseudobroad ligament originating from posterior wall of cervix

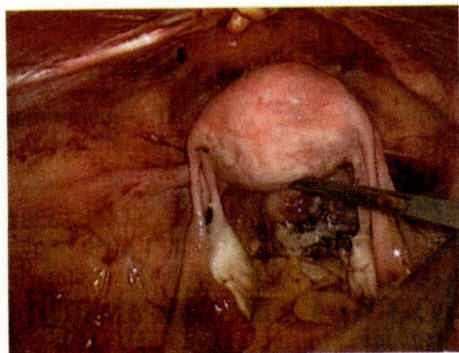

Fig. 16.13: Post enucleation of pseudo broad ligament fibroid

selected cases, fibroid needs to be removed separately before hysterectomy.

COMPLICATIONS

Complication in cervical fibroid are more common than corpus. The near relation of the cervical fibroids to the ureter, bladder, rectum and major blood vessels and the altered anatomy by cervical fibroids increases the risk of injury to these organs.

In high risk group, routine uterine artery ligation and tracing of the ureter. in some cases, stenting will reduce the bleeding complication and ureteric injuries. Routine post procedure cystoscopy in case of anterior wall cervical fibroid will help to diagnose intraoperative injuries and correction at the same sitting.

Surgical management of cervical fibroid is difficult. In view of low incidence and high complications due to distorted anatomy caused by cervical fibroids, we do or cannot have fixed strategy for all kind of cervical fibroid management. But, we can avoid the complications by proper preoperative work up like fibroid mapping (MRI), correction of anaemia.

Thorough counselling and proper informed consent of the patient (regarding complications) is essential.

Intraoperatively identification of distorted anatomy, ligation/clipping of uterine artery and tracing the ureter can reduce complications.

REFERENCES

1. Zaloudek CJ. Hendrickson MR, Soslow RA. Mesenchymal Tumors of the Uterus. In: Kurman RJ, Ellenson LH, Ronnett BM (Eds). Blaustein's Pathology of the Female Genital Tract, 6th edn. New York: Springer; 2011. pp. 455-527.
2. Hiroyuki Takeuchi MD, Mari Kitade MD, Iwaho Kikuchi MD, et al. A new enucleation method for cervical myoma via laparoscopy . Journal of Minimally Invasive Gynecology. 2006;13:334-6.
3. Vollenhoven BJ, Shekleton P, McDonald J, et al. Clinical predictors for buserelin acetate treatment of uterine fibroids: a prospective study of 40 women. Fertil Steril. 1990;54:1032-1038. 18. Lethaby A, Vollenhoven B, Sowter M. Pre-operative GnRH analogue therapy before hysterectomy and myomectomy for uterine fibroids (Cochrane Review). In: The Cochrane Library. Issue 4. Chichester, UK: John Wiley & Sons, Ltd. 2003.
4. Jacqueline N, Gutmann MD, Stephen L. Corson, MD From the Department of Obstetrics and Gynecology, Thomas Jefferson University Medical Center (both authors). Journal of Minimally Invasive Gynecology. 2005;12:529-37.
5. Taipei, Taiwan Chang WC, Chen SY, et al. Strategy of cervical myomectomy under laparoscopy.Fertil Steril. 2010;94:2710-5.
6. Shozo Matsuoka MD, Iwaho Kikuchi MD, Mari Kitade MD, et al. Strategy for Laparoscopic Cervical Myomectomy. Journal of Minimally Invasive Gynecology. 2010;17(3):301-5.
7. Burbank F, Hutchins FL. Uterine artery occlusion by embolization or surgery for the treatment of fibroids: a unifying hypothesis; transient uterine ischemia. J Am Assoc Gyneco Laparosc. 2000;7:S1-S49.
8. Rakesh Sinha MD, Meenakshi Sundaram MD, DNB*, Smita Lakhotia, MD, et al. Cervical Myomectomy with Uterine Artery Ligation at Its Origin Journal of Minimally Invasive Gynecology, 2009;16(5).
9. Shozo Matsuoka, Iwaho Kikuchi, Mari Kitade, et al. From the Department of Obstetrics and Gynecology, Juntendo University School of Medicine, Tokyo, Japan (all authors) Journal of Minimally Invasive Gynecology. 2010;17(3).
10. Robinson AG, Verbalis JG. The posterior pituitary and water metabolism. In: Larsen PR, Kronenberg HM, Melamed S, Polonsky KS (Eds). Williams Textbook of Endocrinology, 10th ed. Philadelphia, PA: WB Saunders. 1998.

11. Monarch Pharmaceuticals, Inc. Pitressin. Available at: http://www. onlinedrugtest.info/generic-pitressin-information.html. Accessed July 19, 2011.

12. Kimura T, Kusui C, Matsumura Y, et al. Effectiveness of hormonal tourniquet by vasopressin during myomectomy through vasopressin V1a receptor ubiquitously expressed in myometrium. Gynecol Obstet Invest. 2002;54:125-31

13. Maggi M, Del Carlo P, Fantoni G, et al. Human myometrium during pregnancy contains and responds to V1 vasopressin receptors as well as oxytocin receptors. J Clin Endocrinol Metab. 1990;70:1142-54.

14. Helmer H. Oxytocin and vasopressin 1a receptor gene expression in the cycling or pregnant human uterus. Am J Obstet Gynecol. 1998;179:1572-8.

15. Scott Chudnoff, Sivan Glazer, Mark Levie. Review of Vasopressin Use in Gynecologic Surgery JMIG. 19(4):422-33.

16. Omaha, Nebraska (Dr Agarwala), Chattanooga Women's Laser Center, Chattanooga, Tennessee (Dr Liu) Journal of Minimally Invasive Gynecology. 2005;12:55-61.

17. Loffer FD. Endoscopy in high-risk patients. In: Martin DC (Ed). Manual of Endoscopy. Santa Fe Springs, CA: American Association of Gynecologic Laparoscopists. 1990. p. 43.

18. McDougall E, Figenshau RS, Clayman RV. J Laparoscopic Surgery. 1994; 4:6.

19. Phillips G, Garry R, Kumar C, et al. How much gas is required for initial insufflation at laparoscopy? Gynaecol Endosc. 1999;8:369-74.

20. Audebert AJ. The role of microlaparoscopy in the diagnosis of peritoneal and visceral adhesions and in the prevention of bowel injury associated with blind trocar insertion. Fertil Steril. 2000;73:631-5. Poindexter AN, Ritter M, Fahim A, et al. Trocar introduction performed during laparoscopy of the obese patient. Surg Gynecol Obstet. 1987;165:57-9.

CHAPTER 17

Measures to Reduce Adhesions Post Myomectomy

● Manjula Anagani

■ INTRODUCTION

Leiomyoma (myoma or fibroids) are the most common monoclonal tumours of the smooth muscle cells found in the human uterus in the reproductive years.[1,2] The global prevalence of leiomyoma varies from 20% to 50%.[3–6] Myomectomy is the standard treatment for symptomatic leiomyoma in women who desire to preserve their fertility. Myomectomy can be carried out via laparoscopy, hysteroscopy, or typically as an open abdominal procedure. The postoperative adhesions are potential morbidity with considerable clinical dilemma after abdominal myomectomy, occurring in 50% to 90% of patients.[7–10] Adhesions are defined as connections between opposite serosal and/or non-serosal surfaces of the internal organs and the abdominal wall, at sites where there should be no connections. Adhesions can be vascular or avascular, filmy or transparent, dense or opaque, or it could be cohesive connections of surfaces without an intervening adhesion band.[11] The aetiology of adhesions is less clearly understood. Surgical management of adhesions is complicated by a high adhesion reformation rate (85%) irrespective of adhesiolysis method or the adhesion type.[12] Despite the conservative approach taken in SCAR study, 1 in 3 post laparotomy patients were readmitted over 10 years.[10,13] The novel surgical techniques and technologies are accessible for prevention and management of adhesions. The clinical complications of adhesions may lead to medico legal consequences for both patients and consultants. Hence adhesion prevention strategies should be the part of routine clinical practice.

■ PATHOPHYSIOLOGY

Hysteroscopic resection of fibroids involves a risk of intrauterine adhesions (IUA). However, the risk of developing intra-abdominal and IUA is very high in open abdominal myomectomy.[7–10]

Intrauterine Adhesions

While the mechanism of tissue repair in the human endometrium is poorly understood, and multiple predisposing factors are probably implicated, the trauma to the endometrium is commonly considered the major factor in the genesis of IUA.[14]

Abdominal Adhesions

At the time of laparoscopic surgery, tissue injury exposes a surface that serves for wound healing. Subsequently, it activates coagulation cascade and deposition of fibrin at site of injury. Under pathological conditions fibrin exudates provide as link between unrelated neighbouring tissues. The inflammatory cells invade the wound and surrounding area. Consequently after 72 to 96 hours, fibrinolytic system is activated which prevents fibrous attachments. The complete repair ensues following 5 to 7 days of trauma. The fibrinolytic system plays essential role in adhesion formation and reformation. The other cellular mediators, plasminogen activator, plasminogen activator inhibitor-1 and matrix metalloproteinase-1 and tissue inhibitor of metalloproteinase also play crucial role in adhesion formation. All of the components interact with fibrinolytic system.[13,15] The suppression of fibrinolytic system by various modifying factors promotes formation of postoperative adhesions (Box 17.1)

Box 17.1: Factors suppressing fibrinolytic activity

Ischemia
Drying of surface owing to dry gas, light and heat
Excessive suturing
Omental patches
Traction of peritoneum
Blood clots retained in peritoneal cavity
Prolong operation time
Adnexal trauma
Infection
Exposure to foreign material (glove powder)

CLASSIFICATION OF ADHESIONS

There is no unified classification of adhesion formation or reformation. Diamond and Nezhat have given a classification of adhesion reformation16.

1. Type I: The de novo adhesions occurring at sites with no previous adhesions:
   • Type 1a: Non-surgical site.
   • Type 1b: At surgical site.
2. Type II: The reformed adhesions occurring at site with previous adhesiolysis:
   • Type 2a: At sites of adhesiolysis only.
   • Type 2b: At sites of adhesiolysis plus sites of another procedure.

CLINICAL COMPLICATIONS OF ADHESIONS

Untreated adhesions may lead to several clinical complications. Adhesion-related morbidity can be divided into two main groups, i.e. physical or treatment related:

1. Physical morbidity includes small bowel obstruction (SBO), infertility and chronic pain:[17]
   a. The incidence of SBO after an abdominal hysterectomy was 16.3 per 1,000 hysterectomies.[18] Indeed, adhesions have been implicated as the cause of 54% to 74% of all cases of SBO.[19] In a study by Stricker B et al, hysterectomy was the most common procedure in patients with adhesion related SBO.[20] Radical hysterectomy with concomitant radiotherapy was the frequent cause of SBO due to peritoneal adhesions in patients with non-adnexal gynecologic malignancy.[21]
   b. Chronic pelvic pain (CPP) is a major gynecologic problem, accounting for 10% of all gynecologic visits and approximately 50% of laparoscopic investigations. 25% to 57% of patients with CPP are estimated to have adhesions, with or without endometriosis.[22,23]
   c. Approximately, 15%–20% of female infertility cases have been associated with adhesions involving the ovaries or fallopian tubes.[24]
2. Treatment-related morbidity includes difficulty with postoperative interventions such as intraperitoneal chemotherapy, radiation, and subsequent complications during repeat operations.[25]

PREVENTION OF POSTOPERATIVE ADHESIONS

The strategies for prevention of adhesion formation comprise several good surgical techniques and application of novel technologies (including antiadhesion adjuvants). The good surgical techniques aim at minimizing tissue trauma, while pharmacological and/or barrier adjutants target to decrease adhesion formation.

TECHNIQUES TO PREVENT ADHESIONS

Microsurgery

The use of microsurgery is fundamental in reducing adhesion formation. These techniques use magnification for precise approximation of tissues. The methods entail gentle tissue handling, prevention of tissue desiccation by constant irrigation, use of non-reactive sutures and meticulous haemostasis. This is because abrasive handling of tissue, combination of blood and tissue drying, lint of suture material used at laparotomy aggravates the inflammatory response.[26] Other surgical aspects to be considered important are increase in vascular permeability, infection control, avoiding GI contamination, limiting the use of cautery and sutures, and use of starch-free gloves. Moreover, avoiding incisions through highly vascularised anatomical structures (muscle layers) and reducing the degree of tissue trauma are the two confirmed basic principles for reducing postoperative adhesions. The formation of adhesions distant from the operative site can be prevented with minimal access, as it limits the exposure of abdominal cavity to air and foreign reactive materials.[26,27] Desiccation can be reduced by the use of humidified gases, which is demonstrated to minimize adhesion formation. Hence, combining controlled intraperitoneal cooling with a rigorous prevention of desiccation might be important for clinical adhesion prevention.

Laparoscopy

Laparoscopy has been thought to encompass an advantage of reducing the formation of postoperative adhesions.[11,27–32] The uncomplicated injuries occurring at laparoscopic site heal without adhesion formation. The decrease in adhesion formation can be attributed to its minimal access to the abdominal cavity reducing the amplitude of peritoneal injury, as the peritoneal injury seems to play a crucial role in the pathophysiology of adhesion formation.[27] Moreover, reduced presence of foreign bodies also reduces risk of adhesions.[33]

The laparoscopic magnified view allows a gentler handling and precise dissection of anatomical structures at the operative site; therefore minimizes the degree of tissue trauma. Furthermore, the laparoscopic environment has been shown to interact directly with the fibrinolytic activity of peritoneum via the inhibition of plasminogen activator inhibitor released by mesothelial cell. This interaction has been shown to reduce postoperative adhesion formation. The advantages over laparotomy are procedure in closed environment; the operative field is not exposed to room air, no tissue drying or lint of suture or surgical gloves.[27,30–32]

Although laparoscopic procedures lead to fewer adhesions compared to laparotomy procedures, adhesions may develop even after laparoscopy. To minimize adhesions, good surgical techniques of microsurgery outlined above should be practiced.

Second Look Laparoscopy

Alternatively, a second look laparoscopy after laparoscopy may be useful for assessing the degree of postoperative adhesion which allows technically easy adhesiolysis, and results in lower adhesion scores shown at third look procedure.[8]

Use of Harmonics

The use of the harmonic scalpel (Fig. 17.1) for laparoscopic myomectomy is associated with low intraoperative blood loss, low postoperative pain, and low total operative time with no change in surgical difficulty.[34,35] The Harmonic scalpel ultracision (Ethicon Endosurgery, Cincinnati, OH) is an ultrasonic surgical instrument, enhances the blade's ability to cut and coagulate blood vessels, and vibrates at 55,000 cycles per second. It dissects with less thermal damage to surrounding tissues and causing no eschar build-up on the blade. It produces no smoke in the operative field and minimizes accidental injury.

Use of preoperative prophylactic antibiotics reduces chance of infection induced adhesions. A high degree of awareness is

necessary for prompt diagnosis of intraoperative complications due to adhesions. The possible intraoperative electrical injuries to the bowel should be conservatively managed, when detected.

■ TECHNOLOGIES TO PREVENT ADHESIONS

According to surveys conducted by the European Society of Human Reproduction and Embryology (ESHRE, 2002) and the European Association of Coloproctology (EACP, 2002), an ideal antiadhesion agent should be safe, efficacious (at the operation site and throughout the cavity), easy to use in all types of abdominal surgery (open and laparoscopic) and economical36. Needless to say, the ideal agent is still elusive.

■ ADJUVANT DRUGS

Many adjuvants drugs have been evaluated in preventing adhesions including Non-steroidal anti-inflammatory drugs (NSAIDS), corticosteroids, and fibrinolytics.

■ INTRA-ABDOMINAL ADHESIONS

1. NSAIDs have been recommended to prevent postoperative pelvic adhesions by blocking the production of thromboxanes, which are known to be involved in the biochemical pathways leading to adhesion formation. The encouraging results have been demonstrated in animal models.[37–39] However, lack of adequate clinical studies evaluating their safety and efficacy has limited their clinical application.[17]
2. The broad-spectrum antibiotics reduce fibrin deposition and subsequent adhesion formation by decreasing inflammation and bacterial load. Cephalosporins were the extensively used antibiotics in the past. However, there is no sufficient evidence to support use of antibiotics in adhesion reduction. In contrast, antibiotics in peritoneal irrigation solution have been found to increase peritoneal adhesion formation in an experimental model. Hence, antibiotics should not be recommended as single agent for adhesion prevention.[40,41]
3. Fibrinolytic agents stimulate plasminogen activator (PA) activity and reduce fibrinous mass. Thrombolytic

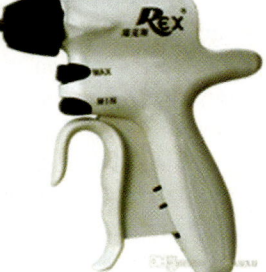

Fig. 17.1: Harmonic scalpel

agents, urokinase, recombinant human tissue PA, and streptokinase, have been found to prevent adhesion formations in majority of animal and clinical studies.[42] Nevertheless, properly designed studies with primary objective as prevention of adhesions are awaited.

Intrauterine Adhesions

1. GnRH administration prior (2–3 month) to myomectomy was found to decrease adhesion formation by increasing peritoneal fibrinolytic activity.[43] Postoperative administration of GnRH agonist has also been suggested.[44]

2. In a review of present literature on intrauterine device (IUD), the IUD was found beneficial in patients with IUA, regardless of stage of adhesions. It is emphasized that, in patients with moderate-to-severe IUA, adjuvant treatment should be combined with IUD to obtain maximal outcomes.

3. The postoperative cyclic administration of oestrogen (dose: 1.25–5 mg/day for 30–60 days) and progestin stimulate endometrial re-epithelialisation of scar surfaces. However, large randomized studies are required to confirm the results.[45]

Adjuvant Agents

Adhesion-reducing agents generally fall within two main categories, physical barriers and solutions. Generally, the physical barriers tend to be site specific, whereas solutions have the advantage of providing broad coverage throughout the cavity.

Physical Barriers

Oxidized Regenerated Cellulose

Oxidized regenerated cellulose (Interceed; Johnson and Johnson) is the most widely used adhesion prevention agent and has been shown to reduce adhesion formation in both animal and human studies.[46,47] It has a mesh-like design placed over or between traumatized surfaces. It is transformed in a viscous gel about 8 h after the application covering the damaged surfaces and forms a barrier, and physically separates the adjacent raw surfaces (Fig. 17.2). It is degraded to monosaccharides and completely absorbed in about 2 weeks. It has been shown to have both barrier and biological effect.[48] Interceed has been used after open as well as laparoscopic myomectomy.[49] In a Cochrane systemic review, Ahmad et al have analysed 11 RCT of Interceed and has shown it as safe and efficacious in reducing the incidence of de-novo adhesions in laparoscopy.[47] In the same review, use of Interceed in laparotomy had a significant reduction in the reformation (or mixture) of adhesions.[50] In a randomized trial, Maias et al have shown that

the Interceed barrier significantly reduces de-novo adhesion formation after laparoscopic myomectomy.[51] Andrea Tinelli et al have shown efficacy of Interceed in reducing adhesions in laparoscopic and abdominal myomectomy.[52] In a randomized trial, Interceed was found to act synergistically with heparin when applied to ovarian surfaces after cystectomy and/or ovariolysis at laparotomy. However, statistically significant difference was not found in adhesion reducing capacity of Interceed after adding heparin.[53] Similar to other site specific agents, application is limited to surgeries where operative surfaces can be completely covered with mesh with benefit limiting to the site of barrier placement. The efficacy of Interceed is reduced in the presence of excess peritoneal fluid and bleeding; hence, thorough haemostasis and removal of excess peritoneal fluid should be attained before application on operative surfaces.[54,55] Besides, Interceed can migrate form the site of application, which reduces its effectiveness.

Hyaluronic Acid Analogues

Seprafilm

Seprafilm (Genzyme) is an absorbable membrane made up of hyaluronic acid (HA) and carboxymethylcellulose. It forms a hydrophilic gel approximately 24 h after application and mechanically separates opposite tissue surfaces. The effect lasts for 7 days and subsequently excreted from the body within 28 days (Fig. 17.3). It is not approved in the USA for laparoscopic use.[56] It does not fit into the shape of pelvic organs and is commonly used to prevent adhesions between the incision of anterior abdominal wall and bowel or omentum.[57] Its use in laparoscopic procedures is difficult. As it is vulnerable to tears and difficult to handle, novel instrument and technique for using Seprafilm in laparoscopic myomectomy has been reported.[58] In another publication, a slurry with the Seprafilm barrier was prepared by mixing 20 cc of sterile saline per 13 × 15 cm sheet of Seprafilm, delivered to the site with back-loading into a leur lock syringe through a 5 mm laparoscopic irrigator.[59] The use of warm saline to create slurry and intraperitoneal delivery by Toumey syringe with Robinson catheter has also been reported.[60,61] A laparoscopic

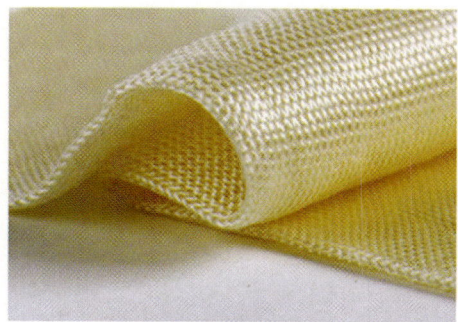

Fig. 17.2: Interceed (oxidised regenerated cellulose)

grasping instrument was used to guide the catheter tip to the operative site for application.[60,61] In a blind prospective, randomized, multicenter study, Seprafilm significantly reduced the incidence, severity, extent, and area of postoperative uterine adhesions.[62] In a prospective study, Seprafilm was highly effective and was superior to Beriplast, Dextran 40 in preventing uterine adhesions after myomectomy.[63] Potential side effects included higher incidence of pulmonary emboli, intra-peritoneal abscess formation, and foreign body reaction; which were not statistically significant in the trials.[64–67] Another limitation of Seprafilm is high cost, as ~4.5 sheets per patient is required for an effective protection from intestinal obstruction.[68]

Expanded Polytetrafluoroethylene Barrier

Expanded polytetrafluoroethylene (PTFE) (Preclude, Gore-Tex Surgical Membrane; Johnson and Johnson) is non-reactive and non-absorbable barrier that inhibits cellular migration and tissue adherence. In a multicenter randomized clinical trial, the PTFE barrier was found effective in reducing post myomectomy adhesion formation.[68] Besides, PTFE was found more effective compared to Interceed in reducing adhesion reformation after adhesinolysis.[69] PTFE has the disadvantages that it is difficult to use in laparoscopic surgery. PTFE being non-absorbable, removal of it necessitates surgery after the injury has healed.[47,70] The use of Preclude in Europe is limited. It has been withdrawn from the market in USA from December 2011.

Polyethylene Glycol

Polyethylene glycol (SprayGel, Confluent Surgical Inc.) consists of two synthetic liquid precursors. They are sprayed together with an air assisted sprayer at the target tissue, rapidly crosslink to form a flexible, solid, and absorbable hydrogel (Fig. 17.4). It can be easily applied at laparoscopic site. The gel remains intact for approximately 5 to 7 days at site of application and then gradually breaks down by hydrolysis and is excreted by the kidneys.[71] The disadvantages of the product are the complexity of preparation and application, and hence the resultant time required to cover the target tissue. Another limitation is the high cost. In a randomized control trial (RCT), Spraygel was found safe efficacious in patients undergoing myomectomy.[72] It has been approved for use in open surgery in USA; while in Europe it is approved for laparoscopic surgery as well.

Polylactide

Polylactide (SurgiWrap, Macropore Biosurgery inc.) is a bioabsorbable film with a long absorption period up to 6 months. It has been approved in May 2005 with intended use in surgeries including gynaecology surgeries. It has to be sutured to avoid its loss from the site. It is metabolised to lactic acid and finally to CO_2 and exhaled. SurgiWrap has been demonstrated efficacious in the reducing adhesion formation in preclinical studies, but there are scarcity of data currently for safety and efficacy in humans.[73–75]

Carboxymethylcellulose Derivatives

Oxiplex is a composite viscoelastic gel of carboxymethylcellulose and polyethylene oxide (Oxiplex; FzioMed). The gel is absorbed by 6 weeks.[76] It has been approved in Europe for use in abdominal and pelvic surgery. In an RCT, Oxiplex produced significant reduction in adhesions in patients of gynecological surgery including adnexal and endometriosis.[77,78] It has ease of application in laparoscopic surgery.

Solutions

Crystalloids

Crystalloid solutions (Ringer lactate, normal saline) get absorbed at a rate of (30–60 mL/h) from the peritoneum causing

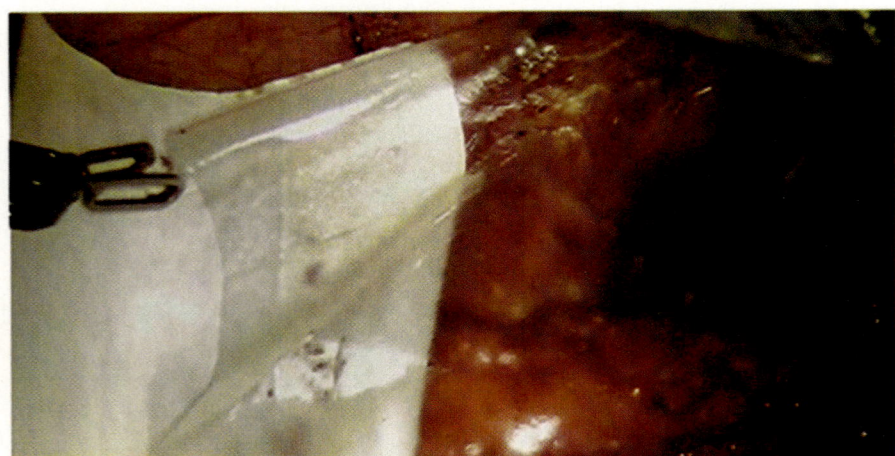

Fig. 17.3: Seprafilm

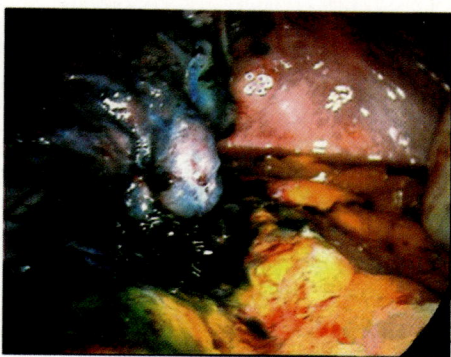

Fig. 17.4: Spraygel

complete assimilation of the fluid in 24–48 hours. They are commonly used since long to produce a hydrofloatation effect though they are not approved as antiadhesive agent. However, Crystalloid instillates did not increase adhesion-free outcome in a meta-analysis of clinical trials.[79]

Icodextrin

Icodextrin 4% (Adept; Shire Pharmaceuticals) is a high molecular weight glucose polymer. Adept has been widely used in peritoneal dialysis. It has a peritoneal residence time of ≥ 4 days and acts to reduce adhesion formation by prolonged hydrofloatation.[80] In a multicenter European registry for use of Adept in general surgery, Adept was found efficacious and safe in adhesion prevention.[81] There was no adhesion related complication found in a randomized study.[82] The preclinical evidence supports efficacy of Adept in gynecological surgery.[83] In a prospective randomized double-blind multicenter study involving laparoscopic gynecological surgery, Adept use resulted in significant reduction in incidence, severity, and extent of adhesions. It was also found to inhibit the deterioration of pre-existing adhesions.[84]

In a recent European, multicenter, double blind, randomized study, Adept was compared to lactate Ringer solution (LRS) for efficacy and safety, in reducing de novo adhesions after laparoscopic gynecological surgery. Adept was safe and efficacious. The study found no difference between Adept and LRS in overall de novo adhesion formation. The study provides future direction that the site specific barrier agent, perhaps in conjugation with Adept may be better strategy to reduce adhesions in site specific surgery like myomectomy.[85] According to the analysis made by a consensus group, low cost is another advantage of Adept. Adept (1.5 litre bags) are about four times cheaper than one Spraygel package and about half the price of each sheet of Interceed or Seprafilm.[36] Disseminated intravascular coagulation after laparoscopic myomectomy with the use of 4% Adept solution has been reported[86]. It has been approved for use in open and laparoscopic surgery in Europe and USA.

Hyaluronic Acid Gels

Hyalobarrier Gel

HA cross-linked to HA (hyalobarrier gel; Baxter) is a highly viscous site-specific gel. In a prospective, RCT, cross-linked HA resulted in significant reduction of adhesions after laparoscopic myomectomy.[87] In another RCT, Hyalobarrier was safe and efficacious in reducing adhesion post myomectomy, though the difference was not significant.[88]

ACP Gel

The ACP gel is an auto cross-linked internal ester of HA (ACP gel; Fidia Advanced Biopolymers). It has higher viscosity and extended residence compared to HA. It was found efficacious in reducing abdominal adhesions in experimental animal models.[88,90] In a prospective RCT, ACP gel significantly reduced the incidence and severity of de novo formation of IUA after hysteroscopic surgery.[91] In another RCT, ACP gel reduced development and severity of adhesions postoperatively in patients with hysteroscopic adhesiolysis.[92]

Sepracoat

Sepracoat is a bioabsorbable macromolecular dilute solution of low-viscosity (Sepracoat; Genzyme). It is a 0.04% HA combined with phosphate-buffered saline. It is cleared from the body in less than 5 days. It is recommended to apply Sepracoat in two phase of surgery. Initially, it is applied before starting the tissue manipulation in the peritoneal cavity to minimize injury from indirect trauma. It has to be again applied finally before end of surgical procedure. In a blind, prospective, randomized, placebo-controlled multicenter study, Sepracoat was found safe and effective in reducing the incidence, extent, and severity of de novo adhesions to multiple sites indirectly traumatized by laparoscopic gynecologic surgery[93]. It has been approved by the FDA for use in open surgery in the USA.

Intergel

Ferric hyaluronate 0.5% gel (Intergel; Gynecare) is a viscous gel that delivers a broader coverage. It was initially approved for use as antiadhesive agent, later on withdrawn from the market in 2003 after reported incidence of late onset postoperative pain and sclerosing peritonitis.

Dextran

The 32% Dextran-70 (Hyskon; Pharmacia Laboratories) is a 1-6-linked dextrose polymer. In two RCTs, Hyskon was found to reduce postoperative adhesion formation effectively in patients requiring an operation for distal tubal disease, endometriosis or pelvic adhesions.[94,95] However, one of the two studies revealed no difference in the adhesion reduction by Hyskon compared to saline.[95] The adverse effects reported were pleural effusion, pulmonary and peripheral oedema caused by its osmotic properties, liver function abnormalities disseminated intra-vascular coagulation and, rarely, allergic reactions or anaphylactic shock. It has not been approved for use as an antiadhesive agent.

Fibrin Glue

Fibrin glue is a biological product. Fibrin glue is made by mixing human fibrinogen with bovine thrombin, factor XIII and calcium. The component solutions are reconstituted in two separate syringes with sterile water immediately before use. Fibrin glue is basically used as sealant used for fistula repair, wound closure or haemostasis, also known as fibrin sealant. The possible mechanism of fibrin glue is the confinement of fibrin, which prevents the development of attachments between opposing tissue surfaces. Commercially prepared fibrin sealants have been used extensively in Europe. Later on, FDA also approved these products. Fibrin glue is available commercially from Tisseel (Baxter, Westlake Village, Calif), Evicel and Evarrest Fibrin Sealant Patch (Johnson & Johnson, Somerville, NJ), and Hemaseel (Hemacure, Sarasota, Fla). They have been approved for haemostasis, sealing of anastomoses in various surgeries, and for topical applications. Fibrin glue has been approved for endoscopic haemostasis in bleeding ulcers and varices in Europe, while the product labeling in the United States does not endorse intravascular application. In a prospective randomized study, fibrin sealants were found to significantly reduce adhesion after laparoscopic myomectomy determined by second look laparoscopy.[96]

Carboxymethylchitosan

N, O-carboxymethylchitosan (Adhes-X, Chitogenics) is a purified chitin derivative, which has similar structure to hyaluronic acid and carboxymethylcellulose. The product includes a clear gel and a solution. A laparoscopic instrument is used to stamp the gel initially at the site of surgical trauma followed by application of solution at the same place. In a prospective RCT, intraperitoneal use of Adhes-X gel and solution was found safe and efficacious for reduction of occurrence, extent, and severity of adhesion recurrence and de novo adhesion formation.[97]

■ COMPARATIVE EVALUATION OF AVAILABLE ANTIADHESIVE AGENTS

A recent review from Cochrane suggests Interceed, Gore-Tex and Seprafilm be more effective than no treatment in reducing the incidence of adhesion formation following pelvic surgery. There has been no conclusive evidence on the relative effectiveness of these interventions. The use of Fibrin sheet was not found more effective compared to no treatment. Moreover, there are no adverse events directly attributed to the use of adhesion agents.[50] A comparative view of basic characteristics of commonly used antiadhesion agents is presented in Table 17.1.

■ OPEN VS LAPAROSCOPIC MYOMECTOMY

Several arguments strongly suggesting that the risk of postoperative adhesions is reduced when myomectomy takes place via the laparoscopic route. In a non-randomized comparative study, there was a statistically significant drop in the degree of post-operative adhesions and the proportion of patients with adhesions connected with use of the laparoscopic route.[98] A prospective collection of data, 45 patients underwent a second look after laparoscopic myomectomy. The rate of adhesions after laparoscopic myomectomy is low and the adhesions rarely involved the adnexa.[99] Although this kind of difference can be explained by differences in the size and number of myomata between cases dealt with by laparoscopy and laparotomy, it is probable nevertheless that the use of the laparoscopic route for myomectomy would reduce the risk of adhesions. Laparoscopic surgery effectively offers the advantage of respecting the principles of microsurgery by

Table 17.2: Comparison of anti-adhesion agents.

Characteristics	Antiadhesion agent				
	Interceed	Seprafilm	Spraygel	Fibrin sealant	Adept
Site specific/broad coverage	Site specific	Site specific	Site specific	Broad coverage	Broad coverage
Composition	Oxidizes regenerated cellulose membrane	Hyaluronic acid/ carboxymeth ylcellulose membrane	Polyethylene glycol	Human fibrinogen with bovine thrombin, factor XIII and calcium	4% icodextrin instillate
Peritoneal residence time	1–2 weeks	7 days	5–7 days	–	3-4 days
Works in presence of bleeding	No	Yes	No	Likely	Not known

its very nature (atraumatic manipulation, fine instruments, thorough washing). In addition, it avoids intraperitoneal contamination and has less effect on the equilibrium of the peritoneum.

■ REFERENCES

1. Parker WH. Etiology, symptomatology, and diagnosis of uterine myomas. Fertil Steril. 2007;87(4):725-36.
2. Kempson RL, Hendrickson MR. Smooth Muscle, Endometrial Stromal, and Mixed Mullerian Tumors of the Uterus. Modern Pathology. 2000;13(3):328-42.
3. Laughlin SK, Baird DD, Savitz DA, et al. Prevalence of uterine leiomyomas in the first trimester of pregnancy: an ultrasound-screening study. Obstet Gynecol. 2009;113(3):630-5.
4. Chen CR, Buck GM, Courey NG, et al. Risk factors for uterine fibroids among women undergoing tubal sterilization. Am J Epidemiol. 2001;153(1):20-6.
5. Borgfeldt C, Andolf E. Transvaginal ultrasonographic findings in the uterus and the endometrium: low prevalence of leiomyoma in a random sample of women age 25-40 years. Acta Obstet Gynecol Scand. 2000;79(3):202-7.
6. Marino JL, Eskenazi B, Warner M, et al. Uterine leiomyoma and menstrual cycle characteristics in a population-based cohort study. Hum Reprod. 2004;19(10):2350-5.
7. Tulandi T, Murray C, Guralnick M. Adhesion formation and reproductive outcome after myomectomy and second-look laparoscopy. Obstet Gynecol. 1993;82(2):213-5.
8. Uğur M, Turan C, Mungan T, et al. Laparoscopy for adhesion prevention following myomectomy. International Journal of Gynecology and Obstetrics. 1996;53(2):145-9.
9. Kubinova K, Mara M, Horak P, et al. Reproduction after myomectomy: comparison of patients with and without second-look laparoscopy. Minim Invasive Ther Allied Technol. 2012;21(2):118-24.
10. Lower AM, Hawthorn RJ, Ellis H, et al. The impact of adhesions on hospital readmissions over ten years after 8849 open gynaecological operations: an assessment from the Surgical and Clinical Adhesions Research Study. Bjog. 2000;107(7):855-62.
11. Hammoud A, Gago LA, Diamond MP. Adhesions in patients with chronic pelvic pain: a role for adhesiolysis? Fertil Steril. 2004;82(6):1483-91.
12. Diamond MP, Freeman ML. Clinical implications of postsurgical adhesions. Hum Reprod Update. 2001;7(6):567-76.
13. Awonuga AO, Fletcher NM, Saed GM, et al. Postoperative Adhesion Development Following Cesarean and Open Intra-Abdominal Gynecological Operations: A Review. Reprod Sci. 182011. p. 1166-85.
14. Revaux A, Ducarme G, Luton D. Prevention of intrauterine adhesions after hysteroscopic surgery. Gynecol Obstet Fertil. 2008;36(3):311-7.
15. Arung W, Meurisse M, Detry O. Pathophysiology and prevention of postoperative peritoneal adhesions. World J Gastroenterol. 2011;17(41):4545-53.
16. MP Diamond FN. Adhesions after resection of ovarian endometriomas. Fertility sterility. 1993;59(4):934-5.
17. Gonzalez-Quintero VH, Cruz-Pachano FE. Preventing adhesions in obstetric and gynecologic surgical procedures. Rev Obstet Gynecol. 2009;2(1):38-45.
18. Al-Took S, Platt R, Tulandi T. Adhesion-related small-bowel obstruction after gynecologic operations. Am J Obstet Gynecol. 1999;180(2 Pt 1):313-5.
19. Menzies D. Peritoneal adhesions. Incidence, cause, and prevention. Surg Annu. 1992;24Pt 1:27-45.
20. Stricker B, Blanco J, Fox HE. The gynecologic contribution to intestinal obstruction in females. J Am Coll Surg. 1994;178(6):617-20.
21. Montz FJ, Holschneider CH, Solh S, et al. Small bowel obstruction following radical hysterectomy: risk factors, incidence, and operative findings. Gynecol Oncol. 1994;53(1):114-20.
22. Hebbar S, Chawla C. Role of laparoscopy in evaluation of chronic pelvic pain. J Minim Access Surg. 12005. p. 116-20.
23. Duffy DM, diZerega GS. Adhesion controversies: pelvic pain as a cause of adhesions, crystalloids in preventing them. J Reprod Med. 1996;41(1):19-26.
24. Ray NF, Denton WG, Thamer M, et al. Abdominal adhesiolysis: inpatient care and expenditures in the United States in 1994. J Am Coll Surg. 1998;186(1):1-9.
25. Van Der Krabben AA, Dijkstra FR, Nieuwenhuijzen M, et al. Morbidity and mortality of inadvertent enterotomy during adhesiotomy. Br J Surg. 2000;87(4):467-71.
26. Luijendijk RW, de Lange DC, Wauters CC, et al. Foreign material in postoperative adhesions. Ann Surg. 1996;223(3):242-8.
27. Gutt CN, Oniu T, Schemmer P, et al. Fewer adhesions induced by laparoscopic surgery? Surg Endosc. 2004;18(6):898-906.
28. Miller CE. Myomectomy. Comparison of open and laparoscopic techniques. Obstet Gynecol Clin North Am. 2000;27(2):407-20.
29. Dubuisso JB, Fauconnier A, Babaki-Fard K, et al. Laparoscopic myomectomy: a current view. Hum Reprod Update. 2000;6(6):588-94.
30. Luciano AA, Maier DB, Koch EI, et al. A comparative study of postoperative adhesions following laser surgery by laparoscopy versus laparotomy in the rabbit model. Obstet Gynecol. 1989;74(2):220-4.
31. Postoperative adhesion development after operative laparoscopy: evaluation at early second-look procedures. Operative Laparoscopy Study Group. Fertil Steril. 1991;55(4):700-4.
32. Lundorff P, Hahlin M, Kallfelt B, et al. Adhesion formation after laparoscopic surgery in tubal pregnancy: a randomized trial versus laparotomy. Fertil Steril. 1991;55(5):911-5.
33. Garrard CL, Clements RH, Nanney L, et al. Adhesion formation is reduced after laparoscopic surgery. Surg Endosc. 1999;13(1):10-3.
34. Litta P, Fantinato S, Calonaci F, et al. A randomized controlled study comparing harmonic versus electrosurgery in laparoscopic myomectomy. Fertil Steril. 2010;94(5):1882-6.
35. Ou CS, Harper A, Liu YH, et al. Laparoscopic myomectomy technique. Use of colpotomy and the harmonic scalpel. J Reprod Med. 2002;47(10):849-53.
36. RCOG. Consensus in adhesion reduction management. The Obstetrician & Gynaecologist. 2015;6(S2):1-16.
37. LeGrand EK, Rodgers KE, Girgis W, et al. Efficacy of tolmetin sodium for adhesion prevention in rabbit and rat models. J Surg Res. 1994;56(1):67-71.

38. LeGrand EK, Rodgers KE, Girgis W, et al. Comparative efficacy of nonsteroidal anti-inflammatory drugs and anti-thromboxane agents in a rabbit adhesion-prevention model. J Invest Surg. 1995;8(3):187-94.

39. Greene AK, Alwayn IPJ, Nose V, et al. Prevention of Intra-abdominal Adhesions Using the Antiangiogenic COX-2 Inhibitor Celecoxib. Ann Surg. 2005;242(1):140-6.

40. Gutmann JN, Diamond MP. Principles of Laparoscopic Microsurgery and Adhesion Prevention. In: Ricardo Azziz AAM, editor. Practical manual of operative laparoscopy and hysteroscopy: Springer New York; 2015. p. 94-107.

41. Nappi C, Sardo ADS, Greco E, et al. Prevention of adhesions in gynaecological endoscopy. Human Reproduction Update. 2007;13(4):379-94.

42. Hellebrekers BW, Trimbos-Kemper TC, Trimbos JB, et al. Use of fibrinolytic agents in the prevention of postoperative adhesion formation. Fertil Steril. 2000;74(2):203-12.

43. Imai A, Sugiyama M, Furui T, et al. Gonadotrophin-releasing hormones agonist therapy increases peritoneal fibrinolytic activity and prevents adhesion formation after myomectomy. J Obstet Gynaecol. 2003;23(6):660-3.

44. Schindler AE. Gonadotropin-releasing hormone agonists for prevention of postoperative adhesions: an overview. Gynecol Endocrinol. 2004;19(1):51-5.

45. Chen FP, Soong YK, Hui YL. Successful treatment of severe uterine synechiae with transcervical resectoscopy combined with laminaria tent. Hum Reprod. 1997;12(5):943-7.

46. Marana R, Catalano GF, Caruana P, et al. Postoperative adhesion formation and reproductive outcome using Interceed after ovarian surgery: a randomized trial in the rabbit model. Hum Reprod. 1997;12(9):1935-8.

47. Ahmad G, Duffy JM, Farquhar C, et al. Barrier agents for adhesion prevention after gynaecological surgery. Cochrane Database Syst Rev. 2008(2):Cd000475.

48. Gago LA, Saed G, Elhammady E, et al. Effect of oxidized regenerated cellulose (Interceed) on the expression of tissue plasminogen activator and plasminogen activator inhibitor-1 in human peritoneal fibroblasts and mesothelial cells. Fertil Steril. 2006;86(4 Suppl):1223-7.

49. Reddy S, Santanam N, Reddy PP, et al. Interaction of Interceed oxidized regenerated cellulose with macrophages: a potential mechanism by which Interceed may prevent adhesions. Am J Obstet Gynecol. 1997;177(6):1315-20; discussion 20-1.

50. Ahmad G, O'Flynn H, Hindocha A, et al. Barrier agents for adhesion prevention after gynaecological surgery. The Cochrane Library:Cochrane Database of Systemic Reviews. 2015(4):1-75.

51. Mais V, Ajossa S, Piras B, et al. Prevention of de-novo adhesion formation after laparoscopic myomectomy: a randomized trial to evaluate the effectiveness of an oxidized regenerated cellulose absorbable barrier. Hum Reprod. 1995;10(12):3133-5.

52. Tinelli A, Malvasi A, Guido M, et al. Adhesion formation after intracapsular myomectomy with or without adhesion barrier. Fertil Steril. 2011;95(5):1780-5.

53. Reid RL, Hahn PM, Spence JE, et al. A randomized clinical trial of oxidized regenerated cellulose adhesion barrier (Interceed, TC7) alone or in combination with heparin. Fertil Steril. 1997;67(1):23-9.

54. Larsson B. Efficacy of Interceed in adhesion prevention in gynecologic surgery: a review of 13 clinical studies. J Reprod Med. 1996;41(1):27-34.

55. Wiseman DM, Gottlick-Iarkowski L, Kamp L. Effect of different barriers of oxidized regenerated cellulose (ORC) on cecal and sidewall adhesions in the presence and absence of bleeding. J Invest Surg. 1999;12(3):141-6.

56. Diamond MP, Burns EL, Accomando B, et al. Seprafilm adhesion barrier: (2) a review of the clinical literature on intraabdominal use. Gynecol Surg. 92012. p. 247-57.

57. Beck DE. The role of Seprafilm bioresorbable membrane in adhesion prevention. Eur J Surg Suppl. 1997(577):49-55.

58. Takeuchi H, Kitade M, Kikuchi I, et al. A novel instrument and technique for using Seprafilm hyaluronic acid/carboxymethylcellulose membrane during laparoscopic myomectomy. J Laparoendosc Adv Surg Tech A. 2006;16(5):497-502.

59. Fenton BW, Fanning J. Laparoscopic application of hyaluronate/carboxymethylcellulose slurry: an adhesion barrier in a slurry formulation goes where the available sheets cannot. Am J Obstet Gynecol. 2008;199(3):325.e1.

60. Ortiz MV, Awad ZT. An easy technique for laparoscopic placement of Seprafilm. Surg Laparosc Endosc Percutan Tech. 2009;19(5):e181-3.

61. Lipetskaia L, Silver DF. Laparoscopic Use of a Hyaluronic Acid Carboxycellulose Membrane Slurry in Gynecological Oncology. Journal of the Society of Laparoendoscopic Surgeons. 2010;14(1):91-4.

62. Diamond MP. Reduction of adhesions after uterine myomectomy by Seprafilm membrane (HAL-F): a blinded, prospective, randomized, multicenter clinical study. Seprafilm Adhesion Study Group. Fertil Steril. 1996;66(6):904-10.

63. Tsuji S, Takahashi K, Yomo H, et al. Effectiveness of antiadhesion barriers in preventing adhesion after myomectomy in patients with uterine leiomyoma. Eur J Obstet Gynecol Reprod Biol. 2005;123(2):244-8.

64. Klingler PJ, Floch NR, Seelig MH, et al. Seprafilm-induced peritoneal inflammation: a previously unknown complication. Report of a case. Dis Colon Rectum. 1999;42(12):1639-43.

65. Becker JM, Dayton MT, Fazio VW, et al. Prevention of postoperative abdominal adhesions by a sodium hyaluronate-based bioresorbable membrane: a prospective, randomized, double-blind multicenter study. J Am Coll Surg. 1996;183(4):297-306.

66. Trickett JP, Rainsbury RM, Green R. Paradoxical outcome after use of hyaluronate barrier to prevent intra-abdominal adhesions. J R Soc Med. 942001. p. 183-4.

67. Tyler JA, McDermott D, Levoyer T. Sterile intra-abdominal fluid collection associated with seprafilm use. Am Surg. 2008;74(11):1107-10.

68. Bristow RE, Santillan A, Diaz-Montes TP, et al. Prevention of adhesion formation after radical hysterectomy using a sodium hyaluronate-carboxymethylcellulose (HA-CMC) barrier: a cost-effectiveness analysis. Gynecol Oncol. 2007;104(3):739-46.

69. Haney AF, Hesla J, Hurst BS, et al. Expanded polytetrafluoroethylene (Gore-Tex Surgical Membrane) is superior to oxidized regenerated cellulose (Interceed TC7+) in preventing adhesions. Fertil Steril. 1995;63(5):1021-6.

70. Farquhar C, Vandekerckhove P, Watson A, et al. Barrier agents

for preventing adhesions after surgery for subfertility. Cochrane Database Syst Rev. 2000(2):Cd000475.

71. Johns DA, Ferland R, Dunn R. Initial feasibility study of a sprayable hydrogel adhesion barrier system in patients undergoing laparoscopic ovarian surgery. J Am Assoc Gynecol Laparosc. 2003;10(3):334-8.

72. Mettler L, Audebert A, Lehmann-Willenbrock E, et al. A randomized, prospective, controlled, multicenter clinical trial of a sprayable, site-specific adhesion barrier system in patients undergoing myomectomy. Fertil Steril. 2004;82(2):398-404.

73. Lee J. Evaluation of Adverse Effects of Polyactic Bioabsorbable Sheet (Surgiwrap®) for the Reduction of Pelvic Adhesion in Gynecologic Surgery. Journal of Minimally Invasive Gynecology. 2008;15(6):147S.

74. Shahmohamady B, Saberi N, LaShay N, et al. Laparoscopic Application of a Polylactic Acid (SurgiWrapMAST) Bioabsorbable Sheet. Journal of Minimally Invasive Gynecology. 2005;12(5):82.

75. Shahmohamady B, Saberi N, Lashay N, et al. To Evaluate Feasibility of Laparoscopy Application of a Polylactic Acid (SurgiWrap™ MAST™) Bioabsorbable Sheet. Fertility and Sterility. 2005;84(1):S469.

76. Young P, Johns A, Templeman C, et al. Reduction of postoperative adhesions after laparoscopic gynecological surgery with Oxiplex/AP Gel: a pilot study. Fertil Steril. 2005;84(5):1450-6.

77. Lundorff P, Donnez J, Korell M, et al. Clinical evaluation of a viscoelastic gel for reduction of adhesions following gynaecological surgery by laparoscopy in Europe. Hum Reprod. 2005;20(2):514-20.

78. diZerega GS, Coad J, Donnez J. Clinical evaluation of endometriosis and differential response to surgical therapy with and without application of Oxiplex/AP* adhesion barrier gel. Fertil Steril. 2007;87(3):485-9.

79. Wiseman DM, Trout JR, Diamond MP. The rates of adhesion development and the effects of crystalloid solutions on adhesion development in pelvic surgery. Fertil Steril. 1998;70(4):702-11.

80. Hosie K, Gilbert JA, Kerr D, et al. Fluid dynamics in man of an intraperitoneal drug delivery solution: 4% icodextrin. Drug Deliv. 2001;8(1):9-12.

81. Menzies D, Pascual MH, Walz M, et al. Use of Icodextrin 4% Solution in the Prevention of Adhesion Formation Following General Surgery: From the Multicentre ARIEL Registry. Ann R Coll Surg Engl. 2006;88(4):375-82.

82. Kraemer B, Wallwiener M, Brochhausen C, et al. A pilot study of laparoscopic adhesion prophylaxis after myomectomy with a copolymer designed for endoscopic application. J Minim Invasive Gynecol. 2010;17(2):222-7.

83. Khani B, Bahrami N, Mehrabian F, et al. Icodextrin reduces adhesion formation following gynecological surgery in rabbits. Iran J Reprod Med. 2011;9(3):187-92.

84. Brown CB, Luciano AA, Martin D, et al. Adept (icodextrin 4% solution) reduces adhesions after laparoscopic surgery for adhesiolysis: a double-blind, randomized, controlled study. Fertil Steril. 2007;88(5):1413-26.

85. Trew G, Pistofidis G, Pados G, et al. Gynaecological endoscopic evaluation of 4% icodextrin solution: a European, multicentre, double-blind, randomized study of the efficacy and safety in the reduction of de novo adhesions after laparoscopic gynaecological surgery. Hum Reprod. 2011;26(8):2015-27.

86. Santos LM, Frenna V, Thoma V, et al. Disseminated intravascular coagulation after laparoscopic multiple myomectomy with use of icodextrin: a case report. J Minim Invasive Gynecol. 2006;13(5):480-2.

87. Pellicano M, Bramante S, Cirillo D, et al. Effectiveness of autocrosslinked hyaluronic acid gel after laparoscopic myomectomy in infertile patients: a prospective, randomized, controlled study. Fertil Steril. 2003;80(2):441-4.

88. Mais V, Bracco GL, Litta P, et al. Reduction of postoperative adhesions with an auto-crosslinked hyaluronan gel in gynaecological laparoscopic surgery: a blinded, controlled, randomized, multicentre study. Hum Reprod. 2006;21(5):1248-54.

89. Belluco C, Meggiolaro F, Pressato D, et al. Prevention of postsurgical adhesions with an autocrosslinked hyaluronan derivative gel. J Surg Res. 2001;100(2):217-21.

90. De Iaco PA, Stefanetti M, Pressato D, et al. A novel hyaluronan-based gel in laparoscopic adhesion prevention: preclinical evaluation in an animal model. Fertil Steril. 1998;69(2):318-23.

91. Guida M, Acunzo G, Di Spiezio Sardo A, et al. Effectiveness of auto-crosslinked hyaluronic acid gel in the prevention of intrauterine adhesions after hysteroscopic surgery: a prospective, randomized, controlled study. Hum Reprod. 2004;19(6):1461-4.

92. Acunzo G, Guida M, Pellicano M, et al. Effectiveness of auto-cross-linked hyaluronic acid gel in the prevention of intrauterine adhesions after hysteroscopic adhesiolysis: a prospective, randomized, controlled study. Hum Reprod. 2003;18(9):1918-21.

93. Diamond MP. Reduction of de novo postsurgical adhesions by intraoperative precoating with Sepracoat (HAL-C) solution: a prospective, randomized, blinded, placebo-controlled multicenter study. The Sepracoat Adhesion Study Group. Fertil Steril. 1998;69(6):1067-74.

94. Group AS. Reduction of postoperative pelvic adhesions with intraperitoneal 32% dextran 70: a prospective, randomized clinical trial. Fertil Steril. 1983;40(5):612-9.

95. Larsson B, Lalos O, Marsk L, et al. Effect of intraperitoneal instillation of 32% dextran 70 on postoperative adhesion formation after tubal surgery. Acta Obstet Gynecol Scand. 1985;64(5):437-41.

96. Takeuchi H, Kitade M, Kikuchi I, et al. Adhesion-prevention effects of fibrin sealants after laparoscopic myomectomy as determined by second-look laparoscopy: a prospective, randomized, controlled study. J Reprod Med. 2005;50(8):571-7.

97. Diamond MP, Luciano A, Johns DA, et al. Reduction of postoperative adhesions by N,O-carboxymethylchitosan: a pilot study. Fertil Steril. 2003;80(3):631-6.

98. Bulletti C, Polli V, Negrini V, et al. Adhesion formation after laparoscopic myomectomy. J Am Assoc Gynecol Laparosc 1996; 3:533-6.

99. Dubuisson JB, Fauconnier A, Chapron C, et al. Second look after laparoscopic myomectorny. Hum Reprod 1998;13:2102-6.

CHAPTER 18

Measures to Reduce Blood Loss During Myomectomy

● Meenakshi Sundaram, Anusha Raaj, Shruthi Nanjundappan

■ INTRODUCTION

Myomas are the most common uterine neoplasms, affecting approximately 20% to 25% of women of reproductive age[1,2] (Figs 18.1 and 18.2). They can develop in any area where there are smooth muscle cells of müllerian origin, such as the fallopian tubes, uterine corpus and cervix. They arise from the benign transformation and proliferation of smooth muscle cells. Increased oestrogen stimulation alone or in concert with growth hormone or human placental lactogen is the major growth regulators. Progesterone appears to inhibit the growth of myomas, but under certain conditions may promote their growth.[3] There are a number of ongoing researches investigating the underlying pathogenesis of these highly prevalent benign tumours linking the latter to high levels of intrinsic aromatase activity, oestrogen and progesterone receptors, and genetic predisposition (aberrations in chromosomes 3,6,7,10,12). They are symptomatic in only 50% of cases, manifesting with a multitude of symptoms and complications.

The standard treatment of symptomatic fibroids is hysterectomy for women who have completed childbearing, and myomectomy for women who wish to preserve fertility. Hysterectomy eliminates both the symptoms and the chance of recurrence. However, many women who suffer from myomas desire future childbearing or want to preserve their uterus. For these women myomectomy with reconstruction and preservation of the uterus is an important option.

Myomectomy can be accomplished by laparotomy, laparoscopy or hysteroscopy. Myomectomy by laparotomy involves the surgical removal of the fibroids through a large incision in the abdominal wall. The laparoscopic approach is a minimal access technique developed to minimize insult to the abdominal wall and to ensure quick recovery of the patient following surgery. For women with submucous myomas, transcervical hysteroscopic myomectomy is a feasible option.

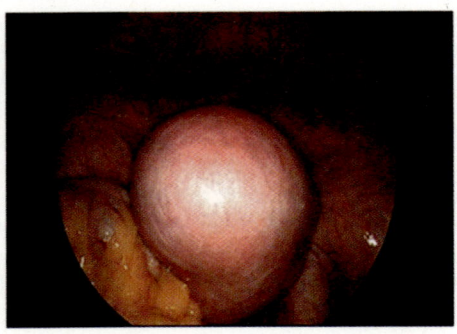

Fig. 18.1: Laparoscopic view of a fundal fibroid

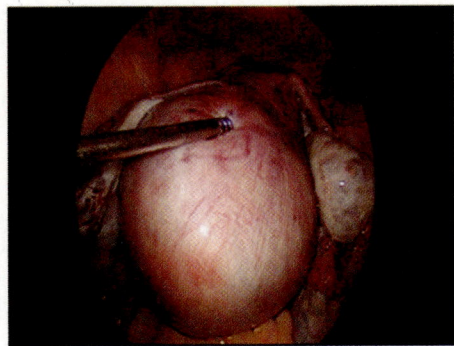

Fig. 18.2: Myoma screw being inserted into myoma

COMPLICATIONS AND ITS INCIDENCE

Myomectomy can lead to both short and long-term complications. Complications of hysteroscopic myomectomy include haemorrhage, uterine perforation, cervical damage and metabolic disturbances from excessive absorption of the distension medium, such as glycine. Laparoscopic myomectomy is associated with the usual risks of laparoscopy, particularly accidents during trocar placement and, additionally, excessive uncontrolled haemorrhage with the need to convert to a laparotomy.

Short-term complications of abdominal myomectomy include bleeding, fever, infection, visceral damage and thromboembolism. A requirement for transfusion in up to 20% of cases following abdominal myomectomy has been reported in the literature.[4] Patients undergoing myomectomy have an unusually high incidence of fever occurring in the first 48 hours following surgery. The incidence of postoperative fever following myomectomy has been reported to be as high as 36%.[4,5] The cause is unknown, but it is believed that 'myomectomy fever' is due to the release of pyrogenic factors during myoma dissection or to haematomas forming in defects left by the removed myomas. In 2% of cases there is a need for conversion of myomectomy to hysterectomy. Long-term complications of abdominal myomectomy include pelvic adhesions in 59% of women after 2 years and recurrent fibroids in 46.0% of women after 1 year. The risk of uterine rupture in subsequent pregnancies varies between 0% and 1%.[5]

Blood loss during myomectomy can be intraoperative or postoperative and with haematoma formation. Massive blood loss associated with the dissection of huge fibroids renders myomectomy a more technically challenging procedure than hysterectomy. Sometimes myomectomy is converted to hysterectomy intraoperatively when bleeding becomes heavy and uncontrollable or when it is impossible to reconstruct the uterus because of the many defects left by the removal of multiple myomas.[6] Excessive bleeding can necessitate emergency blood transfusion.

VASCULAR ANATOMY OF UTERUS AND FIBROIDS (Fig.18.3)

The ascending blood supply of the uterus is from the uterine arteries, which pass through the cardinal ligament at the level of the cervicouterine junction. The descending blood supply is from the ovarian arteries, which pass through the infundibulopelvic ligaments and perfuse the ovaries, fallopian tubes and uterine cornua. The uterine and ovarian vessels anastomose to perfuse the uterus. Arcuate arteries run transversely within the uterine wall and radial arteries penetrate deeply into the myometrium.[7]

The presence of leiomyomas in the uterus distorts normal vasculature.[7] Thus the arcuate arteries may run in any axis, rather than transversely. Thus either vertical or transverse incisions during myomectomy may transect these vessels.

It has been a common teaching that there is a vascular pedicle at the base of each myoma, and that the ligation of this pedicle will achieve complete haemostasis during myomectomy. However, a study using vascular corrosion and electron microscopy revealed that the myomas are surrounded completely by a dense vascular layer supplying the myoma, which is separated from the myometrium by a narrow vascular cleft[8] (Fig. 18.4).

INTERVENTIONS TO REDUCE BLOOD LOSS DURING MYOMECTOMY

The average volume of blood lost during abdominal myomectomy is 200 to 800 mL[8–10] and for laparoscopic myomectomy is 80 to 250 ml.[11,12] Many interventions have been performed to reduce bleeding during myomectomy. Five categories of interventions can be identified:

1. Interventions on uterine arteries such as laparoscopic uterine artery ligation, uterine artery embolisation, pericervical mechanical tourniquet, vasopressin (natural or synthetic), a vasoconstrictive solution of

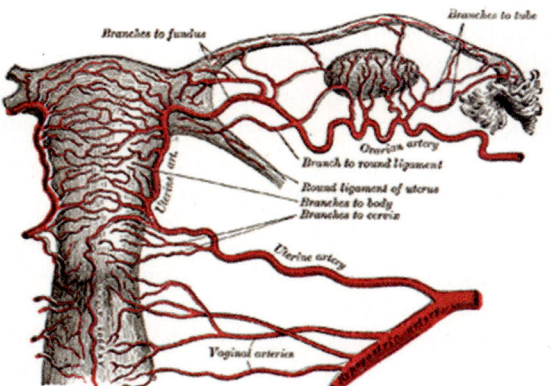

Fig. 18.3: Uterus blood supply

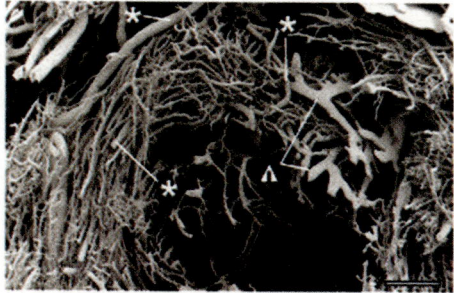

Fig. 18.4: corrosion casting and electron microscopy pictures of vascularity surrounding a fibroid

bupivacaine plus epinephrine, and temporary clipping of the uterine artery.

2. Uterotonics such as Ergometrine, Oxytocin, Misoprostol and Sulprostone.

3. Myoma dissection techniques that include enucleation by morcellation and the use of laser and chemical dissectors such as sodium-2-mercaptoethane sulphonate (mesna).[13]

4. Pharmacologic manipulation of the coagulation cascade with antifibrinolytic agents such as tranexamic acid, aprotinin, aminocaproic acid, recombinant factor VIIa and gelatin-thrombin haemostatic sealant.

5. In developed countries, gonadotrophin-releasing hormone analogues (GnRHa) have been used prior to myomectomy. There is now clear evidence that the use of GnRHa reduces uterine volume and fibroid size and may reduce blood loss and operating time during myomectomy4. In addition, uterine artery embolisation (UAE) has been used as an alternative to myomectomy and to prevent haemorrhage during myomectomy.

This chapter covers preoperative, intraoperative and postoperative measures to decrease bleeding during myomectomy.

■ PREOPERATIVE MEASURES:

Correction of PreOperative Anaemia

Screening for anaemia and iron deficiency should be done as early as possible prior to surgery and should be corrected prior to an elective major surgical procedure. Elective surgery should be scheduled to allow anaemia correction to occur first.

Medical Treatments for Menorrhagia

Medical treatments used for the management of menorrhagia include, tranexamic acid, GnRH antagonists, non-steroidal anti-inflammatories, and other hormonal therapies. These may also be beneficial in decreasing preoperative blood loss and thus facilitating the correction of preoperative anaemia and iron deficiency. The decision to use any of these medical therapies is at the discretion of the treating clinician.

Preoperative Misoprostol

Recommended dose of misoprostol 400 µg intra-vaginally, 1 hour prior to surgery.

■ INTRAOPERATIVE MEASURES

Vasoconstrictor Therapy

Vasopressin

Intramyometrial vasopressin injected into the planned uterine incision site for each fibroid reduces blood loss.

Vasopressin acts by constricting the smooth muscles in the wall of capillaries, small arterioles, and venules. Randomized trial data show that blood loss during myomectomy with vasopressin is significantly less than with placebo 299 mL less[14] and less than or comparable to the use of uterine artery tourniquet.[15–17]

The half-life of intramuscular vasopressin is 10 to 20 minutes and the duration of action is 2 to 8 hours.

Contraindications

1. History of CVS disease, such as hypertension, ischaemic heart disease or other cardiac disease.
2. Caution in smokers or those on nicotine replacement therapy.

Suggested Vasopressin Dilution

Add 20 units of vasopressin (1 ampoule) into 200 mL of saline = 0.1 u/mL (10% solution).

Good Practice Points

1. Surgeons should inform the anaesthetist when injecting.
2. Inject into the base of myomas prior to incision.
3. Aspirate regularly to avoid intravascular injection (Figs 18.5 and 18.6).
4. Vasopressin has a short half-life. A repeat injection in 45 to 60 minutes may be safe.
5. Never exceed the maximum dose of 5 units.
6. Increase the dilution, if more volume is needed for injecting into multiple myomas base.

There are few data about combined use of vasopressin and ligating the myoma pedicle using a loop of suture.[18] Ligation of myoma pedicle merits further study.

Epinephrine

Epinephrine is another vasoconstrictor that is effective in reducing blood loss during myomectomy.

One randomized trial found that intramyometrial injection of Bupivacaine with epinephrine (50 mL bupivacaine 0.25% and 0.5 mL of 1 mg/mL epinephrine) reduced blood loss compared with saline (69 mL less).[19]

Intravascular injection of epinephrine may cause acute cardiovascular adverse events similar to vasopressin. A disadvantage of epinephrine is clinical experience during myomectomy is limited.

Noradrenaline

There is no published literature, but this is still used in some developed countries. The same precautions with regard to potential cardiovascular contraindications and precautions apply.

Suggested Noradrenaline Dilution

Add 2 mg of noradrenaline (1 ampoule) into 1 L of dextrose 5% = 2 µg/mL

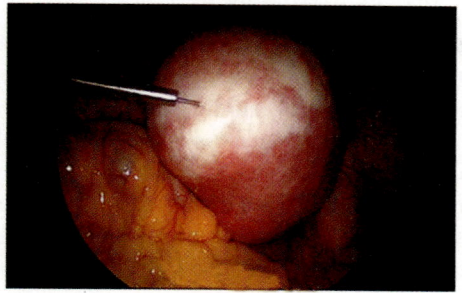

Fig. 18.5: Injection of vasopressin into the myoma

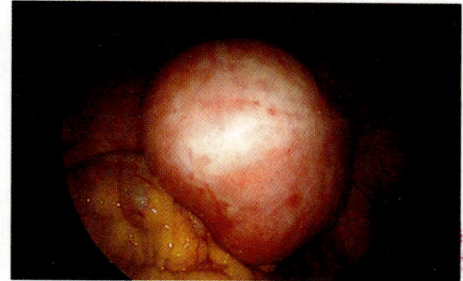

Fig. 18.6: Blanching of uterus

Maximum dose for infiltration is 100 mL of this solution, although more than 60 mL is rarely needed.

Repeat dose in 45 to 60 minutes (probably safe due to short half life).

■ SURGICAL TECHNIQUES

Surgical Techniques to Reduce Blood Loss During Open Myomectomy

Pericervical Tourniquet

This can be achieved by passing and tying a Foley's catheter around the cervix and the infundibular pelvic ligaments as low as possible compressing the uterine and ovarian vessels.

The best way to achieve a tight seal is to throw one knot on the catheter and then use a clip to hold this tight. This technique may not be feasible, if the location of the fibroids prevents the catheter from encircling the cervix.

Ovarian Artery Clamps

The addition of ovarian artery clamps to a peri-cervical tourniquet (the triple tourniquet technique) has shown the greatest benefit in decreasing overall blood loss. Specific ovarian artery clamps designed to avoid damage to the fallopian tubes are available for this purpose.[20]

Surgical Techniques to Reduce Blood Loss During Laparoscopic Myomectomy

Anatomical Considerations of Blood Supply of the Uterus and Myomas

The uterus is primarily supplied by the uterine artery, which is a branch from the anterior division of the internal iliac artery. The vascularity of the uterus is rich as it also receives its blood supply from other sources. Myometrium has an extremely rich blood supply. First, blood reaches the uterus primarily through the uterine arteries whose sizes are in the range of 2 to 6 mm diameter.[21,22] Second, small (0.5 mm) communicating arteries connect the uterus with ovarian arteries.[22] Third, many named arteries have potential to supply blood to the uterus—inferior

mesenteric, lumbar, vertebral, middle sacral, deep iliac circumflex, inferior epigastric, medial femoral circumflex, and lateral femoral circumflex arteries.[23] Fourth, innumerable very small, unnamed arteries reach the uterus from the broad ligament and retroperitoneum. Unlike the uterus that has various blood supplies, the vascular supply to the fibroids comes exclusively from the uterine arteries.

Effects of Uterine Artery Occlusion on the Myometrium and Myoma

As most blood enters the uterus through the uterine arteries, it was postulated that after occluding the arteries by catheter or laparoscopic technique, transient uterine ischemia occurs. The hypothesis proposes that soon after occlusion, blood within myometrium clots, myometrium becomes hypoxic, and metabolism shifts from oxidative pathways to anaerobic glycolysis. The hypothesis further postulates that hours later clot within myometrium lyses and the uterus is reperfused through collateral arteries.[24]

Burbank and colleagues put forward this 'transient uterine ischemia' hypothesis to explain the mechanism of uterine artery occlusion. They proposed that after uterine artery occlusion, both myometrial and myoma vessels were occluded by clotting, resulting in organ ischemia.[25] Work on uterine artery occlusion found that necrosis in the myoma, contributed to the shrinkage of tumours, which was shown both through pathological observations and with magnetic resonance imaging (MRI).

The major advantage of ligating the uterine vessels before myomectomy is that blood loss during the procedure is considerably reduced. Studies have also shown that there is shrinkage of very small fibroids that are not removed during the surgery and prevents recurrence of new fibroids.

Laparoscopic Myomectomy with Uterine Artery Ligation

In our centre, we ligate the uterine vessels before myomectomy in all large myomas. Laparoscopic ligation of uterine arteries has been combined with myomectomy with a successful reduction in blood loss.[26] Most cases of large myomas can be devascularized before myomectomy by laparoscopic intracorporeal suturing of uterine artery. The uterine arteries can be ligated by anterior approach or posterior approach depending on the location of the myoma. In case of lower segment myomas or cervical myomas, the uterine artery can be ligated at its origin from the anterior division of the internal iliac.

We prefer to ligate the ascending branch of the uterine artery anteriorly during most laparoscopic myomectomies. The uterovesical fold of peritoneum is opened and the bladder is pushed down. This moves the ureters laterally and prevents them being included in the suture. The uterine vessels are identified on either side and ligated. We use No. 1 delayed absorbable sutures for ligating the uterine vessels. We always prefer to suture intracorporeally by contralateral suturing using two needle holders. There can be technical difficulties in approaching the uterine vessels in cases of large myomas. There can be some venous bleeding, if the uterine vein is accidentally punctured. In such cases, the suturing is completed and the venous bleed stops by itself. Once the uterines are occluded bilaterally, the myoma turns pale. This devascularises the myoma and decreases the blood loss during the procedure.

The myoma capsule is then opened with harmonic ultracision or with monopolar hook or bipolar and scissors.

Incision on myoma using a monopolar cautery to delineate the capsule of the myoma. Enucleation is made along the cleavage plane separating the myoma and surrounding myometrium (Fig. 18.7).[27] It is facilitated by traction with a 5-mm myoma screw and countertraction on the cervix with a tenaculum held by the assistant (Figs 18.8 and 18.9). A degenerated myoma may be too friable to allow a firm grip with a myoma screw. Haemostasis is ensured. The myoma bed is obliterated with mattress sutures. The myoma capsule is closed with interrupted intracorporeal sutures with No. 1 polyglyconate in one or two layers depending on the depth of the myoma in the uterine wall. If the uterine cavity is opened, the endometrium is reposited and the uterine wall is closed excluding the endometrium. The myoma is retrieved through the 15 mm port by morcellation.

In cases of lower segment myomas or cervical myomas, we ligate the uterine vessels at its origin from the anterior division

of the internal iliac.[28] Before dissection, diluted vasopression is infiltrated (Fig. 18.10). We start the dissection for the vessel ligation from the anterior leaf of the broad ligament. The triangle enclosed by the round ligament, external iliac artery and infundibulopelvic ligament is opened with the harmonic ultracision. The areolar space is dissected and the origin of the uterine artery from the internal iliac is identified. It is important at this point to also identify the ureter and its relation to the uterine artery in order to avoid inadvertent ligation. The uterine artery is isolated from the surrounding structures and sutured with No. 1-0 delayed absorbable suture, especially in cases of multiple fibroids (Figs 18.11 and 18.12). Suturing can be done with a free tie or with a needle. The myoma turns pale after the bilateral suturing of the uterine arteries. The myoma is enucleated from its bed by traction and counter traction. The myoma capsule is closed with interrupted intracorporeal sutures. The myoma is retrieved by morcellation.

The other major advantage of ligating the uterine vessels is in cases of degenerated myomas where the morcellation is done, while the myoma is still attached to its bed. This is especially the case when dealing with large, softened, degenerated myomas that do not allow adequate grip. There can be profuse bleeding, if the myoma is morcellated without enucleation. This can be prevented by ligating the uterine vessels bilaterally before myomectomy.[29]

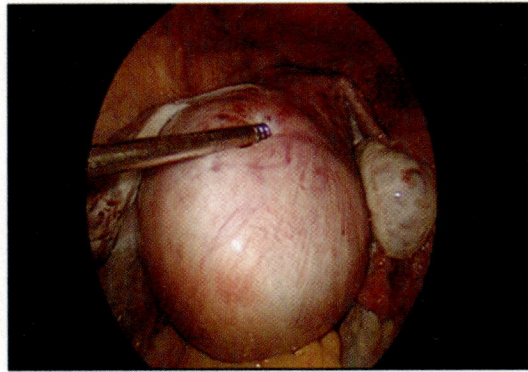

Fig. 18.8: Insertion of myoma screw into the uterus

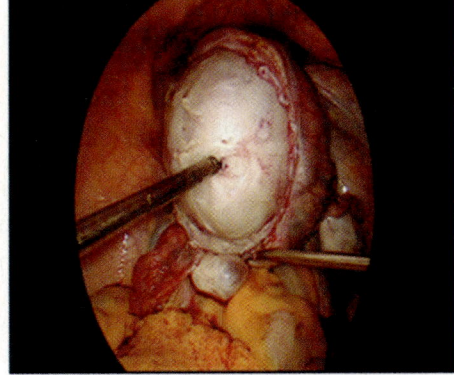

Fig. 18.9: Enucleation of fibroid using the myoma screw

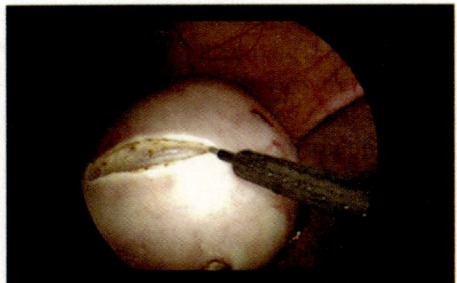

Fig. 18.7: Incision on myoma with monopolar hook

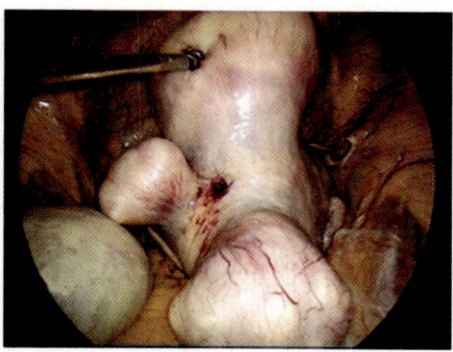

Fig. 18.10: Injection of vasopressin into the fibroid uterus

Leiomyomas derive their blood supply almost totally from the uterine arteries. Devascularisation of the myomas by selective uterine artery ligation is the basis for many treatment modalities used for symptomatic myomas, namely, laparoscopic bipolar coagulation of uterine arteries30 and uterine artery embolisation. The author has also reported that ligation of uterine vessels as the first step in total laparoscopic hysterectomy considerably reduces the blood loss during the procedure especially in cases of large myomas.[31]

Uterine artery embolisation (UAE) for the treatment of uterine myomas was first reported in 1995.[32] Since then, the long-term efficacy of UAE was indicated for the treatment of heavy uterine bleeding and for the reduction of uterine volume. A complication associated with UAE was postembolisation syndrome, characterized by fever, pain, nausea and vomiting, and leukocytosis, which affects up to 26% of patients and contributes to prolonged institutional stays (including readmission), heavy analgesic use, and delayed return to normal activities.[33]

Clinical results similar to those obtained with UAE were revealed using laparoscopically directed uterine artery occlusion (UAO) with bipolar coagulation/desiccation or surgical clips. Cheng et al[34] studied the effect of laparoscopic uterine artery occlusion combined with myomectomy for uterine myomas and stated that though haemostasis does not appear to be a problem after artery occlusion, anatomic apposition is the main target of suturing under laparoscopy. Peng Hui et al[35] studied the necessity of laparoscopic myomectomy in the treatment of women with symptomatic uterine myomas who are undergoing laparoscopic uterine vessel occlusion. They concluded that uterine vessel occlusion with laparoscopic myomectomy is better compared to only uterine artery occlusion without myomectomy.

Concerns of Uterine Artery Ligation During Laparoscopic Myomectomy

Technical difficulties of ligating the uterine vessels especially in large myomas may be a restricting factor. But with adequate training and the skill of the surgeon, it is not impossible. The other issue is that injecting vasopressin may per say be adequate to control the bleeding during myomectomy. But in large myomas injecting large amount of vasopressin can also be detrimental. If it is possible technically to ligate the uterine vessels before myomectomy especially in large myomas, then bleeding during the procedure would not be a major concern. Including the ureters in the suture is another concern. If the uterovesical fold of peritoneum is opened and bladder pushed down, the ureters move laterally and the chance of including them in the suture is less.

Fertility after Uterine Artery Ligation

Studies on uterine artery embolisation have clearly stated the possibility of ovarian failure following the procedure. Tulandi et al[36] have described that due to transient ovarian ischemia, some degree of ovarian reserve appears to be lost when ovaries are inadvertently embolised. In most women, the ovarian blood supply is dual. Blood flow reaches the ovary either from the ipsilateral ovarian artery or from the ipsilateral uteroovarian communicating arteries, and does so depending on local arterial and arteriolar resistances.[37] Most utero-ovarian communicating arteries are 0.5 mm or greater in diameter. Consequently, when UAE is performed with sufficiently small embolic particles, approximately 60% of ovaries are vulnerable to embolisation. Pathology

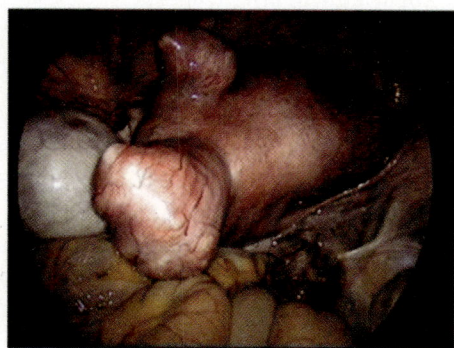

Fig. 18.11: Multiple fibroid uterus

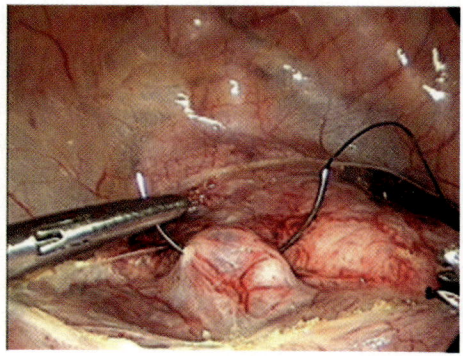

Fig. 18.12: Uterine artery ligation

examinations of ovaries following UAE demonstrate embolic particles in the ovaries following UAE.

In our technique, we selectively isolate the uterine arteries and ligate them. This excludes the possibility of ligating the utero-ovarian communicating artery and does not cause decreased ovarian reserve or ovarian failure. Xiaoyan Qu et al38 have done a study to assess the effect on ovarian reserve function after laparoscopic uterine artery occlusion (LUAO) compared with laparoscopic myomectomy (LM).Blood samples were collected before surgery, and at 1, 3 and 6 months postoperatively. Concentrations of follicle-stimulating hormone (FSH), leuteinizing hormone (LH) and estradiol (EZ) were determined using an immunoassay, and serum inhibin B (INHB) concentration was evaluated using an enzyme-linked immunosorbent assay. The study concluded that at short-term follow-up, no significant effect on ovarian reserve in patients with myoma who underwent laparoscopic uterine artery occlusion was found. There are no long-term randomized trials on this effect published so far. We are conducting a study in our institute to assess the effects of uterine artery ligation on ovarian reserve and future pregnancy.

Pregnancy after Uterine Artery Ligation

Successful pregnancy rates have been reported in literature following bilateral internal iliac ligation.[39] Fertility and pregnancy following selective ligation of the uterine arteries has also been reported in literature. Between 1964 and 1980, nearly two dozen full-term, successful pregnancies in women who had uterine artery ligation performed were recorded in the world's medical literature.[40,41] From this we can conclude that following selective ligation of the uterine arteries, pregnancy is possible. Reports on pregnancy rates after uterine artery embolisation has been variable as most of these women were in the older age group.

Given that the uteroplacental arteries are formed by the retrograde invasion of trophoblasts into and around arterioles in the decidua, trophoblasts encountering PVA particles or the like in and around these arteries might be expected to present a dilemma. Embolisation with temporary materials such as Gelfoam or clotted autologous blood might be superior at preserving reproductive potential. Similarly, surgical methods that temporarily occlude the uterine arteries, such as ligation of the uterine arteries with resorbable suture material or a temporary paracervical clamp, might allow more successful future pregnancies than small, permanent embolic particles.

Holub et al[42] assessed pregnancy outcomes and deliveries after laparoscopic uterine artery transsection in symptomatic women with fibroids. About 153 patients underwent laparoscopic transection of uterine vessels during a 4-year period. The study concluded that laparoscopic transection of uterine vessels is a minimally invasive operative procedure that preserves the uterus and ovarian blood supply and allows for the achievement of pregnancy in women with symptomatic fibroids. Fetal growth and umbilical Doppler findings remained normal in all cases. An increased risk for preterm delivery and caesarean section was found in this small series.

Laparoscopic myomectomy with uterine artery is a technically feasible procedure. Ligating the uterine arteries bilaterally, either the ascending branch or at its origin from the internal iliac considerably reduces blood loss during myomectomy. It also helps to shrink small fibroids and prevent the recurrence of fibroids.

■ ANAESTHESIA TECHNIQUES

Controlled Hypotension/Intraoperative Blood Pressure Control

There is good evidence that there is a linear relationship between mean arterial blood pressure and blood loss. Most of the evidence for controlled hypotension/deliberate hypotension comes from spinal surgery, ENT/maxillofacial surgery, orthopaedic joint replacement surgery and some papers in gynae oncologic surgery showing benefit. The major risk is organ ischaemia or hypoperfusion and caution should be exercised in patients with cardiovascular disease. It is probable that the risks of a MAP < 65 mm Hg may outweigh any benefit, but it is a recommended practice to avoid hypertension. Aiming for a MAP 65 to 70 mm Hg (e.g. low normal) seems reasonable in patients without pre-existing cardiovascular disease. Any method can be used, e.g. thoracic epidural, spinal + GA, Remifentanil, or deepening the volatile anaesthesia depth. If infusing vasoactive drugs (e.g. GTN or phentolamine), the insertion of an arterial line is considered prudent.

It is not advisable to use deliberate hypotension if the patient has poorly controlled hypertension, cardiovascular or cerebrovascular disease. To ensure the surgeons have obtained good haemostasis before closing, the anaesthetist should allow the BP to return to normal levels first. This reveals any bleeding points, which may not be obvious at the lower blood pressure, but which may lead to concealed postoperative bleeding, if not dealt with prior to closure.

Regional Anaesthesia

There is evidence that regional techniques decrease intraoperative blood loss, possibly through their ability to lower blood pressure and sympathetic responses. When discussing merits of thoracic epidural analgesia with patients, this additional benefit should be included in the discussion.

Another acceptable alternative for patients not keen on an epidural is a single shot spinal with intrathecal morphine in addition to general anaesthesia.

Avoidance of Hypothermia

Aggressive intraoperative warming and avoidance of hypothermia will decrease blood loss. Wrapping the patient's head and warming all irrigation and intravenous fluids also helps.

Intravenous Fluid and Coagulation Management

Monitor coagulation and treat abnormalities accordingly. Colloid solutions can interfere with fibrinogen polymerisation, and potentially increase blood loss. Consider avoiding or minimising colloid use, if possible.

■ TRANEXAMIC ACID

This treatment is contraindicated in women with a history of, or risk factors for, thromboembolic disease.

Suggested Tranexamic Acid Regimen

Tranexamic acid 10 mg/kg (maximum 1 g) loading dose over 10 min followed by infusion of 1 mg/kg/min to stop at the end of surgery.

Postoperative Anaemia Correction

Women undergoing myomectomy are usually relatively young and fit with minimal comorbidities. They are likely to be able to tolerate lower levels of haemoglobin (Hb) for short periods of time compared to other elderly patients or those with CVS/respiratory disease. Consider enhancing their own ability to replace the lost Hb with intravenous iron, if there is significant postoperative anaemia (or oral iron if mild). This is important, if they were iron deficient preoperatively and this has not been corrected, as they will have no iron stores to help them correct their postoperative anaemia. In the stable non-bleeding patient, a reasonable aim should be to transfuse only if Hb < 60 to 70 g/L and give only one unit at a time, while assessing the patient's response.

■ CONCLUSION

Myomectomy is a technical challenging procedure especially if it is done by minimal access. The major concern is the vascularity of the fibroid and the blood loss associated with the procedure. Meticulous techniques followed during the surgery and adequate precautions and preparations taken before the surgery can reduce the total amount of blood loss. Understanding the ways of reducing the blood loss makes minimal access myomectomy a techniqually feasible procedure.

■ REFERENCES

1. Buttram VC, Reiter RC. Uterine leiomyomata: Etiology, symptomatology, and management. Fertil Steril. 1981;36:433.
2. Vollenhoven BJ, Lawrence AS, Healy DL. Uterine fibroids: A clinical review. Br J Obstet Gynaecol. 1990;97:285.
3. Cramer SF, Robertson AL, Ziatas NP, et al. Growth potential of human uterine leiomyomas: Some in vitro observations and their implications. Obstet Gynecol. 1990;97:393.
4. Freidman AJ, Rein NS, Harrison-Atlas D, et al. A randomized, placebo-controlled, blind study evaluating leuprolide acetate depot treatment before myomectomy. Fertil Steril. 1989;52:728.
5. Lumsden MA, West CP, Baird DT. Goserelin therapy before surgery for uterine fibroids. Lancet. 1987;1:36.
6. Fedele L, Vercellmi P, Bianchi S, et al. Treatment with GnRH agonists before myomectomy and the risk of short-term myoma recurrence. Br J Obstet Gynaecol. 1990;97:393.
7. West S, Ruiz R, Parker WH. Abdominal myomectomy in women with very large uterine size. Fertil Steril. 2006;85:36.
8. Sampson, JA. The blood supply of uterine myomata. Surg Gynecol Obstet. 1912;14:215.
9. Sawin SW, Pilevsky ND, Berlin JA, et al. Comparability of perioperative morbidity between abdominal myomectomy and hysterectomy for women with uterine leiomyomas. Am J Obstet Gynecol. 2000;183:1448.
10. Paul GP, Naik SA, Madhu KN, et al. Complications of laparoscopic myomectomy: A single surgeon's series of 1001 cases. Aust N Z J Obstet Gynaecol. 2010;50:385.
11. Sinha R, Hegde A, Mahajan C, et al. Laparoscopic myomectomy: do size, number, and location of the myomas form limiting factors for laparoscopic myomectomy? J Minim Invasive Gynecol. 2008;15:292.
12. Benassi L, Lopopolo G, Pazzoni F, et al. Chemically assisted dissection of tissues: an interesting support in abdominal myomectomy. J Am Coll Surg. 2000;191:65.
13. Kongnyuy EJ, Wiysonge CS. Interventions to reduce haemorrhage during myomectomy for fibroids. Cochrane Database Syst Rev. 2011;CD005355.
14. Ginsburg ES, Benson CB, Garfield JM, et al. The effect of operative technique and uterine size on blood loss during myomectomy: a prospective randomized study. Fertil Steril. 1993;60:956.
15. Fletcher H, Frederick J, Hardie M, et al. A randomized comparison of vasopressin and tourniquet as hemostatic agents during myomectomy. Obstet Gynecol. 1996;87:1014.
16. Zhao F, Jiao Y, Guo Z, et al. Evaluation of loop ligation of larger myoma pseudocapsule combined with vasopressin on laparoscopic myomectomy. Fertil Steril. 2011;95:762.
17. Nezhat F, Admon D, Nezhat CH, et al. Life-threatening hypotension after vasopressin injection during operative laparoscopy, followed by uneventful repeat laparoscopy. J Am Assoc Gynecol Laparosc. 1994;2:83.
18. Zullo F, Palomba S, Corea D, et al. Bupivacaine plus epinephrine for laparoscopic myomectomy: a randomized placebo-controlled trial. Obstet Gynecol. 2004;104:243.
19. Patient Blood Management Guidelines: Module 2 – Perioperative, - http://www.nba.gov.au/guidelines/module2/

20. Browning RM, Trentino K, Nathan EA, et al. Preoperative anaemia is common in patients undergoing major gynaecological surgery and is associated with a fivefold increased risk of transfusion. Aust N Z J Obstet Gynaecol. 2012:52(5):455-9.

21. Lipshutz B. A compsite study of the hypogastric aretry and its branches. Ann Surg. 1918;67:584-608.

22. Borell U, Fernstrom I. The adnexal branches of the uterine artery. An arteriographic study in human subjects. Acta Radiol. 1953;40:561-82.

23. Burchell RC. Arterial physiology of the human female pelvis. Obstet Gynecol. 1968;31:855-60.

24. Lichtinger M, Burbank F, Hallson L, et al. The time course of myometrial ischemia and reperfusion after laparoscopic uterine artery occlusion—Theoretical implications. J Am Assoc Gynecol Laparosc. 2003;10:553-63.

25. Burbank F, Hutchins Jr FL. Uterine artery occlusion by embolization or surgery for the treatment of fibroids: a unifying hypothesis–transient uterine ischemia. J Am Assoc Gynecol Laparosc. 2000;7:S1–49.

26. Liu WM, Tzeng CR, Yi-Jen C, et al. Combining the uterine depletion procedure and myomectomy may be useful for treating symptomatic fibroids. Fertil Steril. 2004;82:205-10.

27. Rakesh Sinha, Aparna Hegde, Neeta Warty et al. Laparoscopic. Excision of Very Large Myomas. J Am Assoc Gynecol Laparosc 2003;10(4):461-8.

28. Rakesh Sinha, Meenakshi Sundaram, Smita Lakhotia, et al. Cervical Myomectomy with Uterine Artery Ligation at Its Origin. Journal of Minimally Invasive Gynecology. 2009;16:604-8.

29. Rakesh Sinha, Aparna Hegde, Neeta Warty, et al. Laparoscopic myomectomy: Enucleation of the myoma by morcellation while it is attached to the uterus. Journal of Minimally Invasive Gynecology. 2005;12:284-9.

30. Liu WM. Laparoscopic bipolar coagulation of uterine vessels to treat symptomatic leiomyomas. J Am Assoc Gynecol Laparosc. 2000;7:129-31.

31. Rakesh Sinha, Meenakshi Sundaram, Yogesh A Nikam, et al. Total Laparoscopic Hysterectomy with Earlier Uterine Artery Ligation. J Minim Invasive Gynecology. 2008;15(3):355-9.

32. Ravina JH, Merland JJ, Ciraru-Vigneron N, et al. Arterial embolization: a new treatment of menorrhagia in uterine fibroma [in French]. Presse Med. 1995;24:1754.

33. Edwards RD, Moss JG, Lumsden MA, et al. Uterine-artery embolization versus surgery for symptomatic uterine fibroids. N Engl J Med. 2007;356:360-70.

34. Zhongping Cheng, Weihong Yang, Hong Dai, et al. Laparoscopic Uterine Artery Occlusion Combined with Myomectomy for Uterine Myomas. Journal of Minimally Invasive Gynecology. 2008;15:346-9.

35. Peng-Hui Wang, Wei-Min Liu, Jong-Ling Fuh, et al. Laparoscopic Uterine Vessel Occlusion in the Treatment of Women with Symptomatic Uterine Myomas with and without adding Laparoscopic Myomectomy: 4-Year Results. Journal of Minimally Invasive Gynecology. 2008;15:712-8.

36. Tulandi T, Sammour A, Valenti D, et al. Ovarian reserve after uterine artery embolization for leiomyomata. Fertil Steril. 2002;78:197-8.

37. Ryu RK, Chrisman HB, Omary RA, et al. The vascular impact of uterine artery embolization: prospective sonographic assessment of ovarian arterial circulation. J Vasc Interv Radiol. 2001;12:1071-4.

38. Xiaoyan Qu, Zhongping Cheng, Weihong Yang, et al. Controlled Clinical Trial Assessing the Effect of Laparoscopic Uterine Arterial Occlusion on Ovarian Reserve. Journal of Minimally Invasive Gynecology. 2010;17:47-52

39. Shinagawa S. Extraperitoneal ligation of the internal iliac arteries as a life- and uterus-saving procedure for uncontrolled postpartum hemorrhage. Am J Obstet Gynecol. 1964;88:130-1.

40. Lenzi G. Pregnancy after ligation of uterine arteries. Attual Ostet Ginecol. 1969;15:31-5.

41. Liberman G. Normal labor after ligation of major vessels of the uterus. Akush Ginekol. 1966;12:45-46.

42. Z Holub, J Lukac, L Kliment, et al. Pregnancy outcomes and deliveries following laparoscopic transsection of uterine vessels: A pilot study. European Journal of Obstetrics & Gynecology and Reproductive Biology. 2006;125:165-70.

CHAPTER 19

Complications of Laparoscopic Myomectomy

● Aswath Kumar R, Lola Ramachandran

Nowadays patients demand minimum period of hospitalisation and faster return to work. Hence laparoscopic myomectomies are becoming more and more common.[3] Therefore, it is imperative that we understand the various complications that can occur during a laparoscopic myomectomy and learn how best to avoid them or at least manage those if at all they occur. The main complications that can occur in a laparoscopic myomectomy are (Table 19.1).

Table 19.1: Complications of laparoscopic myomectomy

Complications	Incidence
Haemorrhages requiring blood transfusion	0.14%
Postoperative hematomas	0.48%
Bowel injury	0.04%
Postoperative acute kidney failure	0.04%
Unexpected sarcomas	0.09%
Failure to complete planned surgery/conversion to open surgery	0.34%
Hysterectomy	0.26%
Spontaneous uterine rupture during pregnancy	4%–30%
Recurrence	23–25

1. Intraoperative and immediate post operative:
   a. Haemorrhage and haematoma formation.
   b. Conversion to laparotomy.
   c. Hysterectomy (very rare).
   d. Morcellator injury.
   e. Lost needles and myomas.
   f. Dilutional coagulopathy.[12]
   g. Minor complications like pyrexia, abdominal pain, vaginitis, metrorrhagia, dysuria, etc.
2. Late:
   a. Recurrence of myomas
   b. Scar dehiscence during pregnancy.
   c. Port site hernia.

In an Italian study, which included 2,050 laparoscopic myomectomies, the total complication rate was 11.1% out of which 9.1% were minor and 2.02% were major.[1] The most serious events were haemorrhages requiring blood transfusions in three cases. There were 10 postoperative haematomas, one in the broad ligament and nine in the myomectomy scar itself, one bowel injury, one post operative kidney failure, two unexpected sarcomas and failure to complete planned surgery in seven cases. This study, one of the largest done so far, shows that even in experienced hands complications can occur. In that study two patients were readmitted for surgery—one had a laparoscopic hysterectomy because of severe blood loss and the other had drainage of a haematoma in the broad ligament. One patient who became pregnant had a spontaneous uterine rupture at 33 weeks gestation.

The odds ratio to estimate the risk of complications significantly rises with an increase in number and with the intramural or the intraligamentous location of the myomas whereas the myoma size seems to influence particularly the risk of major complications.[1]

Other complications generally associated with laparoscopy like shoulder pain, subcutaneous emphysema, atelectasis, gas embolism, pnuemothorax, rarely diaphragmatic rupture can also occur.

■ HAEMORRHAGE

Control of bleeding during myomectomy has multiple purposes:

1. Most of the surgeons find it difficult to perform myomectomy when it bleeds during the procedure as it becomes difficult to get into the correct plane of dissection. If this bleeding or blood staining of tissues is prevented it will be easier to get into the correct plane of dissection.
2. Suturing becomes difficult laparoscopically when the myoma bed keeps bleeding. If this can be controlled it becomes easier to suture the myoma bed.
3. If there is no bleeding then the use of energy sources is minimized and tissue necrosis is prevented, and this leads to better healing.
4. Small haematomas that can occur in the myoma bed lead to a weaker scar. This is considerably reduced, if there is less bleeding and this leads to better scar integrity. Several methods have thus been devised to decrease blood loss at myomectomy (Figs 19.1 to 19.2A and B).

Preoperative Methods

Gonadotropin-releasing Hormone Agonists

Gonadotropin-releasing hormones (GnRH) agonists preoperatively cause degeneration within the fibroid, which interferes with the enucleation of the myoma.

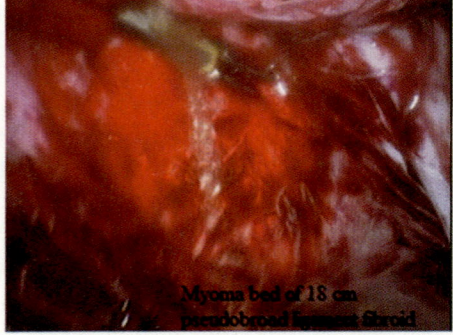

Fig. 19.1: Intraoperative haemorrhage at myoma bed after large myoma excision

Intraoperative Methods

Vasopressin

The use of vasopressin was first reported by Dillon in 1962, for open myomectomy. It has been available in India, since 2003. Vasopressin is a synthetic anti-diuretic hormone, which induces local vasoconstriction lasting for approximately 30 minutes, and thus helps in the control of bleeding from the incised sites.

Procedure

After the primary trocar is introduced, three accessory trocars are introduced under vision as previously discussed. A laparoscopic injection needle is then introduced through the left accessory port and inserted at the junction of the myoma and myometrium.

Vasopressin Injection

About 200 mL of saline with 20 units of vasopressin is then introduced through the laparoscopic injection needle, after first aspirating and ruling out accidental venous entry of the needle (Figs 19.3 and 19.4). Blanching of the myoma is then observed. The needle should not be removed from the first site of entry because if multiple sites of entry are created by the needle then the vasopressin and saline fluid will start leaking from the other sites. The purpose of this injection is not to create planes, but to reduce vascularity. The large amount of fluid injected also produces a compartment effect and helps to reduce bleeding. When the vasopressin saline solution is injected, care has to be taken that the needle does not penetrate so deep as to be inside the endometrial cavity. In such cases, it is noticed that the pressure of injecting will be lesser than normal, the fluid will then leak through the vagina and there will be failure of the vasoconstricting effect of vasopressin.

Caution

It has to be used with caution in patients suffering from cardiovascular diseases and hypertension as it can lead to a sudden increase in blood pressure (BP) and can also precipitate angina.

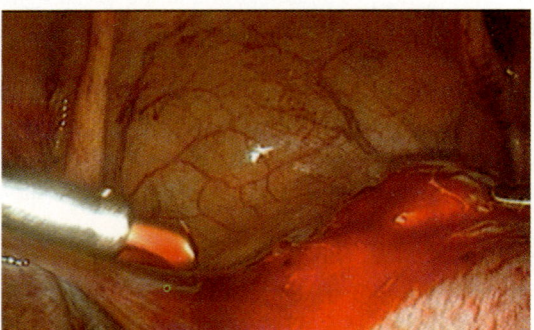

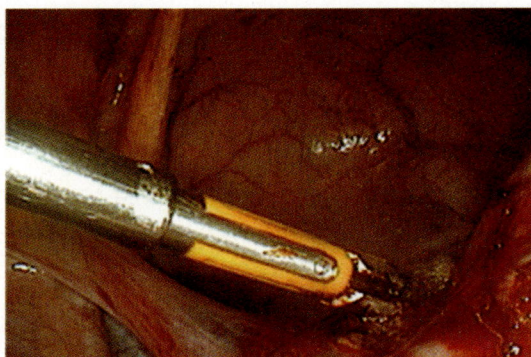

Figs 19.2A and B: A. Active bleeding from feeding vessel of myoma; **B.** Bleeding managed using bipolar energy source.

It is also associated with the adverse affect of water intoxication when used in very concentrated forms/inadvertent intravenous use.

Bilateral Uterine Artery Ligation

The skeletonized uterine artery is coagulated and cut using any of the energy sources. It is better if a 5 mm clip applicator is used to clip the vessel instead of cutting it. Damage to the underlying vein has to be avoided during clipping. The procedure is then repeated on the opposite side. We use No. 1 vicryl to ligate the vessel (Fig. 19.5):

1. In several studies, it is found that bilateral uterine artery ligation, at origin, does not interfere with future fertility as the end vessels and collaterals of the uterus are not interfered with.[17]
2. In multiple fibroid uterus, the very small myomas that are not tackled at the time of myomectomy, have been seen to shrink in size in the long-term studies, after uterine artery ligation.
3. It is also seen that this procedure prevents the recurrence of fibroids for a longer period than when myomectomy is done alone.

Other Methods

To reduce bleeding during myomectomy, the use of misoprostol in the vagina[9] vaginal insertion of dinoprostone, a

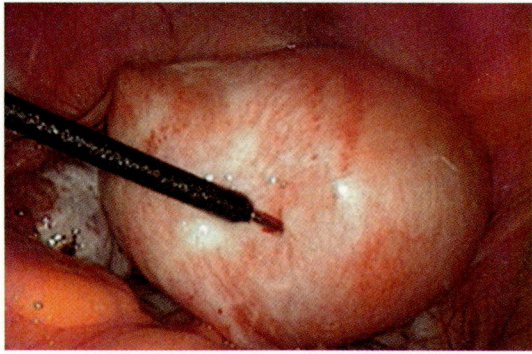

Fig. 19.3: Vasopressin being injected

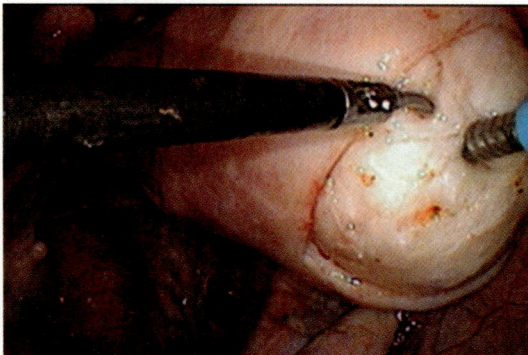

Fig. 19.4: Bloodless field after vasopressin injection

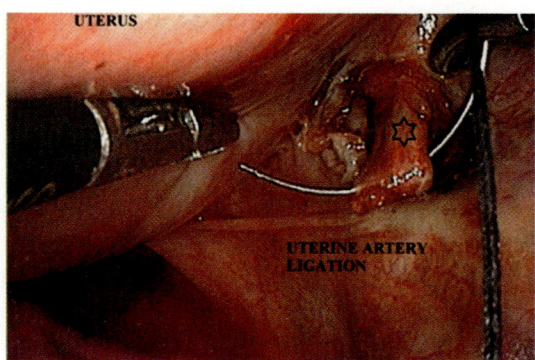

Fig. 19.5: Uterine artery ligation by posterior approach

gelatin-thrombin matrix, tranexamic acid, infusion of vitamin C, infiltration of a mixture of bupivacaine and epinephrine into the uterine muscles, or the use of a fibrin sealant patch has been mentioned. There is less evidence supporting the usefulness of this methods.

■ MORCELLATOR INJURIES

The first specimen removal during laparoscopic surgery was done in 1973. Despite this innovation, it took extensive amounts of time to remove even small specimens due to the manual force necessary. In 1993, the Steiner morcellator revolutionized laparoscopic specimen removal.

In contrast, the electromechanical morcellator makes it easy to remove even relatively large sections of tissue from the abdomen within a short period through the existing incisions.

It is very important to close the bigger port site laparoscopically to avoid incidence of Reiter's hernia. A special port closure needle is used and the rest closed laparoscopically. After removing the morcellator, port closure needle enters the abdomen through one end of the 15 mm incisions, carrying No.1 vicryl suture along with it (Figs 19.6A to E). The suture is released and the needle withdrawn. It is reintroduced from the other end of the incision. The first free end of suture in the peritoneal cavity is grasped and brought out over the abdomen. When the suture is tied the defect in the peritoneum and the rectus sheath gets adequately closed and eliminates the risk of bowel and omental herniation. Care should be exercised during introduction of morcellator. Vital tissue damage can be sustained by inadvertent morcellation beyond the myoma or uterus.

In the article 'A Laparoscopic Morcellator-Related Inuries' Magdy P Milad, MD, et al have reported in the journal of American Association of Gynecologic Laparoscopists, August 2003 that they are unable to locate any references to morcellaltor-related visceral injuries in the medical literature. Of 17 cases identified from the Food Drug Administration (FDA) data-base, three were excluded based on the trivial nature of the event (e.g. instrument did not function). The remaining 14 visceral injuries were to small and large bowel (11) kidney (2), pancreas (1), and major vascular structures (3). Identification of the complication was immediate in 10 patients, but was delayed until 4 days postoperatively in 1 woman. Three patients died. No device manufacturer or surgical specialty was responsible for a preponderance of the injuries. They did not locate any literature references to morcellator related visceral injuries. Obviously there may be bias against publishing such potentially catastrophic complications. Surgeon inexperience appeared to play an important role. Proper surgical technique may also lower the risk of visceral and major vascular injury.

Tips to Avoid Morcellator Injuries (Figs 19.7A to C)

1. The removing blade should always remain as anterior as possible. (Fig. 19.7).

2. Excellent pneumoperitoneum should be maintained.
3. Adequate panoramic view, and allowing the operator to visualize the blade at all times (Fig. 19.7).
4. The specimen should be completely separated from surrounding structures and vessels.
5. Specimen should always be pulled into the morcellator rather than pushing the morcellator into the specimen.
6. The individual holding the hand-piece should also be responsible for its activation.
7. Use of a laparoscopic bag to retain the specimen should not create a false sense of security with vital structures located in such close proximity. If the bag is torn during morcellation, the surgeon should immediately deactivate the morcellator and consider carefully inspecting surrounding viscera for injury.
8. It is very important to close the morcellator port site laparoscopically using a port closure needle to avoid incidence of Reiter's hernia.

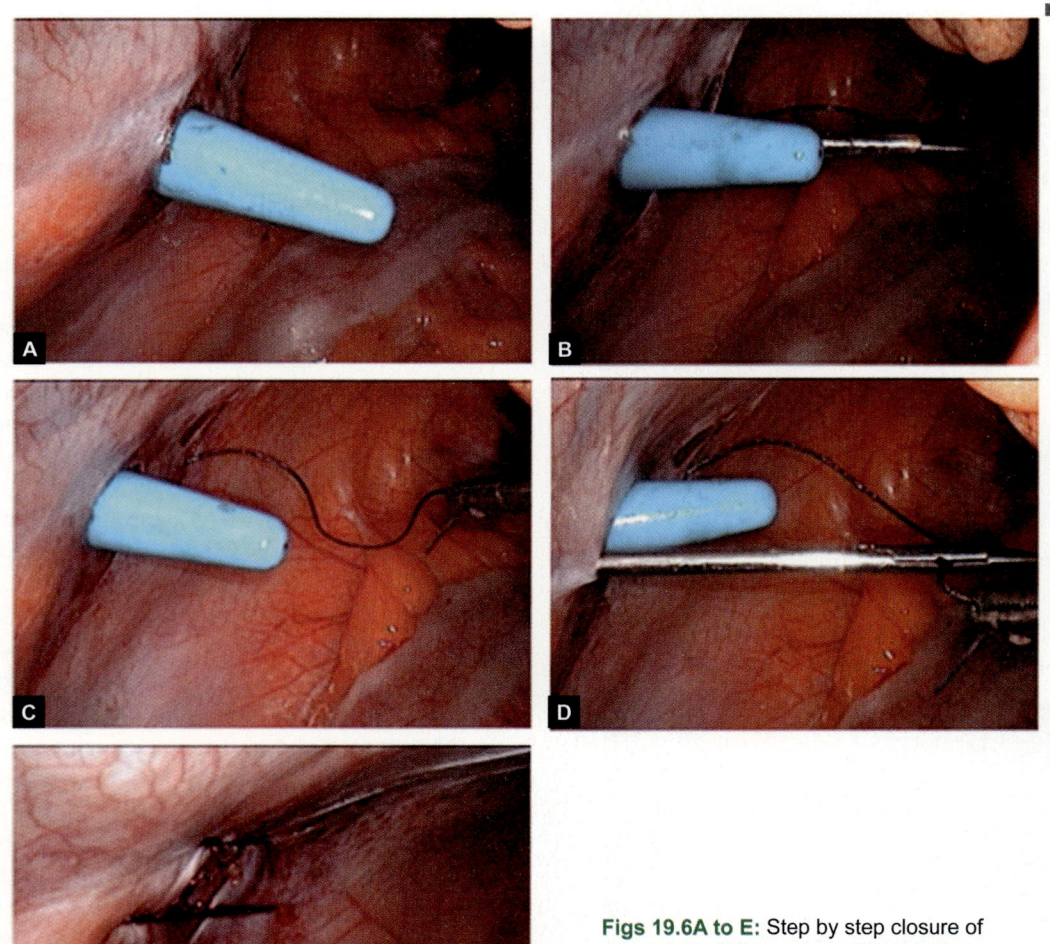

Figs 19.6A to E: Step by step closure of port site (15 mm morcellator port)

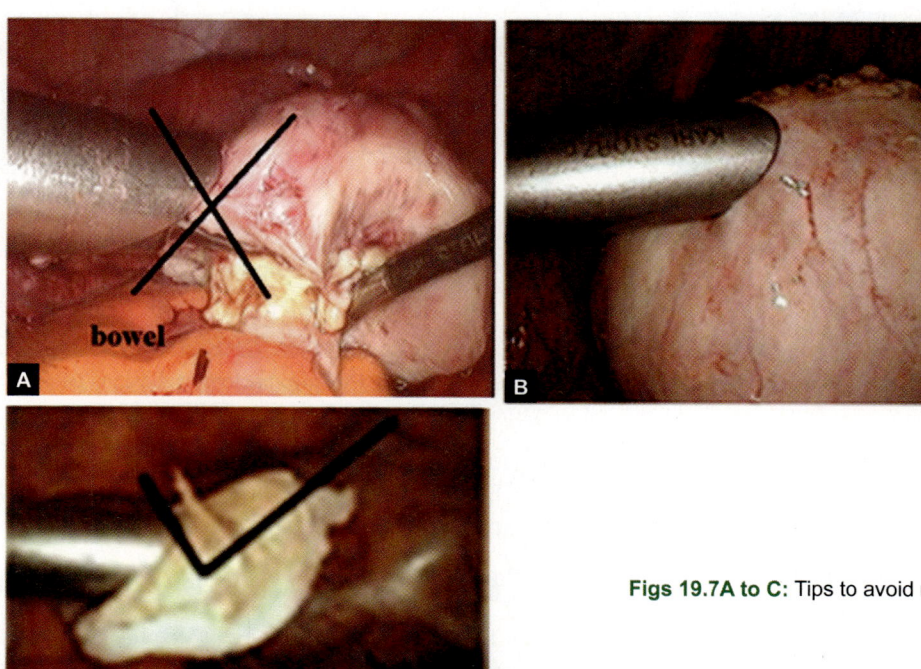

bowel

Figs 19.7A to C: Tips to avoid morcellator injuries

It is ideal, if morcellation can be done inside a bag so that pieces of the myoma do not get left out in the abdomen. Also in the rare case of an unsuspected sarcoma, the chance of disseminating it is minimized. The tip of the morcellator should always be visible and the mocellation should be like the peeling of an onion so that you do not create holes in the myoma.

The FDA's current recommendations discourage the use of power morcellators during hysterectomy or myomectomy for fibroids and that if, after carefully weighing the available options. If the doctor feels that laparoscopic power morcellation is the best option for the patient, then the doctor should inform the patient that the fibroid may contain unexpected cancerous tissue and that lap. Power morcellator may spread the disease significantly worsening their prognosis.

PELVIC ADHESIONS POST LAPAROSCOPIC MYOMECTOMY

Incidence: Varies from 18% to 30%.[6] When the incision on the myoma is posterior, the incidence rises. The incidence also rises when the patient also already had adhesions at initial surgery (Figs 19.8 and 19.9).

Prevention

Use Minimum Cautery

Avoid using posterior incisions and multiple incisions as far as possible. The initial incision should be placed such that

you can enucleate most of the myomas through it. For this proper fibroid mapping prior to the procedure by the surgeon will help. Transvaginal sonography and hysteroscopy may be used.

Thorough haemostasis and use of barriers like interceed has been shown to prevent adhesions at second look laparoscopy. One must not allow the tissues to become charred. Frequent irrigation to keep the tissue moist also helps in preventing adhesions

UTERINE RUPTURE DURING PREGNANCY

Exact incidence not known. But it is rare.

Cause is the integrity of myometrium compromised badly.

Prevention

Huge myomas especially intramural reaching submucous plane are more likely to give way. There should be good approximation of the tissues with no dead space. When the myoma cavity is deep it should be closed in layers. There should be no dead space to allow a haematoma to form there when the action of vasopressin wears off. Barbed sutures and baseball suturing technique will help. Preferably do not violate the endometrial cavity, if possible during myomectomy.

The risk of uterine rupture in pregnancy post laparoscopic myomectomy is there when intramural myomas are excised. Studies by Hasson,[7] Romeich and Nezhat[8] as well as one study by Miller[9] revealed no uterine rupture either pre- or

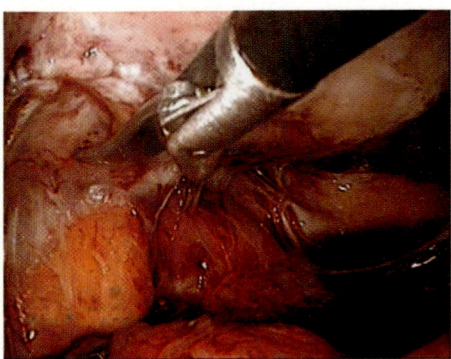

Fig. 19.8: Postmyomectomy adhesions being released

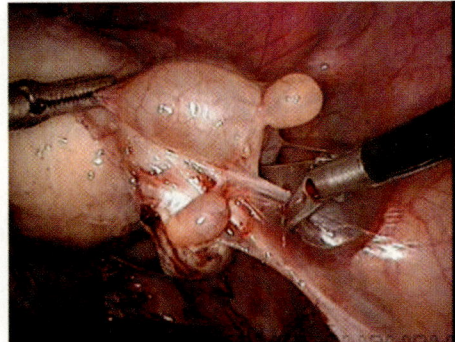

Fig. 19.9: Postmyomectomy adhesions causing hydrosalpinx of right tube

intra-partum, but Miller recommends caesarean section for all post myomectomy patients.

RECURRENCE OF MYOMAS

Incidence

Approximately 23%–25%.

Cause

Missing small myomas and deep intramural myomas at original surgery. Recurrence risk increases after preoperative GnRH agonist usage.

Prevention

1. Thorough mapping of all myomas by transabdominal as well as transvaginal sonography, if necessary, hysterosonogram, MRI, etc.
2. Do not use GnRH agonists prior to laparoscopic myomectomy. It makes dissection more difficult also by shrinking the myomas makes them more likely to be missed.

    Mean time of recurrence was 42 months with 4.08% of patient requiring repeat surgery.[10]

Lost Needles/Myoma Bits in Peritoneal Cavity

Leaving needles is rare. Suturing technique should be good. Do not hold the needle too close to swaging. The needles should be removed from the peritoneal cavity after each sequence of suturing. If you need to suture in another place it can be reintroduced.

Management

If, even after thorough inspection of the peritoneal cavity, one is unable to find the needle, it can be removed using a C arm.

Small myoma bits are sometimes missed (Figs 19.10A and B). To prevent this morcellation should preferably be done in endobags (Fig. 19.11). Orange peel method of morcellation should be used. It should be done under vision. When small pieces do fall off they should be picked up and removed

immediately before starting another bout of morcellation. Some surgeons prefer to keep a gauze piece below, so that the pieces may be later picked off it.

ROLE OF TRANSVAGINAL SONOGRAPHY

Transvaginal sonography (TVS) has a very important role to play in laparoscopic myomectomy. The exact site, size and number of myomas should be known to the operating surgeon prior to surgery, so that all of them get removed. The distance from endometrium, cornu as well as relative position from one another in case of multiple myomas is important. It is ideal if the surgeon himself does this on the day prior to surgery. This is of immense importance since the tactile findings are minimal during laparoscopic surgery. This also helps in planning port selection and incisions.

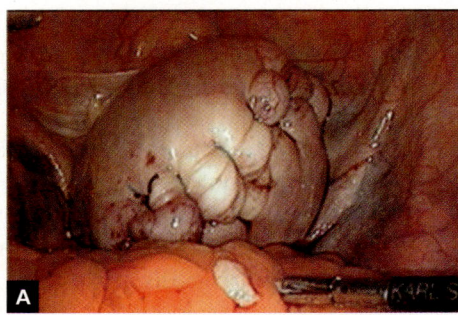

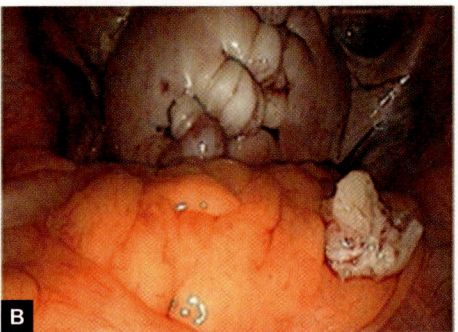

Figs 19.10A and B: Removing bits of myoma after morcellation using toothed grasper

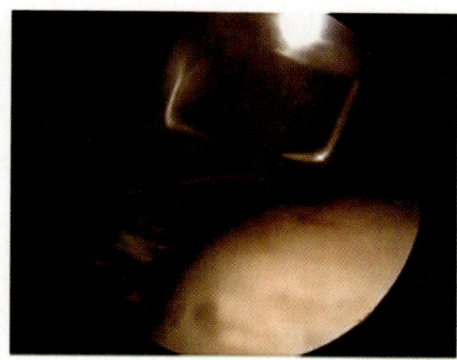

Fig. 19.11: Morcellation inside the endobag

INTRAOPERATIVE ULTRASOUND IN LAPAROSCOPIC MYOMECTOMY

Use of high frequency ultrasound (10–12 MHZ) transducer placed directly on the surface of an organ provides sharper images than might be obtained through the abdominal wall.[13–15]

In a study done by David Levine et al laparoscopic ultrasound transducer was placed through a 10–12 mm port to map the uterus and then identify the location, type, size and number of myomas to be treated via radiofrequency thermal ablation. Gynaecologic surgeon performed the scan.

The transducer was passed over each wall systematically (anterior, right, posterior, left and fundus). Scanning was done from lower segment up to the fundus. Laparoscopic ultrasound (LUS) enabled imaging of the entire extent of the myoma in all planes. When a myoma was identified, the surgeon could determine its location and anatomical relationship to the serosa, the myometrium and endometrium. These parameters enabled proper classification of the myoma. LUS could identify more myomas when compared with contrast enhanced MRI. So the conclusion is that LUS should be used at the time of myoma treatment to maximize detection of their number and location, and therefore enable treatment of most if not all myomas. Thus recurrences can be prevented.

Thromboembolism Prevention

American College of Obstetricians and Gynaecologists (ACOG)[19] recommends that until more evidence is accumulated patients undergoing laparoscopic surgery should be stratified by risk category and should receive prophylaxis similar to that provided in patients undergoing open surgery.[16]

Early ambulation and/or pneumatic compression stockings may be adequate if the patient is not obese and the surgery does not last more than 30 minutes.

All other patients especially if obese, aged more than 40 years, have been immobilised recently or have been prescribed oestrogens or progestogens recently should receive low molecular weight heparin 40 mg administered subcutaneously 12 hours before surgery and once a day postoperatively till discharge.[18]

◼ BOWEL INJURY[20] (Figs 19.12 and 19.13)

Incidence

0.5%–2%.

Causes

Thermal/Trauma by entry technique instruments/instruments of myomectomy procedure.

Prevention

High degree of suspicion, cold scissors for dissection. Avoid electrical energy source for cauterisation directly on the bowel rather suturing using No. 3-0 delayed absorbable suture material is preferred. Previous surgical history be prepared for difficult surgery and dense adhesions.

Diagnosis

Stormy postoperative period with fever, rising erythrocyte sedimentation rate (ESR) and C-reactive protein (CRP), evidence of peritonitis like fever, abdominal distension, vomiting, absent or sluggish bowel sounds and passage of purulent stools. Can be diagnosed by computed tomography (CT) abdomen/diagnostic laparoscopy.

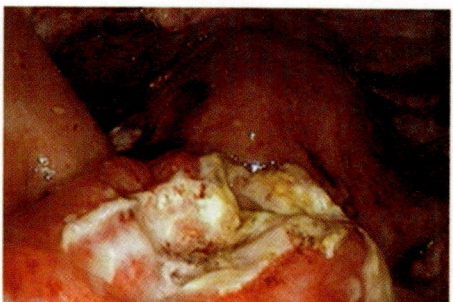

Fig. 19.12: Evidence of bowel necrosis on postoperative day 5, was associated with localised peritonitis

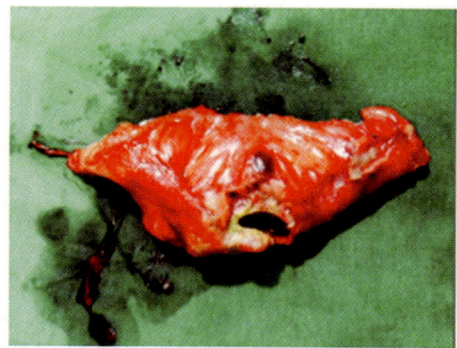

Fig. 19.13: Specimen of wide segmental bowel resection by laparoscopic assisted minilaparotomy

Management

Timely detection wide segmental resection with coverage of broad spectrum antibiotics.

■ CONCLUSION

Since laparoscopy and laparoscopic myomectomy has come to stay, it is imperative that the surgeons know the possible complications and have a very good idea regarding the management of these complications. Of course it goes without saying that prevention is better than cure.

■ REFERENCES

1. Omella Sizzi, Alfonso Rosetti, Mario Malzoni, et al. Italian multicentric study on complications of laparoscopic myomectomy JMIG. 2007;14(4):453-62.
2. Gerard S Letterie. Surgery, Assisted Reproductive Technology and Infertility 2nd ed. Taylor and Francis, 2006. p. 237.
3. Nezhat C, Nezhat F, Bess O, et al. Laparoscopically assisted myomectomy: a report of a new technique in 57 cases. Int J Fertil Menopausal Stud. 1994;39:39-44.
4. Stringer NH, Strassner HT, Lawson L, et al. Pregnancy outcomes after laparoscopic myomectomy with ultrasonic energy and laparoscopic suturing of the endometrial cavity. J Am Assoc Gynecol Laparosc. 2001;8:129-36.
5. Dubuisson JB, Faucontier A, Deffarges JV, et al. Pregnancy outcome and deliveries following laparascopic myomectomy. Hum Reprod. 2000;15:869-73.
6. Dubisson JB, Faucontier A, Chapron C, et al. Second look after laparoscopic myomectomy. Human Reprod. 1998;13:2102-6.
7. Hasson H M, Rotman C, Ramans N. Laparoscopic myomectomy. Obstet Gynecol. 1992;80:884-88.
8. Roemisch M, Nezhat F R, Nezhat C. Pregnancy after laparoscopic myomectomy. JMIG. 1996;3:s42.
9. Miller C, Jhonston M, Rundell M. Laparoscopic myomectomy in the infertile woman. J Am Assoc Gynecol laparosc. 1996;3(4):525-32.
10. Doridot Y, et al. J American Assoc. Gynae Laparoscopists (AAGL). 2001:8(4):495-500.
11. Yoo EH, LeePI, Huh CY, Kim DH, et al. J Minim Invasive Gynecol. 2007;14(6):690-7.
12. Kamath MS, Acharya M, Kamath V, et al. Disseminated Intravascular Coagulation after Myomectomy: A case report and review of literature. Int J Infertility Fetal Med. 2013;4(1):31-3.
13. SChimer BD. Intraoperative laparoscopic ultrasound. In: Holzheimer RG, Mannick JA (Eds). Surgical treatment: Evidence based and Problem oriented. Munich Germany: W Zuckschwerdt Verlag GMBH. 2001.
14. CritiniA, Lin PC. Applications of itraoperative ultrasound in gynaecological surgery. Curr Opin Obstet Gynecol. 2005;17:339-42.
15. Angioli R, Battista C, Terranova C, et al. Intra operative contact ultrasonography during open myomectomy for uterine fibroids. Fertil Sterili. 2010;94:1487-90.
16. Cheng Z, Yang W, Dai H, et al. Laparoscopic uterine artery occlusion combined with myomectomy for uterine myomas. J Minim Invasive Gyneacol. 2008;15:346-9.
17. Lichtinger M, Hallson L, CalvoP, et al. Laparoscopic uterine artey occlusion for symptomatic leiomyomas. J Am Assoc Gynecol Laparosc. 2009;9:191-8.
18. Howard A Shah; Chief Editor Kris Srohbehn, et al. Thromboembolism prophylaxis in Gynecologic Surgery. Medscape English Edition updated Aug 28, 2014.
19. ACOG practice bulletin No:84: Prevention of Deep vein thrombosis and pulmonary embolism. Obstet Gynecol. 2007;110(2Pt1):429-40.
20. Magrina JF. Complications of laparoscopic surgery. Clin Obstet Gynecol. 2002;45:469-80.

CHAPTER 20

Open Myomectomy

● L Fahmida Banu

Open or abdominal myomectomy is still considered as major surgical procedure in which uterine fibroids are removed by laparotomy and the uterus is then repaired. The primary objective of myomectomy is to preserve the uterus and fertility, so it is considered as the current treatment of choice for the women who are desired to have children or who wants to conserve their uterus.

This is generally preferred for women with symptomatic fibroids, which are either too large or too numerous to be removed under minimal-invasive or laparoscopic modalities.

Traditionally, open myomectomy thought to be a procedure with excessive blood loss, but the use of injection vasopressin and dissection in the correct tissue plane of myoma has changed it into a safe and successful technique with least blood loss.

Though we perform many myomectomy operations through operative laparoscopy or hysteroscopy open myomectomy also retains its district role with definite indications. In many fibroid uterei cases every surgeon cannot perform laparoscopic myomectomy because of its limitations like long learning curve, surgical expertise in endosuturing, expensive equipment and cost involved. Controversial laparoscopic morcillation can be avoided in open technique there by litigations associated with it.

Open myomectomy can be learned, practiced and performed in a much easier way provided one understands the anatomy and surgical principles and has the passion for perfection.

■ HISTORY

The first successful abdominal myomectomy was performed in the USA by the Atlee brothers, Washington and John, in Lancaster, Pennsylvania in 1844. The first abdominal multiple myomectomy was performed by William Adam Alexander of Liverpool in 1898. However, the doyen of abdominal myomectomy is Victor Bonney, generally considered the father and pioneer of modern gynaecological surgery.[1]

Victor and Annie met each other, while he was a resident and she is sister at the Chelsea Hospital for women in London and got married in 1905. 2 years later, Annie developed profuse bleeding in her periods and on consultation, majority of the doctors suggested that she would need hysterectomy to prevent further heavy bleeding and complications. This loss of hope for the family stimulated Bonney to improve the technique by avoiding these complications and limitations.[1]

'In my early years as a gynaecological surgeon, a case occurred, which profoundly affected my outlook. A lady, recently married, wishing above all things to have a child underwent a subtotal hysterectomy on account of a single submucous fibroid. Being a woman of strong character and reticent fortitude, she accepted the blow without complaint and by assuming a proud indifference to children held her insistent mother instinct at bay and none, but those who knew her well perceived the tragedy. I was among them and the grief of it is still keen in me today.'[2]

Victor Bonney

Bonney's Myomectomy Clamp and Hood Technique

With his early experience that myomectomy involved heavy preoperative blood loss, Bonney's two contributions to myomectomy were will appreciated. The myomectomy clamp and the hood technique. Bonney had introduced the indigenous surgical instrument, myomectomy clamp (Fig. 20.1) in 1922, which will compress the uterine arteries on both sides and could temporarily cut-off the blood supply to the uterus, and proved its efficacy in reducing the blood loss. He also put rubber-covered clamps on each fallopian tube to occlude the arteries from ovarian artery. The hood technique was designed to reduce the risk of adhesion formation, which involves a serosa flap that covers the base of the defect left after removal of the fibroid.[3]

Patient Selection and Indications

Myomas are of different sizes, variety of shapes and variable in the number. Their location could be any where in the uterus or cervix can extended in any direction ex broad ligament fibroid.

One of the patient was 35 years nulliparous with mass per abdomen, which is extending up to epigastrium. She has multiple (12) myomas enucleation and the largest was 40 × 40 cm weighed 4.74 kg (Figs 20.2A to D). Open myomectomy can be performed successfully on any myoma irrespective of the size, number and location (Figs 20.3A and B).

In our series of open myomectomy I have enucleated 80 fibroids in one sitting in a nulliparous woman suffering from intractable menorrhagia leading to severe anaemia (refer Figs 20.3 Aand B).[4,6]

Abdominal myomectomy is preferred mostly for women with large intramural or subserosal leiomyomas and in big intracavitary myomas. More commonly, it is performed in patients with too many fibroids, and in cases where hysteroscopic or laparoscopic myomectomy is not feasible in view of any contraindications. It is not recommended in women in whom uterine conservation are contraindicated because of medical comorbidities or cervical and uterine malignancies. One has to remember that myomectomy is not required in asymptomatic women who were diagnosed incidentally with myomas less than 12 weeks size, and in perimenopausal women with minimal symptoms.[3,5]

Among open myomectomy patients treated in our series over the past 8 years, 50% are nulliparous, 20% are uniparous, 20% are biparous, 10% are triparous and above. Infertility is the common indication accounting in 50% of cases, menorrhagia in 37.5% of cases, abdominal mass in 15% of cases, dysmenorrhoea in 12.5% of cases and severe anaemia in 12.5% of cases (Figs 20.4 and 20.5).

■ INDICATIONS

1. Most common:
   - Abnormal uterine bleeding (menorrhagia)
   - Discomfort and mass per abdomen
   - Infertility
   - Anaemia and its manifestations
   - Asymptomatic large size fibroids incidently diagnosed
   - Dysmenorrhoea
   - Pressure symptoms on adjacent organs
   - Pressure on urinary tract (e.g. urinary frequency, urinary incontinence, hydroureter)
   - Pressure on gastrointestinal tract (GIT) (e.g. constipation).
2. Rare:
   - Torsion of fibroid
   - Retention of urine
   - Acute pain with degeneration of fibroids, etc.

■ PREOPERATIVE EVALUATION

Gynaecological History

A detailed obstetric and gynaecological history is very important to analyse and plan the surgery. History of menstrual rhythm, infertility, pain abdomen, pressure symptoms, etc. should be documented.[3,7]

Medical History

Detailed medical history should especially include medical comorbid conditions like diabetes, hypertension and obesity which could affect the possible safety concerns of the surgery.[3,7] The personal and family history of fibroids (genetic predisposing is seen in fibroids), genital malignancies, bleeding disorders were noted.

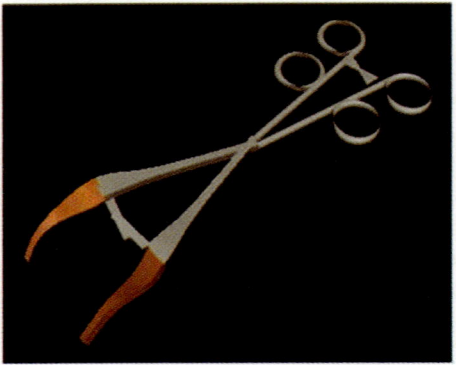

Fig. 20.1: Bonney's myomectomy clamp

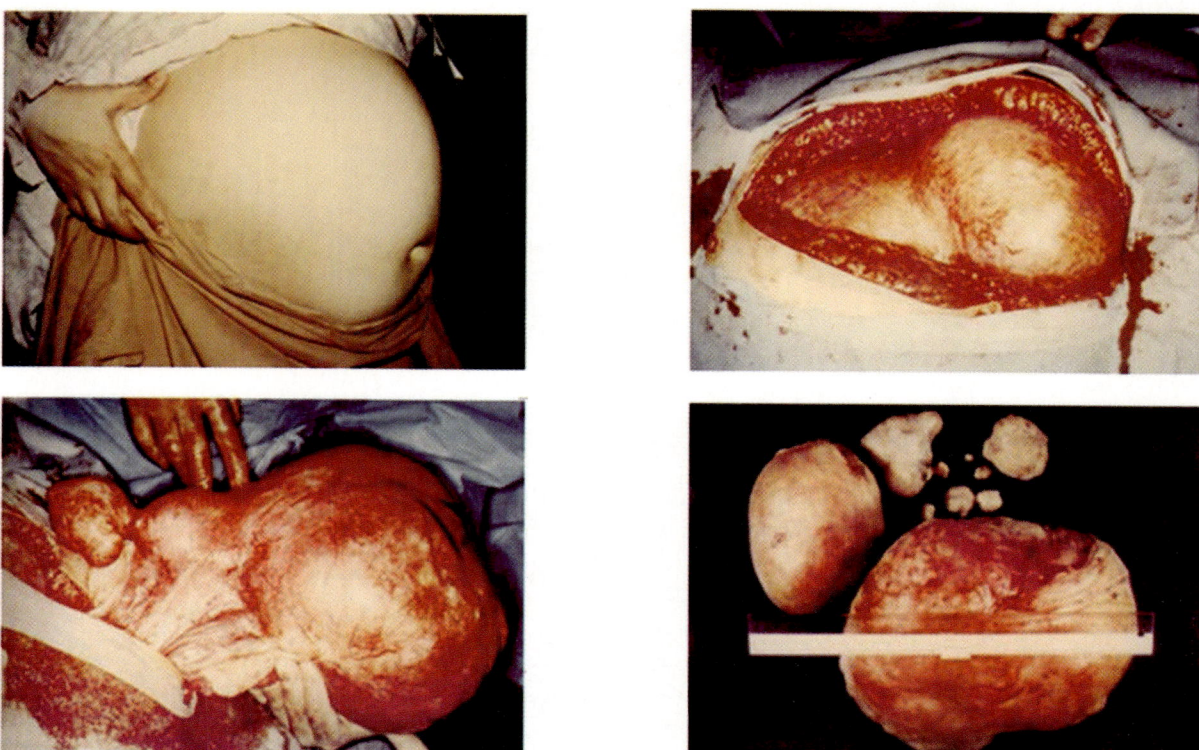

Figs 20.2A to D: A. Nulliparous lady with myoma uteri extending up to epigastrium; **B.** Vertical incision near xiphisternum to symphysis pubis; **C.** Huge myoma 40 cm × 40 cm total 12 fibroids; **D.** Largest myoma weight 4.74 kg.

Counselling

Proper counselling of the women about their medical condition, available surgical options, possible risks and outcome should be explained. Potential complications of the surgical procedure and the likelihood of recurrence of fibroids and other long-term complications should also be reviewed.[3,7]

Physical Examination

A thorough pelvic examination and uterus examination should be carried out, which helps the surgeon to suggest on

the investigations required and plan for the feasible surgical procedure.

Imaging an Laboratory Investigation

Ultrasound imaging is generally recommended to confirm the findings of the physical examination and mapping of the fibroids. A detailed ultrasound examination of abdomen and pelvis depicts the number of fibroids, their size and location and its proximity to the endometrial cavity and vascularity. It also evaluates kidney-ureters-bladder (KUB) area, and the

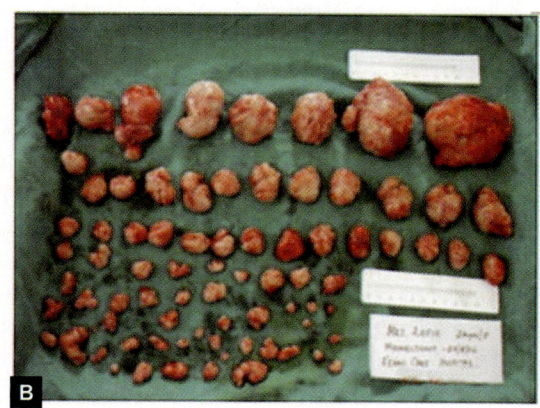

Figs 20.3A and B: A. Varieties of myoma uterus; **B.** Total 80 myomas enucleated in single operation.

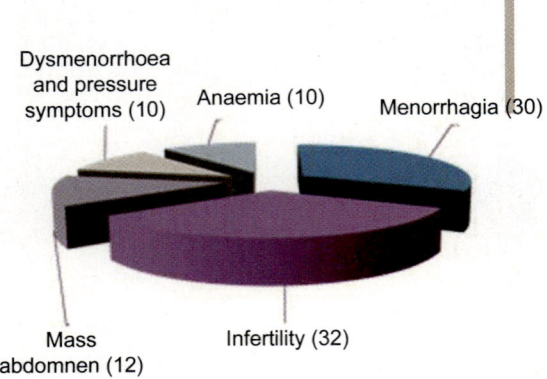

Dysmenorrhoea and pressure symptoms (10) Anaemia (10) Menorrhagia (30)

Mass abdomnen (12) Infertility (32)

Fig. 20.4: Distribution of symptoms

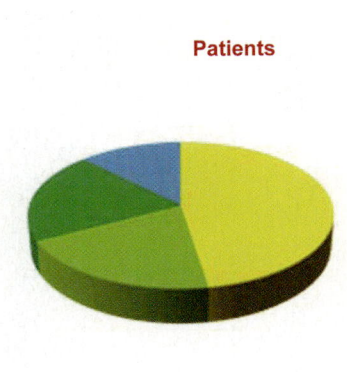

Patients

Fig. 20.5: Distribution of parity

pressure-related effects can be detected pre-operatively. Also to confirm the presence or absence of other intraabdominal pathology.

All these factors help to plan the surgery accordingly. Magnetic resonance imaging (MRI) can be performed in selected cases keeping its cost effectiveness especially in complex cases like suspected degenerations and malignancies.

Routine pre-operative investigations are suggested as performed in all surgical cases.

■ PREOPERATIVE PATIENT PREPARATION

Preparation for Potential Blood Loss

Though not usually results in significant blood loss, at least in advert of latest methodologies and techniques, preoperative measures such as correction of anaemia with intravenous (iv) iron infusion may reduce the risk of complications and the need for blood transfusions.[3]

Role of Reduction of Uterine Size with GnRH Agonists

It is not mandatory to treat the patients by gonadotropin-releasing hormone (GnRH) agonists to reduce the size of fibroids. In spite of common observation that GnRH agonists reduces the blood loss and the risk of blood transfusion, these have various disadvantages (Box 20.1), like intraoperative difficulty in enucleation as it causes fibrosis and the cleavage plane is distorted. It also increases the risk of persistent myomas as small seedling fibroids may shrink and not detected intraoperatively thus majority of the surgeons are against their use in routine myomectomy. Also, their treatment is expensive and not cost-effective, the similar reduction of blood loss could be achieved by injection of vasopressin and tranexamic acid, which are effective and cheaper.[3,7,8]

Box 20.1: Disadvantages of GnRH agonists in preoperative preparation of open myomectomy

Difficulty in rendering surgical enucleation due to destruction of tissue planes
Risk of persistant myomas/risk of recurrence (smaller myomas are missed and regrow aggressively after their effects wear off)
Significant menopausal side effects
Expensive and not cost effective

Prophylactic Antibiotics

There is no substantial evidence to support the use of prophylactic antibiotics in women undergoing myomectomy surgery. One school of surgeons recommend their use considering the prevention of pelvic infection regard to preservation of fertility, whereas others do not routinely recommend considering the surgery as clean procedure with no vaginal or intestinal incision.[7]

Thromboprophylaxis

Patients especially with obesity and comorbid pathology require either mechanical stockings, application of pneumatic calf compressions or pharmacologic low-molecular-weight/fractioned heparin measures of thromboprophylaxis.[7]

■ PROCEDURE

The key steps involved in the procedure are:
1. Incision on abdomen.
2. Adequate exposure.
3. Application of measures to reduce blood loss.
4. Uterine incision.
5. Myoma enucleation.
6. Closure of uterine defects.
7. Adhesions Prevention.

Incision on Abdomen

Most appropriate and accessible incision should be chosen based on the size of the uterus, and the location and size of the fibroids. More commonly for primary myomectomy, the transverse incisions, e.g. Pfannenstiel or Maylard incision prefered. Vertical incisions reserved for larger myomas, which are extended above the umbilicus and for secondary myomectomy operations, as bowel adhesions are anticipated and the access can be severely compromised with multiple transverse incisions.[9]

Secondary myomectomies are procedures with history of previous operations performed for myomas enucleation. Frederick J, Hardie M, et al in their prospective study showed a high operative morbidity and a poor fertility outcome after a repeat myomectomy. The factors affecting successful outcome in a logistic regression model were age, tubal adhesions and number of uterine fibroid.

Adequate Exposure

The uterus with the fibroid is exteriorized (Fig. 20.6). For large fibroids or multiple fibroids, a myoma screw is used so that uterus is stabilised. The intestines are pushed up into the upper abdominal cavity using warm moist abdominal swabs. The uterus is kept elevated either by packing the pouch of Douglas with warm moist gauze or by abdominal retractors.[3]

Application of measures to reduce blood loss multiple factors that accounts for the increased risk of intraoperative blood loss include:[3,7]

1. Increased vascularity of fibroid uterus.
2. Mechanical obstruction of venous drainage of myometrium and endometrium due to fibroids.
3. Brisk bleeding from the adjoining blood vessels after enucleation of the intramural fibroids from the pseudocapsule.
4. Potential accumulation of haematomas at the site of enucleation.

Different range of measure that are employed to reduce the risk of blood loss are listed in Box 20.2.[3,7,8]

Tourniquet Techniques

Tourniquet techniques are implemented to achieve haemostasis by interrupting the blood supply to the uterus. The main feeding vessels supplying blood to uterus are compressed. In the single tourniquet technique, a single tourniquet is applied around the cervix to compress both uterine arteries. In the triple tourniquet technique, three tourniquets are applied, one to occlude each of the ovarian arteries, and one around cervix to occlude the uterine arteries.[8]

Table 20.2: Measures applied to reduce risk of blood loss[3,7,8]

Physical occlusion of blood flow: • Use of clamps/tourniquets (single or triple tourniquets) • Ligation of uterine arteries • Pre-myomectomy uterine artery embolisation
Pre-operative drugs: • Use of pre-operative GnRH analogues
Chemical haemostatics: • Intramyometrial vasopressin • Intravenous tranexamic acid • Intravaginal misoprostol • Intravenous oxytocin
Chemical dissection techniques: • Use of mesna
Surgical dissection techniques: • Use of electrocautery • In situ morcellation

Injection Vasopressin

Vasopressin 20 units in 100 cc normal saline injected routinely prior to making an incision in the into the pericapsular plane of myoma. This has revolutionized myomectomy operation along with dissection in the correct tissue planes (Fig. 20.7). This is the best and favoured technique for achieving blood less field with the caution to inform anaesthetist, while infiltrating and relative contraindication in hypertensive women.

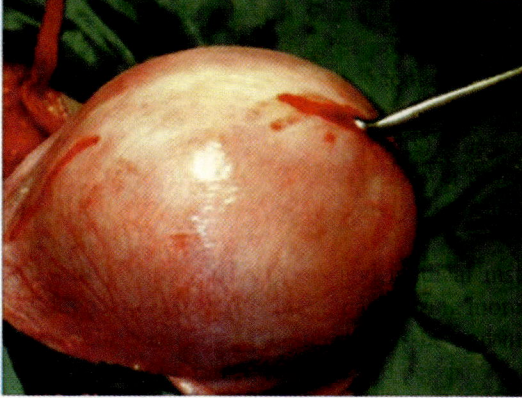

Fig. 20.6: Exteriorisation of the uterus

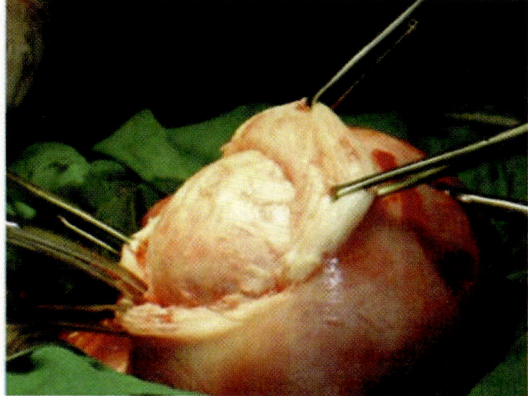

Fig. 20.7: Dissection in correct cleavage of tissue planes

Chemical Dissection with Mesna

Sodium 2 mercaptoethanesulfonate (mesna) is a thiolic drug, which has been used in the chemical separation of tissue connections. Mesna is injected locally at the dissection zone (from incision of visceral peritoneum to complete enucleation of the myoma). The operation time was significantly shorter than the control group and with significantly less reduction in haemoglobin attributed by higher levels of haematocrit levels.[3,8]

Uterine Incision

The uterine serosal incision is generally determined by the size, number and location of myomas and by their proximity to the uterine vessels and fallopian tubes. Generally, a single, anterior, transverse or in some cases, midline vertical incision is given or at location to access and remove the myomas without breaching the uterine cavity. Alternatively, an incision can be made directly over each myoma especially the posterior incisions are required to remove posterior myomas.[3,9]

The number of incisions determines the chances of adnexal and bowel adhesions and all the possible attempts to be made to minimize the number of incisions with prompt closure of uterine defects and secure haemostasis.[3]

Electrocautery

Effective usage of electrocautery for incision, coagulation and haemostasis will shorten the surgical time and reduces the blood loss (Fig. 20.8).[3]

Myoma Removal

Incision should be extended through the serosa, myometrium and into the pseudo capsule of the myoma. The myoma will be clearly visible and may bulge slightly after extending the incision into little deeper into the capsule through planes of least vascularity (Figs 20.9A and B).[3]

Myometrial edges are put under traction with Allis clamps and the myoma is held in position with myoma screw (if myoma is large) or with single tooth tenaculum (bullet forceps) (if myoma is small) to facilitate enucleation.[3]

After accurately achieving the plane of cleavage between the myoma and surrounding myometrium (refer Fig. 20.9A), it is dissected bluntly (e.g. using a peanut sponge or the back end of an empty knife handle or a finger) (Fig. 20.10) from its bed. From one incision other fibroids are enucleated through tunnelling incisions to minimise number of incisions (Fig. 20.11).[3,7]

Closure of Uterine Defects

The myometrium defects are closed with sutures in layers, with suture material number 1—polyglactin. Interrupted mattress sutures or continuous running (Fig. 20.12) or locking

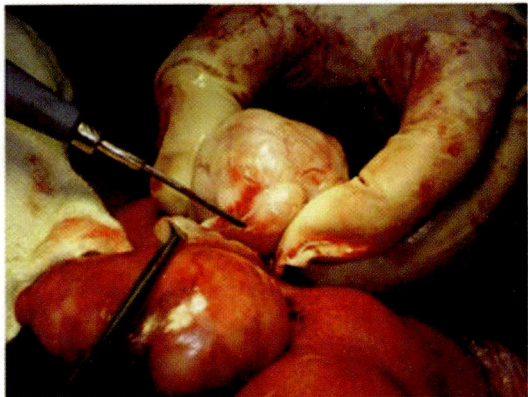

Fig. 20.8: Judicial use of electrocautery

sutures are applied depending upon the vascularity and the location of the myoma in myometrium or subserosal suture or in the serosa.

If the myometrial defect is too deep, it is sutured in two layers to reapproximate the tissue and attain haemostasis. The sutures should have sufficient tensile strength. Later, an adhesion barrier can be applied over the wound and the peritoneal cavity is lavaged with warm saline to remove any remnant collection of blood or body fluids.[3,7]

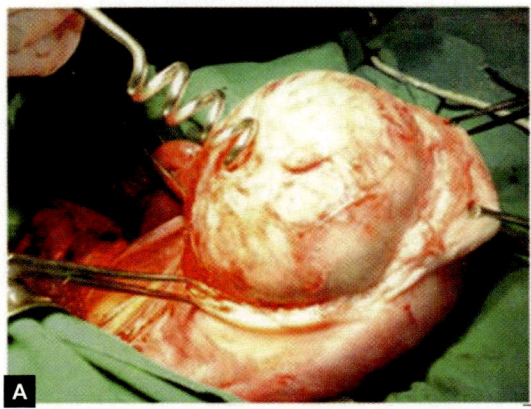

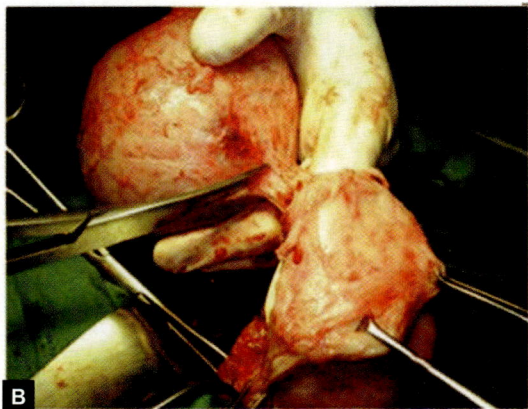

Figs 20.9A and B: A. Dissection in least vascular planes of myometrium; **B.** Enucleation of myoma.

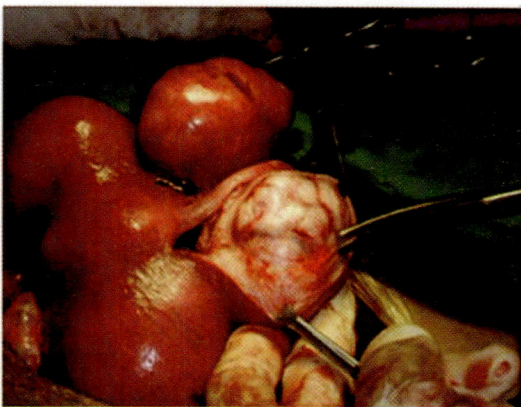

Fig. 20.10: Multiple enucleation from single incision

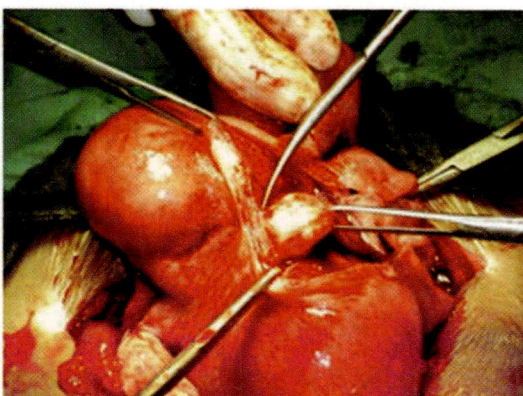

Fig. 20.11: Tunnelling incisions

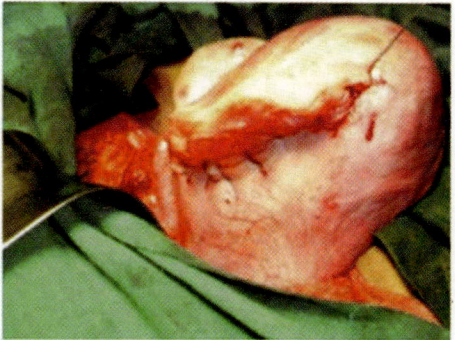

Fig. 20.12: Running sutures of the uterine serosal layer

Drains and Abdominal Closure

It is always recommended to insert intra-abdominal drain into the peritoneal cavity, especially for large and multiple myoma enucleated cases and it could be removed after 48 to 72 hours after surgery.

▮ POSTOPERATIVE CARE AND FOLLOW-UP

Routine postoperative care in regards with haemodynamic status, pain control, diet management and ambulation should be followed. Regular follow-up visits at 2 weeks then at 8 weeks is recommended to evaluate the wound condition and potential complications.

▮ OPERATIVE CHALLENGES IN REMOVAL OF MYOMAS IN SPECIAL SITUATIONS

Broad Ligament Myomas

Close proximity to ureters and the possibility of alteration of course of ureters due to broad ligament myomas, identification of ureters is most important before any attempt made to secure haemostasis and myoma removal. In cases of difficulty, the myoma should be approached directly and enucleation performed from within the capsule.[3,7]

Cervical Myomas

Cervical myomas often have a complex blood supply, may involve the distal part of the ureter. It is difficult to remove myomas, which are centrally or circumferentially located, with the uterus apparently sitting perched on the myoma. However, careful identification and incision of peritoneum should be done, followed by myoma removal with traction and blunt dissection in the proper surgical plane away from the vital structures.[3,7] Indicated cases preoperative demarcation of ureter course with computed tomography (CT) will give anatomical details and enables safe dissection planes.

Caesarean Myomectomy

Open myomectomy can be performed along with caesarean section to avoid another interval surgery. Under epidural anaesthesia technique, myomectomy after lower segment caesarean section (LSCS) is preferred, if needed uterine arteries could be ligated (Figs 20.13A and B).

▮ MALIGNANT TRANSFORMATION

Uterine leiomyosarcoma (LMS) is a rare gynaecologic malignancy, comprising about 1% of all uterine malignancies and 25% to 36% of uterine sarcomas.[1–3] LMS is generally considered a highly malignant neoplasm with 5-year survival rate of 18.8% to 65% for all stages of disease.[18–20] Unexpected histopathological confirmation of sarcomatous changes in myoma is reported to be 1:1000 cases. High degree of suspicion, detailed history of rapidly growing mass, ultrasound evaluation of increased vascularity on Doppler flow studies and degenerative changes in USG/MRI and intraoperative specimen on cut section observation are important clues to find the possibility of malignant transformation. All enucleated fibroids without exception should be subjected for histopathological examination.

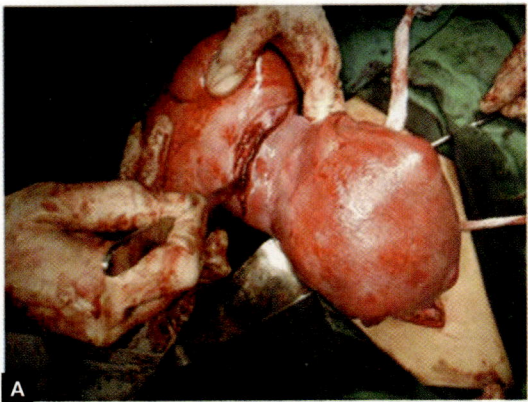
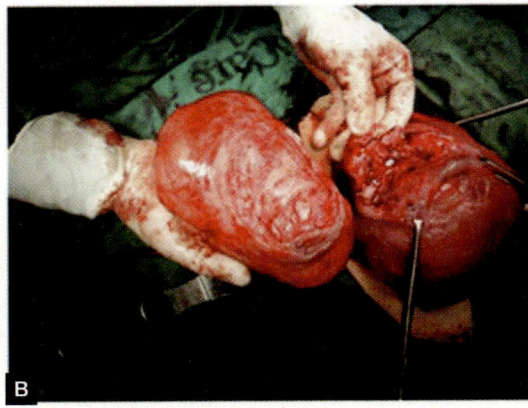

Figs 20.13A and B: Caesarean myomectomy

In our series a 27 years women with primary infertility with asymptamatic fibroid corresponding to 18 weeks size incidentally diagnosed in clinical examination and confirmed by USG as single large fibroid had myomectomy (Figs 20.14A to D). She had uneventful surgery with least blood loss (refer Figs 20.14B and C). The cut section of the specimen appeared as degenerated fibroid (refer Fig. 20.14D) and hope reported as leiomyosarcoma (Fig. 20.15A) and further studies of histochemistry was performed (Figs 20.15B and C).

RISK FACTORS

Nulliparity, increasing age and obesity are some of the risk factors for uterine sarcomas. A history of pelvic radiation has also been identified as an aetiological factor, as well as exposure to tamoxifen. The most frequent symptoms of uterine LMS are abnormal vaginal bleeding and palpable mass followed by weight loss and weakness. Intraoperative visual distinction between leiomyosarcoma and large leiomyoma is nearly impossible, therefore leimyosarcoma is often diagnosed at postoperative histologic evaluation of hysterectomy or myomectomy specimens.

HISTOPATHOLOGY

Leiomyosarcomas are composed of malignant uterine smooth muscle cells. The cells are elongated with tapered ends. Microscopically, these tumours may histologically resemble the normal uterine musculature. As the cellularity increases, nuclear atypism increases, the cytoplasm becomes more eosinophilic and the number of giant cells increase. Evans was the first to document this information in 1920. He divided his cases into high, moderate, and low mitotic counts, depending on the number of mitotic figures per cubic millimeter of tissue. Most authors now accept 10 mitotic figures per 10 high-powered fields (HPF) as diagnostic feature.

IMMUNOHISTOCHEMISTRY

The CD10 is a reliable and sensitive immunohistochemical marker of normal endometrial stroma. Positive staining with CD10, when strong and diffuse, may be useful in distinguishing these tumours (Figs 20.15A to C). CD10 should be used as part of a panel, which might include desmin and alpha-inhibin depending on the differential diagnosis considered.

SURGICAL MANAGEMENT OF LEIOMYOSARCOMA

The treatment of choice for uterine LMS is surgical removal such as total hysterectomy and bilateral salpingo-oophorectomy and appropriate surgical staging, including peritoneal washings and sampling of suspicious nodules, should be carried out.

Pelvic Lymphadenectomy

The role of lymphadenectomy is unclear because of the limited number of studies in this area. The incidence of lymph node metastasis from uterine leiomyosarcomas is very low. Giuntoli et al, stated in their study 7 of 208 women with uterine leiomyosarcomas, 36 had lymph node dissection, of whom 4 (11%) had positive nodes. Lymph node status may, however, have a role as a staging procedure as well as in determining the need for adjuvant pelvic radiotherapy.

RISKS AND COMPLICATIONS OF OPEN MYOMECTOMY

Intraoperative Complications Haemorrhage

The average volume of blood loss varies across studies from approximately 50 to 200 mL and the blood transfusion rate varies widely in various studies from 2 to 28%.[7]

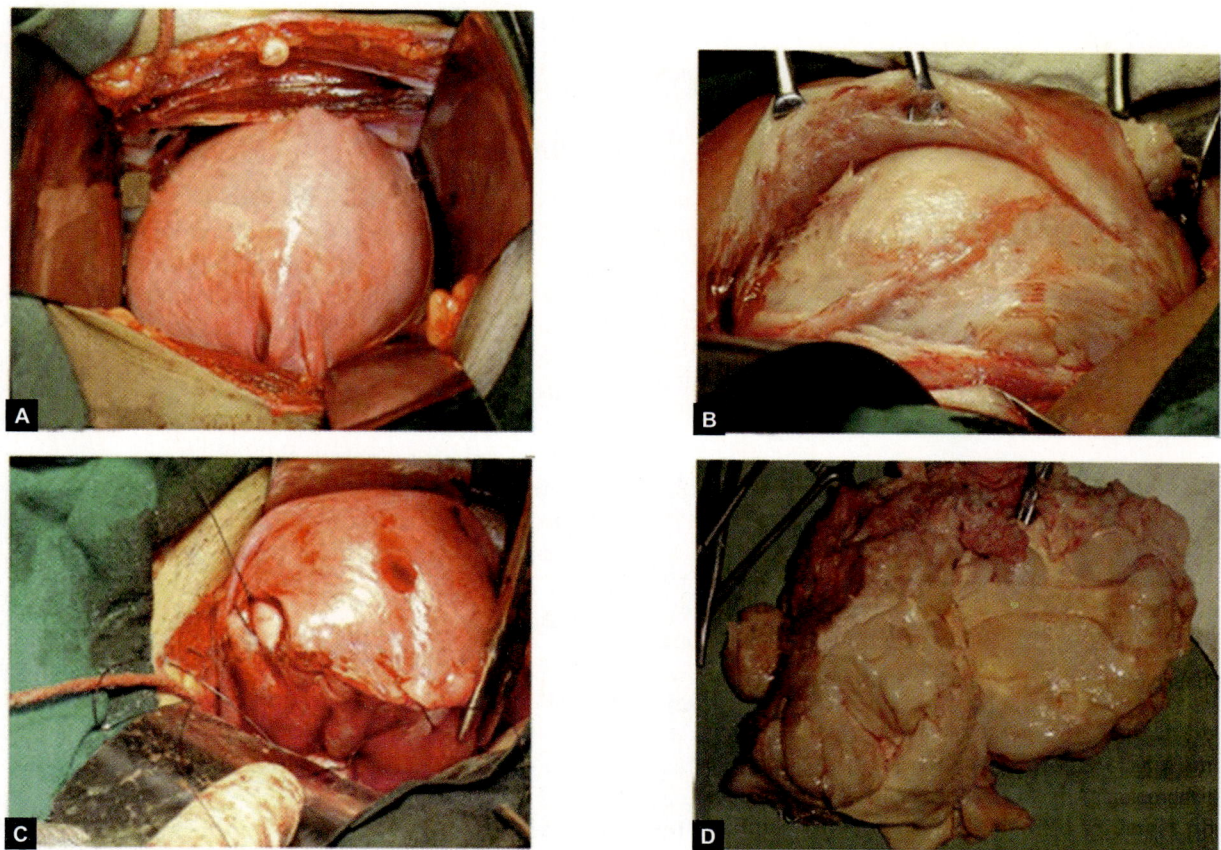

Figs 20.14A to D: A. 27 years lady with Infertility came for myomectomy; **B.** Intra operative picture with clean avascular plane; **C.** The same patient end of surgey with least blood loss and uneventful procedure; **D.** The cut section appearance was like degenerated fibroid sent for HPE.

Considering all the techniques, vasopressin injection show the most impact on blood loss especially when higher number of fibroid are removed during surgery. A randomized controlled trial conducted by Taylor A et al, also showed that triple tourniquets are effective in reducing bleeding and transfusion rates with no obvious adverse effect on uterine perfusion or ovarian function.[8,10] In our series blood transfuction rate is intraoperative 2.5% and postoperatively 6%.

Conversion to Hysterectomy

Risk of conversion to hysterectomy due to uncontrolled bleeding is considered earlier to be 1% to 2% in primary myomectomy (removal of uterine fibroid for the first time) and slightly higher, 2% in secondary myomectomy (for recurrent symptomatic uterine fibroid).[11] But, in recent times, with vasopressin injection, perfect plane enucleation conversion has become a rarity. In our study also none of the case got converted to intraoperative hysterectomy.

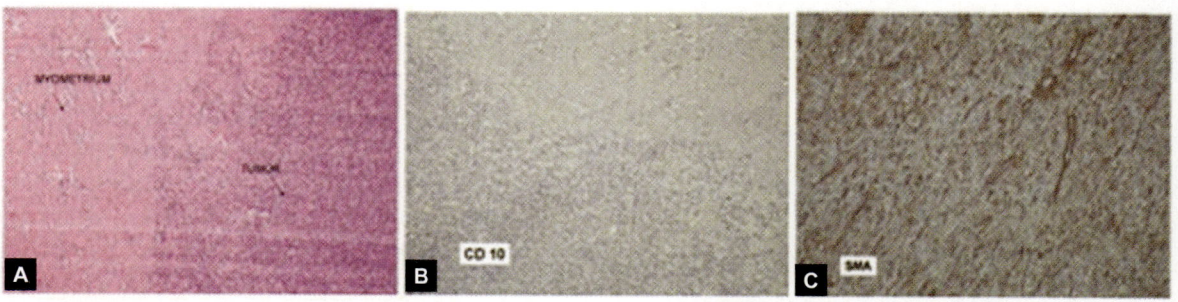

Figs 20.15A to C: A. The HPE staining of above specimen; **B and C.** Immune Histochemistry staining of above specimen.

Infection and Pyrexia

Post-myomectomy pyrexia affects 12%–38% of women and that wound infection affects less than 2% of women.[12,13] Sometimes, pyrexia may be reactionary or is due to haematomas collected within uterine defects, rather due to true infection of tissues. Good haemostasis and the use of prophylactic antibiotics will minimize the risk of post myomectomy febrile morbidity.[3]

Visceral Injury

Visceral injury (like injury to ureters, cystostomy, bowel obstruction, etc.) is rare in open myomectomy.

Long-term Complications

Adhesive Disease

Open myomectomy is associated with increased risk of adhesions when compared with other minimal invasive surgeries. Adhesions increases the risk of infertility, ectopic gestation, and bowel obstruction.[14]

Use of various antiadhesion agents like, hyaluronic acid carboxymethylcellulose film, Dextran, Beriplast (factor 13 with fibrinogen), Seprafilm, Interceed (Fig. 20.16), Gore-Tex, steroids, icodextrin 4%, SprayGel, etc. are used, however more research is required to explore effective approaches for adhesion prevention. The best adhesion preventive measure is gentle handling of the tissue, perfect haemostasis and preventing drying of the tissue.[3]

◼ OUTCOMES OF OPEN MYOMECTOMY

Quality of Life

Majority of the patients report improved quality of life after myomectomy as menorrhagia is relived and haemoglobin levels are improved. Despite lack of prospective research the available evidence suggest that open myomectomy is

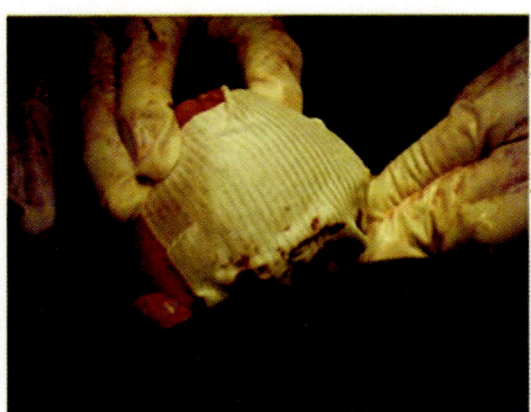

Fig. 20.16: Adhesion barriers

associated with improvements in health-related quality of life.[3] In our series, 94% of the patients reported satisfactory outcome with relief of menorrhagia and dysmenorrhoea.[6]

Fertility

Often, submucosal and intramural myomas distort the uterine anatomy significantly, and therefore presumably alter uterine physiology as well, leading to decreased fertility. So, removal of myomas help in gaining the normal anatomy and physiology, thereby improving the reproductive function.[3]

A study by Machupalli S et al, showed that open myomectomy resulted in increase in the chances of successful pregnancy (with 49% and 58%, respectively) and live births (with 27% and 55%, respectively).[15,18]

In our series, many parous women also opted for myomectomy for various social reasons there by carry home baby results in infertility group alone was 50%.

Miscarriage

Risk of miscarriage is also reduced with open myomectomy. Pregnancy and live-birth rates per cycle, and time to achieve first pregnancy and live-birth are improved with the removal of myomas.[3]

Obstetric Complications

Various complications like pain associated with red degeneration, preterm labour, malpresentation, placental abruption, intrauterine growth restriction, increased operative delivery, postpartum haemorrhage and postpartum are associated with myomas, which will be decreased after myomectomy. However, myomectomy appears to be associated with higher risk of uterine rupture when compared with minimal/laparoscopic myomectomy, though these have certain rate of risk.[3,16,17]

◼ CONCLUSION

Open myomectomy is a successful and promising approach for symptomatic, large, and multiple fibroids, especially with the application of recent methodologies and techniques to minimize the potential intraoperative and postoperative complications. It is a valuable surgical option to remove myomas, conserve the uterus and to restore the fertility in young nulliparous women. Also, open myomectomy is still considered in the parous women who prefers to undergo conservative surgery. This technique can be mastered easily compared to laparoscopic suturing technique. It is cheaper, cost effective, replicable and effective procedure with excellent patient satisfactory results. It is very rewarding both for patient and surgeon.

■ REFERENCES

1. Chamberlain G. The master of myomectomy. J R Soc Med. 2003;96(6):302-4.
2. Bonney V. The fruits of conservation. J Obstet Gynaecol Br Emp. 1937;44:1-12.
3. Mukhopadhaya N, De Silva C, Manyonda IT. Conventional myomectomy. Best Pract Res Clin Obstet Gynaecol. 2008;22(4):677-705.
4. Data on File. FehmiCare Hospital, 2010.
5. Iftikhar R. Outcome of abdominal myomectomy. Journal of Surgery Pakistan (International). 2009;14 (2):85-8.
6. Data on File. Surgical Management of Fibroid Uterus. FehmiCare Hospital, 2010.
7. Parker WH. Abdominal myomectomy. UpToDate Website. Available at http://www.uptodate.com/contents/abdominal-myomectomy. Last Updated Mar 03, 2014. Accessed November 05, 2015.
8. Conforti A, Mollo A, Alviggi C, et al. Techniques to reduce blood loss during open myomectomy: a qualitative review of literature. Eur J Obstet Gynecol Reprod Biol. 2015;192:90-5.
9. Stewart EA. Abdominal Myomectomy. In: Uterine Fibroids. The Complete Guide. A John Hopkins Press Health Book. Baltimore, MA. 2007: 75-83. Best Pract Res Clin Obstet Gynaecol. 2008;22(4):677-705.
10. Taylor A, Sharma M, Tsirkas P, et al. Reducing blood loss at open myomectomy using triple tourniquets: a randomised controlled trial. BJOG. 2005;112(3):340-5.
11. Frederick J, Hardie M, Reid M, et al. Operative morbidity and reproductive outcome in secondary myomectomy: a prospective cohort study. Hum Reprod. 2002;17:2967-71.
12. LaMorte AI, Lalwani S, Diamond MP. Morbidity associated with abdominal myomectomy. Obstet Gynecol. 1993;82:897-900.
13. Olufowobi O, Sharif K, Papaionnon S, et al. Are the anticipated benefits of myomectomy achieved in women of reproductive age? A 5-year review of the results at a UK tertiary hospital. J Obstet Gynaecol. 2004;24:434-40.
14. Conforti A, Krishnamurthy GB, Dragamestianos C, et al. Intrauterine adhesions after open myomectomy: an audit. Eur J Obstet Gynecol Reprod Biol. 2014;179:42-5.
15. Machupalli S, Norkus EP, Mukherjee TK, et al. Abdominal Myomectomy Increases Fertility Outcome. Gynecol Obstet. 2013;3(2):1-4.
16. Claeys J, Hellendoorn I, Hamerlynck T, et al. The risk of uterine rupture after myomectomy: a systematic review of the literature and meta-analysis. Gynecological Surgery. 2014;11(3):197-206.
17. Vilos GA, Allaire C, Laberge PY. The management of uterine leiomyomas. J Obstet Gynaecol Can. 2015;37(2):157-81.
18. Frederick J1, Hardie M, Reid M, et al Operative morbidity and reproductive outcome in secondary myomectomy: a prospective cohort study. Hum Reprod. 2002;17(11):2967-71.
19. Livi L, Paiar F, Shah N, et al. Uterine sarcoma: twenty-seven years of experience. Int J Radiat Oncol Biol Phys. 2003;57:13661373.
20. Major FJ, Blessing JA, Silverberg SG, et al. A Gynecologic Oncology Group study. Prognostic factors in early-stage uterine sarcoma. Cancer. 1993;71(4 Suppl):17021709.

CHAPTER 21

Embolisation for Uterine Fibroids

● Indusekhar Subbanna, Rajesh V Helavar

INTRODUCTION

Many methods of treatment for uterine fibroids have evolved since the last 2 decades. Whilst the exact incidence of fibroids is not known, it is said to occur in approximately 40% of women above the age of 40, commonly detected by ultrasound examination, although many are asymptomatic. Embolisation is now a recognized option for treatment in symptomatic women. In this chapter we will review the indications, contraindications, preprocedure evaluation, procedure, outcomes and complications related to uterine fibroid embolisation.

HISTORY

Dr Jacques Ravina from Paris in 1990s noted that patients undergoing uterine artery embolisation for uterine bleeding also had reduction in size of the uterine fibroids. He requested interventional radiologists to perform preoperative embolisation of the uterine artery to reduce intraoperative blood loss. He later realised that uterine artery embolisation alone was able to reduce the symptoms related to fibroids. Today, uterine artery embolisation is a widely accepted, less invasive method of treating uterine fibroids.

ANATOMY

Uterine fibroids predominantly derive their blood supply from the uterine artery, which is a branch of the anterior division of the internal iliac artery. The internal iliac artery divides into anterior and posterior divisions. The anterior division divides into three parietal branches (obturator, inferior gluteal and internal pudendal arteries) and three visceral arteries (vesical, uterovaginal and middle rectal arteries).[1] The uterine artery is best visualised on the contralateral anterior oblique view. The uterine artery has descending, transverse and ascending course. There are anastamoses between the uterine artery and the branches of the ovarian artery. There are anastamoses between uterine arteries of both sides. The cervicovaginal branches of the uterine artery are usually visualised during angiography.

INDICATIONS

Menorrhagia is the most common indication for embolisation of uterine fibroids. Other indications include dysmenorrhoea, pelvic pain, pelvic pressure and urinary frequency.

CONTRAINDICATIONS

Pregnancy is an absolute contraindication to uterine artery embolisation. Other contraindications include uncorrectable coagulopathy, renal disease with elevated serum creatinine. Presence of uterine malignancy (uterine, cervical, endometrial) is also an absolute contraindication. Routine Pap smear before every uterine artery embolisation to rule out cervical pathologies is a safe method of assessment. Small intracavitary fibroids are best managed by hysteroscopy. In case of pedunculated fibroids surgery produces best results. With massively enlarged uterus, the degree of reduction in uterine size may not be optimal.

PREPROCEDURE WORK UP

Presence of uterine fibroids, size, and location is confirmed with ultrasound, but MRI is preferred due to superior spatial and contrast resolution. Serum creatinine, coagulation profile (PT, APTT, INR, platelet count) and routine urine examination are obtained at the time of out patient visit. In case of inter menstrual bleed, an endometrial biopsy is necessary. Patient is typically admitted the evening prior to study or in the morning on the day of procedure. On the day of procedure, urine pregnancy test is performed. Broad-spectrum antibiotics are administered prior to start of procedure.

INSTRUMENTATION AND TECHNIQUE

Right common femoral artery access is obtained with an arterial introducer set. An initial pigtail catheter angiogram can be performed with the tip of the catheter in the infrarenal abdominal aorta. This also helps to localize the ovarian arteries. The uterine arteries can be catherised using variety of catheters. We prefer Cobra or RUC type catheters either 4Fr or 5Fr. Generally, the contralateral internal iliac artery is catheterised first (contralateral to the site of femoral access). With the tip of the catheter in the internal iliac artery angiograms are obtained in the contralateral anterior oblique position. The catheter is then progressed distally into the uterine artery up to the horizontal segment. Microcatheters can be used if there is spasm or if there is difficulty in progressing the catheter to the horizontal segment. Tip of the catheter is beyond the origin of the cervical and vaginal branches before commencing embolisation. The uterine arteries supplying the fibroids are often hypertrophied and tortuous. The fibroids are identified as dense staining of contrast.

Variety of materials can be used to embolise uterine fibroids. Our preference is PVA particles with size between 700 and 900 microns. Gelfoam pledgets can be used at the end of the procedure, but is not usually necessary as we prefer to complete the procedure with PVA particles alone. Use of coils is not necessary for the occlusion of the arteries. The endpoint of embolisation is near stasis in the uterine artery. Embolisation of the uterine artery on the other side is similarly completed.[2,3]

PAIN RELIEF

Severe pelvic cramping pain can last up to 12 to 24 hours after the procedure. It is important to start pain management either before or during the procedure.[2] We prefer to start patients on opiates during the procedure and continue the same till the time of discharge. On discharge, the patient is transferred to oral non-steroidal anti-inflammatory drugs (NSAIDs). Sometimes pain due to embolisation can be severe and not controlled on opiates and may necessitate patient controlled analgesia pump with morphine. In patients not controlled on opiates, apprehensive patients we prefer to obtain the help of anesthetists for pain management.

OUTCOMES

Technical success is achieved in up to 95% to 99% of patients. Menorrhagia is controlled in about 85% to 95% of patients3. Response of pressure symptoms is marginally less than menorrhagia. Fibroids shrink in volume by about 50% to 60%. The REST trial, a multicenter trial from the United Kingdom compared patients randomly assigned to either embolisation or surgery. 106 patients underwent embolisation and 51 underwent surgery (43 hysterectomies and 8 myomectomies). Hospitalisation was shorter in embolisation group (1 day vs 5 days for surgery), and a shorter time before returning to work. At 1 year, symptom scores were better in the surgical group (P=0.03). During the first year of follow-up, there were 13 major adverse events in the embolisation group (12%) and 10 in the surgical group (20%) (P=0.22). 10 patients in the embolisation group (9%) required repeated embolisation or hysterectomy for inadequate symptom control. There was a greater likelihood of reintervention with uterine embolisation, with 20% of patients undergoing reintervention after embolisation by the median initial follow-up interval of 32 months. By 5 years after treatment, symptoms, quality of life and satisfaction were very high in both groups.[4]

FERTILITY AFTER UTERINE ARTERY EMBOLISATION

There is absence of large, randomized controlled trials evaluating the results of fertility after uterine artery embolisation. Mara et al studied 121 women with fibroids having reproductive plans. They were randomly assigned to embolisation or myomectomy. 58 embolisations and 63 myomectomies were performed. There were no significant differences between the two groups in the rate of technical success, symptomatic effectiveness, post procedural follicle-stimulating hormone levels or complication rates. There were more pregnancies and labours and fewer abortions[5] after surgery than after embolisation (17 pregnancies, 5 labours, 9 abortions). Obstetrical and perinatal results were similar in both groups. They concluded that UAE is less invasive and as symptomatically effective and safe as myomectomy, but myomectomy appears to have superior reproductive outcomes in the first 2 years after treatment.[4] In patients with reproductive plans in the near future we advise myomectomy unless a compelling indication against surgery and for embolisation is present.

COMPLICATIONS

Pain is the most common complaint after procedure and can be managed with analgesics, requiring PCA sometimes. Passage of uterine fibroids can happen in case of submucosal/intracavitary fibroids. It usually occurs 3 to 6 months after embolisation. Infections can result after embolisation and patients need to be informed to obtain medical care in case of any warning symptoms. Uterine fibroid embolisation is thought to induce a hypercoagulable state with about 0.25% of rate of venous thrombosis in patients undergoing embolisation. Prophylactic compression devices on the legs and in patients with other risk factors for venous thrombosis, low-molecular-weight heparin can be used.

Puncture site complications are rare and not different from any other procedure in patients of similar age.

CONCLUSION

Uterine artery embolisation is a safe and effective method to treat symptomatic uterine fibroids. Patients planning to conceive are best treated with myomectomy. With careful patient selection, multidisciplinary involvement of gynaecologists and anaesthetists, adequate symptom relief is obtained while minimizing complications.

REFERENCES

1. Jean-Pierre Pelage, Oliveier Le Dref, Philippe Soyer, et al. Arterial anatomy of the female genital tract: Variations aand relevance to transcatheter embolization of the uterus. American Journal of Roentgenology. 1999;172:989-94.
2. Kauffman, John A. Abdominal aorta and pelvic arteries. Michael J Lee John A Kauffman. Vascular and Interventional Radiology: The requisites. s.l. : Elsevier Saunders, 2014.
3. James B Spies, Ferenc Czeyda-Pommersheim. Uterine fibroid embolization. Kieran P J Murphy, Kenneth R Thomson, Anthony C Venbrux, Robert A Morgan Mathew A Mauro. Image guided interventions. s.l. : Elsevier, 2014.
4. L E Lampmann, P N Lohle, A Smeets, et al. Pain Management During Uterine Artery Embolization for Symptomatic Uterine Fibroids. Cardiovascular and Interventional Radiology, 2007;30:809-11.
5. Uterine artery embolization versus surgery for symptomatic uterine fibroids. trial, The REST. The new England jornal of medicine. 2007;356:360-70.

CHAPTER 22

Magnetic Resonance-guided High Intensity Focused Ultrasound

● Sudhir Kale

■ INTRODUCTION

Magnetic resonance-guided high intensity focused ultrasound (MR-HIFU) is a break through in the medical field. Its novel concept of combining high intensity focused ultrasound and MRI (Fig. 22.1) has opened up a new non-invasive treatment option for fibroid management. MR-HIFU is also called MR-guided focused ultrasound surgery (MRgFUS) and are interchangeably used in this chapter.

Fibroids are benign growths in the uterus, which are symptomatic in up to 25% of women of childbearing age.[1] Clinical studies demonstrate that MRgFUS is a safe and effective treatment for symptomatic uterine fibroids.[2-4]

■ HISTORY AND BACK GROUND OF HIFU

The first investigations of HIFU for non-invasive ablation were reported by Lynn et al, in the early 1940s. Extensive important early work was performed in the 1950s and 1960s by William Fry and Francis Fry at the University of Illinois and Carl Townsend, Howard White and George Gardner at the Interscience Research Institute of Champaign, Ill, culminating in clinical treatments of neurological disorders.

Until recently, clinical trials of HIFU for ablation were few perhaps due to the complexity of the treatments and the difficulty of targeting the beam noninvasively. With recent advances in medical imaging and ultrasound technology, interest in HIFU ablation of tumours has increased.

The first commercial HIFU machine, called Sonablate 200, was developed by the American company Focus Surgery, Inc. (Milipitas, CA) and launched in Europe in 1994 after receiving CE approval, bringing a first medical validation of the technology for benign prostatic hyperplasia (BPH).

Use of magnetic resonance-guided focused ultrasound was first cited and patented in 1995.

The InsighTec ExAblate 2000 was the first MRgFUS system to obtain Food Drug Administration (FDA) market approval in the United States (US). ExAblate was approved by the US FDA in October 2004 to treat symptomatic uterine fibroids. InSightec has begun clinical trials to study the technology's use for other indications including breast, bone, liver and brain tumours. The device received the European CE mark and ISO 13485 and is commercially available in the US, Israel, Europe, and Asia.

Philips Sonalleve MR-HIFU system is available for volumetric ablation of uterine fibroids. The Sonalleve is approved for treating uterine fibroids in Europe, most of Asia, the Middle East and South America. Philips has received CE marking for its Sonalleve MR-HIFU system. The device is also approved for the treatment of bone metastasis and is undergoing development for the treatment of prostate cancer and breast cancer.

■ PRINCIPLES

The use of ultrasound in clinical practice is no longer limited to diagnostic imaging or to simple needle guidance in the performance of percutaneous procedures such as amniocentesis or tumour biopsy. Ultrasound technology now allows the use of focused ultrasound energy for therapeutic purposes such as tissue ablation and haemostasis.

High intensity focused ultrasound causes tissue ablation by delivery of acoustic energy into the target tissue using focused ultrasound (Fig. 22.2). Ultrasound transducer is the source of this ultrasound energy, which gets converted to heat energy at the focal point in the target tissue. Generally, a temperature rise of 60°C to 75°C is required for tissue ablation. This induces necrosis leading to protein denaturation, irreversible cell damage and coagulative necrosis (Fig. 22.9). A single exposure of focused US energy is called sonication. The volume ablated in the target tissue by each sonication is called focal target volume. The fibroid can be ablated in a sequential manner by selecting multiple focal target volumes. Two sonication techniques are available point-by-point ablation technique using pencil beam and volumetric ablation technique using cone beam in spiral trajectories.

The MRI plays a vital role in accurate targeting of this ultrasound beam and monitoring temperature rise in the fibroid. Specialised softwares have been developed to provide real time temperature colour maps during each sonication. This enables the operator to manually abort the sonication based on the temperature maps. The MRI machine is also programmed to abort the sonication automatically when the temperature rise or thermal dose exceeds the desired limit.

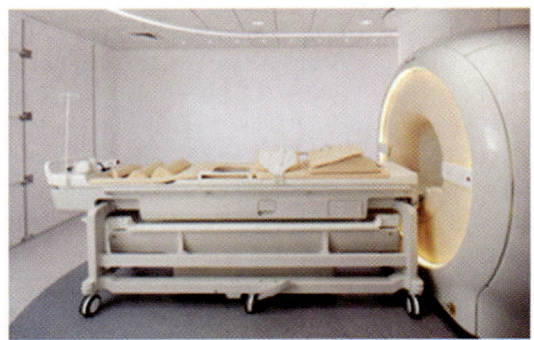

Fig. 22.1: Detachable HIFU table integrated into MRI machine

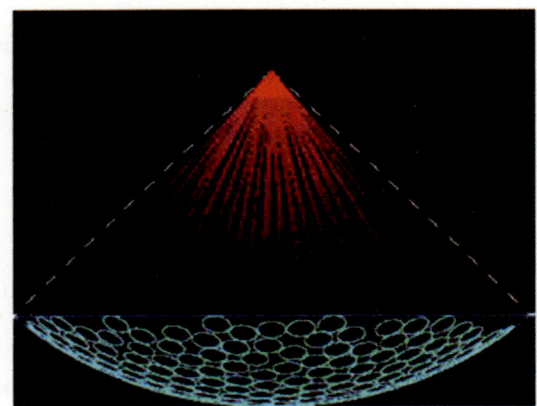

Fig. 22.2: Schematic diagram shows cone beam emanating from transducer converging on a focal point

INDICATIONS FOR MR-HIFU

1. Perimenopausal women with symptomatic fibroids—who want to avoid surgery and want to get symptomatic relief for few years up to menopause.
2. Anterior wall and fundal fibroids—optimal for HIFU.
3. Lateral Wall fibroids, posterior wall fibroids up to 10 cm depth, submucous fibroids and subserosal symptomatic fibroids, if accessible by HIFU beam.
4. Fibroids in patients desiring for pregnancy
5. Those who want to preserve their uterus
6. Where surgery is not possible or could be harmful.
7. Anaesthesia is high risk.
8. Adenomyosis can also be treated by HIFU similar to fibroids.

HIFU SCREENING

All patients with fibroid who have chosen for HIFU treatment have to undergo HIFU screening MRI. Screening is done to confirm the diagnosis and localize the fibroid. The size, location and number of fibroids are mapped. The depth of the fibroids from skin surface is calculated. Currently, the HIFU beam used for sonication has its focal point at 10 cm from the skin surface. The fibroids beyond this are not amenable for therapy. Presence of bowel loops or abdominal wall scar tissue along the beam path are considered as limting factors for therapy. The air in the bowel loops randomly scatter ultrasound beam, thereby not allowing focus the beam at the desired point. It can even cause abnormal heating of the bowel wall and thereby increase chance of bowel perforation. The scar tissue being avascular fibrotic zones cause cumulative heating and thereby increase chance of skin burns. HIFU screening test helps in carefully selecting the optimal patients for therapy.

FIBROID CATEGORISATION BASED ON MRI SIGNAL INTENSITY

The fibroids are categorized based on signal intensity in T2Wt sequence11 as follows (Figs 22.3A to C):
1. Type 1: Low signal intensity on T2 Wt sequence. It is hypointense to skeletal muscle or myometrium (refer Fig. 22.3A).
2. Type 2: Intermediate intensity and it has signal intensity higher than skeletal muscle, but lower than the myometrium (refer Fig 22.3B).
3. Type 3: High intensity and it has a signal intensity equal to or greater than the myometrium (refer Fig. 22.3C).

Procedure

The MR-HIFU procedure generally takes 3 to 4 hours. Patients are instructed to be nil orally 4 to 6 hours prior to

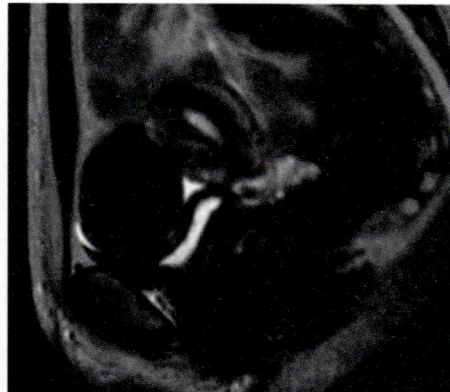

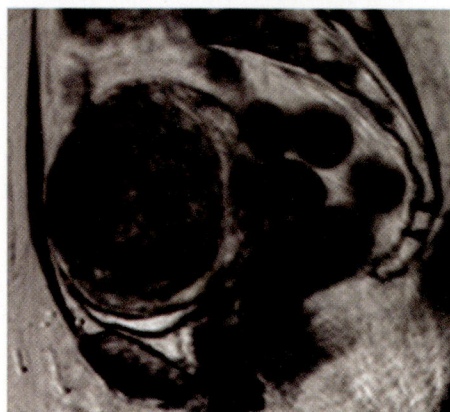

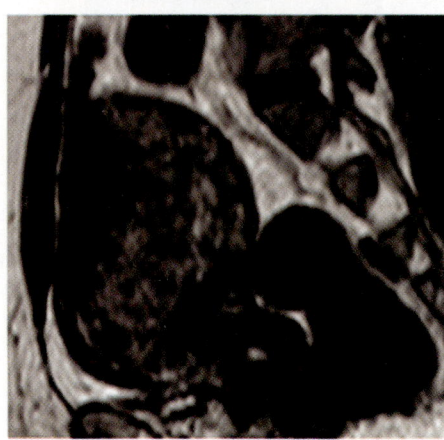

Figs 22.3A to C: A. Type 1 Fibroid: Dark, a very low-intensity image comparable to skeletal muscle; **B.** Type 2 Fibroid: an image intensity lower than that of the myometrium and higher than that of skeletal muscle; **C.** Type 3 Fibroid: Bright, an image intensity equal to or higher than that of myometrium.

the procedure. All patients who are contraindicated for MRI are also contraindicated for this procedure, as this done under MRI guidance Ex. Patients with cardiac pacemakers, cochlear implants, implanted medical electronic devices, etc. No anaesthesia is required. Simple analgesic as a premedication can be given.

Patient is conscious through out the procedure and can interact. Patient lies down in prone position on the MRI gantry (Fig. 22.4). The anterior abdominal wall is facing the HIFU transducer hosed in the gantry (Fig. 22.5). The gel pad is used as a coupling agent in between abdominal wall and transducer for smooth transmission of high frequency ultrasound beam. Emergency STOP button switch is given in patient's hand, which can be pressed to abort sonication if patient feels excessive heating.

MRI sequence is then performed to localize the fibroid. The fibroid for which HIFU procedure will be performed is called target fibroid. The MR-HIFU trained radiologist/specialist then plans the target volume and verifies beam path. The treatment cell is placed and test sonication is done to assess fibroid tissue's thermal response to HIFU. The treatment cell sizes generally range from 4 to 16 mm (Fig. 22.6). Multiple treatment cells are planned within the fibroid in the form of honey comb.

Based on the data obtained from test sonication, appropriate power is selected for sequential sonications of treatment cells.

Then sequential therapeutic sonications are initiated on each of the treatment cell planned within the fibroid. Each sonication displays real time dynamic images of the treating fiboid (Fig 22.7).

Data analysis of each sonication is automatically done by machine software in the form of graph and table (Fig. 22.8).

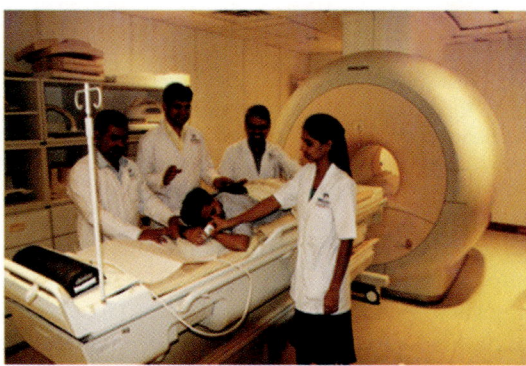

Fig. 22.4: Patient is placed in prone position on MR-HIFU table with emergency stop button given in hand. On site photograph at Clumax Medall diagnostic centre Bangalore

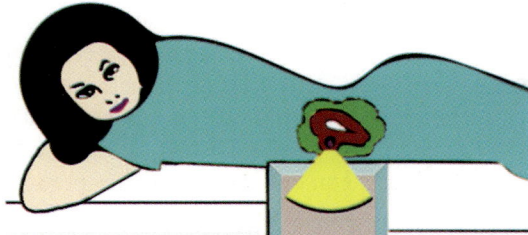

Fig. 22.5: Schematic representation of patient, Hifu transducer and HIFU beam focussed on fibroid

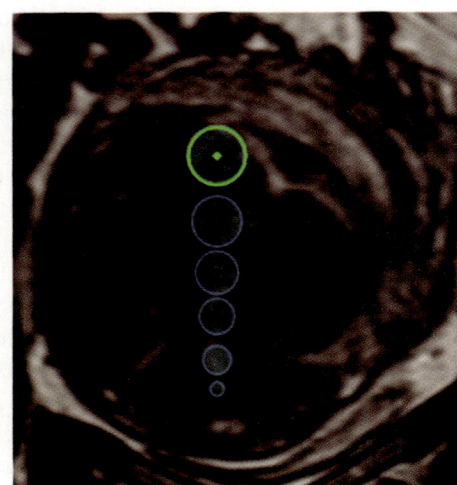

Fig. 22.6: Treatment cell size range from 4 mm to 16 mm used for HIFU

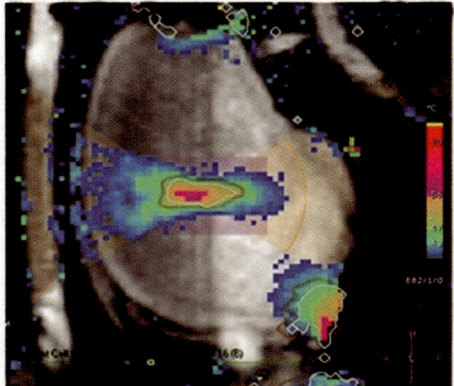

Fig. 22.7: Taken during the HIFU procedure on the HIFU monitor showing beam path, focal sonication point, colour thermal map with real time visualisation of fibroid. The central pink area at the sonication point indicates necrotic area induced in the fibroid.

It gives information of maximum temperature attained during sonication, duration, dose volume, sonication efficiency, recommended power, cooling time, etc. Generally each sonication time varies from 15 to 30 seconds. Cooling time extends from 1 to 4 minutes. Multiple sonications are required on the planned treatment cells on the fibroid for obtaining better tissue necrosis. The treated fibroid volume can be assessed during the procedure by the automated software.

Multiple planned sonications induces coagulative necrosis within the fibroid (Fig. 22.9). Once all the sonications are completed. Contrast enchanced study is performed to assess the treated volume in the fibroid. This is assessed as non-perfused volume (NPV) (Figs 22.10A and B, 22.11A and B). The NPV is the non-enhancing necrotic portion within the fibroid, which correlates with the ablated portion of the fibroid.

The percentage of treated fibroid volume is measured and defined as NPV as a percentage of the total fibroid volume (%NPV, or simply 'NPV'). For the best outcomes, as much of the fibroid as possible should be ablated4. A minimum NPV of 60% produced significantly more sustained symptom relief over 24 month study length.[4] The primary objective of the HIFU procedure is to ablate more than 60% of the fibroid volume for better clinical outcome (Figs 22.12A and B).[4]

HIFU Beam Path

Cone shaped emanating from transducer meet at a focal point called sonication focus. The triangular beam between the transducer and sonication focus is called near field and diverging beam beyond the focus is called far field (Fig. 22.13). The heating occurs along the beam path and important structures like bowel, nerves, etc. should be avoided to prevent any adverse complications. This information is accurately provided on the monitor during the procedure.

Information during and after sonication

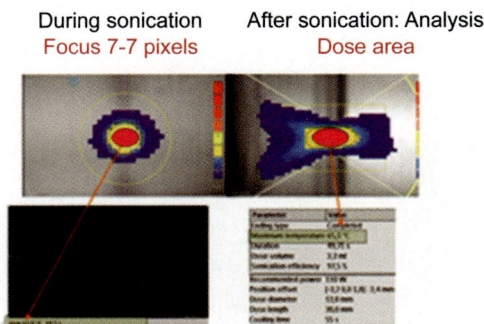

Fig. 22.8: Analysis of each sonication by machine software in the form of graph and table. Sonication volume and recommended power values information is given by machine.

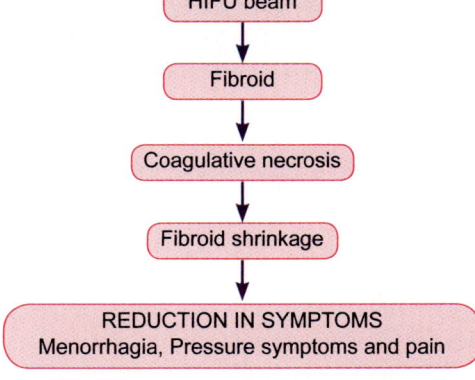

Fig. 22.9: Flow chart showing cascade of events after HIFU therapy.

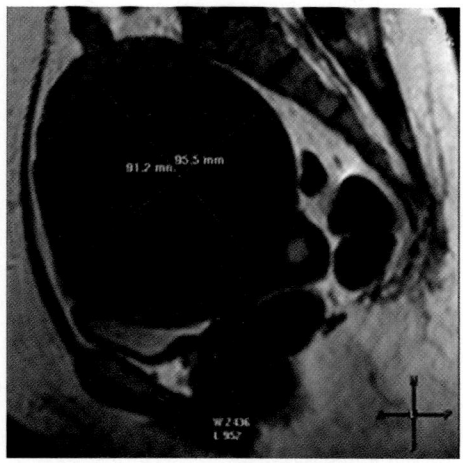 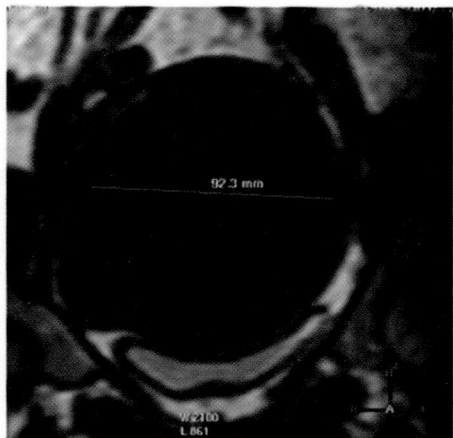

Figs 22.10A and B: Pre-HIFU. MRI sagittal and coronal T2 wt image showing large fibroid (white arrow) involving the fundus and body of uterus. Pre-HIFU volume of fibroid (523 cc).

Table 22.1: UPS-QOL scores for patients undergoing MRgFUS before treatment (baseline) nand at 3 and 6 months after treatment

	Baseline, n = 108, Mean (SD)	Month 3, n = 108, Mean (SD)	Mean change in score	P-value	Month 6, n = 108, Mean (SD)	Mean change in score	P-value
SSS HRQL scales	61.7 (15.2)	41.2 (21.8)	−20.5	<.0001	37.7 (21.2)	−24.0	<.0001
Concern	46.1 (26.7)	62.9 (27.0)	16.8	<.0001	63.1 (26.5)	17.0	< .0001
Activities	47.3 (21.8)	66.4 (24.9)	19.1	<.0001	70.3 (23.8)	23.0	< .0001
Energy/Mood	48.5 (22.6)	67.7 (23.3)	19.2	<.0001	69.7 (22.1)	21.2	< .0001
Control	48.7 (24.1)	68.1 (26.6)	19.4	<.0001	70.1 (25.6)	21.4	< .0001
Sett-consciousness	39.2 (26.6)	60.7 (29.3)	21.5	<.0001	61.6 (28.0)	22.4	< .0001
Sexual function	51.2 (28.0)	66.8 (28.2)	15.7	<.0001	69.3 (29.6)	18.1	< .0001
Total HRQL score	47.0 (18.6)	65.9 (22.4)	18.9	<.0001	67.9 (21.7)	21.0	< .0001

■ FIBROID TYPES BASED ON SIGNAL INTENSITY IN T2 WT MRI SEQUENCE (PICTORIAL PRESENTATION)

Monitoring Outcomes Post HIFU

Uterine fibroids are associated with most common symptoms like menorrhagia, pain, bulk-related pressure symptoms on urinary bladder or rectum, infertility issues, etc. The symptoms generally correlate with the size and location of the fibroids. The intramural fibroids and submucosal fibroids are generally associated with menorrhagia, pain and infertility in some cases. Larger fibroids and subserosal fibroids may be associated with pressure related symptoms. Hence, monitoring of outcome of HIFU can be done assessing fibroid symptom response and morphologic volumetric reduction of fibroid in the post HIFU follow ups.

The uterine fibroid symptom and health related quality of life questionnaire (UFS-QOL) is a uterine fibroid-specific questionnaire developed specifically to evaluate the symptoms

of uterine fibroids and their impact on health-related quality of life.[6] The UFS-QOL appears to be a useful evaluative tool for assessing symptoms in studies among patients with uterine fibroids.[6] Monitoring treatment outcome using these criteria to assess response is recommended (Table 22.1).

Symptom severity scale (SSS) of the UFS-QOL questionnaire pre- and post-HIFU 6 months follow-up after treatment. The SSS assesses both symptoms of menorrhagia and bulk-related symptoms on a single 100-point scale.

This measure is the only validated instrument for assessing symptoms specific for quality of life (QOL) due to uterine fibroids. The SSS discriminates between women with symptomatic fibroids, who have a mean score of approximately 40, and normal women, who have a score of approximately 20. Thus, a 10-point improvement is consistent with the clinical data from validation studies.[35]

Uterine fibroid symptoms were reduced to 53% and the degree of menstrual pain was reduced to 50% as reported by Yoon et al. Bulk related and menstrual symptoms diminished in 51% of patients after 6 months of HIFU treatment.

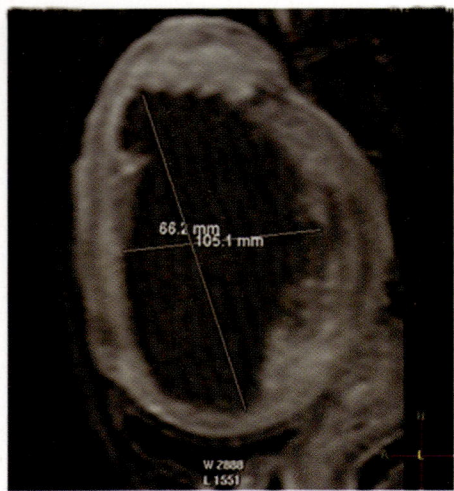 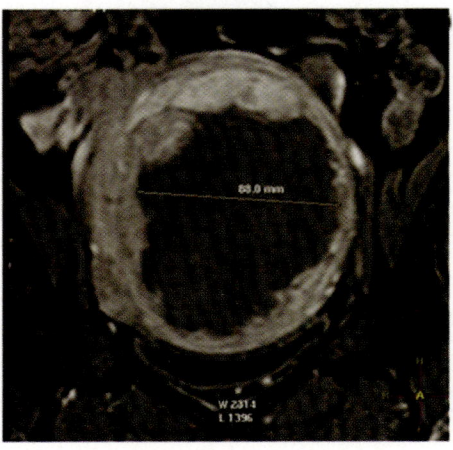

Figs 22.11A and B: Post-HIFU Treatment Day. Contrast-enhanced MRI sagittal and coronal images showing non-enhancing non-perfused volume (NPV) within the fibroid (arrow Head). NPV is 463 cc.

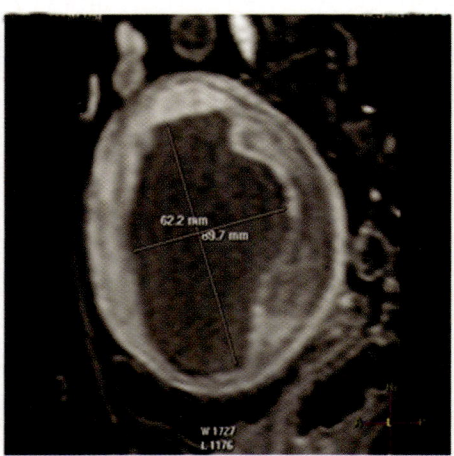 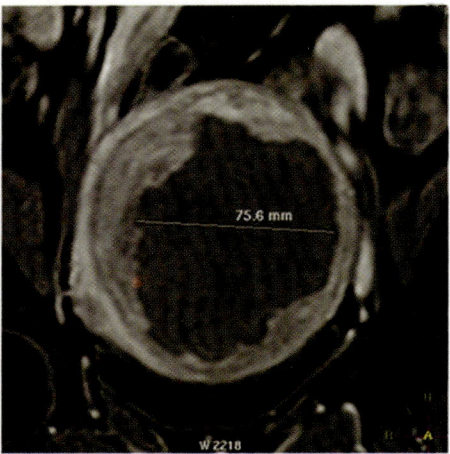

Figs 22.12A and B: Post-HIFU one month follow-up. Contrast-enhanced MRI sagittal and coronal images showing reduction in the volume of non-enhancing non-perfused volume (NPV) within the fibroid. NPV is 203 cc.

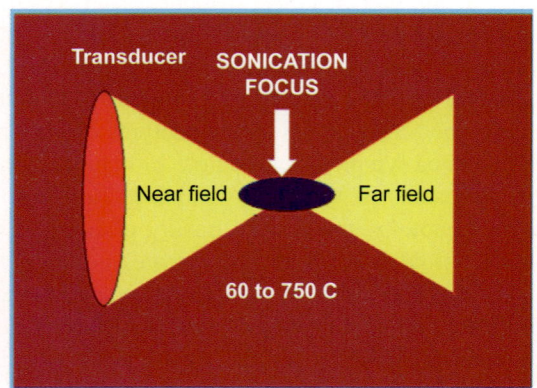

Fig. 22.13: HIFU beam Path showing sonication focus, Near field and Far field

Several studies have shown that MRgFUS significantly improves clinical symptoms in 70% to 80% of women with uterine myomas.[5,7,8] Studies have also demonstrated a correlation between the treated volume of the myomas, improvement in symptoms, and lesion shrinkage (Table 22.2).[3,4,5,7,8,9]

Table 22.2: Mean fibroid shrinkage 6 months after MRI-guided focused ultrasound for three ranges of non-perfused volume ratios. Greater shrinkage was found for fibroid treatments resulting in greater non-perfused volume ratios (n = number of fibroids).[20]

Number of fibroids (n)	NPV ratios range (%)	Mean Shrinkage at 6 months (%)
30	0–50	18
30	50–75	35
21	75–100	50

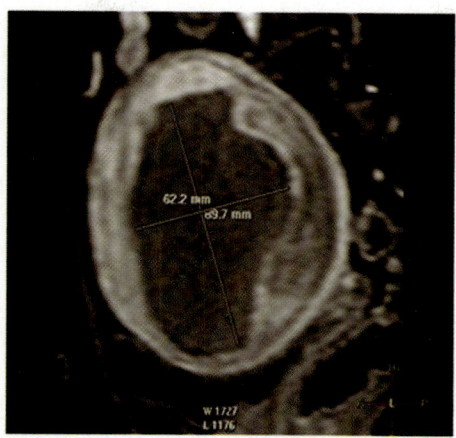 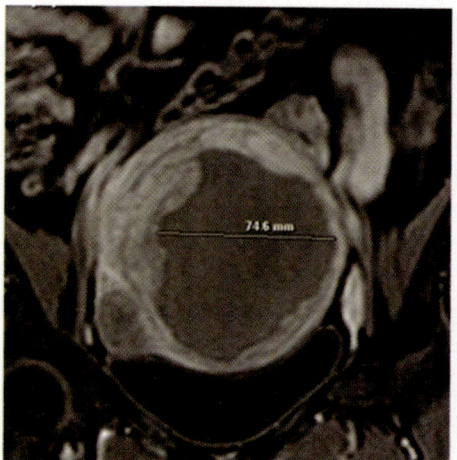

Figs 22.14A and B: Post-HIFU three month follow-up. Contrast-enhanced MRI sagittal and coronal images showing reduction in the volume of non-enhancing non-perfused volume (NPV) within the fibroid (white arrow). NPV is 190 cc.

Volumetric quantification of the fibroid size reduction is assessed by follow-up MRI scan, which is done at 3 months, 6 months and 1 year post HIFU therapy. The fibroid volume is calculated and assessed for the size regression. The fibroid shrinkage and symptom reduction were directly proportionate to the NPV obtained post treatment.

Suzanne D LeBlang et al, reported the average shrinkage of fibroids 6 months after treatment was slightly greater than 30% in a study group of 80 patients (Fig. 22.14A and B). The greater non-perfused volume ratio correlates with greater shrinkage and has been found to correlate with decreased symptoms.[10]

A relation was found between fibroid volume and posttreatment NPV and 6-month shrinkage. For all groups of fibroids (independent of size) it was possible to achieve a nonperfused volume ratio of at least 50%, yet larger NPV ratios (> 60%) were achieved in the management of smaller fibroid volumes. These larger NPV ratios also resulted in greater 6-month fibroid shrinkage.[10]

The MRI-guided focused ultrasound therapy for leiomyoma can result in NPV ratio and shrinkage that exceed those in previous clinical trials because the treatment guidelines have been relaxed to allow a greater amount of tissue ablation. The results suggest that a larger NPV ratio can be achieved, resulting in greater shrinkage and improved relief of symptoms.[10]

A study by Funaki et al, evaluated the signal intensity of the T2-weighted images and the therapeutic results. They treated 95 fibroids in 63 patients. Before treatment the fibroids were categorized on the basis of the signal intensity of the T2-weighted images.[11] The type I fibroids had the best results with 31% volume reduction, type 2 was 20.5%, and type 3 was 16.5%. They also found that the panic button was pushed more frequently in patients with type 3 fibroids than type 1 or type 2.[11]

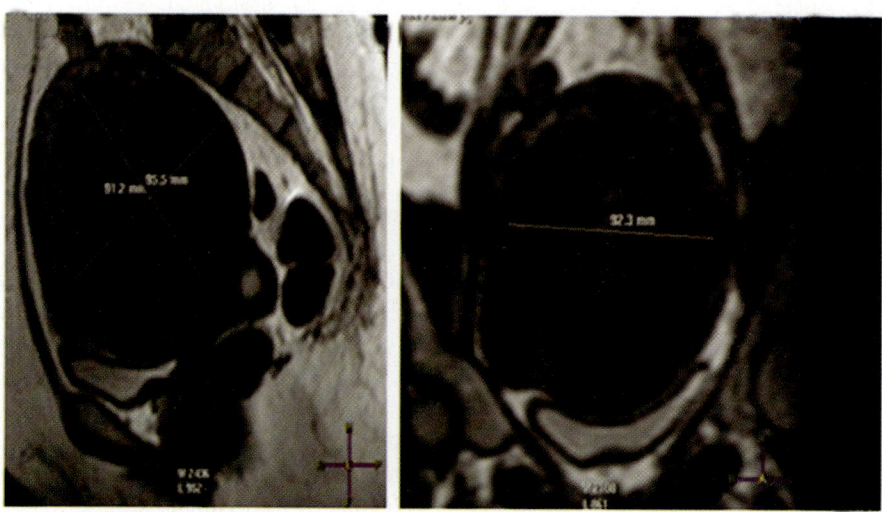

Figs 22.15A and B: Large intramural fibroid along the fundus and posterior wall. Pre-Hifu. Pre-treatment volume of fibroid 523 cc.

A study by Mikami et al, also demonstrated a higher technical success (treatment of the planned target zone) in patients with low-intensity fibroids when compared with high-intensity fibroids.

Fibroids with low signal intensity on pre-treatment T2-wt images were more likely to shrink than were ones with high signal intensity.[12]

■ ROLE OF HIFU IN LARGE FIBROIDS, MULTIPLE FIBROIDS AND DEGENERATIVE FIBROIDS

All types of fibroids intramural, submucosal and subserosal types can be treated by HIFU.

Fibroids of varying sizes from 1 to 15 cm have been treated. Size has no bar. Since for better clinical out comes, the NPV of 60% should be achieved, very large fibroids can be treated by two or more sittings within an interval of 1 to 4 weeks.

Multiple fibroids may also require more than one sitting depending on the number and size of fibroids. This assessment can be done to a greater extent during pre-HIFU screening. But, final decision on the next sitting can be taken only after assessing NPV of the first hifu procedure.

In degenerative fibroids, HIFU has a limited role. If fibroids already show more than 50% degeneration, then performing MR HIFU in such patients may not yield favourable results as volume shrinkage may not be significant enough to better the clinical out come.

■ ADVANTAGES OF MR-HIFU

It is an outpatient, non-invasive procedure not requiring any anaesthesia. Patients walks out from MRI table immediately after procedure. MR-HIFU recovery time is short in comparison to other uterine fibroid therapies. In contrast to hysterectomy where a typical full recovery time is 6 to 8 weeks, the majority of patients treated with MR-HIFU return to normal activity and/or work in 1 to 2 days post-treatment. It has excellent safety profile with no reported major complications. Only minor complaints like, pain or low grade fever for 1 to 2 days. There is no exposure to radiation. It is an uterus sparing surgery. It can be performed in women with fibroid desiring pregnancy. Future pregnancy is promising.

■ COMPLICATIONS OF MR-HIFU

In general, MR-HIFU is regarded to be a safe method for the treatment of uterine fibroids. Discomfort and pain are the most common side effects of MR-HIFU treatment of uterine fibroids and are considered minor.

Treatment-related fatigue and backache are possible, yet they typically require only over-the-counter pain medication.[10] Less common minor complications include diarrhea in 3 of the

42 patients in Hesley and colleagues 2006 study and nausea, both presumed to be related to post-treatment opioids.[10]

The most serious, but uncommon complications include sustained leg and buttock pain, and skin burns. Hindley et al, (2004) reported the first sustained leg and buttock pain were this event was linked to the heating of the sciatic nerve. Despite initial concern and patient discomfort, according to MR neurography and electromyography there was no intrinsic nerve damage caused. This case lead to a change in operator practices. In all reported cases, these symptoms have resolved.

Although infrequent, skin burns have occurred through the course of the use of MR-HIFU.[7] Generally, mild skin burns have been reported by several groups. Most of the cases were mild first degree burns that were often caused by imperfect hair removal or air bubbles trapped between the gel pad and skin of the patient. The majority of the reported burns occurred in the early phases of the technology. Damage to adjacent organs, such as bowel perforation, is also possible during treatment but rare.[9]

■ CONTRAINDICATIONS AND LIMITATIONS OF MR-HIFU

1. All those contraindicated for MRI are contraindicated for MR-HIFU, e.g. cardiac pacemakers, electronic implants, non compatible metallic implants, etc.
2. Abdominal wall scar in the beam path.
3. Bowel loop interposition in-between the fibroid and HIFU transducer along the beam path.
4. Fibroid localised beyond target area.
5. Acute pelvic infection.
6. Documented m yocardial infarction or cerebrovascular accident in the recent past 6 months. Unstable cardiac status.
7. Individuals who are not able or willing to tolerate the required prolonged stationary prone position during treatment (approximately 3 hours).
8. Obese patient > 110 kg who will not fit in MRI gantry bore.

■ MR-HIFU AND PREGNANCY

Fibroids may reduce the possibility of successful implantation by promoting abnormal contractility, altering endometrial blood supply and inducing localised endometrial inflammation and changes in biochemistry of the intrauterine fluid.

Uterine fibroids alone may even lead to infertility. In many cases, increase in fertility rates has been observed in patients following fibroid therapies. Submucosal fibroids reduce implantation rate increasing possibility of spontaneous abortion. Intramural fibroids can at times lead to pregnancy loss due to abnormal uterine contractility and altering endometrial blood supply. Subserosal fibroids have no stastically significant effect on infertility.

Myomectomy is most often considered the current standard of care for patients with fibroids seeking to become pregnant. There are enough evidence showing improved pregnancy outcomes following myomectomy. Nevertheless, myomectomy has known risks, both directly related to procedure and for patients who do become pregnant. They have increased risk of uterine rupture, intraoperative conversion to hysterectomy, fibroid recurrence and adhesion. Some people who conceive may have risks of miscarriage, uterine rupture during pregnancy fibroid, caesarean section and pre term delivery.

Uterine artery embolisation in women desiring future pregnancy is absolutely contraindicated Lee et al. The procedure can cause ovarian failure, higher incidence of miscarriages, preterm term delivery, abnormal placentation, malpresentaion and post partum haemorrhage. However, number of successful pregnancies have been reported in the past post UAE procedure.

The MR-HIFU has been used for treatment of uterine fibroid patients who want to preserve fertility and pursue future pregnancy.

In Europe, patients who desire further fertility have been allowed to undergo MRgFUS, since 2007 under the device's CE mark. With expanded experience in the field of MRgFUS FDA changed the labeling of the device to take into account desire for future pregnancy, but not to have this as an absolute contraindication.

Based on the prospective registry of all known pregnancies occurring after MRgFUS, and maintained by the device manufacturer and reported to the FDA, 54 pregnancies in 51 women have occurred. The mean time to conception was 8 months after treatment.[13] Live births occurred in 41% of pregnancies. There was a 28% spontaneous abortion rate, an 11% rate elective pregnancy termination rate and 20% ongoing pregnancies beyond 20 gestational weeks. The mean birth weight was 3.3 kg and the vaginal delivery rate was 64%.[10]

Hanstede et al, reported a case in which treatment of two uterine fibroids by MR-HIFU resulted in restoration of normal shape of endometrial cavity, which possibly facilitated subsequent pregnancy.[14]

Yoon et al, reported a case in which the patient conceived 4 months post treatment of two intramural fibroids. She continued her pregnancy to term and delivered a healthy baby through vaginal delivery.

Zaher et al, (2011) described a case of successful in vitro fertilisation and pregnancy following MR-HIFU therapy.[15]

In selected patients, MR-HIFU can be tried as a non-invasive alternative for treating fibroids desiring pregnancy.

CURRENT OTHER APPLICATIONS IN MR-HIFU

Currently, MR-HIFU has been used for adenomyosis, prostate cancer, breast tumours, painful bony metastases and liver tumours. For the brain, it has been used for the ablation of glioblastomas and for functional neurosurgery. Future applications for acute stroke treatment are being explored

ROLE OF MR-HIFU IN ADENOMYOSIS

Adenomyosis is a non-neoplastic condition, characterized by benign invasion of ectopic endometrium into the myometrium with hyperplasia of adjacent smooth muscle. It is pathology at the interface of the endometrium and myometrium. Its definition is based on histology findings. Siegler and Camilien[33] define adenomyosis as the presence of endometrial glandular cells and cells of the chorion more than 2.5 mm from the endometrium-myometrium interface. It manifests with uterine myoma-mimicking symptoms such as heavy menstrual bleeding, pain and diffuse uterine enlargement.

Magnetic resonance imaging is an accurate, nonsurgical diagnostic modality used preoperatively to distinguish uterine myoma from adenomyosis.[16,17,18,37] T2-weighted MR images of adenomyosis disclose either focal or diffuse thickening of the junctional zone, and show areas of low signal that are often poorly defined. At MRI, a junctional zone (inner myometrium) 12 mm thick or thicker is highly predictive of adenomyosis.[20,21] Diffuse adenomyosis is defined as a diffuse ectopic growth of the endometrium into the myometrium with either diffuse or focal widening of the endometrial-myometrial junctional zone, whereas focal adenomyosis is defined as an actual circumscribed mass within the myometrium.[22]

Focal adenomyosis (adenomyoma) forms a round or oval mass that is poorly distinguishable from the adjacent myometrium. At MR imaging, myometrial adenomyoma typically exhibits low signal intensity on T2-weighted images[23,24] an appearance indistinguishable from that of the more common leiomyoma. When the lesion is accompanied by small foci of high signal intensity representing ectopic endometrial tissue, adenomyoma can be considered in the differential diagnosis.

Clear-cut surgical excision of the whole adenomyosis lesion is difficult because of its ambiguous boundary. Alternatively, there are minimally invasive modalities for the management of adenomyosis, such as hormonal therapy,[25–30] endometrial ablation therapy,[31–34] and uterine artery embolisation (UAE). Hormonal treatment with gonadotropin-releasing hormone analog provides only temporary relief because it cannot be administered for more than 6 months because of the risk of inducing a hypoestrogenic status and discontinuation of the therapy results in prompt regrowth of adenomyosis tissue.[15]

A danazol- or levonorgestrel-releasing intrauterine device provides encouraging results;[17–19] however, side effects of its long-term use remain to be clarified. Endometrial ablation is an alternative to hysterectomy when the depth of myometrial penetration is limited,[20,21] and UAE has elicited mixed responses

The MRgFUS has been used in ablating adenomyosis. The patient selection criteria, principle, technique and treatment is similar to fibroid. The non perfused volume after the treatment and symptom analysis is done in periodic interval follow-up up to 1 year to assess the benefits of the procedure.

The symptom severity score (SSS), which primarily assesses symptoms related to menorrhagia and bulk, was converted to create a total score comparable with a 0- to 100-point scale. The higher score indicated more severe symptoms.

Analysis of 20 cases, early results of magnetic resonance guided focused ultrasound surgery of adenomyosis showed significant improvement in symptom severity scale during follow-up for 1 to 6 months after treatment.[36]

The MRgFUS can safely and effectively ablate adenomyosis sufficiently to produce a decrease in mean uterine volume and significant improvement in SSS values for up to 6 months post-treatment. The results suggest that MRgFUS is a promising minimally invasive option for patients seeking treatment of symptomatic adenomyosis.

■ SONOGRAPHY-GUIDED HIFU THERPAY

Sonography can also be used for guidance and monitoring during HIFU therapy. Temperature mapping with sonography is not available at present in most of the countries. Sonography also has other limitations related to bowel loop interference,

relation to adjoining viscera and limited information in obese patients.

Guidance and monitoring of acoustic therapy is most important to ensure that the desired region is treated and to minimize damage to adjacent structures. Monitoring using real-time imaging, such as with sonography or MRI, ensures that the targeting of the HIFU beam is maintained on the correct area throughout the procedure.

Transrectal HIFU is being widely used for ablating prostate malignancy.

Currently for fibroids, MRI is being used for guidance and monitoring of HIFU therapy.

■ UTERINE ARTERY EMBOLISATION

Uterine artery embolisation (UAE) is a procedure where an interventional radiologist uses a catheter to deliver small particles that block the blood supply to the uterine body. The procedure is done for the treatment of uterine fibroids and adenomyosis. Given that this minimally invasive procedure is commonly used in the treatment of uterine fibroids it is also called uterine fibroid embolisation (UFE).

Indication

Uterine artery embolisation is used to treat bothersome bulk-related symptoms or abnormal or heavy uterine bleeding due to uterine fibroids or for the treatment of adenomyosis

The UAE can also be used to control heavy uterine bleeding for reasons other than fibroids, such as postpartum obstetrical haemorrhage and adenomyosis.

Table 22.3: Shows comparison of patient factors by various treatment modalities for fibroid

SL No.	Patient factors	Hysterectomy	Myomectomy	UFE	HIFU
1	General anaesthesia	Yes	No	No	No
2	Future fertility	No	Preserved	Preserved	Preserved
3	Risk of haemorrhage requiring blood transfusions	Can occur	Can occur	No	No
4	Post procedure infection	Can occur	Can occur	No	No
5	Post procedure pain nausea and vomiting	Can occur	Can occur	Generally occurs	Less likely
6	Requires hospitalisation	Yes	Short stay	Short stay	Not required
7	Recovery time to return to normal activity	4 to 6 weeks	1 week	4 To 7days	1 to 2 days
8	Risk of symptom recurrence	No	Can occur	Can occur	Can occur
9	Mental stress with uterine loss	Can be present	No	No	No
10	Hormonal imbalance & side effects	Can be present	No	Can be present	No
11	Accelerated menopause	Yes	No	Some times	No
12	Non-invasive	It is invasive	It is invasive	Minimally invasive	Non-invasive

Limitations and Complications

1. Iliac artery or aortic dissection.
2. Severe ischaemic pain like heart attack.
3. Normal adjacent myometrium and other uterine ischemia.
4. Misplaced embolisation elsewhere.
5. Post embolisation syndrome or sever secondary infection.
6. Ovarian failure due to ovarian artey embolisation.
7. Not performed in women desiring for pregnancy.
8. Placental implantation problems.
9. Anaesthesia-related problems.

For women with symptomatic uterine fibroids, UAE improves symptoms and total health-related quality of life more than MR-HIFU, Froeling and colleagues evaluated and compared the long-term reintervention rate and changes in symptom severity, as well as total health-related quality of life scores, among 77 patients undergoing UAE or MR-HIFU for symptomatic uterine fibroids. Reintervention was significantly lower after UAE than after MR-guided HIFU at long-term follow-up, the researchers found.[38] They also observed relatively better improvement in symptom severity in post UAE patients when compredto post MR-HIFU patients.

■ RADIOFREQUENCY ABLATION (RFA)

Radiofrequency ablation (RFA) is a medical procedure in which part of the electrical conduction system of the heart, tumour or other dysfunctional tissue is ablated using the heat generated from high frequency alternating current (in the range of 350–500 kHz). 1 RFA is generally conducted in the outpatient setting, using either local anesthetics or conscious sedation anaesthesia RFA procedures are performed under image guidance (such as X-ray screening, CT scan or ultrasound).

The RFA is a minimally invasive procedure, so procedure pain and risk are significantly decreased. This technique avoids hysterectomy and the early onset of menopause, and may preserve a woman's fertility.

The RFA is being investigated to treat uterine fibroids. The device is inserted via a laparoscopic probe and guided inside the fibroid tissue using an ultrasound probe. The prongs deliver electrical energy to the fibroid and keep the ablation catheter firmly in place during treatment. In about 10 to 15 minutes, targeted tissue is heated to 105°C, killing tumour cells. Because the heat dissipates rapidly, surrounding normal tissue is not affected. Most procedures are completed in 2 to 3 hours and patients discharged the same day or the day following the procedure. Complications, such as bleeding and post-operative pain, are minimal.

■ OUR CLINICAL EXPERIENCE ON MR-HIFU

We performed MR-guided HIFU procedure at Clumax-Medall diagnostic centre, a unit of Medall Healthcare private limited at Bangalore, India. We used Philips sonalleve MR-HIFU system for uterine fibroid ablation. We performed MR-HIFU procedure on about 30 patients treating about 45 uterine fibroids. Post HIFU follow-up after 1 month, 3 months, 6 months and 1 year was done. The treatment response was assessed based on the shrinkage of fibroid NPV volume and symptom severity index. No immediate emergency surgical interventions, unexpected short-term adverse events or long-term complications were observed in our clinical practice so far. We illustrate few of these cases in a pictorial presentation for better understanding in the following pages (Figs 22.16A and B to 22.25A and B).

Case Study 1

46-year-old female with symptomatic fibroids. She had predominantly pressure symptoms, increased frequency of urination, heaviness, pelvic pain and menorrhagia screening

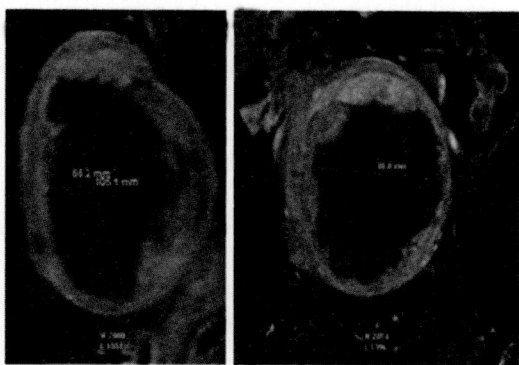

Figs 22.16A and B: Post-HIFU (day 1), contrast-enhanced MRI reveals non-enhancing central area suggesting non-perfused volume. The NPV measured 463 cc. Approximately 90% of the fibroid was treated.

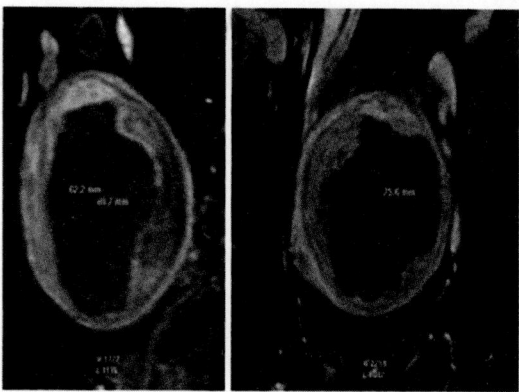

Figs 22.17A and B: Post-HIFU (1 month follow-up), contrast enhanced MRI reveals interval reduction in the non-perfused volume. The NPV measured 203 cc. Approximately 44% reduction in the NPV.

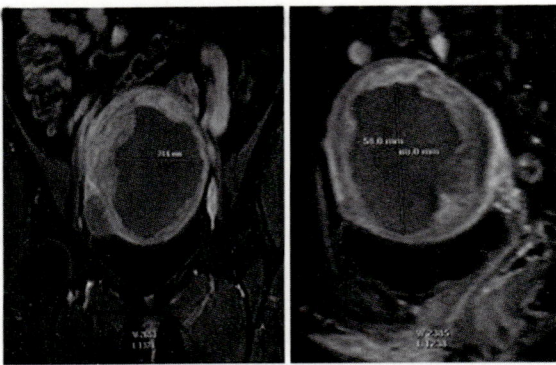

Figs 22.18A and B: Post-HIFU (3 month follow-up), contrast-enhanced MRI reveals interval reduction in the non-perfused volume. The NPV measured 190 cc.

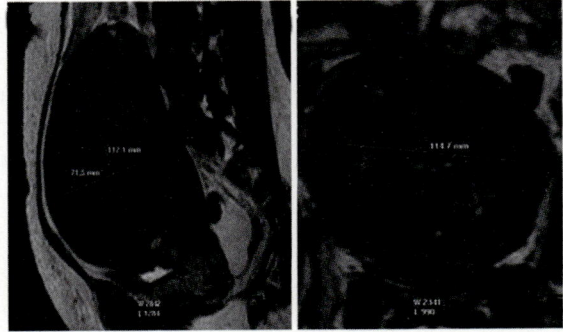

Figs 22.19A and B: Large intramural fibroid along the anterior wall. Pre-HIFU. Pre treatment volume of fibroid (618 cc).

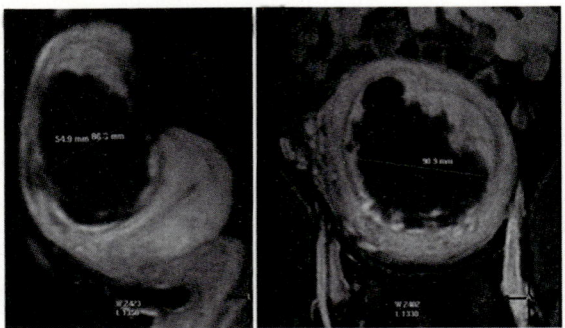

Figs 22.20A and B: Post-HIFU (day 1), contrast-enhanced MRI reveals non-enhancing central area suggesting non-perfused volume. The NPV measured 494 cc. Approximately 80% of fibroid was treated.

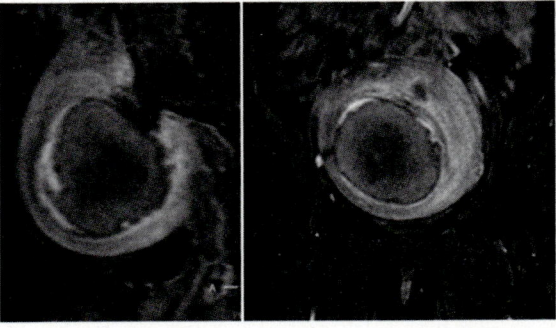

Figs 22.21A and B: Post-HIFU (1 month follow-up), contrast-enhanced MRI reveals interval reduction in the non-perfused volume. The NPV measured 360 cc.

Case Study 2

43-year-old female with symptomatic fibroids. She had menorrhagia, 2 days heavy bleed, passing clots, severe back pain restricting her movements, mild crampy abdominal pain, not able to do household work and increased frequency of urination. Screening MRI revealed a large Fundal and post wall dark signal intensity fibroid and three more smaller 2 to 4 cm lateral wall fibroids.

By 3rd month follow-up post-HIFU, menorrhagia reduced and dysmenorrhoea reduced by 50%. Low backache reduced by 80%. Quality of life much improved, felt her abdomen very lighter and quite active through the day.

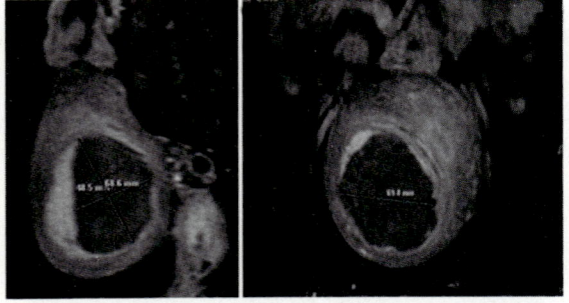

Figs 22.22A and B: Post-HIFU (3 month follow-up), contrast-enhanced MRI reveals interval reduction in the non-perfused volume. The NPV measured 212 cc.

MRI revealed a large fundal and post wall dark signal intensity fibroid and three more smaller 2 to 4 cm lateral wall fibroids.

By 3rd month follow-up post-HIFU, her back pain had reduced by 70%, pelvic pain/discomfort had reduced almost completely, frequency of micturition had reduced. Menorrhagia was not assessed as she did not have any menstrual cycle after HIFU procedure.

Case Study 3

This patient had large anterior wall Bright fibroid (type 3) with poor response to HIFU sonication.

In our study, the temperature rise was only up to 520 celsius, far below the desired level (about 60°–70°) for tissue necrosis. We had to abort the procedure after few sonications.

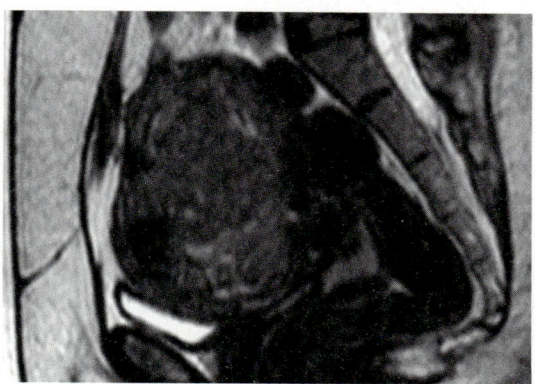

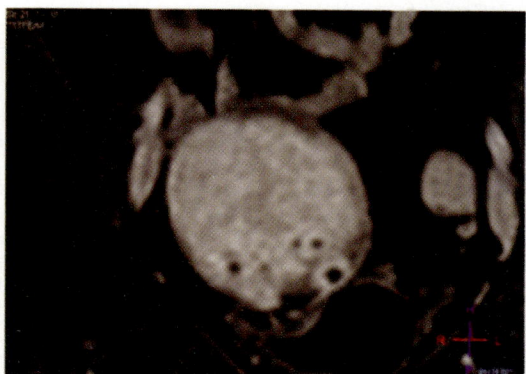

Fig 22.23A and B: A. Large anterior wall bright intramural fibroid along the anterior wall. Pre-HIFU; **B.** Post-HIFU (day 1): Only few tiny areas of NPV. HIFU procedure was aborted after few sonications as the desired temperature rise for fibroid ablation was not achieved due to hypervascular nature of fibroid.

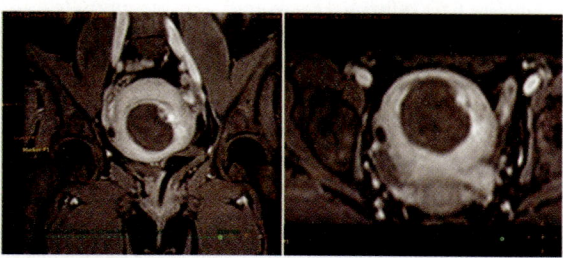

Fig 22.24A and B: Post-HIFU T1-Wt gadolinium-enhanced images. The volume was measured at 69 cm³, giving 92% non-perfused volume (NPV) based on a total fibroid volume of 75 cm³.

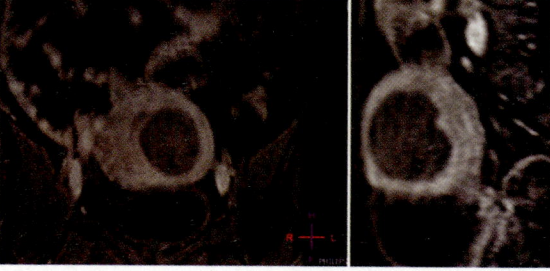

Figs 22.25A and B: T1-weighted gadolinium-enhanced images were showing the reduction of the NPV to 58 cc. QOL score pre-HIFU 111, now 46. This patient had good clinical outcome.

The fibroid signal intensity is brighter than the skeletal muscle and myometrium in T2 wt images. These are considered as type 3 or bright fibroids. They are considered to be hypervascular as compared the dark fibroids. The hypervascular nature of the tissue prevents optimal temperature rise for coagulative necrosis. Due to this, these fibroids are not suitable for ablation.

Case Study 4

38-year-old mother of 2 children presents with severe menorrhagia and pelvic pain. Ultrasound shows anterior intramural fibroid, 6 cm × 5 cm. Patient non-responsive to conservative management, not a surgical candidate due to pre-existing cardiac condition (pulmonary hypertension). With her cardiac illness, the patient was a high risk surgical candidate. Treating physician did not want to pursue a surgical procedure. So, referred to MR-HIFU.

▪ SUMMARY

The MR-HIFU integrated systems with recent technological advances is a promising modality as an alternative non-invasive imaging modality for treating uterine fibroids and adenomyosis. Its an outpatient, non-invasive procedure not requiring anaesthesia. MR-HIFU can be offered to the majority of patients suffering from symptomatic uterine fibroids. Currently due to broader inclusion criteria as well as the technological advances it is possible to offer MR-HIFU to a much larger subset of patients than previously believed. In case, if the treatment results are not satisfactory, still all other treatment options are available for treating fibroid and can be planned as per the merit of the case. It has excellent safety profile. It is a uterus sparing treatment option. It can be performed in women desiring pregnancy with symptomatic fibroids.

▪ ABBREVIATIONS

1. HIFU: High intensity focused ultrasound.
2. MRgFUS: Magnetic resonance-guided focused ultrasound surgery.
3. MR-HIFU: Magnetic resonance-guided high intensity focused ultrasound.
4. MRI: Magnetic resonance imaging.
5. NPV: Non-perfused volume.
6. RFA: Radiofrequency ablation

7. SSS: Symptom severity scale
8. T2 wt: T2 weighted MRI sequence.
9. UAE: Uterine artery embolisation.
10. UFE: Uterine fibroid embolisation.
11. UFS-QOL: The uterine fibroid symptom and health related quality of life questionnaire.

■ REFERENCES

1. Ryan GL, Syrop CH, Van Voorhis BJ. Role, epidemiology, and natural history of benign uterine mass lesions. Clin Obstet Gynecol. 2005;48(2):312-24.
2. Hesley GK, Felmlee JP, Gebhart JB, et al. Noninvasive treatment of uterine fibroids: early Mayo Clinic experience with magnetic resonance imaging-guided focused ultrasound. Mayo Clin Proc. 2006;81(7):936-42.
3. Stewart EA, Gostout B, Rabinovici J, et al. Sustained relief of leiomyoma symptoms by using focused ultrasound surgery. Obstet Gynecol. 2007;110(2 Pt 1):279-87.
4. Stewart EA, Rabinovici J, Tempany CM, et al. Clinical outcomes of focused ultrasound surgery for the treatment of uterine fibroids. Fertil Steril. 2006;85(1):22-9.
5. Hynynen K, Damianou C, Darkazanli A, et al. "On-line MRI monitored noninvasive ultrasound surgery". Proceedings of the Annual International Conference of the IEEE Engineering in Medicine and Biology Society. 1992, doi :10.1109/IEMBS. 1992.5760999. ISBN 0-7803-0785-2.
6. Harding G, Coyne KS, Thompson CL, et al. The responsiveness of the uterine fibroid symptom and health-related quality of life questionnaire (UFS-QOL) Health Qual Life Outcomes. 2008;6:99.
7. Hindley J, Gedroyc WM, Regan L, et al. MRI guidance of focused ultrasound therapy of uterine fibroids: early results. AJR Am J Roentgenol. 2004;183(6):1713-9.
8. Fennessy FM, Tempany CM, McDannold NJ, et al. Uterine leiomyomas: MR imaging-guided focused ultrasound surgery--results of different treatment protocols. Radiology. 2007;243(3):885-93.
9. Hesley GK, Gorny KR, Henrichsen TL, et al. A clinical review of focused ultrasound ablation with magnetic resonance guidance: an option for treating uterine fibroids. Ultrasound Q. 2008;24(2):131-9.
10. Suzanne D LeBlang1 Katherine Hoctor Fred L. Steinberg, et al. Leiomyoma Shrinkage After MRI-Guided Focused Ultrasound Treatment: Report of 80 Patients. AJR. 2010;194:274-80
11. Kaoru Funaki, et al. Magnetic resonance-guided focused ultrasound surgery for uterine fibroids: relationship between the therapeutic effects and signal intensity of preexisting T2-weighted magnetic resonance imagesajog. 2006.08.030..
12. Lénárd ZM, et al. Uterine leiomyomas: MR imaging-guided focused ultrasound surgery--imaging predictors of success. Radiology. 2008, 10.1148/radiol.2491071600.
13. Rabinovici J, David M, Fukunishi H, et al. Pregnancy outcome after magnetic resonance-guided focused ultrasound surgery (MRgFUS) for conservative treatment of uterine fibroids. Fertil Steril. 2010;93(1):199-209.
14. MM Hanstede, CM Tempany, EA Stewart. 'Focused ultrasound surgery of intramural leiomyomas may facilitate fertility: a case report,' Fertil Steril. 2007;88:497.
15. S Zaher, D Lyons, L Regan. 'Uncomplicated term vaginal delivery following magnetic resonance-guided focused ultrasound surgery for uterine fibroids,' Biomed Imaging Interv J. 2010;6(2):28.
16. Bazot M, Cortez A, Darai E, et al. Ultrasonography compared with magnetic resonance imaging for the diagnosis of adenomyosis: correlation with histopathology. Hum Reprod. 2001;16:2427-33.
17. Ascher SM, Arnold LL, Patt RH, et al. Adenomyosis: prospective comparison of MR imaging and transvaginal sonography. Radiology. 1994;190:803-6.
18. Arnold LL, Ascher SM, Schruefer JJ, et al. The nonsurgical diagnosis of adenomyosis. Obstet Gynecol. 1995;86:461-5.
19. Reinhold C, McCarthy S, Bret PM, et al. Diffuse adenomyosis: comparison of endovaginal US and MR imaging with histopathologic correlation. Radiology. 1996;199:151-8.
20. Reinhold C, Tafazoli F, Wang L. Imaging features of adenomyosis. Hum Reprod Update. 1998;4:337-49.
21. Kang S, Turner DA, Foster GS, et al. Adenomyosis: specificity of 5 mm as the maximum normal uterine junctional zone thickness in MR images. AJR Am J Roentgenol. 1996;166:1145-50.
22. Byun JY, Kim SE, Choi BG, et al. Diffuse and focal adenomyosis: MR imaging findings. Radiographics. 1999;19(Suppl):S161-S170.
23. Reinhold C, Tafazoli F, Mehio A, et al. Uterine adenomyosis: endovaginal US and MR imaging features with histopathologic correlation. Radio Graphics. 1999;19:S147-S160.
24. Outwater EK, Siegelman ES, Van Deerlin V. Adenomyosis: current concepts and imaging considerations. AJR Am J Roentgenol. 1998;170:437-41.
25. Grow DR, Filer RB. Treatment of adenomyosis with long-term GnRH analogues: a case report. Obstet Gynecol. 1991;78:538-9.
26. Freundl G, Go¨ dtke K, Gnoth C, et al. Steroidal 'add-back' therapy in patients treated with GnRH agonists. Gynecol Obstet Invest. 1998; 45(Suppl1):22-30.
27. Imaoka I, Ascher SM, Sugimura K, et al. MR imaging of diffuse adenomyosis changes after GnRH analog therapy. J Magn Reson Imaging. 2002;15:285-90.
28. Igarashi M. A new therapy for pelvic endometriosis and uterine adeno- myosis: local effect of vaginal and intrauterine danazol application. Asia Oceania J Obstet Gynaecol. 1990;16:1-12.
29. Fong YF, Singh K. Medical treatment of a grossly enlarged adenomyotic uterus with the levonorgestrel-releasing intrauterine system. Contraception. 1999;60:173-5.
30. Bragheto AM, Caserta N, Bahamondes L, et al. Effectiveness of the levonorgestrel-releasing intrauterine system in the treatment of adenomyosis diagnosed and monitored by magnetic resonance imaging. Contraception. 2007;76:195-9.
31. Smith SJ, Sewall LE, Handelsman A. A clinical failure of uterine fibroid embolization due to adenomyosis. J Vasc Interv Radiol. 1999;10:1171-4.
32. Pelage JP, Jacob D, Fazel A, et al. Midterm results of uterine artery embolization for symptomatic adenomyosis: initial experience. Radiology. 2005;234:948-53.

33. Lohle PN, De Vries J, Klazen CA, et al. Uterine artery embolization for symptomatic adenomyosis with or without uterine leiomyomas with the use of calibrated tris-acryl gelatin microspheres: mid term clinical and MR imaging follow up. J Vasc Interv Radiol. 2007;18:835-41.

34. Mikami K, Murakami T, Okada A, et al. Magnetic resonance imaging-guided focused ultrasound ablation of uterine fibroids: early clinical experience. Radiat Med. 2008;26(4):198-205.

35. Mara M, Fucikova Z, Kuzel D, et al. Hysteroscopy after uterine fibroid embolization in women of fertile age. J Obstet Gynaecol Res. 2007;33: 316–324

36. Stewart EA, et al. Clinical outcomes of focused ultrasound surgery for the treatment of uterine fibroids Fertil Steril. 2006;85(1):22-9.

37. Hidenobu Fukunishi, et al, Early Results of Magnetic Resonance-guided Focused Ultrasound Surgery of Adenomyosis: Analysis of 20 Cases. JMIG. 2008;15(5):571-9.

38. Froeling V, et al, Outcome of uterine artery embolization versus MR-guided high-intensity focused ultrasound treatment for uterine fibroids: Long-term results Eur J Radiol. 2013;82(12):2265-9.

CHAPTER 23

Laparoscopic Uterine Artery Occlusion in Myomectomy

● Alphy S Puthiyidom

■ INTRODUCTION

Surgical myomectomy is currently regarded as the standard conservative treatment for patients who wish to preserve their fertility and uterus. However, it presents two main problems, i.e. the intra- or post-operative risk of bleeding and the risk of recurrence of leiomyomas. Several methods are employed to reduce blood loss during the operation and these include preoperative use of gonadotrophin-releasing hormone (GnRH) agonist, injection of diluted vasopressin into the myometrium, intraoperatively uterine artery embolisation and bilateral uterine artery occlusion. Preventive occlusion of bilateral uterine arteries during laparoscopic myomectomy is a promising procedure in reducing the blood loss and improving the quality of suturing during myomectomy. Other expected long-term benefits are an improvement in the effectiveness of the treatment, both clinical symptoms and the recurrences of leiomyomas. In this chapter we will be discussing on different techniques of uterine artery occlusion, its effect on pregnancy, recurrence, benefits and its possible disadvantages of laparoscopic uterine artery occlusion (LUAO).

■ ANATOMICAL CONSIDERATIONS AND PROPOSED MECHANISM OF ACTION OF UTERINE ARTERY OCCLUSION ON THE MYOMETRIUM AND MYOMA

The uterus is primarily supplied by the uterine artery, which is a branch from the anterior division of the internal iliac artery. The blood reaches the uterus primarily through the uterine arteries, whose sizes are about 2 to 6 mm in diameter and small (0.5 mm) communicating arteries connect the uterus with the ovarian arteries.[1,2] Many named arteries have the potential to supply blood to the uterus, i.e. inferior mesenteric, lumbar, vertebral, middle sacral, deep iliac circumflex, inferior epigastric, medial femoral circumflex and lateral femoral circumflex arteries.[3] Innumerable very small, unnamed arteries reach the uterus from the broad ligament and retroperitoneum. Unlike the uterus, which has various blood supplies, the vascular supply to the fibroids comes exclusively from the uterine arteries.

As most of the blood enters the uterus through the uterine arteries, it was postulated that after occluding the arteries with a laparoscopic technique, transient uterine ischemia occurs. The hypothesis proposes that soon after occlusion, the blood within the myometrium clots, the myometrium becomes hypoxic, and the metabolism shifts from oxidative pathways to anaerobic glycolysis.[4] After several hours of ischaemic-clotted stasis, the uterus is able to lyse clotted blood and is reperfused by blood flow from ovarian and collateral arterial circulation. Myomas do not have mechanisms to lyse clotted blood and reperfuse, and eventually infarct and die.[5]

To test the above hypothesis, Lichtinger et al,[4] studied the time courses of myometrial ischaemia and reperfusion after LUAO in a small group of women with fibroids. The pH was measured with a catheter electrode embedded in the endometrium and myometrium. The pH reached its minimum by a median time of 36 minutes. The pH returned to base line after 2 to 8 hours of UAO. The uterus escaped ischaemia within 6 hours of UAO in 80% of women. Dubuisson JB et al,[6] in their comparative study with Doppler vascularisation before and after occlusion of uterine arteries in 43 patients did not show significant differences in the resistance index of the uterine arteries and the homogeneity of the myometrial vasculature. The same results were found at 3, 6 and 12 months postoperatively by Liu et al.[7]

Burbank and colleagues[8] put forward the 'transient uterine ischemia' hypothesis, and they mentioned that childbirth and myoma treatment by uterine artery occlusion share a common biology. On the basis of the above theory, it is assumed that uterine artery occlusion allows the preservation of the uterus and the achievement of pregnancy, and, also, following childbirth, it may help to treat fibroids through mechanisms of transient ischaemia.

■ TECHNIQUES OF LAPAROSCOPIC UTERINE ARTERY OCCLUSION

Based on the course of uterine artery, three different approaches are used for laparoscopic uterine artery occlusion:
1. Lateral approach.
2. Anterior approach.
3. Posterior approach.

Lateral Approach

The line of dissection is in the triangle bounded by the round ligament anteriorly, infundibulopelvic ligament medially and pelvic sidewall (external iliac vessels) laterally. The peritoneum opened and paravesical and obturator space developed by a blunt dissection. Start dissecting retrograde on medial aspect of obliterated umbilical artery in the paravesical space and continue till it gets obstructed by uterine artery, which traverses from lateral to medial side. Subsequently, distancing uterine vessels from the ureter, uterine artery is occluded either by coagulation and cutting or clipping or ligating uterine artery just medial to the origin from the hypogastric artery.

The advantages of lateral approach is that there is less risk of damage of uterine vein as it is farthest from artery at this point and dissection is easy because of the loose plain compared to further course where the fascia starts getting more condensed and the uterine vein starts approaching close to the artery after crossing the ureter.

Anterior Approach

In cases with very large myomas filling the pelvic cavity, access to the posterior broad ligament and lateral pelvic side wall can be difficult, and in such cases anterior approach to the uterine artery through the anterior broad ligament makes ligation feasible. In this approach uterine artery can be occluded at the transverse or the ascending part of uterine artery (Fig. 23.1).

Surgical Method

Careful inspection of the anterior broad ligament over the paravesical area can often reveal pulsation of the uterine artery to assist in mapping its course. This peritoneum is elevated, then incised transversely using monopolar scissors over the avascular window between the limit of the paravesical fat and the round ligament. The potential space between the leaves of the broad ligament is opened using a combination of pneumodissection and blunt dissection, thus enabling access to the base of the broad ligament (Fig. 23.2). Care is taken to coagulate any small bleeding points as the space is explored because even a small amount of bleeding makes it difficult to identify structures. The space opened up has the posterior peritoneum as its floor, which is not incised because it forms a helpful 'platform' to work on; otherwise, the ureter and UA would retract caudad with the incised posterior broad ligament peritoneum. The external iliac vessels lie laterally, and extra vigilance is vital to avoid inadvertent injury. The uterine artery and the ureter run at the base of the broad ligament surrounded by accompanying fat and lymphatic loose tissue (Figs 23.3 and 23.4).

The preferred site of UA ligation is lateral to its crossing over the ureter because it is away from the ureter and is less intimately intertwined with the uterine vein. At times, especially when there is a large amount of fatty tissue covering

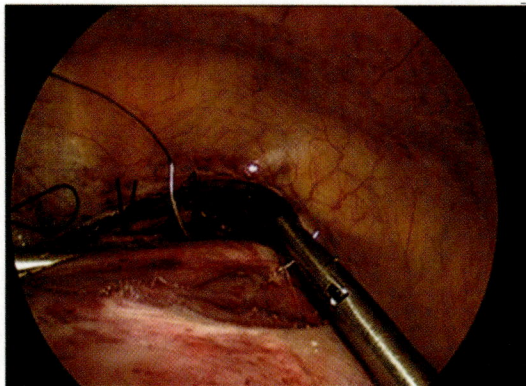

Fig. 23.1: Ligation of ascending part of uterine artery

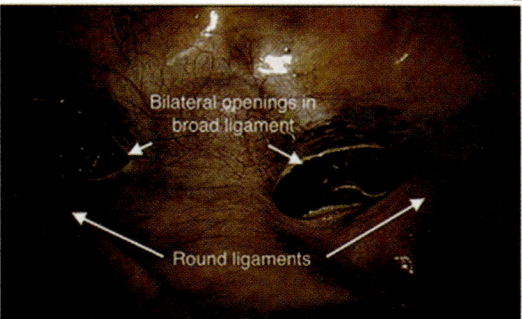

Fig. 23.2: Bilateral opening of the anterior broad ligament

the UA, the anatomy is extremely distorted, or access to the area is limited, it can be helpful to dissect laterally into the paravesical space. The UA can be identified more proximally as it branches off the internal iliac artery. Once the artery has been sufficiently skeletonized, including a segment of artery for proximal control of the vessel in case of unexpected bleeding, a single clip can be applied (Fig. 23.5).

Differentiating the UA and the ureter relies on observation of pulsation or vermiculation, although it is also possible for the ureter to exhibit transmitted pulsation when lying over an artery. It is also possible to expose the superior vesical artery, which is often of smaller caliber than the UA, and the 'water under the bridge' relationship with the ureter is not present.

When uterine artery is ligated at the ascending part there is increased chance that uterine vein can get damaged and should be very careful, while using electrical energy in this region as bladder and ureter is quite near.

Posterior Approach

In posterior approach, the pelvic parietal peritoneum is incised over 15 mm under the ovarian fossa opposite the uterine artery, whose path runs parallel to the path of the ureter located just below. The ureter, therefore, has to be previously identified by transparency by its crawling movement, so that the peritoneal incision is carried out parallel to its path 10 mm above it. Occlusion of the artery is performed by inserting

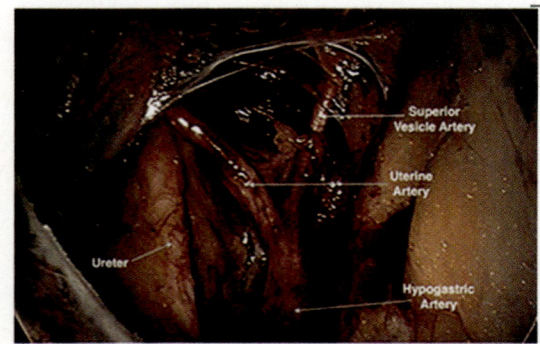

Fig. 23.3: Retroperitoneal Anatomy showing origin of right uterine artery from Internal iliac artery

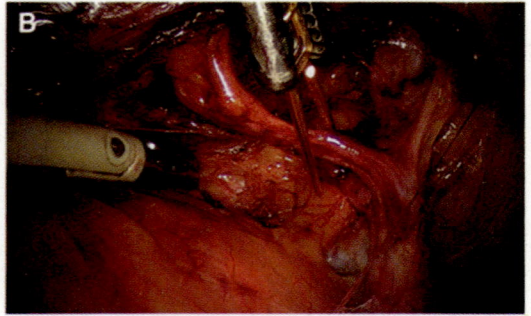

Fig. 23.4: Vascular clip applied on right uterine artery

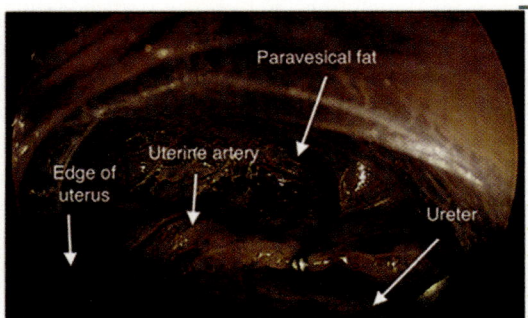

Fig. 23.5: Right sided dissection—clip applied to the uterine artery with the ureter seen at the base of the dissection

10 mm vascular clip across the 10 mm accessory trocar. The technique can be facilitated by temporarily fixing the ovary to the abdominal wall ipsilaterally.

■ LAPAROSCOPIC TEMPORARY CLIPPING OF UTERINE ARTERY DURING LAPAROSCOPIC MYOMECTOMY

Some authors remove the occluding clips at the end of myomectomy procedure. But the potential disadvantage described in this method is that an intraoperative dry field may start bleeding at the end of the procedure compared to myomectomy without occluding uterine artery where every potential source of bleeding can be discovered intra operatively and taken care of. But compared to vasoconstrictors such as vasopressin whose duration of action is not controllable and with a vasoconstriction lasting longer than the operation may lead to postoperative haemorrhage. In these respect the use of vascular clip have a definite advantage, allowing an immediate restart of the physiological blood supply after the clip removal.[9]

■ CONCERNS OF UTERINE ARTERY LIGATION DURING LAPAROSCOPIC MYOMECTOMY

Technical difficulties of ligating the uterine vessels, especially in large myomas may be a restricting factor. Ureter and iliac vessels can be damaged due to its proximity to the uterine artery. Holub Z et al,[10] has reported about neuritis of the obturator nerve, which subsided with anti-inflammatory and electrostimulative convalescence therapy. However, with adequate training and the skill of the surgeon, it is not impossible.

■ UTERINE ARTERY OCCLUSION AND BLOOD LOSS DURING MYOMECTOMY

Generally, it is shown that LUAO reduces the intraoperative and postoperative blood loss in myomectomy. Holub et al,[11] analysed blood loss in a small sample by comparing the

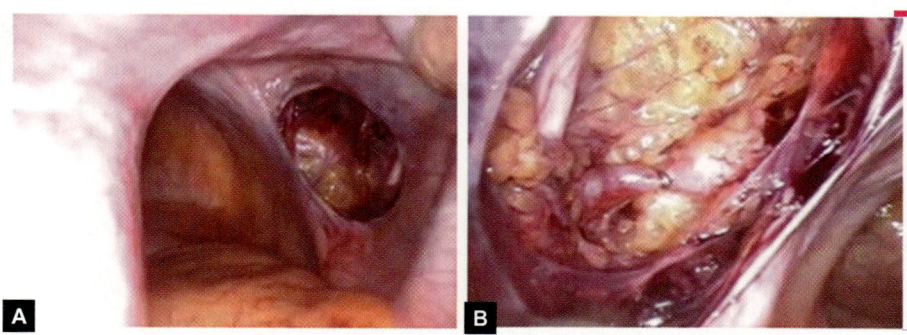

Figs 23.6A and B: Clip applied to uterine artery. **A.** On right side; **B.** On left side.

'occlusion + myomectomy' (n=16) and 'myomectomy only' (n = 15) groups. The results did not reach statistical significance for intraoperative bleeding, with an average blood loss estimated at 93.7 mL in the first group versus 134 mL in the second group. However, postoperative bleeding, evaluated by drainage of the abdominal cavity, was significantly reduced in the LUAO + M group (46 versus 92.4 mL). Similarly, the measurement of changes in haemoglobin on the 3rd postoperative day is in favour of preventive uterine artery occlusion.

UTERINE ARTERY OCCLUSION AND RESULTS ON SYMPTOMS

Even though there are no prospective randomized studies comparing the improvement of symptoms in case of myomectomy alone or combined with preventive occlusion of uterine arteries, all observational comparative series show a significant improvement in symptoms in the cases associated with uterine artery occlusion. Liu et al, demonstrated a 99.1% improvement in symptoms in the 'occlusion + myomectomy' group compared to 81.5% in the 'myomectomy only' group for a minimum postoperative follow-up of 3 months.[12]

Holub et al,[11] found a 100% improvement in symptoms after 3 months in the 'occlusion + myomectomy' group versus 85.7% in the myomectomy only group. Finally, Alborzi et al,[13] confirm these data in a 24 month follow–up with an improvement in symptoms of 98.1% in the 'occlusion + myomectomy' group versus 83.1% in the myomectomy only group.

UTERINE ARTERY LIGATION AND RECURRENCE OF MYOMA

In 2007, Liu et al,[14] evaluated the myoma recurrence rate in LUAO-M compared with traditional myomectomy. During 41.5 months of follow-up, the recurrence rate with LUAO-M was 5.8%, and with traditional myomectomy was 36.7%. In patients who did not use contraception, the pregnancy rate was 19.2% in the LUAO-M group compared with 22.4% in the traditional myomectomy group; pregnancy outcomes were similar in the two groups. The low recurrence rate in this study demonstrated that the blood supply to leiomyoma may be primarily from the uterine artery. Preexisting small myomas would be necrotic after uterine artery occlusion,[15] however, uterine physiologic functions (menses, pregnancy, and delivery) would be sustained by the blood supply from the collateral circulation.

Thus, LUAO has a great advantage for treatment of symptomatic uterine myomas. The need for re-intervention is markedly greater in patients after uterine artery embolisation (up to 35% within 5 years compared to myomectomy[16]).

LAPAROSCOPIC UTERINE ARTERIAL OCCLUSION ON OVARIAN RESERVE

The LUAO procedure was developed from the UAE technique. But studies on uterine artery embolisation have clearly stated the possibility of ovarian failure following the procedure. Tulandi et al,[17] have described that due to transient ovarian ischemia, some degree of ovarian reserve appears to be lost when the ovaries are inadvertently embolised. Most researchers believe three causes are responsible for ovarian failure after UAE. First, the ovarian arteries may be embolised by polyvinyl alcohol between the uterine and ovarian arteries. Second, in patients aged 40 to 45 years, the incidence of amenorrhea is higher than in patients younger than 40 years, and patients younger than 35 rarely develop amenorrhea. Third, long exposure to radiation during interventional radiotherapy could injure ovarian function.[18]

But in case of uterine artery occlusion, the uterus receives enough blood to meet its physiologic functions because there is plentiful vascular anastomosis between the uterine artery and the round ligament, ovarian, inferior epigastric, and median sacral arteries. In theory, the blood supply to the ovaries would be affected after LUAO, and ovarian function would be impaired. However, the ovaries continue to obtain adequate blood supply via the ovarian arteries because the hilum of the ovaries were not injured, and it was also possible to receive blood via natural vascular anastomosis.

Arthur et al (2014) compared the long-term impact on ovarian reserve after UAE and LM. Showed that median serum AMH levels and median AFC per ovary were significantly lower in reproductive-aged women who have undergone UAE over the long term (> 12 month) than women with LM.[19]

Cheng et al reported that 4 of 348 patients (1.3%) treated with LUAO-M had postoperative amenorrhea, compared with 3 of 172 patients (2.1%) treated with laparoscopic myomectomy (LM) and was no significant difference in the incidence of postoperative amenorrhea between these 2 groups.[20] Qu X et al, have conducted a study to assess the effect on ovarian reserve function after LUAO compared with LM. Blood samples were collected before surgery and at 1, 3, and 6 months postoperatively. Concentrations of the follicle-stimulating hormone (FSH), leuteinizing hormone (LH), estradiol (EZ) and serum inhibin B (INHB) were determined using an immunoassay. The study concluded that at a short-term follow-up, no significant effect was found on ovarian reserve in patients with myoma, who underwent laparoscopic uterine artery occlusion.[21]

Even though there are no long-term randomized trials on this effect published so far based on the results of retrospective studies. Preventive uterine artery occlusion during myomectomy does not appear to alter hormones of the pituitary-ovarian feedback loop compared with myomectomy alone.

PREGNANCY AFTER UTERINE ARTERY LIGATION

Fertility and pregnancy following selective ligation of the uterine arteries has also been reported in literature since ages. Between 1964 and 1980, nearly two dozen full-term, successful pregnancies in women who had uterine artery ligation performed have been recorded in the world's medical literature.[22,23]

Holub et al,[24] assessed pregnancy outcomes and deliveries after laparoscopic uterine artery transection in symptomatic women with fibroids. About 153 patients underwent laparoscopic transection of uterine vessels during a 4 year period. The study concluded that laparoscopic transection of uterine vessels is a minimally invasive operative procedure that preserves the uterus and ovarian blood supply and allows for the achievement of pregnancy in women with symptomatic fibroids. Fetal growth and umbilical Doppler findings remained normal in all cases. An increased risk for preterm delivery and caesarean section was found in this small series.

Even though no randomized study has examined long-term fertility, observational comparative studies have shown comparable pregnancy rates in LUAO-M group compared with LM alone.

OUR EXPERIENCE

In our centre we are routinely doing LUAO along with myomectomy in all patients with symptomatic multiple fibroids, who have completed the fertility function. We have noticed a good symptomatic relief in 96% of patients with reduction of size in those few deep seated fibroid, which were not removed during the procedure. In patients with future child-bearing desire we prefer to do LUAO as a stand alone procedure in selected cases with large and multiple fibroids after explaining the benefits and the possible risk. Lateral approach to occlude the uterine artery from origin is the preffered method in our centre.

In cases with large fibroid uterus where access to uterine artery is difficult due to the location of fibroid, we inject vasopressin first followed by myomectomy and then uterine artery occlusion done before the myoma bed suturing. We have done a retrospective analysis of women with large uterine size (24–30 weeks) who have undergone laparoscopic myomectomy.

In study group women underwent vasopressin injection followed by myomectomy then uterine artery ligation at its origin before closure of myoma bed. In control group, women underwent laparoscopic myomectomy with vasopressin alone or uterine artery ligation. In control group, uterine artery ligation was done before myomectomy. The need for blood transfusion (intra and post-operative period) was significantly less in study group (nil) compared with control group (12.9%). The length of hospital stay (3 or more days) was lesser in study group compared with control group (nil v/s 12.9%). During laparoscopic myomectomy for large uteri, combined use of vasopressin and uterine artery ligation before myomectomy bed closure is very useful method for haemostasis especially in large fibroid uterus.

MYOLYSIS

Myolysis refers to the use of temperature to destroy tissue by thermal coagulation or cryoablation (cryomyolysis) of leiomyoma tissue to reduce myoma size (by approximately 50%) by means of myoma destruction and interference with local vascular supply (Fig. 23.7A to D).[25–27] Despite reports of apparently successful outcomes, these techniques have not enjoyed widespread popularity and use. The techniques require placement of probes into the fibroid, usually via laparoscopy, and the fibroid tissue is destroyed by heat (unipolar or preferably, bipolar), cold coagulation (cryomyolysis) or laser.[28–30]

Laparoscopic myolysis was developed and performed in Germany by Gallinat in 1986 and reported in the United States by Goldfarb in 1992.[31] Myolysis is done using heat energy delivered by a neodymium: yttrium-aluminum garnet laser fibre or monopolar or bipolar electrode, the aim is to disrupt, diminish, or abolish the blood supply to the myoma, depriving it of dependent nutrients, sex hormones, and growth factors and causing it to shrink. Initially, the energy was delivered through numerous punctures to the myoma in contiguous fashion. However, multiple puncture on uterine surface with localised tissue destruction without repair may increase the chance of subsequent adhesion formation (in one study, dense adhesions were found in 6 of 15 women).[32] Subsequently, the blood supply was coagulated at the periphery of the myoma without puncturing the fibroid itself. The latter technique may result in less post-operative adhesion formation over the myoma site, although randomized, prospective studies have not been reported.

Laparoscopic electromyolysis can be considered an alternative to myomectomy in certain cases because it is effective, easier to master than laparoscopic myomectomy, since it does not require laparoscopic suturing. In general, after 3 months of therapy with a GnRH agonist the myoma volume deceases by 30% to 50%.[33,34] A myoma that increased in size after 1 month of GnRH agonist treatment should raise the suspension of a leiomyosarcoma.[35] 6 months after myolysis, myomas shrink by an additional 30% to 50% beyond the effects of the GnRH agonist, and overall reduction appears to be permanent.[36] Since myolysis reduces or replaces the myoma by scar tissue, which might compromise integrity and tensile strength of the uterine wall, concern exists that the uterus may rupture during subsequent pregnancies. It has been reported in only a limited number of women who wish to preserve fertility.[37] Three patients conceived within 3 months after laparoscopic electromyolysis. In two of them the uterus

ruptured at 32 and 39 weeks' gestation, respectively. Therefore, if pregnancies occur after myolysis, great caution should be exercised and intensive surveillance of both mother and fetous must be applied. Caesarean section should be performed at the earliest signs and symptoms of uterine rupture and at term before onset of labour.[38]

Lee Y, Cho HH, Kim JH, et al, reported on transvaginal radiofrequency myolysis (RFM). RFM can be performed in premenopausal post childbearing patients with symptomatic submucosal leiomyomas who desired preservation of their uterus. RFM has several advantages—it does not require admission care, is associated with low postoperative bleeding and pain, and patients may rapidly resume daily activities within a few hours after RFM. Furthermore, after RFM, myoma cells and feeding vessels are coagulated, which ensures minimal bleeding during subsequent hysteroscopic myomectomy.[39]

In women with menorrhagia, myolysis combined with endometrial ablation may be more effective therapy than either procedure alone, but this is investigational. An observational study comparing ablation alone versus with the combined procedure found that the risks of a second surgery were 38 and 13%, respectively (Figs 23.8A and B).[40]

■ OUR EXPERIENCE

We have limited experience in myolysis. In our centre, we prefer to do myolysis only for subserosal fibroid of less than 1–2 cm with bipolar or monopolar needle in coagulation mode.

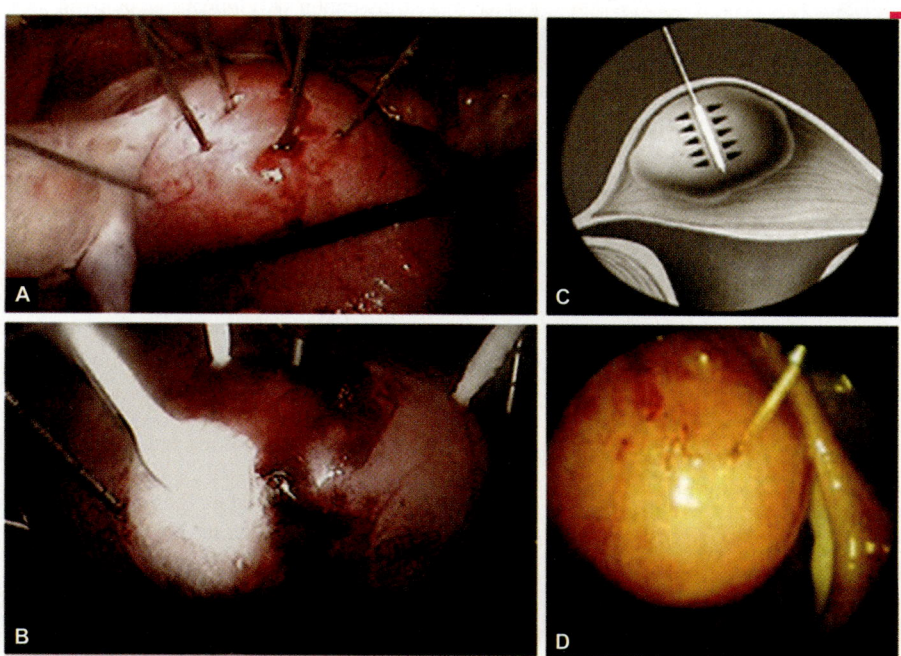

Figs 23.7A to D: A and B. Needle placement in fibroid before and after freezing (Cryomyolysis); **C and D.** Monopolar needle in fibroid.

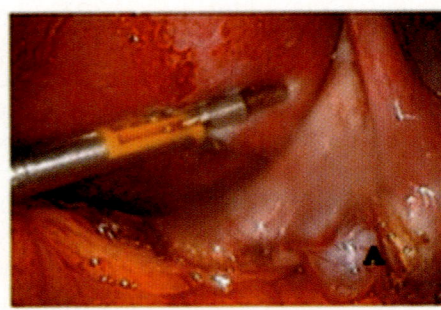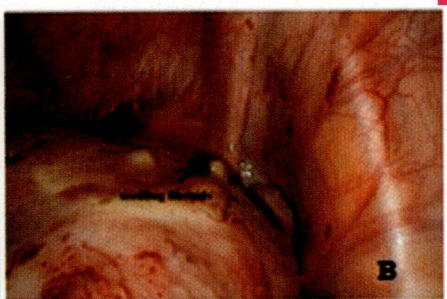

Figs 23.8A and B: A. Myolysis of seedling fibroids using bipolar coagulation; **B.** Myomas at the end of myolysis.

■ CONCLUSION

Laparoscopic myomectomy with uterine artery occlusion is a technically feasible procedure. Ligating the uterine arteries bilaterally with either the ascending branch or at its origin from the internal iliac, considerably reduces intraoperative and postoperative blood loss in myomectomy. In the absence of excessive bleeding in myometrium improves the quality of the uterine suturing there by improved uterine healing and reduces the risk of scarring necrosis.

It should be considered in patients with symptomatic multiple fibroids, as this promots involution by ischemia of deeper and smaller leiomyomas left in place and reduces the risk of symptomatic recurrence. Although the current data are reassuring, it is not recommended to use this technique routinely in patients who wish to become pregnant.

As myolysis is easy to master and perform than laparoscopic myomectomy, it can be used in selected candidates. Most experts do not recommend myolysis for women who wish future fertility due to the risk of uterine rupture during subsequent pregnancy. Candidates for myolysis are further limited to women with fewer than four leiomyomas with the largest leiomyoma less than 10 cm in diameter. As per the literature myolysis is not an alternative to laparoscopic myomectomy, it should be done only in selected patients who have completed fertility function with no suspicion of leiomyosarcoma.

■ REFERENCES

1. Lipshutz B. A composite study of the hypogastric artery and its branches. Ann Surg. 1918;67:584-608.
2. Borell U, Fernstrom I. The adnexal branches of the uterine artery. An arteriographic study in human subjects. ActaRadiol. 1953;40:561-82.
3. Burchell RC. Arterial physiology of the human female pelvis. Obstet Gynecol. 1968;31:855-60.
4. Lichtinger M, Burbank F, Hallson L, et al. The time course of myometrial ischemia and reperfusion after laparoscopic uterine artery occlusion-Theoretical implications. J Am Assoc Gynecol Laparosc. 2003;10:553-63.
5. Lichtinger M, Hallson L, Calvo PAG. The course of uterine myometrial perfusion after laparoscopic occlusion of uterine arteries for symptomatic leiomyomas. J Am AssocGynecolLaparoscop. 2002;9:32-3.
6. Dubuisson JB, Jacob S, Chapron C, et al. Preventive artery occlusion combined with laparoscopic myomectomy: a valid procedure to prevent bleeding. J GynecolSurg. 2004;20:105-12.
7. Liu WM, et al. Efficacy of combined laparoscopic uterine artery occlusion and myomectomy for symptomatic uterine myoma. Fertilsteril. 2007;95(1):254-8.
8. Burbank F. Childbirth and myoma treatment by uterine artery occlusion: do they share a common biology? J Am AssocGynecolLaparosc. 2004;11:138-52.
9. Giuseppe E, Evrim Erdemoglu, Aries Joe. Laparoscopic temporary clipping of uterine artery during laparoscopic myomectomy. Arch Gynecol Obstet. 2012;286:1181-1186
10. Hald K, Langebrekke A, Klow NE, et al. Laparoscopic occlusion of uterine vessels for the treatment of symptomatic fibroids: Initial experience and comparison to uterine artery embolization. Am J Obstet Gynecol. 2004;190:37-43.
11. Holub Z, Jabor A, Lukac J. The effect of lateral uterine artery dissection on clinical outcomes in laparoscopic myomectomy: a prospective randomized study. Gynecol Surg. 2004;1:253-8.
12. Liu WM, et al. Combining the uterine depletion procedure and myomectomy may be useful for treating symptomatic fibroids. FertilSteril. 2004;82(1):205-10.
13. Alborzi S, et al. A comparison of combined laparoscopic uterine artery ligation and myomectomy versus laparoscopic myomectomy for symptomatic uterine myoma. Fertile Steril. 2009;92(2):742-7.
14. Lui WM, Wang PH, Chou CS, et al. Efficacy of combined laparoscopic uterine artery occlusion and myomectomy via minilaparotomy in the treatment of recurrent uterine myomas. FertilSteril. 2007;87:356-61.
15. Cheng Z, Xie Y, Dai H, et al. Unequaltissue expression of proteins from the PA/PAI system, myoma necrosis, and uterus survival after uterine artery occlusion. Int J Gynaecol Obstet. 2008;102:55-9.
16. Goldberg J1, Pereira L. Pregnancy outcomes following treatment for fibroids: uterine fibroid embolization versus laparoscopic myomectomy. CurrOpinObstet Gynecol. 2006;18(4):402-6.
17. Tulandi T, Sammour A, Valenti D, et al. Ovarian reserve after uterine artery embolization for leiomyomata. FertilSteril. 2002;78:197-8.
18. Nikolic B, Spies JB, Lundsten MJ, et al. Patient radiation

dose associated with uterine artery embolization. Radiology. 2000;214:121-5.

19. Arthur R1, Kachura J2, Liu G3, et al. Laparoscopic myomectomy versus uterine artery embolization: long-term impact on markers of ovarian reserve. J ObstetGynaecol Can. 2014;36(3):240-7.

20. Cheng Z, Yang W, Dai H, et al. Laparoscopic uterine artery occlusion combined with myomectomy for uterine myomas. J Minim Invasive Gynecol. 2008;15:346-9.

21. Qu X, et al. Controlled clinical trial assessing the effect of laparoscopic uterine arterial occlusion on ovarian reserve.J Minim Invasive Gynecol. 2010;17(1):47-52.

22. Lenzi G. Pregnancy after ligation of uterine arteries. AttualOstetGinecol. 1969;15:31-5.

23. Liberman G. Normal labor after ligation of major vessels of the uterus. AkushGinekol. 1966;12:45-6.

24. Holub Z, Lukac J, Kliment L, et al. Pregnancy outcomes and deliveries following laparoscopic transsection of uterine vessels: A pilot study. Eur J ObstetGynecolReprod Biol. 2006;125:165-70.

25. Goldfarb HA. Laparoscopic coagulation of myoma (myolysis). Obstet Gynecol Clin North Am. 1995;22:807.

26. Zupi E, Piredda A, Marconi D, et al. Directed laparoscopic cryomyolysis: a possible alternative to myomectomy and/or hysterectomy for symptomatic leiomyomas. Am J Obstet Gynecol. 2004;190:639.

27. Visvanathan D, Connell R, Hall-Craggs MA, et al. Interstitial laser photocoagulation for uterine myomas. Am J Obstet Gynecol. 2002;187:382.

28. Nisolle M, Smets M, Malvaux V, et al. Laparoscopic myolysis with the Nd:YAG laser. J Gynecol Surg. 1993;9:95.

29. Zupi E, Marconi D, Sbracia M, et al. Directed laparoscopic cryomyolysis for symptomatic leiomyomata: one-year follow up. J Minim Invasive Gynecol. 2005;12:343.

30. Bradley S Hurst, Mollie Elliot, BSN, Michelle et al. Ultrasound-directed transvaginal myolysis: J of Minim Invasive Gynecol. 2007;14:502-5.

31. Goldfarb HA. Nd:YAG laser laparoscopic coagulation of symptomatic myomas. J Reprod Med. 1992;36:636-8.

32. Donnez J, Squifflet J, Polet R, Nisolle M. Laparoscopic myolysis. Hum Reprod Update. 2000;6:609.

33. Friedman AJ, Hoffman DI, Cominet F, et al. Treatment of leiomyomata uteri with leuprolide acetate depot: A double-blind placebo-controlled multicentre study. Obstet Gynecol. 1991;77:720-5.

34. Kiltz RJ, Rutgers J, Phillips J, et al. Absence of a doseresponse of leuprolide acetate in leiomyomatauterine size. Fertil Steril. 1994;61:1021-6.

35. Goldfarb HA. Bipolar laparoscopic needles for myoma coagulation. JAm Assoc Gynecol Laparosc. 1995;2:175-9.

36. Phillips DR, Milim SJ, Nathanson HG, et al. Experience with laparoscopic leiomyoma coagulation and concomitant operative hysteroscopy. J Am Assoc Gynecol Laparosc. 1997;4:425-433.

37. Arcangeli S, Pasquarette MM. Gravid uterine rupture after myolysis. Obstet Gynecol. 1997;89:857.

38. GA Vilos, LJ Daly, BM Tse. Pregnancy Outcome after Laparoscopic Electromyolysis.JAm Assoc Gynecol Laparosc. 1998;5(3):289-92.

39. Lee Y, Cho HH, Kim JH. Outpatient Multimodality Management of Large Submucosal Myomas Using Transvaginal Radiofrequency Myolysis, Journal of Minimally Invasive Gynecology. 2014;21:1049-54.

40. Goldfarb HA. Combining myoma coagulation with endometrial ablation/resection reduces subsequent surgery rates. JSLS. 1999;3:253.

SECTION 4

Fibroids in Fertility and Pregnancy

CHAPTER 24

Fibroids and Pregnancy Outcome

● Sandip Datta Roy, Shyjus Puliyathinkal

■ INTRODUCTION

Uterine fibroids (leiomyomas) are benign smooth muscle tumours of the uterus. Since these tumours are quite common in women of reproductive age, the potential effects of fibroids on pregnancy and effects of pregnancy on fibroids are a frequent clinical concern for the present day obstetrician. Most pregnant women with fibroids do not develop any fibroid-related complication during pregnancy. Pain is the most common problem, and there may be a slightly increased risk of obstetrical complications such as miscarriage, preterm labour and delivery, abnormal fetal position and placental abruption.

■ PREVALENCE

The prevalence of uterine fibroids in pregnancy varies between 1.6% and 10.7%, depending upon the trimester of assessment and the size threshold used.[1,2] In one study, 1.6% of 12,600 consecutive pregnant patients had fibroids > 1 cm.[3] In another study, 4% of 12,708 pregnant patients had fibroids with a diameter > 3 cm.[4] A third series in over 15,000 women with non-anomalous singleton pregnancies undergoing routine second trimester ultrasonography reported that 2.7% had fibroids ≥ 1 cm. A fourth series of 4271 first trimester or post-miscarriage ultrasound examinations observed 10.7% of women had a fibroid of ≥ 0.5 cm.

The prevalence of fibroids increases with age and is higher in African-American women than in white or Hispanic women.[5] Increase in parity and prolonged duration of breastfeeding are associated with a small, but statistically significant, reduction in prevalence.[6]

■ DIAGNOSIS OF FIBROID IN PREGNANCY

The diagnosis of fibroids in pregnancy is neither simple nor straight forward. Only 42% of large fibroids (> 5 cm) and 12.5% of smaller fibroids (3–5 cm) can be diagnosed on physical examination.[7] The ability of ultrasound to detect fibroids in pregnancy is even more limited primarily due to the difficulty of differentiating fibroids from physiologic thickening of the myometrium. The prevalence of uterine fibroids during pregnancy is therefore likely to be underestimated.

■ EFFECTS OF FIBROID ON CONCEPTION, PREGNANCY AND LABOUR

Approximately 10% to 30% of women with uterine fibroids develop complications during pregnancy.[8] Although there are inconsistencies as far as available evidence is concerned, decreased uterine expansibility or mechanical obstruction may explain some of the adverse pregnancy outcomes.

Miscarriage

Spontaneous miscarriage rates are greatly increased in pregnant women with fibroids compared with control subjects without fibroids (14% vs 7.6%, respectively).[9] Available evidences suggest that multiple fibroids may increase the miscarriage rate in comparison to a single fibroid (23.6% vs 8.0%). The location of the fibroid may be more important than its size. Submucous fibroids or intramural fibroids with submucous component are known to be the culprits. Increased uterine irritability, the compressive effect of fibroids, and compromise to the blood supply of the developing placenta and fetous have all been implicated as possible reasons.[10]

Preterm Labour and Preterm Premature Rupture of Membranes

Pregnant women with fibroids are significantly more likely to develop preterm labour and to deliver preterm than women without fibroids (16.1% vs 8.7% and 16% vs 10.8%, respectively).[8] Multiple fibroids and retroplacental fibroids appear to be independent risk factors for preterm labour.[11,12] In contrast, fibroids do not appear to be a risk factor for preterm premature rupture of membranes (PPROM).

Placental Abruption

Although reports are conflicting, pooled cumulative data suggest that the risk of placental abruption is increased 3-fold in women with fibroids.[13] Submucosal fibroids, retroplacental fibroids and fibroid volumes > 200 cm^3 are independent risk factors for placental abruption.[14] One retrospective study reported placental abruption in 57% of women with retroplacental fibroids in contrast with 2.5% of women with fibroids located in alternate sites. One possible mechanism of placental abruption may be diminished blood flow to the fibroid and the adjacent tissues with resultant partial ischemia and decidual necrosis in the placental tissues overlying the leiomyoma.[15]

Placenta Previa

The presence of fibroids is associated with a 2-fold increased risk of placenta previa, after adjusting for prior surgeries such as caesarean section or myomectomy.[16]

Fetal Growth Restriction and Fetal Anomalies

Fetal growth does not appear to be affected by the presence of uterine fibroids. Although cumulative data and a population-based study suggested that women with fibroids are at slightly increased risk of delivering a growth-restricted infant, these results were not adjusted for maternal age or gestational age.[17] Rarely, large fibroids can compress and distort the intrauterine cavity leading to fetal deformities. A number of fetal anomalies have been reported in women with large submucosal fibroids, including dolichocephaly (lateral compression of the fetal skull), torticollis (abnormal twisting of the neck), and limb reduction defects.[18]

Labour and Delivery

Malpresentation, Labour Dystocia and Caesarean Delivery

The risk of fetal malpresentation increases in women with fibroids compared with control subjects (13% vs 4.5%, respectively).[13,17] Large fibroids, multiple fibroids and fibroids in the lower uterine segment have all been reported as independent risk factors for malpresentation.

Numerous studies have shown that uterine fibroids are a risk factor for caesarean delivery. In a systematic review, women with fibroids were at a 3.7-fold increased risk of caesarean delivery (48.8% vs 13.3%, respectively).[13] This is due in part to an increase in labour dystocia, which is increased 2-fold in pregnant women with fibroids. Malpresentation, large fibroids, multiple fibroids, submucosal fibroids, and fibroids in the lower uterine segment are considered predisposing factors for caesarean delivery. Despite the increased risk of caesarean, the presence of uterine fibroids, even large fibroids (> 5 cm), should not be regarded as a contraindication to a trial of labour.[17]

Postpartum Haemorrhage

Reports on the association between fibroids and postpartum haemorrhage are conflicting. Pooled cumulative data suggest that postpartum haemorrhage is significantly more likely in women with fibroids compared with control subjects (2.5% vs 1.4%, respectively).[13] Fibroids may distort the uterine architecture and interfere with myometrial contractions leading to uterine atony and postpartum haemorrhage.[19] The same mechanism may also explain why women with fibroids are at increased risk of puerperal hysterectomy.

Retained Placenta

Available evidence suggests that retained placenta is more common in all women with fibroids compared with control subjects, regardless of the location of the fibroid (1.4% vs 0.6%, respectively).[13]

Effects of Pregnancy on Fibroid

Pregnancy associated increase in oestrogen and progesterone levels and uterine blood flow are believed to affect fibroid growth. There was a commonly held belief that fibroids increase in size throughout gestation. Studies, which sonographically monitored the size of fibroids throughout the pregnancy have refuted the belief,[20] with a few exceptions. It appears that fibroid size reasonably remains stable across gestation in 50% to 60% of cases, increases in 22% to 32% and decreases in 8% to 27%.[11,21]

Inconsistency in the data on the effect of pregnancy on fibroid may be due to the difference in trimester of assessment and for the fact of fibroid growth not being linear in pregnancy. For example, in those fibroids that increase in size, most of the growth occurs in the first trimester, with little if any further increase in size during the second and third trimesters. Larger fibroids (> 5 cm in diameter) are more likely to grow, whereas smaller fibroids are more likely to remain stable in size.[3] The mean increase in fibroid volume during pregnancy is 12%, and very few fibroids increase by more than 25%.[21]

Majority of women with fibroids detected in the first trimester will have regression in total fibroid volume when re-evaluated 3 to 6 months postpartum, but almost 10 percent will have an increase in volume.[22] Regression may be less in women who use progestin-only contraception.

■ MANAGEMENT

During Pregnancy

It is almost always a conservative line of approach as far as management of fibroid in pregnancy is concerned. It is a rarity for fibroids to be treated surgically in the first half of pregnancy. If necessary, however, several studies have reported that antepartum myomectomy can be safely performed in the first and second trimester of pregnancy.[23,24] Acceptable indications include intractable pain from a degenerating fibroid especially if it is subserosal or pedunculated, a large or rapidly growing fibroid, or any large fibroid (> 5 cm) located in the lower uterine segment. Obstetric and neonatal outcomes in women undergoing myomectomy in pregnancy are comparable with that in conservatively managed women,[25] although women who had a myomectomy during pregnancy were far more likely to be delivered by caesarean due to concerns about uterine rupture.

During Labour

Most of the fibroids do not hinder the descent of the presenting part or cervical dilatation and hence do not interfere with the progress in labour. And hence the presence of uterine fibroids, even large fibroids (> 5 cm), should not be regarded as a contraindication to a trial of labour. Fibroids occupying the lower uterine segment or cervical fibroids may be the only varieties, which warrant a caesarean section.

Most authorities still recommend that every effort should be made to avoid performing a myomectomy at the time of caesarean delivery due to the substantial risk of severe haemorrhage requiring blood transfusion, uterine artery ligation, and/or puerperal hysterectomy.[26] But there has been numerous case reports from around the world over the last few years on successful caesarean myomectomies with hardly any untoward outcome even with intramural myomas. Use of haemostatic agents like vasopressin in dilution and effective use of uterine artery ligation seems to have greatly helped to reduce the amount of blood loss and thereby reduce the related morbidity. Occasionally, a caesarean myomectomy may also be indicated to facilitate baby delivery or to enable a good closure of the hysterotomy. Pedunculated subserosal fibroids can always be safely removed at the time of caesarean delivery without any increase in the risk of haemorrhage.[27]

Caesarean Myomectomy: Tips and Tricks

The basic approach for a caesarean myomectomy does not differ much from myomectomy in a non-pregnant uterus. The only difference being the fact that the gravid uterus is much more vascular than the non-pregnant one.

Methods to reduce intraoperative blood loss should be given due importance in the setting of a caesarean myomectomy. Infiltration of temporary haemostatic agents like vasopressin in dilution (10 units in 100 mL of normal saline), the use of bilateral uterine artery ligation or uses of tourniquets are the available options. All the techniques mentioned above, can be used alone or in combination. Incision is made over the most prominent part of the myoma. An intramural myoma with a submucous component could be approached through the uterine cavity also, avoiding a scar on the surface of the uterus. A transverse incision may be preferred over a vertical incision on the uterine wall, since it has been shown to cause disruption of less number of muscle fibres. Whichever the incision, haemostasis and good approximation of myometrium at closure is of utmost importance. This primarily decides the quality of the uterine scar and its behavior in next pregnancy (Figs 24.1 to 24.4).

Pain Management of Fibroid in Pregnancy: Practical Points

Most fibroids are asymptomatic. However, severe localised abdominal pain can occur if a fibroid undergoes 'red degeneration', torsion (seen most commonly with a pedunculated subserosal fibroid), or impaction. Pain is the most common complication of fibroids in pregnancy, and is seen most often in women with large fibroids (> 5 cm) during the second and third trimesters of pregnancy.[8,15]

In a study of 113 pregnant women, 9% of fibroids showed a heterogeneous echogenic pattern or cystic changes on

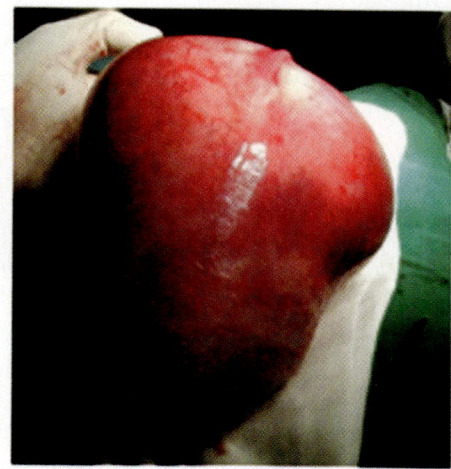

Fig. 24.1: An intramural fundal myoma encountered at Caesarean section

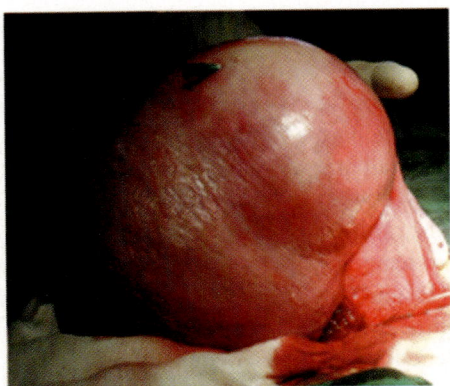

Fig. 24.2: Intraoperative picture after vasopressin infiltration. Note the blanching of the myometrium prior to a caesarean myomectomy.

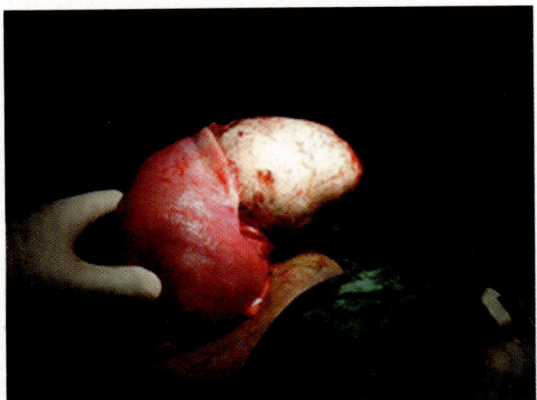

Fig. 24.3: The intramural myoma popping out through the incision. Due respect to the planes of dissection can help to reduce the intraoperative blood loss.

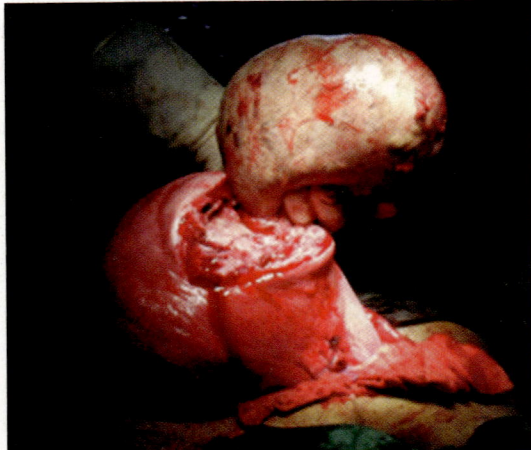

Fig. 24.4: Myoma removal in Caesarean myomectomy

ultrasound indicating the development of red degeneration. Three main theories have been proposed to explain the severe pain associated with red degeneration. First, that rapid fibroid growth results in the tissue outgrowing its blood supply leading to tissue anoxia, necrosis and infarction. Second that the growing uterus results in a change in the architecture

(kinking) of the blood supply to the fibroid leading to ischemia and necrosis even in the absence of fibroid growth. Third that the pain results from the release of prostaglandins from cellular damage within the fibroid. This is supported by the observation that ibuprofen and other prostaglandin synthetase inhibitors effectively and rapidly control fibroid pain.[8]

Fibroid pain during pregnancy is usually managed conservatively by bed rest, hydration and analgesics. Prostaglandin synthase inhibitors (non-steroidal anti-inflammatory drugs) should be used with caution considering the possibility of both fetal and neonatal adverse effects, including premature closure of the fetal ductus arteriosus, pulmonary hypertension, necrotizing enterocolitis, intracranial haemorrhage or oligohydramnios.[28] Rarely, severe pain may necessitate additional pain medication (narcotic analgesia including morphine), epidural analgesia or surgical management (Figs 24.5 to 24.9).[29]

■ PREGNANCY AFTER LAPAROSCOPIC MYOMECTOMY

Fertility after Laparoscopic Myomectomy

Laparoscopic myomectomy in infertile patients complicated with uterine myoma is expected to improve the postoperative pregnancy rate as observed with laparotomy. The pregnancy rate after laparoscopic myomectomy have been reported to be between 33.3% to 65.7%,[30–32] although various factors like patient's age, duration of infertility, diameter of the largest myoma, and number of enucleated myomas etc can have variable influence on outcome. Although there is no effect of myoma location, women with a larger volume (>100 mL) of myomas removed tend to have higher pregnancy rates.[33] In a prospectively randomized study of 131 women with myomectomy by laparoscopy versus laparotomy, pregnancy rates were almost comparable (55.9% in the laparotomy group vs 53.6% in the laparoscopy group).[34] Hence, the individual patient's infertility characteristics are probably the most important factors.

Seracchioli et al,[35] reported 27.2% spontaneous abortion among 158 pregnancies achieved after laparoscopic myomectomy (43/158), a rate very similar to that reported by Dubuisson et al (26.2%).[36] The majority of these abortions occurred during the first trimester.[33,36,37] Li et al,[38] observed a reduction in the miscarriage rate from 60% before myomectomy to 24% after myomectomy. The same results have been reported by Buttram and Reiter (from 41% to 19%) quite a long time back.[39]

Women with submucous myomas experience significantly lower implantation rate, clinical pregnancy rate, and ongoing pregnancy/live birth rate compared with infertile women without such myomas.[60] There were significantly higher spontaneous abortion rates in women with submucous

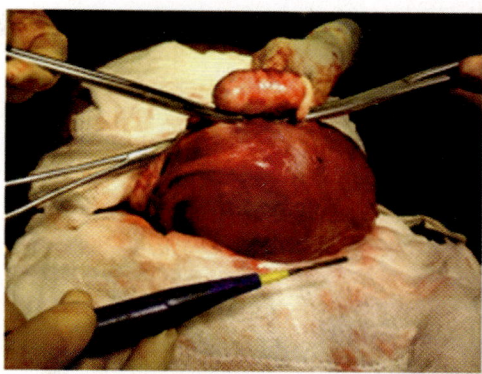 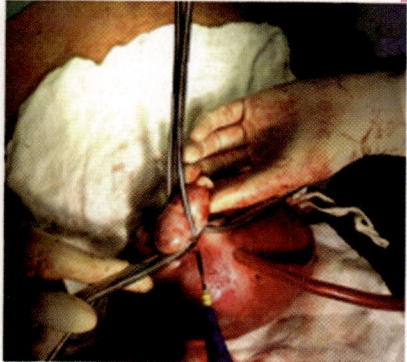

Fig. 24.5: Subserous fibroid removal at caesarean delivery

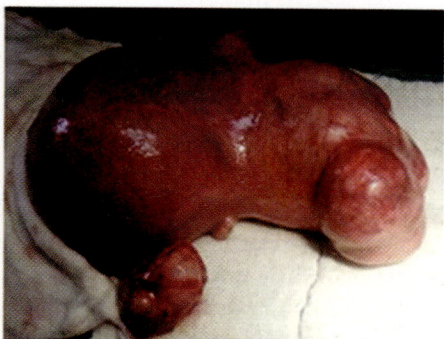

Fig. 24.6: Second trimester pregnancy with fibroid uterus

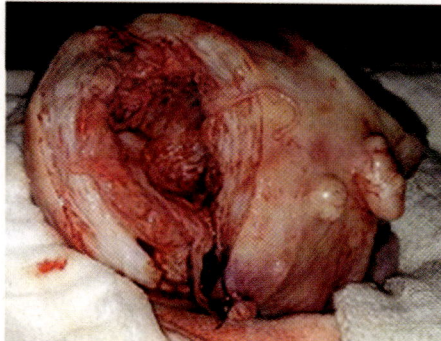

Fig. 24.7: Picture of myomectomy in a multiple fibroids

myomas, a difference that seemed to vanish after resectoscopic myomectomy. The author concluded that submucous myomas lower fertility rates and their removal enhances the rates of conception and live births.[60] Fertility rates improve better after transcervical resectoscopic myomectomy for type 0 and type 1 myomas, but no significant difference was noted between the groups for type II myomas.[61]

■ DELIVERY AFTER LAPAROSCOPIC MYOMECTOMY

Despite the heterogeneity of methodologies in the published studies, it has been suggested that, compared with abdominal myomectomy, laparoscopic myomectomy (LM) is associated with increased rates of caesarean delivery and uterine rupture. However, a recent meta-analysis has shown that the rate of successful vaginal delivery was as high as 93% after laparoscopic myomectomy and was 88% after abdominal myomectomy among women who attempted vaginal birth.[40] Two RCTs that compared laparoscopic and laparotomic myomectomy, reported caesarean rates of 65% and 72% after laparoscopic myomectomy, and 78% and 64% after laparotomic approach, with no cases of uterine rupture.[34,41] The high caesarean delivery rate is mostly due to elective cases rather than due to intrapartum complications. Factors that prompt the surgeons

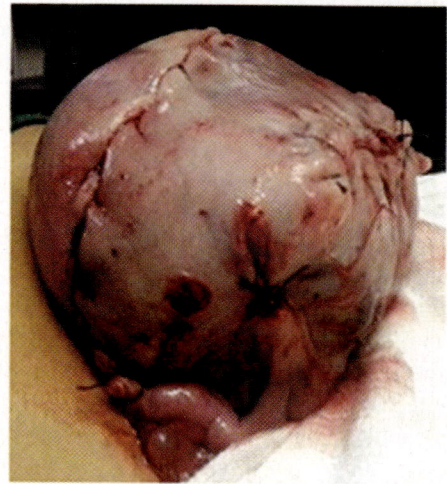

Fig. 24.8: Myomectomy incision closure gravid uterus

to perform caesarean section are presence of uterine scars, infertility length, patient age, malpresentations and the fact that pregnancy and delivery is strongly influenced by worries of the patient and defensive attitude of her gynaecologist, which is perhaps unnecessary. Probably, the few cases of uterine rupture reported in the literature in last few years may have led to an excessive use of caesarean section. In women with a history of previous caesarean section, the prevalence

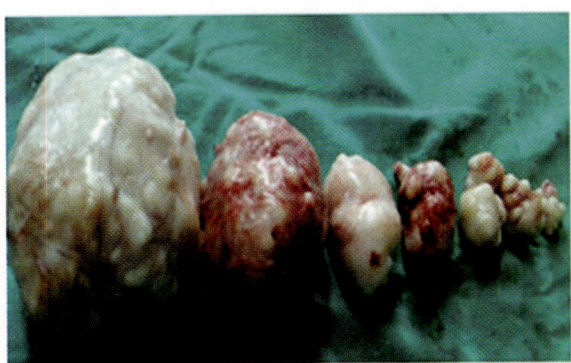

Fig. 24.9: Multiple fibroids removed from a in a gravid uterus

of uterine rupture is estimated to be approximately 1%.[42] Claeys et al,[40] in their meta-analysis reported that the risk of uterine rupture during labour and delivery was low (0.75%) among women who had prior myomectomy, but it was higher after laparoscopic myomectomy (1.2%) than after abdominal myomectomy (0.4%), although not significant statistically. In the event of pregnancy after LM, vaginal birth is possible in 42.9% to 80.6% of patients according to some reports.[43,44,30] Although it has been reported that uterine rupture occurred at a frequency of 5.3% (95% CI 0.5–14.8) during delivery after open myomectomy30, the picture is not clear for LM. In a retrospective series, vaginal birth after laparoscopic myomectomy (VBALM) was successful in 82.6% who attempted it (19/23 pregnancies) and the authors were of the opinion that vaginal delivery can be accomplished safely without uterine rupture after LM, provided that delivery is managed as in VBAC.[45]

■ UTERINE RUPTURE AFTER LAPAROSCOPIC MYOMECTOMY

One of the main concerns raised about laparoscopic myomectomy is the theoretical increased risk of uterine rupture in pregnancy. Although uterine rupture occurs very rarely, it may lead to extremely unfavourable outcomes including foetal and/or maternal death, thus making even a small risk unacceptable.

Uterine rupture during pregnancy or delivery as a consequence of abdominal myomectomy is very rare. Two studies comprising 2,36,454 deliveries reported 209 instances of uterine rupture, but only 4 were attributable to previous myomectomy.[46,47] However, the total number of women who had a previous myomectomy was not known, so the incidence of rupture could not be determined.

A realistic estimation of the rate of uterine rupture after laparoscopic myomectomy is difficult as most of the data comes from small case series and isolated case reports. Nevertheless, several studies have demonstrated a 0 to 1% risk of uterine rupture following laparoscopic myomectomy.[35,48,30]

The rate of uterine rupture after abdominal myomectomy has been estimated to be less than 1% in most, but not all studies.[30] Although these comparison data appears reassuring, the integrity of the myometrial scar and the risk of uterine rupture during pregnancy and labour following a laparoscopic myomectomy is still a topic of debate. Recently, a meta-analysis of 56 articles published from 1970 to 2013 regarding myomectomy reflected a trend towards an increasing occurrence of uterine rupture after laparoscopic myomectomy (1.2%) compared to abdominal myomectomy (0.4%).[40] However, a more recent large retrospective review of 523 women with completed pregnancy data after laparoscopic myomectomy reported a uterine rupture rate of 0.6% (3 of 523 deliveries), consistent with the previous studies.[49] Although uterine rupture does not appear to correlate with factors such as the number, size, location and type of the myoma, variations in surgical technique and surgeon's skill can be a conflicting factor. Because a randomized trial comparing the obstetrical outcomes following abdominal versus laparoscopic myomectomy is unlikely, this large retrospective data is quite informative with regard to the risk of rare events like uterine rupture and it also helps to establish laparoscopic myomectomy as a safe approach with uterine rupture risk comparable to that of caesarean section or abdominal myomectomy. So the presence of a uterine scar due to a laparoscopic myomectomy need not excessively increase the risk of uterine rupture during pregnancy.

As of now, no study has specifically examined the risk factors of uterine rupture after laparoscopic myomectomy. A large Italian multicenter study[48] on complications of laparoscopic myomectomy found that myoma size (> 5 cm), number (> 3), and location (intraligamentous) were significantly linked to an increased risk of major complications like haemorrhage, bowel injury, etc. but not with uterine rupture (1 rupture out of 386 patients conceived after laparoscopic myomectomy). Therefore, it is uncertain whether these risk factors can also predict uterine rupture in pregnancy. Some authors have indicated various potentially related factors, such as myoma types, endometrial cavity entry, intramural haematomas, indentations, postoperative infection and uterine fistulas based on their experience.[50] Some experts recommend caesarean section if > 50% of the myometrium has been disrupted, because the myometrium, and not the endometrium, is primary responsible for uterine integrity.[51]

The major challenge in laparoscopic myomectomy remains on the surgeon's ability to suture and reconstruct the uterus. There are reports of myometrial incision being left un-sutured after myomectomy,[52–54] whereas some authors used only a thin thread.[36,55] Consequently, conflicting results were published on the role of sutures and electrocoagulation in uterine rupture. Indeed, a proper suturing of the uterine incision is essential for adequate haemostasis and anatomical reconstruction.

Especially when myoma is deeply situated or when the uterine cavity has been opened, the suture must be performed deeply, at myometrium level, and on or between the myometrium and serosa.[36] There are several reports of uterine rupture in women with subserosal myomas being removed without suturing with coagulation being applied for dissection and/or haemostasis. All ruptures occurred between 29 and 35.5 weeks.[53,54,56] In a review article, the authors have recommended applying sutures even in pedunculated or subserosal myomas because of the risk of uterine rupture after laparoscopic myomectomies being performed using only electrosurgery[50] (Figs 24.10A and B).

Cases of uterine rupture have been reported after technical mistakes like sub-optimal myometrial suturing and excessive use of electrocoagulation.[57] However, a recent study with relatively long study period have shown that cases of uterine rupture occurred after the surgeons have performed > 100 cases of laparoscopic myomectomies.[49] So the occurrence of uterine rupture may not always be related to surgeon's experience and learning curve. The site of the incision and the direction (vertical/horizontal) does not seem to contribute to the potential for rupture. However, no precise data exists regarding this point.

There is a concern about the risk of beginning pregnancy too soon after laparoscopic myomectomy, such as 2 months[54] or 3 months,[55] but some authors did not express this risk in their findings.[53,56] However, spontaneous uterine rupture in pregnancy has been reported as late as 8 years after laparoscopic myomectomy.[53] Therefore, the absolutely safe time interval between laparoscopic myomectomy and pregnancy is still not clear. Rupture, though a very rare event can occur anytime during pregnancy.

The 22 articles published on uterine rupture after laparoscopic myomectomy describe a total of 37 events.[49] Most of the ruptures (90.6%) were reported when a single myoma was removed. In 52.8% cases of rupture, the removed myomas were either pedunculated or subserosal and in 47.2% cases, it was intramural. Majority of the fibroids were located on posterior wall (47.1%). Endometrial cavity entry was reported in only 20% of the events of uterine rupture. Majority of the cases of rupture (91.7%) occurred before the onset of labour, and the time of rupture ranged widely, from 17 to 40 weeks of gestation. Rupture during labour occurred in only 8.3% of cases. A meta-analysis[40] on risk of uterine rupture after laparoscopic myomectomy showed that rupture occurred before labour in all reported cases except one in which the mode of myomectomy was not known. These reports strongly point that labour is not an indispensable prerequisite for uterine rupture after laparoscopic myomectomy.

Several intraoperative strategies have been proposed to minimize the risk of uterine rupture after laparoscopic myomectomy. Although there are no comparative studies, it is prudent to choose a multi-layer closure over a single layer suturing. Theoretically, a multilayer closure can improve the strength of the wound and decrease the risk of postoperative haematoma formation, which can interfere with optimal tissue healing. Use of barbed suture is a novel approach and can facilitate a multilayer closure of the defect with ease. The application of electrosurgery should be minimized owing to the risk of tissue devascularisation. When possible, use of a cold scissor or an alternative energy source like the ultrasonic energy may be preferred (Figs 24.11A and B).

In a review of 19 cases of uterine rupture after laparoscopic myomectomy, only three cases involved multilayered closure of myometrial incisions, and electrosurgery was used for haemostasis in all but two cases.[58] Similar concerns were raised about lack of a proper multilayer closure and the widespread use of bipolar electrocoagulation for haemostasis in a recent case report of seven uterine ruptures after laparoscopic myomectomy.[59] Surgeons should adhere to the principles of limited use of electrosurgery and multilayered suturing for repair of the myometrial defect in cases of intramural and subserosal myomas with deep intrusion. Entry into the endometrial cavity should be avoided and any inadvertent entry should be recognized and repaired. Nevertheless,

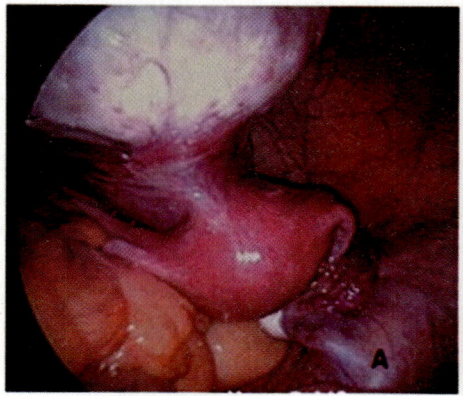 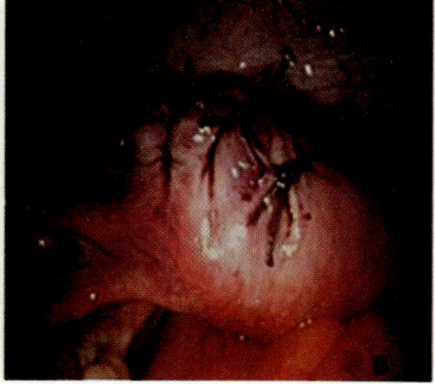

Figs 24.10A and B: Large subserous fibroid with broad base. Suturing must be done after removal of such fibroids even if the defect is superficial.

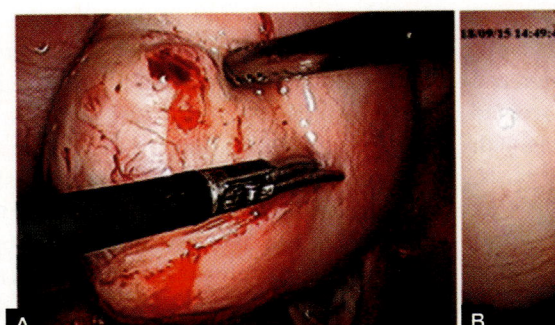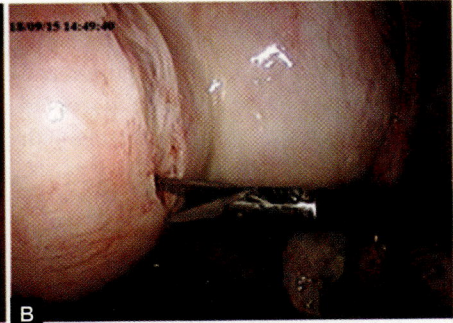

Figs 24.11A and B: Myometrial incision with cold scissors without using any energy source

individual wound healing characteristics may predispose a particular patient to uterine rupture.

Isolated reports of uterine rupture in subsequent pregnancies continue to raise doubts about the safety of laparoscopic myomectomy. Although uterine rupture is probably not completely preventable, following long-established and standard surgical principles may reduce the risk to a great extent. Careful counselling and monitoring is indicated well before the onset of labour as most reported cases of rupture occurred before 36 weeks' gestation. Data from several recent studies have shown that laparoscopic myomectomy is a safe surgical option in women who desire pregnancy.[49] Uterine rupture is extremely rare and concern over rupture based on preoperative findings of myomas must not deter expert surgeons from performing laparoscopic myomectomy. As new technologies evolve constantly for better haemostasis and tissue approximation, more favourable outcome can be expected in future.

■ CONCLUSION

1. The prevalence of uterine fibroids in pregnancy varies between 1.6% and 10.7%.
2. Approximately 10% to 30% of women with uterine fibroids develop complications during pregnancy.
3. Miscarriage, preterm labour, preterm premature rupture of membranes, placental abruption, placenta previa and fetal growth restriction are the common problems encountered in women with fibroids in pregnancy.
4. Malpresentation, labour dystocia, need for caesarean delivery, postpartum haemorrhage and retained placenta are the intrapartum and postpartum complications encountered in these women.
5. Fibroid size reasonably remains stable across gestation in 50% to 60% of cases, increases in around 20% and decreases in the remaining.
6. It is almost always a conservative line of approach as far as the management of fibroid in pregnancy is concerned. Only in the rarest of circumstances, a surgical management may have to be considered in these women.

7. Most of the fibroids do not hinder with the descent of the presenting part or cervical dilatation and hence is not a contraindication for a trial of labour.
8. Numerous case reports and case series from around the world support the use of caesarean myomectomies with hardly any untoward outcome. Use of haemostatic agents like vasopressin in dilution and effective use of uterine artery ligation seem to have greatly helped to reduce the amount of blood loss and thereby reduce the related morbidity.
9. Pain is the most common complication of fibroids in pregnancy, and is seen most often in women with large fibroids (> 5 cm) during the second and third trimesters of pregnancy. It is usually managed conservatively by bedrest, hydration, and analgesics.
10. The pregnancy rates after laparoscopic myomectomy have been reported to be between 33.3% and 65.7%. Pregnancy rates appear to be almost comparable between the laparotomy and the laparoscopy group. Individual patient's infertility characteristics are probably the most important factors.
11. The high caesarean delivery rate after laparoscopic myomectomy is mostly due to elective indications rather than due to intrapartum complications. The presence of uterine scars, infertility length, patient age, malpresentations, patient's worry and defensive attitude of her gynaecologist often influence the decision for caesarean delivery. Probably, the few cases of uterine rupture reported in the literature in last few years may have led to an excessive use of caesarean section.
12. One of the main concerns raised about laparoscopic myomectomy is the theoretical increased risk of uterine rupture in pregnancy. However, a realistic estimation of this risk is difficult as most of the data is derived from case reports and small case series. Nevertheless, several studies have demonstrated a 0% to 1% risk of uterine rupture following laparoscopic myomectomy.
13. Recent studies have reported higher rates of successful vaginal delivery after laparoscopic myomectomy and abdominal myomectomy among women who attempted

vaginal birth. Vaginal delivery can be accomplished safely without uterine rupture after laparoscopic myomectomy, provided that delivery is managed as in VBAC.

14. Uterine rupture does not appear to correlate with factors such as the number, size, location and type of the myoma.

15. Suboptimal myometrial suturing and excessive use of electrocoagulation may result in a poor scar and predispose to rupture during pregnancy and labour.

16. The absolutely safe time interval between laparoscopic myomectomy and pregnancy is still not clear. Rupture, though rare, can occur anytime during pregnancy.

17. Endometrial cavity entry was reported in only 20% of the events of uterine rupture.

18. Most of the cases of rupture occur before the onset of labour and the time of rupture range widely, from 17 to 40 weeks of gestation. Rupture during labour is reported in only 8.3% of cases. These reports strongly point that labour is not an indispensable prerequisite for uterine rupture after laparoscopic myomectomy.

19. Limited use of electrosurgery and multilayered suturing of the myometrial defect is likely to result in optimal wound healing. Use of a cold scissor or an alternative energy source like the ultrasonic energy may be preferred. Entry into the endometrial cavity should be avoided and any inadvertent entry should be recognized and repaired. Nevertheless, individual wound healing characteristics may predispose a particular patient to uterine rupture.

20. Laparoscopic myomectomy is a safe surgical option in women who desire pregnancy. Uterine rupture, though not completely predictable and preventable, is extremely rare.

■ REFERENCES

1. Qidwai GI, Caughey AB, Jacoby AF. Obstetric outcomes in women with sonographically identified uterine leiomyomata. Obstet Gynecol. 2006;107:376.

2. Stout MJ, Odibo AO, Graseck AS, et al. Leiomyomas at routine second-trimester ultrasound examination and adverse obstetric outcomes. Obstet Gynecol. 2010;116:1056.

3. Strobelt N, Ghidini A, Cavallone M, et al. Natural history of uterine leiomyomas in pregnancy. J Ultrasound Med 1994;13:399.

4. Exacoustòs C, Rosati P. Ultrasound diagnosis of uterine myomas and complications in pregnancy. Obstet Gynecol. 1993;82:97.

5. Laughlin SK, Baird DD, Savitz DA, et al. Prevalence of uterine leiomyomas in the first trimester of pregnancy: an ultrasound-screening study. Obstet Gynecol. 2009;113:630.

6. Terry KL, De Vivo I, Hankinson SE, et al. Reproductive characteristics and risk of uterine leiomyomata. Fertil Steril. 2010;94:2703.

7. Muram D, Gillieson M, Walters JH. Myomas of the uterus in pregnancy: ultrasonographic follow-up. Am J Obstet Gynecol. 1980;138:16-9.

8. Katz VL, Dotters DJ, Droegemueller W. Complications of uterine leiomyomas in pregnancy. Obstet Gynecol. 1989;73:593-6. [PubMed]

9. Benson CB, Chow JS, Chang-Lee W, et al. Outcome of pregnancies in women with uterine leiomyomas identified by sonography in the first trimester. J Clin Ultrasound. 2001;29:261-4.

10. Wallach EE, Vu KK. Myomata uteri and infertility. Obstet Gynecol Clin North Am. 1995;22:791-9.

11. Lev-Toaff AS, Coleman BG, Arger PH, et al. Leiomyomas in pregnancy: sonographic study. Radiology. 1987;164:375-80.

12. Winer-Muram HT, Muram D, Gillieson MS. Uterine myomas in pregnancy. J Can Assoc Radiol. 1984;35:168-70.

13. Klatsky PC, Tran ND, Caughey AB, et al. Fibroids and reproductive outcomes: a systematic literature review from conception to delivery. Am J Obstet Gynecol. 2008;198:357-66.

14. Exacoustòs C, Rosati P. Ultrasound diagnosis of uterine myomas and complications in pregnancy. Obstet Gynecol. 1993;82:97-101.

15. Burton CA, Grimes DA, March CM. Surgical management of leiomyomata during pregnancy. Obstet Gynecol. 1989;74:707–709.

16. Vergani P, Locatelli A, Ghidini A, et al. Large uterine leiomyomata and risk of cesarean delivery. Obstet Gynecol. 2007;109:410-4.

17. Coronado GD, Marshall LM, Schwartz SM. Complications in pregnancy, labor, and delivery with uterine leiomyomas: a population-based study. Obstet Gynecol. 2000;95:764-9.

18. Romero R, Chervenak FA, DeVore G, et al. Fetal head deformation and congenital torticollis associated with a uterine tumor. Am J Obstet Gynecol. 1981;141:839-40.

19. Szamatowicz J, Laudanski T, Bulkszas B, Akerlund M. Fibromyomas and uterine contractions. Acta Obstet Gynecol Scand. 1997;76:973-6.

20. Neiger R, Sonek JD, Croom CS, Ventolini G. Pregnancy-related changes in the size of uterine leiomyomas. J Reprod Med 2006; 51:671.

21. Rosati P, Exacoustòs C, Mancuso S. Longitudinal evaluation of uterine myoma growth during pregnancy. A sonographic study. J Ultrasound Med. 1992;11:511.

22. Laughlin SK, Hartmann KE, Baird DD. Postpartum factors and natural fibroid regression. Am J Obstet Gynecol. 2011;204:496.

23. De Carolis S, Fatigante G, Ferrazzani S, et al. Uterine myomectomy in pregnant women. Fetal Diagn Ther. 2001;16:116-9.

24. Wittich AC, Salminen ER, Yancey MK, Markenson GR. Myomectomy during early pregnancy. Mil Med. 2000;165:162-4.

25. Mollica G, Pittini L, Minganti E, et al. Elective uterine myomectomy in pregnant women. Clin Exp Obstet Gynecol. 1996;23:168-72.

26. Ehigiegba AE, Ande AB, Ojobo SI. Myomectomy during cesarean section. Int J Gynaecol Obstet. 2001;75:21-5.

27. Hasan F, Arumugam K, Sivanesaratnam V. Uterine leiomyomata in pregnancy. Int J Gynaecol Obstet. 1991;34:45-8.

28. Norton ME, Merril J, Cooper BA, et al. Neonatal complications after administration of indomethacin for preterm labor. N Engl J Med. 1993;329:1602-7

29. Seki H, Takizawa Y, Sodemoto T. Epidural analgesia for painful myomas refractory to medical therapy during pregnancy. Int J Gynaecol Obstet. 2003;83:303-4.

30. Dubisson JB, Fauconnier A, Deffarges JV, et al. Pregnancy outcome and deliveries following laparoscopic myomectomies. Hum Reprod. 2000;15:869-73.

31. Dubuisson JB, Chapron C, Chavat X, et al. Fertility after laparoscopic myomectomy of large intramural myomas: preliminary results. HumReprod. 1996;11:518-22.

32. Malzoni M, Rotond M, Perone C, et al. Fertility after laparoscopic myomectomy of large uterine myomas: operative technique and preliminary results. Eur J Gynaecol Oncol. 2003;24:79-82.

33. Gary N Frishman, Marcus W Jurema. Myomas and myomectomy. J Minim Invasive Gynecol. 2005;12:443-56.

34. Seracchioli R, Rossi S, Govoni F, et al. Fertility and obstetric outcome after laparoscopic myomectomy of large myomata: a randomized comparison with abdominal myomectomy. Human Reprod. 2000;15:2663-8.

35. Seracchioli R, Manuzzi L, Vianello F, et al. Obstetric and delivery outcome of pregnancies achieved after laparoscopic myomectomy. Fertil Steril. 2006;86:159-65.

36. Dubuisson JB, Fauconnier A, Chapron C, et al. Reproductive outcome after laparoscopic myomectomy in infertile women. J Reprod Med. 2000;45:23-30.

37. Vercellini P, Maddalena S, De Giorgi O. Determinants of reproductive outcome after abdominal myomectomy for infertility. Fertil Steril. 1999;72:109-14.

38. Li TC, Mortimer R, Cooke ID. Myomectomy: a retrospective study to examine reproductive performance before and after surgery. Hum Reprod. 1999;14:1735-40.

39. Buttram VC, JrReiter RC. Uterine leiomyomata: etiology, symptomatology, and management. Fertil Steril. 1981;36:433-45.

40. Claeys J, Hellendoorn I, Hamerlynck T, et al. The risk of uterine rupture after myomectomy: a systemic review of the literature and meta-analysis. Gynecol Surg, 2014; 11: 197-206.

41. Palomba S, Zupi E, Falbo A, et al. A multicenter randomized controlled study comparing laparoscopic versus minilaparotomic myomectomy:reproductive outcomes. Fertil Steril. 2007;88:933-41.

42. Hoffmeyer G, Say L, Gulmezoglu A, et al. WHO systematic review of maternal mortality and morbidity; the prevalence of uterine rupture. BJOG. 2005;112:1221-8.

43. Riberio SC, Reich H, Rosenberg J, et al. Laparoscopic myomectomy and pregnancy outcome in infertile patients. Fertil Steril. 1999;71:571-4.

44. Darai E, Dechaud H, Benifla JL, et al. Fertility after laparoscopic myomectomy: preliminary results. Hum Reprod. 1997;12:1931-4.

45. Kumakiri J, Takeuchi H, Kitade M, et al. Pregnancy and delivery after laparoscopic myomectomy. J Minim Invasive Gynecol. 2005;12:241-6.

46. Palerme GR, Friedman EA. Rupture of the gravid uterus in the third trimester. Am J Obstet Gynecol. 1966;94:571-6.

47. Garnet JD. Rupture of the uterus in pregnancy. Postgrad Med. 1964;36:28-33.

48. Sizzi O, Rossetti A, Malzoni M, et al. Italian multicenter study on complications of laparoscopic myomectomy. J Minim Invasive Gynecol. 2007;14:453-62.

49. Koo YJ, Lee JK, Lee YK, et al. Pregnancy outcome and risk factors for uterine rupture after laparoscopic myomectomy: a single-center experience and literature review. J Minim Invasive Gynecol. 2015;22:1022-8.

50. Desai P, Patel P. Fibroids, infertility and laparoscopic myomectomy. J Gynecol Endosc Surg. 2011;2:36-42.

51. Alessandri F, Lijoi D, Mistrangelo E, et al. Randomized study of laparoscopic versus minilaparoscopic myomectomy for uterine myomas. J Mimim Invasive Gynecol. 2006;13:92-97.

52. Pelosi MA III, Pelosi MA. Spontaneous uterine rupture at thirty three weeks after previous superficial laparoscopic myomectomy. Am J Obstet. 1997;177:1547-9.

53. Özgür Ö, Gökaslan H, Durmusoglu F. Spontaneous uterine rupture in pregnancy 8 years after laparoscopic myomectomy. J Am Assoc Gynecol Laparosc. 2001;8:618-20.

54. Lieng M, Olav I, Langebrekke A. Uterine rupture after laparoscopic myomectomy. J Am Assoc Gynecol Laparosc 2004;11:92-3.

55. Harris WJ. Uterine dehiscence following laparoscopic myomectomy. Obstet Gynecol. 1992;80:545-6.

56. Hasbargen U, Summerer-Moustaki M, Hillemanns P, et al. Uterine dehiscence in a nullipara, diagnosed by MRI, following use of unipolar electrocautery during laparoscopic myomectomy: case report. Human Reprod. 2002;17:2180-2.

57. Dubuisson JB, Chapron C, Chavet X. Uterine rupture during pregnancy after laparoscopic myomectomy. Hum Reprod. 1995;10:1475-7.

58. Parker W, Einarsson J, Istre O, et al. Risk Factors for Uterine Rupture after Laparoscopic Myomectomy. J Minim Invasive Gynecol. 2010;17:551-4.

59. Pistofidis G, Makrakis E, Balinakos P, et al. Report of 7 Uterine Rupture Cases After Laparoscopic Myomectomy: Update of the Literature. J Minim Invasive Gynecol. 2012;19:762-7.

60. Pritts EA, Parker WH, Olive DL. Fibroids and infertility: an updated systematic review of the evidence. Fertil Steril. 2009;91:1215-23.

61. Shokeir T, El-Shafei M, Yousef H, et al. Submucous myomas and their implications in the pregnancy rates of patients with otherwise unexplained primary infertility undergoing hysteroscopic myomectomy: a randomized matched control study. Fertil Steril. 2010;94:724-9.

CHAPTER 25

Fibroid and Infertility

● Nirmala Sadasivam, Haritha Desai

■ INTRODUCTION

Leiomyoma (fibroid) is a benign smooth muscle tumour arising from myometrium or mesenchymal cells of coelomic origin. Fibroid is an important health care concern because it is one of the most common indication for the performance of hysterectomy and of late is an important cause for infertility due to delayed child bearing by the women of modern era. Fibroid is common in reproductive age group (20%–40%) rarely seen before puberty and after menopause. Fibroids grow dramatically during pregnancy. Serum E2 level is the same both in women with and without fibroids but there is increased number of oestrogen receptors in a leiomyoma than in a normal myometrium. Fibroids greatly vary in size and shape. Largest fibroid on record is 63.6 Kg.

■ AETIOLOGY

Fibroids are monoclonal in origin and 40% have chromosomal abnormalities that include translocation between 12% and 14%, deletion of chromosome 7 and trisomy of 12. African-Americans have highest incidence with peak around 35 years (60%). Factors that increase overall oestrogen exposure like obesity and early menarche increase the incidence . Anti oestrogen measures like smoking and increased parity reduce the incidence. First degree relatives of women with fibroid have 2.5 times increased risk. Growth factors play an important role—transforming growth factor (TGF), bFGF (fibroblast growth factor), EGF (epidermal growth factor), platelet-derived growth factor, vascular endothelial growth factor—increase mitogenesis, angiogenesis and stimulate the synthesis of extracellular matrix.

■ CLINICAL IMPACT OF FIBROID

- Menorrhagia
- Dysmenorrhoea
- Infertility
- Recurrent pregnancy loss
- Pressure symptoms
- Mass effect
- Asymptomatic (50%)
- Fibroid > 5 cm—degeneration
- Poor obstetric outcome.

■ RISKS OF OBSTETRIC OUTCOME WITH FIBROID

- Preterm labour: 1%–4 %
- Malpresentation: 1.5%–4 %
- Placenta previa: 1.8%–3.9 %
- Abruption placenta: 0.5%–16.5 %
- Lower segment caesarean section (LSCS): 1.1%–6.7 %
- Postpartum haemorrhage (PPH): 1.6%–4 %
- Retained placenta: 2%–2.7 %

■ CONDITIONS ASSOCIATED WITH FIBROID

- Follicular cysts of ovary
- Endometrial hyperplasia
- Endometrial carcinoma
- Adenomyosis
- Endometriosis
- Salpingo-oophoritis.

ROLE OF FIBROID IN INFERTILITY

Fibroid causing infertility is 5% to 10% directly/indirectly, but fibroid being the sole cause of infertility is only around 3%. Fibroid is commonly seen in women who delay childbearing. Reasons for subfertility in women with fibroid are as follows:

- Greater distance for sperms to travel
- Encroachment of tubal ostium
- Uterine cavity distortion
- Endometrial vascular changes
- Interferes with normal rhythmic uterine contractions
- Impaired implantation
- Abnormal endometrial maturation because of altered vascularity
- Alteration of oxytocinase activity (coutino maia hypothesis). Action of prostaglandin derived from seminal plasma, which induce rhythmic uterine contractions facilitating transuterine sperm transport is hampered by the presence of large uterine fibroids. Large posterior wall fibroids may alter the normal relationship between cervical os and vaginal pool of semen by elevating cervix into anterior position behind symphysis pubis.

ROLE OF FIBROID IN RECURRENT PREGNANCY LOSS

- Atrophy of endometrial glands and stroma due to pressure effect
- Altered vascularity of endometrium
- Venous distension of endometrium adjacent to fibroid results in disordered placentation.

MECHANISM OF INFERTILITY IN SUBMUCOUS AND INTRAMURAL LEIOMYOMA

1. Number of caveolae in host myometrium is conceivably decreased compared to normal myometrium—this specific structural abnormality affects calcium metabolism increasing intracellular calcium thereby causing myometrial irritability and hyperactivity. This causes disruption of rhythmical contractions of junctional zone.
2. Submucous fibroids result in endometrial erosion, which causes inflammation and alters the nature of intrauterine fluid making the environment hostile.
3. Because of hostile intrauterine environment nidation and sustenance of early embryo is affected.
4. Intramural myoma possibly by disrupting junctional zone affects embryonic invasion and placentation.

Effect of Large Intramural Myoma > 5 cm

- Implantation rate: Decreased from 20% to 11%
- Pregnancy rate: Decreased from 34% to 23%.

Large intramural myoma > 5 cm negatively affects IVF results, reduces success rate by 40%, therefore should be removed before IVF. (Hart R et al and Khalaj Y et al).

Effect of Small Intramural Myoma < 5 cm

- Check et al, found no difference in implantation and pregnancy rate but they found a lower delivery rate and increased miscarriage rate
- Live birth rate dropped from 24% to 15%.

Further Classification of Intramural Myoma

1. Outer myometrial fibroid.
2. Junctional zone fibroid.

Need for myomectomy should be individualised because of risk of adhesion formation (50% for laparoscopy and 90% for laparotomy).

Junctional zone of myometrium is ontogenetically, structurally and hormonally different from outer myometrium. MRI can successfully distinguish junctional zone myometrium from outer zone myometrium determining the precise location of intramural myoma. MRI also identifies associated conditions like endometrial polyps, adenomyosis and endometriosis.

Subgroup analysis failed to indicate any effect of fibroids on fertility that did not have a submucous component conversely women with submucous myoma demonstrated lower pregnancy rate and lower implantation rate. Current data suggests that only fibroids with a submucous or an intracavitary component are associated with reduced reproductive outcome and that of hysteroscopic myomectomy may be of benefit. Subserosal fibroid is not found to have significant negative effect on fertility. Fibroids in general are associated with 30% reduced live birth rate and 67% increased miscarriage rate. Submucous fibroid—64% reduced pregnancy rate, 67% increased miscarriage rate.

Intramural Fibroid (22% Reduced Live Birth Rate)

Cause

Effect relationship was identified between submucous fibroid and infertility fibroid has a malignant transformation risk of 1 in 1,000.

Investigations

- Ultrasonography (USG)
- Magnetic resonance imaging (MRI)
- Saline infusion sonohysterography (SIS)
- Hysterosalpingogram (HSG)
- Diagnostic hysterolaparoscopy.

There is insufficient evidence to prove the role of myomectomy for intramural myoma.

Role of myomectomy is approved for infertile women with submucous and cavity distorting intramural myoma. Following myomectomy 40%–60% become pregnant.

Casini et al, has proved that patients who underwent myomectomy for submucous fibroid had higher clinical pregnancy rate compared to patients who did not undergo surgery.

CRITERIA FOR TREATMENT OF ASYMPTOMATIC FIBROID

- Uterine size > 12 weeks
- Rapidly growing
- Fibroids with pressure effects (hydroureter/hydronephrosis)
- Subserous pedunculated fibroid.

Recent studies have shown that there is no role of treating a fibroid based on size alone. All that a fibroid of >12 weeks size needs is only frequent monitoring .It needs to be operated only if is symptomatic.

Treatment for a Fibroid Depends Upon

- Age
- Parity
- Pregnancy status
- Desire for future pregnancy
- General health
- Symptoms
- Size
- Location.

ACOG Criteria for Myomectomy in Infertile Patients

- Patients in the reproductive age group and desirous of fertility
- Unexplained infertility with distortion of uterine cavity when no more likely explanations exist for failure to conceive
- Unexplained recurrent abortions
- Fibroid located in the lower part of uterus and likely to complicate delivery.

PREOPERATIVE REQUISITES BEFORE MYOMECTOMY

- Other causes for infertility should be evaluated
- Husband semen analysis should be normal unless planned for donor procedures
- HSG/Hysteroscopy to detect cavity encroaching fibroids/polyps/tubal block

- Map all fibroids by USG/MRI
- Surgery is planned in preovulatory phase
- Counsel the patient about the risk of recurrence and need for resurgery
- Remote chance of hysterectomy in uncontrollable bleeding should also be explained.

SURGICAL MANAGEMENT

Pritts et al proved that the removal of submucous myoma increases conception rate. Submous myoma extending to uterine serosa is not appropriate for hysteroscopic surgery (type 2-5/2-6). Abdominal morcellation increases the risk of parasitic fibroids.

Vaginal myomectomy can be done for submucous pedunculated fibroid, which prolapses through cervix. Preoperative assessment of submucous fibroid is essential to decide the type of approach. For women with infertility adequately classify fibroids particularly those impinging on the cavity by TVS/MRI/SIS/diagnostic hysteroscopy. Mode of approach is always determined not only by fibroid size and location, but also by surgeon's skill.

For a submucous myoma, preoperative assessment of thickness of residual myometrium to serosa should be done (combination of hysteroscopy + TVS). Submucous fibroid < 5 cm—hysteroscopy is ideally done. Submucous fibroid > 5 cm—needs repeat procedures. HSG is not useful to classify fibroids.

In women with unexplained infertility there is a role in removing intramural myoma, but not a subserosal myoma to enhance conception rate. If there is a hysteroscopically confirmed intact endometrium there is no role of removal of intramural myoma. If fibroids are removed abdominally efforts are made to use an anterior wall uterine incision to minimize post operative adhesions.

Pretreatment with GNRHa is given if fibroid > 16 weeks size. GNRHa reduces cell size but not cell number, so it tends to regrow following discontinuation of therapy.

Majority of blood vessels tend to be compressed to the sides of fibroid, thereby avoidance of blunt dissection reduces amount of bleeding associated with extirpation of leiomyoma. For these reasons a leiomyoma is grasped with tenaculum and raised. Using either a contact ND:YAG laser/electrocautery needle/scalpel a shallow incision is made across adventitial layer allowing vessels to retract under tension or with gentle pressure without cutting across vessels. Once leiomyoma is removed large vessels in resulting cavity are ligated individually, cavity is closed in layers using absorbable suture material making sure not to leave a potential space for subsequent fluid/blood collection. Myometrium is sutured using 1-0 vicryl and serosa using 3-0 vicryl. Serosa is closed using baseball stitch technique to invert the edges and to expose

Table 25.1: Leiomyoma classification system

Leiomyoma Subclassification system	Submucosal (SM)	0	Pedunculated intracavitary
		1	< 50% intramural
		2	> 50% intramural
	Other (O)	3	Contacts endometrium; 100% intramural
		4	Intramural
		5	Subserosal > 50% intramural
		6	Subserosal < 50% intramural
		7	Subserosal pedunculated
		8	Other (specify, e.g. cervical, parasitic)
	Hybrid leiomyomas (impact both endometrium and serosa)	Two numbers are listed separated by a hypen. By convention, the first refers to the relationship with the endometrium, while the second refers to the relationship to the serosa. One example is given below.	
		2–5	Submucosal and subserosal, each with less than half the diameter in the endometrial and peritoneal cavities, respectively.

minimal suture material. Some prefer to use INTERCEED (antiadhesion barrier), but it has no proven value.

LAPAROSCOPIC MYOMECTOMY

Serosa overlying myoma is injected with a dilute solution of pitressin and then incised with a electrocautery needle/laser/scissors. Excessive use of electrocautery results in necrosis, which causes poor healing and subsequently uterine dehiscence. Small fibroids are removed from peritoneal cavity via lap port. Larger myomas require a posterior colpotomy/morcellation for extirpation.

Laparoscopic myolysis coagulates blood supply to myoma resulting in shrinkage using electrocautery/laser/cryotherapy. This procedure carries a high risk of postoperative adhesions and poor uterine wall integrity. Cryomyolysis using liquid N2 probes remains under investigation. There are 2 RCT comparing open vs laparoscopic myomectomy and they found no evidence for a significant effect on live birth rate/clinical pregnancy rate / recurrence risk. Laparoscopic myomectomy is found to have less postoperative pain and shorter hospital stay.

Role of Abdominal Myomectomy in Infertile Women

Now a days most of the fibroids can be removed laproscopically, It depends on the skills of the surgeon, When laproscpic route is contraindicated or the surgeon is not skilled one can opt for open myomectomy. Subumblical midline vertical incision is used for large fibroids and Pfannensteil incision is used for fibroid < 10 cm.

Risk of postoperative adhesion formation is 90% with posterior wall incision and 55% with anterior wall incision. These adhesions adversely affect fertility outcome. Uterine incision should be such that it affords removal of maximum number of fibroids through single incision. Comparing the laparotomy and laparoscopic approach both have similar cumulative pregnancy rate at the end of 12 months. Febrile morbidity and postoperative drop in haemoglobin is found to be low with laparoscopic approach. The advantage of laparotomy is gentle tissue handling, appropriate selection of incision site and atraumatic repair with perfect haemostasis.

Interventions to Reduce Haemorrhage During Myomectomy

- GnRH agonist to reduce vascularity and shrink the size of myoma
- Timing the surgery in postmenstrual phase
- Use of vasopressin 20 units in 100 mL NS
- Mechanical methods: Tourniquet/Myomectomy clamp (these should be released every 15 minutes to prevent potential hypoxic injury and release of toxic substances into circulation that can lead to circulatory collapse).

Scar of myomectomy can be assessed on 30th postoperative day to asses healing process, a high resistance index suggest an abnormal healing and an increased area of fibrosis.

HYSTEROSCOPIC MYOMECTOMY

Bipolar electrodes can be passed through instrument channel of standard hysteroscopic sheaths 5 mm or greater. Small submucous fibroids can be dissected with such sources.

Bipolar resectoscope use normal saline as distension media (conducting media). Monopolar resectoscope uses 1.5% glycine (non-conductive distension media).

Myomectomy Techniques

- Morcellation
- Cutting (electrogical loop/radiofrequency)
- Vaporisation.

Radiofrequency based hysteromyomectomy has minimal thermal damage. Loop should not touch the myometrium. Loop electrosurgical resection is performed with electrode activated with low voltage current to allow repetitive creation of strips of myoma with periodic interruption to allow removal of tissue fragments. Chips can be left behind until they obstruct visualisation of uterine cavity for later removal with grasper or suction. Bulk electrosurgical vaporisation is performed with a large surface area electrode with low voltage current to vaporize relatively large volume of tissue. Such vaporisation results in no tissue fragments. Compared to loop resection, vaporisation with these electrodes result in less systemic absorption of distension media. Single pilot RCT is available to show mechanical device was more efficient than radiofrequency resectoscope.

Removal of T0/T1—straightforward hysteroscopic procedure deep T1/T2 (that extends to serosa)—there is a role to perform concomitant laparoscopy to reduce perforation. Alternatively, USG can be used when performing dissection of leiomyoma close to uterine serosa. Fluid contrast in endometrial cavity may allow the surgeon to determine the amount of myometrium between electrode and the uterine serosa.

Complications

- Perforation of uterus
- Bowel injury
- Cervix laceration
- Fluid overload (pulmonary, cerebral edema, heart failure).

Goals Of Fluid Management

- Prevention of excess absorption
- Early recognition of excess absorption
- Choosing the distension media least likely to cause complications in the event of excess absorption.

Intracervical injection of vasopressin and PGF2alpha have shown to reduce fluid absorption. 1000 mL—maximum allowable amount of absorption.

Recent studies have proven that there is no role for posthysteroscopic myomectomy placement of Foley's catheter/LNG IUCD for prevention of adhesions.

Hysteroscopic Morcellation

Aims to remove leiomyoma during single insertion of hysteroscope into uterus and tends to reduce the risk of traumatic injury to uterus and risk of inadvertent fluid overload associated with traditional procedures. Procedure is done under spinal/general anaesthesia. Saline is used as distension media. Specially designed morcellator is introduced via hysteroscope and used to cut and simultaneously aspirate myoma tissue. It has less intraoperative time compared to the traditional hysteroscopic resection.

Casini et al, proved in his study that patients with submucous fibroid who underwent myomectomy had higher clinical pregnancy rate compared to those who did not undergo surgery.

Effects of Myomectomy on ART Outcome

Intramural fibroid > 5 cm—myomectomy before invitro fertilisation (IVF) shows a positive impact on pregnancy outcome (surgical 33% vs non surgical 15%). This study suggests that myomectomy before ART is likely to improve pregnancy outcome in infertile patients with submucous and intramural fibroid > 5 cm. Subserous fibroid myomectomy before ART do not affect pregnancy outcome. GnRh agonist pretreatment increases the risk of recurrence with negligible effect on blood loss and operating time.

Alternatives to Myomectomy

- MRIgFUS
- Uterine artery embolisation
- Myolysis
- Radiofrequency ablation.

MRI-guided Focussed Ultrasound Therapy

Food Drug Administration (FDA) approved in 2004. Outcomes are enhanced by GnRh agonist pretreatment. Rabinovici et al, reported 51 pregnancies in 54 women following MRIgFUS with a mean time to conception of 8 months after the procedure with 41% live birth rate. Of women who conceived 64% delivered vaginally. 6.7% risk of preterm births and 9% risk of placenta previa. Women who conceive after MRIgFUS should be carefully followed during pregnancy. Furthermore RCTs are needed to confirm the role of MRIgFUS in infertile women. As per the available data uterine artery embolisation is not recommended for women desiring to become pregnant because of the following reasons (Fig. 25.1):

- Transient and permanent amenorrhea
- Post embolisation syndrome—(due to release of inflammatory mediators from fibroid) low grade fever, pelvic pain, nausea, vomiting
- Abnormal placentation
- Reduced ovarian function
- Preterm births
- Caesarean section
- Malpresentations

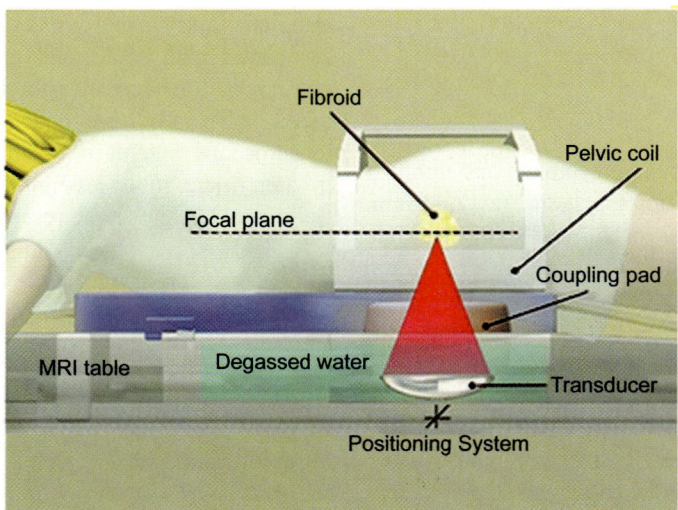

Fig. 25.1: MRIgFUS—magnetic resonance imaging-guided focussed ultrasound therapy

- Miscarriage
- Intrauterine growth restriction (IUGR)
- Intrauterine synechiae
- Fistula between uterine cavity and intramural fibroid UAE results in an abnormal endometrium with tissue necrosis. High rate of intrauterine pathologies explain increased risk of pregnancy loss.

Reproductive Impact of MRIgFUS for Fibroid

Minimally invasive treatment for fibroids, which improves quality of life. It is now proposed as a treatment of choice for women desiring fertility. It uses MRI to direct ultrasonic energy to a focal point within a fibroid resulting in tissue necrosis with minimal damage to surrounding tissues. It is afforded through quantitative temperature mapping allowing for detection of small temperature elevation in surrounding tissue prior to irreversible damage.

The MRIgFUS is integrated in a table docked with a compatible MRI scanner. Patient lies prone on a gel pad coupled to a water tank that propagates USG beam. Prior to procedure, T2 weighed image identifies target fibroid and asses as proximity to critical structures including bowel, spine and neurovascular bundle. After treatment completion, repeat contrast MRI is used to determine the area of non-perfusion volume, which is represented as percentage ablation of targeted fibroid.

It is Not Suitable for Women

- Weighing more than 100 Kg
- Uterine size > 24 weeks
- Pedunculated/Heavily calcified fibroid.

About 58% of women experienced vaginal expulsion of necrotic tissue after MRIgFUS that resolved within 2–3 months.

T2 weighed image prior to treatment classifies fibroid as hyperintense/hypointense. Hyperintense correlates with vascularisation and responsive to GnRH agonists potentially improving MRIgFUS success rate. Hypointense fibroids carry better success rate compared to hyperintense fibroid.

■ LAPAROSCOPIC MYOMECTOMY AND FERTILITY OUTCOMES

Association of infertility and fibroids is not evident in all cases. So questions arise whether myomectomy should be done or not? Few studies say that myomectomy can lead to postoperative adhesions and increased rate of uterine rupture. Further studies say only submucus and large fibroids should be removed. But recent studies have shown that there is a lower fertility rate in woman presenting with a myoma.[1,2] Association between myoma and infertility is seen in observational studies.[3] Rate of implantation for pregnancy obtained by IVF is lower in women with intramural myomas.[1]

If we decide to operate then which method be done— laparoscopy or laparotomy? More chances of recurrence, more conversion rate to laparotomy, prolonged surgery, more bleeding are the complications attributed to laparoscopy. So this study was undertaken to find answers to these dilemmas related to myomectomy.

It is a retrospective observational study at advanced laparoscopic division of Altius Hospital, we had 605 operated cases from January 2011 to February 2015. The study was done in two groups. 208 (34.3%) patients were treated solely for infertility and 397 (65.6%) were operated for AUB and dysmenorrhoea. We present the study of infertility group here, 124 patients in that group had follow-up.

All patients underwent preoperative workup. Hysteroscopy was done in all cases. Uterine artery ligation was done in five cases with multiple fibroids, posterior approach was preferred, bilateral arteries ligated with vicryl No. 1. Patients were counselled to avoid pregnancy for 3 months and later reassessed for natural, induction, IUI or IVF conception.

Fibroids typically occur in women of reproductive age as they are hormone dependant tumours as seen in our study. Conception rate decreased after 35 years, majority conceived with IVF. Fibroids mostly cause infertility, interference with pregnancy is less common, only 14% had previous abortions. 50% patients with fibroid size 4 to 6 cm conceived. Large 15 cm fibroid was also removed by laparoscopy. Only 1 patient with endometriosis conceived, two patients with septal resection and no patients with tubal disease conceived. 54% patients that conceived had single fibroid. Need for blood transfusion is rare, except with multiple fibroids.

About 43 patients with primary infertility conceived. In our study, postmyomectomy pregnancy rate is 45.96%. In a study by Bulleti et al, pregnancy rate in operated cases of fibroid was 42% and in unoperated cases 11%.[3] Conception rates are good after myomectomy if no associated infertility factors are present.

The cumulative pregnancy rate was 27% at the end of 6 months, 50% at 12 months and 15% at 36 months. Maximum patients conceived naturally or with induction. All were delivered by LSCS because of increased age and years of infertility. Due to fear of uterine rupture in these cases LSCS is often preferred. In a study by Tulandi et al of 26 patients undergoing myomectomy most patients conceived between 12 and 36 months after operation, the cumulative pregnancy rate was 33.4% at 6 months and 66.7% at 12 months after the procedures (Table 25.2 and 25.3).[4]

Table 25.2: Distribution of data (Altius Hospital data)

Type of infertility	Primary 77.8%	Secondary 22.2%	
Age	24–38 years 85%	> 39 years 6.7%	
Gravida	Nulligravida 77.8%	Abortions 14%	Primipara 1.7%
Size of fibroids	4–6 cm 40%	7-9 cm 13%	10–18 cm 7.9%
Number of fibroids	Single 41%	> 2 21%	
Procedure	Laparoscopy 64.6%	Hysteroscopy 2%	
Intraoperative findings	Endometriosis 4%	Tubal block 1.4%	Uterine septum 1.4%

Table 25.3: Pregnancy outcomes after myomectomy (Altius Hospital data). Total conceived 57 patients (45.96%) out of 124 follow-ups.

Treatment modality received	No. of patients	Percentage %
Ovulation induction with timed intercourse	48	84.2%
IUI	2	3.4%
Invitro fertilisation (IVF)	7	12.2%
Not tried	35	28.22%
Failed IVF	6	4.83%
Ongoing treatment	29	23.38%

No patient had preterm birth or abortion, no neonatal intensive care unit (NICU) admissions. Other studies found abortion rate of 8% to 10% post myomectomy. In a study by Buttram and Reiter reveals that 30% of patients had spontaneous abortion rate before myomectomy and 19% after myomectomy5. In our study conversion rate was 0.96% mainly for multiple fibroids. In other studies conversion rates have increased with large fibroids.[2] In a study by Sizzi of 2050 laparoscopic myomectomies and study of complications, conversion rate is 1.51% (Table 25.4).[12]

Table 25.4: Complications of myomectomy (Altius Hospital data)

Complications	No of patients
Intraoperative haemorrhage	1
DVT	1
Wound sepsis	1
Conversion to laparotomy conservatively managed	2 (0.96%)
Recurrence	7 (6.4%), only 1 was symptomatic, no reoperation done
Blood transfusion	3

In our study, there were no cases of rupture. In one study by Roopnarinesingh S on obstetric outcomes after open myomectomy rupture rate was 5.3%.[6] Dubuisson et al, (2000) study of 100 patients following laparoscopic myomectomy had three cases of uterine rupture, though only one involving the myomectomy scar.[7] In a study by PG Paul of 115 pregnancies after laparoscopic myomectomies there were no cases of rupture.[8]

In our study ,1 patient with uterine artery ligation conceived. Holub et al, assessed pregnancy outcomes and deliveries after laparoscopic uterine artery transection in symptomatic women with fibroids. 153 patients underwent laparoscopic transection of uterine vessels during a 4-year period. The study concluded that laparoscopic transection of uterine vessels is a minimally invasive operative procedure that preserves the uterus and ovarian blood supply and allows for the achievement of pregnancy in women with symptomatic fibroids.[9] In a study by Lenzi on pregnancy after uterine artery ligation successful pregnancies have been recorded.[10]

The 3 patients continued to have dysmenorrhoea, 4 had chronic pelvic pain treated conservatively, no patients had menorrhagia. The recurrence rate was 6.4% after 1 to 4 years of follow up which is significantly less than other studies. In a multicenter study[11], the recurrence rate of leiomyomas was estimated to be 11.7%, 36.1%, 52.9% and 84.4%, respectively, after 1, 3, 5, and 8 years following laparoscopic myomectomy. However, the probability of a reoperation is 6.7% after 5 years and 16% after eight years. When done with experienced surgeon chance of missing fibroids in laparoscopy is negligible.

As ours is a laparoscopy and infertility referral centre, the population number is large but as it is a retrospective study, preoperative and postoperative data collected is less. Male factor, hormonal levels, ovulatory dysfunction are not available. As patients were lost to follow-up, precise outcomes cannot be obtained.

Laparoscopic myomectomy is a safe procedure with good reproductive outcome and very low conversion rate to laparotomy even with large fibroids, low recurrence. Multiple fibroids > 10 should be dealt with caution and decision individualised.

■ REFERENCES

1. Bernard G, Darai E, Poncelet C, et al. Fertility after hysteroscopic myomectomy: effect of intramural myomas associated. European Journal of Obstetrics, Gynecology, and Reproductive Biology. 2000;88:85-90.

2. Bulletti C, Ziegler D, Levi SP, et al. Myomas, pregnancy outcome, and in vitro fertilization. Annals of the New York Academy of Sciences. 2004;1034:84-92.

3. Bulletti C, Polli V, Negrini V, et al. Adhesion formation after laparoscopic myomectomy. J. Am. Assoc. Gynecol. Laparosc. 1996;3;533-6.

4. Buttram VC, Jr, Reiter RC. Uterine leiomyomata: Etiology, symptomatology, and management. Fertil Steril. 1981;36:433-45.

5. Campo S, Campo V, Gambadauro P. Reproductive outcome before and after laparoscopic or abdominal myomectomy for subserous intramural myomas. European Journal of Obstetrics, Gynecology, and Reproductive Biology. 2003;110:215-9.

6. Casini M L, Rossi F, Agostini R, et al. Effects of the position of fibroids on fertility. Gynecological Endocrinology. 2006;22(2):106-9.

7. Chang WC, Chou LY, Chang DY, et al. Simultaneous laparoscopic uterine artery ligation and laparoscopic myomectomy for symptomatic uterine myomas with and without in situ morcellation. Human Reproduction. 2011;26(7):1735-40.

8. Donnez J, Jadoul P. What are the implications of myomas on fertility? A need for a debate? Hum Reprod. 2002;17:1424-30.

9. Dubuisson JB, Fauconnier A, Chapron C, et al. Reproductive outcome after laparoscopic myomectomy in infertile women. J Reprod Med. 2000;45:23-30.

10. Dubuisson J B, Fauconnier A, Chapron C, et al. Reproductive outcome after laparoscopic myomectomy in infertile women. The Journal of Reproductive Medicine. 2000;45(1):23-30.

11. Fauconnier A, Dubuisson J, Ancel P, et al. Prognostic factors of reproductive outcome after myomectomy in infertile patients. Human Reproduction. 2000;15(8):175-7.

CHAPTER 26

Uterine Fibroids and Invitro Fertilisation Outcomes

● Shwetha Pramodh

The correlation between uterine fibroids and fertility in women has been of substantial concern in obstetric outcome. The underlying mechanisms and relationship between fibroids and infertility is still unclear, with possible reasons suggested as interference with sperm or ovum migration, endometrial vascular disturbance, inflammation, production of vasoactive substances. etc.[1] Focal vascular lesions in the endometrium covering submucosal fibroids and local production of inflammatory and vasoactive cytokines altering the endometrial environment have been hypothesized to impair women's fertility.[2] Fibroids occur in both normally fertile and infertile women. However, a history of infertility prior to pregnancy is observed in 43% of pregnant women with fibroids.[3]

Uterine fibroids vary in size, location, composition and number, thereby have dissimilar effect on fertility. While it is clear from studies that subserosal fibroids have no effect on pregnancy outcomes and submucosal fibroids whether or not impinging uterine cavity space significantly decreases the outcomes, the intramural fibroids have variable effect based on size, number and location. It is now apparent that intramural myomas may indeed have an unfavourable effect on conception and outcome of pregnancy. However this is not largely supported by hysteroscopic findings indicating the compromise of intrauterine space.[4]

In a single-centre retrospective study by Antonella, 51 women with fibroids who underwent 97 treatment cycles, 63 women with previous myomectomy who underwent 127 cycles, and 106 infertile women without fibroids who underwent 215 cycles were included. The results indicated that implantation rates were comparable in the three groups, whereas a higher ongoing pregnancy rate was observed in women with previous myomectomy compared to women with fibroids. Further comparison between the type of fibroid (subserosal, submucosal and intramural) revealed no difference in implantation, miscarriage and pregnancy rates. The submucous or intramural fibroid with cavity distortion, intramural and subserous fibroids were compared to assess the number of cycles required to achieve an ongoing pregnancy. There was no observed difference between the types of fibroids and number as well. Only size of the fibroid was observed to have a direct impact on the fertility of women in the group. The result from this study only supported a pre-IVF myomectomy in women with uterine fibroids larger than 4 cm.[5] In another study by Surrey ES et al, neither ongoing pregnancy nor implantation rates were significantly different among either oocyte donor recipients of invitro fertilisation-embryo transfer (IVF-ET) in comparison with controls[6] as shown in Figures 26.1 and 26.2.

In another retrospective study by Flávio et al, 245 women with subserosal and intramural fibroid not compromising intrauterine space were compared with 245 women with no evidence of fibroids for IVF-ICSI outcomes. Implantation rates were similar in the normal infertile women and women with fibroids. Women with subserosal fibroids and intramural fibroids < 4 cm mean diameter had IVF-ICSI outcomes (pregnancy, implantation and abortion rates) similar to normal infertile women. Women with fibroids > 4 cm had a lower implantation and pregnancy rate compared to women with fibroids < 4 cm.[7]

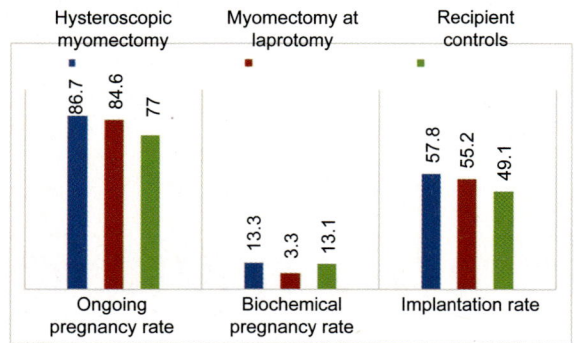

Fig. 26.1: Cycle outcomes of patients undergoing oocyte donation[6]

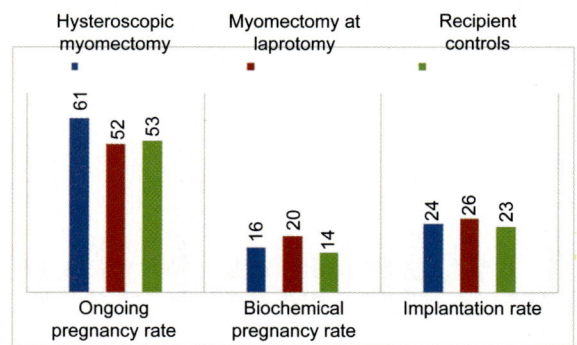

Fig. 26.2: Cycle outcomes of patients undergoing in vitro fertilisation-embryo transfer[6]

Another retrospective study by Talia EG et al, compared 88 women with uterine fibroids who underwent 106 antiretroviral therapy (ART) cycles with 249 age-matched women without fibroids undergoing 318 ART cycles. In the fibroid group 33 presented with subserosal fibroids (categorized as SS fibroids), 46 with either intramural or mixed intramural and subserosal fibroids (categorized as IM fibroids), and 9 with submucosal or mixed submucosal and other fibroids, all with cavity distortion (categorized as SM fibroids). The implantation and pregnancy rates were lower in women with IM (without deformation of the uterine cavity) and SM fibroids compared to SS fibroids and age-matched women without fibroids8.

Farhi et al, analysed data retrospectively comparing results of IVF cycles in 18 women (55 cycles) with uterine cavity distortion due to fibroids to those of 28 women (86 cycles) with fibroids not resulting in cavity distortion, and a control group of 50 age-matched women (127 cycles) with infertility. It was observed that the pregnancy and implantation rates were significantly lower in the fibroid group with cavity distortion than in the controls and in the group with fibroids and a normal uterine cavity.[9]

Ramzy AM et al, conducted a retrospective analysis in 39 women with fibroids ≤ 7 cm not encroaching uterine cavity and 367 women without fibroids undergoing IVF treatment. The results from this study did not indicate a significant difference in implantation and pregnancy rates following IVF-ICSI.[10] In a prospective matched study by Check JH, 61 women with intramural fibroids ≤ 5 cm undergoing first IVF cycle were compared with women not presenting any fibroids undergoing first IVF cycle. Positive pregnancy tests and clinical pregnancy were reported by 52.4% and 47.5% women without fibroids and 42.6% and 34.4% of women with intramural fibroids. There were no significant difference between the two groups for pregnancy rates or implantation rates.[11]

A prospective study by Hart R and Khalaf Y evaluated the effect of small intramural fibroids on outcome of assisted conception. The study enrolled 322 women without fibroids and 112 women with fibroids not encroaching uterine space who underwent 606 IVF cycles. The study results indicate a significant reduction in cumulative pregnancy, ongoing pregnancy and live birth rate in women with intramural fibroids irrespective of the size.[12,13]

A systematic review was performed by Pritts et al in 2009 to investigate the effects of subserosal, intramural and submucosal fibroids on fertility outcomes. The results from this study indicated a significantly lower clinical pregnancy (relative risk = 0.849, P = 0.029), implantation (relative risk = 0.821, P = 0.002), And ongoing pregnancy/live birth rate (relative risk = 0.679, P < 0.001) in women with fibroids (irrespective of the location) compared to women without fibroids. When further evaluated for type of fibroid, women with submucosal fibroids, demonstrated a significantly lower pregnancy (relative risk = 0.363, P = 0.005), Implantation rate (relative risk = 0.283, P = 0.003), And ongoing pregnancy/live birth rate (relative risk = 0.318, P < 0.001) compared with women without fibroids. Even in women with fibroids not encroaching uterine cavity, implantation rate (relative risk = 0.792, P < 0.001) And ongoing pregnancy/live birth rate (relative risk = 0.780, P < 0.001) was reduced significantly compared with nonfibroid control women (Table 26.1). Myomectomy does not significantly increase the clinical pregnancy and live birth rates, but the data are scarce (Table 26.2). Subserosal fibroids did not demonstrate any difference in comparison with women without fibroids. Results from the study demonstrated undesirable effect of fibroids encroaching uterine cavity. The study also indicated that intrmural fibroids whether or not encroaching uterine cavity has a deleterious effect on fertility with poorer reproductive outcomes.[4]

In 2009, another systematic review analysed 19 observational studies including 6087 cycles to evaluate the association between non-cavity-distorting intramural fibroids and IVF outcome. Of the 19 studies 14 were retrospective and 5 were prospective studies. The systematic review reported live births as primary outcome followed by clinical pregnancy, implantation rate and miscarriage rate as secondary outcomes.

Table 26.1: Effect of various fibroids on fertility[4]

Outcome	All location		Submucosal		No cavitary involvement		Intramural	
	Relative risk	Significance	Relative risk	Significance	Relative risk	Significance	Relative risk	Significance
Clinical pregnancy rate	0.849	P = 0.029	0.363	P = 0.005	0.897	Not significant	0.81	P = 0.006
Implantation rate	0.821	P = 0.002	0.283	P = 0.003	0.792	P < 0.001	0.684	P < 0.001
Ongoing pregnancy/live birth rate	0.697	P < 0.001	0.318	P < 0.001	0.78	P < 0.001	0.703	P < 0.001
Spontaneous abortion rate	1.678	P < 0.001	1.678	P = 0.022	1.891	P < 0.001	1.747	P = 0.002
Preterm delivery rate	1.357	Not significant	Not available	Not available	2.767	Not significant	6	Not significant

Table 26.2: Effect of myomectomy on fibroids[4]

Outcome	Controls: Fibroids in situ (no myomectomy)		Controls: Infertile women with no fibroids		Intramural fibroids (fibroids in situ controls)	
	Relative risk	Significance	Relative risk	Significance	Relative risk	Significance
Clinical pregnancy rate	2.034	P=0.028	1.545	Not significant	3.765	Not significant
Implantation rate	Not available	Not available	1.116	Not significant	Not available	Not available
Ongoing pregnancy/live birth rate	2.654	Not significant	1.128	Not significant	1.671	Not significant
Spontaneous abortion rate	0.771	Not significant	1.241	Not significant	0.758	Not significant
Preterm delivery rate	Not available	Not available	Not available	Not available	Not available	Not available

Live birth rate was reduced by 21% in women with non-cavity-distorting intramural fibroids compared to women without fibroids (relative risk = 0.79, P = 0.0001). When results from two prospective studies that reported live birth as an outcome were pooled for analysis a 40% reduction in live birth rate in women with intramural fibroids was observed (relative risk = 0.60, P = 0.007). Pooling results from various studies demonstrated that the clinical pregnancy rate was reduced by 15% (relative risk = 0.85, P = 0.002), Implantation was reduced by 13% (relative risk = 0.87, P = 0.11) And miscarriage rate was reduced by 24% (relative risk = 1.24, P = 0.07) in women with non-cavity-distorting intramural fibroids compared to women without fibroids. When only prospective studies were pooled, clinical pregnancy rate was reduced by 11% (relative risk = 0.89, P = 0.41) And miscarriage rate was increased by

10% (relative risk = 1.10, P = 0.80) in women with intramural fibroids following IVF treatment compared to women without fibroids (Table 26.3). The results clearly demonstrated a significant decrease in the live birth and clinical pregnancy rates in women with non-cavity-encroaching intramural fibroids compared with those without fibroids, following IVF treatment.[14]

For women with small intramural/subserous fibroids a more conservative technique is suggested, as there are several complications associated with laparoscopic myomectomy prior to IVF cycles. Outcome of IVF cycles are affected by secondary infection, damage to internal organs, adhesions and uterine scars (Pritts, 2001). Thus, ART treatment could be considered as an option in patients with small intramural/subserosal fibroids, but not in patients with intramural or

Table 26.3: Effect of intramural fibroids without uterine cavity involvement on the outcome of IVF treatment[14]

Outcome	All studies			Prospective studies		
	No. of studies	Relative risk	Significance	No. of studies	Relative risk	Significance
Live birth rate	11	0.79	P < 0.0001	2	0.6	P = 0.007
Clinical pregnancy rate	18	0.85	P = 0.002	4	0.89	P = 0.41
Implantation rate	19	0.87	P = 0.11	Not available	Not available	Not available
Miscarriage rate	19	1.24	P = 0.07	3	1.1	P = 0.80

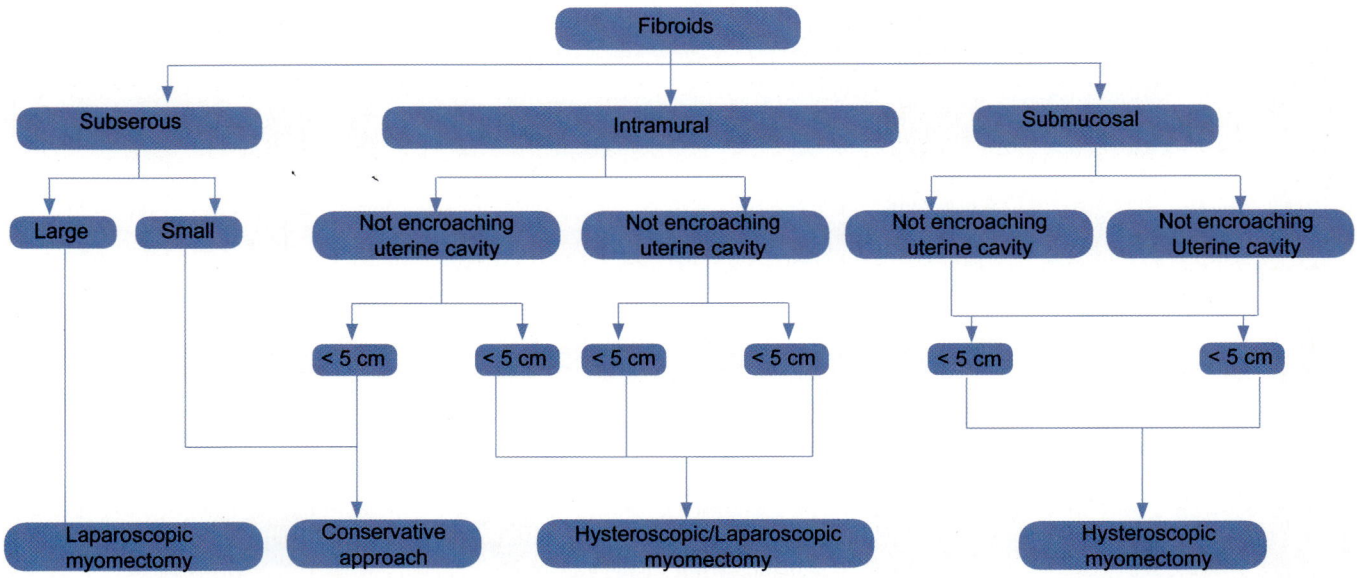

Fig. 26.3: Fibroids management algorithm in IVF treatment

submucosal fibroids. In intramural fibroids not encroaching uterine space > 5 cm in size and all intramural fibroids encroaching uterine space myomectomy is recommended prior to IVF treatment to improve outcomes. Pregnancy outcomes in women with submucosal fibroids following resection increase demonstrating an overall benefit following IVF (Table 26.4 and Fig. 26.3).

Table 26.4: Effect of fibroids on fertility and IVF outcome[14]

Type of fibroid	Size	Uterine cavity distortion	Effect on fertility and IVF outcome
Subserosal	Small	NA	No
	Large	NA	No
Intramural		Yes	Likely
		No	Unlikely
	< 5 cm	Yes	Yes
		No	Yes
Submucosal	Any	Yes	Yes
		No	Yes

◼ INDICATIONS FOR SURROGACY IN FIBROIDS

1. Multiple fibroid that are difficult to remove.
2. Recurrent implantation failure after myomectomy.
3. Intrauterine adhesions post hysteroscopic submucosal resection of fibroids.
4. Women more than 50 years of age with fibroids who desire for pregnancy.

5. In the event of emergency hysterectomy during fibroid removal.

REFERENCES

1. Donnez J, Jadoul P. What are the implications of myomas on fertility? A need for a debate? Hum Reprod. 2002;17(6):1424-30.
2. Deligdish L, Loewenthal. Endometrial changes associated with myomata of the uterus; J Clin Pathol. 1970;23(8):676-80.
3. Vollenhoven BJ, Lawrence AS, Healy DL. Uterine fibroids: a clinical review. Br J Obstet Gynaecol. 1990;97:285-98.
4. Pritts EA, Parker WH, Olive DL. Fibroids and infertility: an updated systematic review of the evidence. Fertil Steril. 2009;91(4):1215-23.
5. Vimercati A, et al. Do uterine fibroids affect IVF outcomes? Reprod Biomed Online. 2007;15(6):686-91.
6. Surrey ES1, Minjarez DA, Stevens JM, Schoolcraft WB. Effect of myomectomy on the outcome of assisted reproductive technologies. Fertil Steril. 2005;83(5):1473-9.
7. Flavio GO, et al. Impact of subserosal and intramural uterine fibroids that do not distort the endometrial cavity on the outcome of in vitro fertilization–intracytoplasmic sperm injection. Fertil Steril. 2004;81(3):582-7
8. Eldar-Geva T, Meagher S, Healy DL, et al. Effect of intramural, subserosal, and submucosal uterine fibroids on the outcome of assisted reproductive technology treatment. Fertil Steril. 1998;70(4):687-91.
9. Farhi J, Ashkenazi J, Feldberg D, et al. Effect of uterine leiomyomata on the results of in-vitro fertilization treatment. Hum Reprod. 1995;10:2576.
10. A M Ramzy, M Sattar, Y Amin, et al. Uterine myomata and outcome of assisted reproduction; Hum. Reprod. 1998;13(1):198-202.

11. Check JH, Choe JK, Lee G, et al. The effect on IVF outcome of small intramural fibroids not compressing the uterine cavity as determined by a prospective matched control study. Hum Reprod. 2002;17(5):1244-8.

12. Hart R1, Khalaf Y, Yeong CT, et al. A prospective controlled study of the effect of intramural uterine fibroids on the outcome of assisted conception. Hum Reprod. 2001;16(11):2411-7.

13. Khalaf Y1, Ross C, El-Toukhy T, et al. The effect of small intramural uterine fibroids on the cumulative outcome of assisted conception. Hum Reprod. 2006;21(10):2640-4.

14. Sunkara SK, Khairy M, El-Toukhy T, et al. The effect of intramural fibroids without uterine cavity involvement on the outcome of IVF treatment: a systematic review and meta-analysis. Hum Reprod. 2010;25(2):418-29.

SECTION 5

Controversies and Recent Advances

CHAPTER 27

Controversies with Myoma Morcellation—an Update

● Dipanwita Banerjee, Bhaskar Pai

BACKGROUND

After the introduction of endoscopic surgery way back in 1980s, the first laparoscopic hysterectomy was performed by Harry Reich in Pennsylvania in 1988. Minimally invasive surgery (MIS) has been validated as a better approach than open techniques in day to day gynecological practices. As part of the rapid technological advances in the field of MIS, the first electrical morcellator was introduced in 1993. Morcellation refers to the division of large tissues into smaller pieces or fragments and is often used during laparoscopic surgeries. Previously morcellation was commonly performed using devices, which had to be squeezed; there was also the practice of inserting a scalpel inside the abdomen to make the specimen small. With a few modifications, today's power morcellator has a fast rotating cylindrical knife, which divides the tissue into smaller pieces or fragments that are amenable to retrieval through less than 2 cm surgical incision on the abdomen.

Despite the decades of usage of this device the understanding of the short- and long-term sequel of this instrument remains under scrutiny. The case reports of relatively benign conditions like intravenous leiomyomatosis, benign metastasizing leiomyoma and even highly malignant leiomyosarcoma following morcellation has raised the controversy on its safety in day-to-day surgical practices.[1] The objective of the present review is to look at the present status of this method and its future perspectives.

INCIDENCE OF MYOMA

In reproductive age group women, uterine fibroid is a common concern causing bleeding problems and pain, which can have a negative impact on quality of life. Worldwide prevalence of uterine fibroid ranges from 4% to 10%. The prevalence is almost 15% in age group 40 years and older.[2] Zimmermann et al reported that the mean age of diagnosis of uterine fibroid is between 33.5 and 36.1 years.[3] The changing paradigm of today's women with regards to delayed child birth and subfertility has made the use of MIS in the management of myoma more popular. Laparoscopic surgery is also advantageous due to less blood loss, shorter hospital stay and quicker return to daily activities when compared to open surgical procedures.[4] According to estimates by United States (US) Food and Drug Administration (FDA), annually approximately 60,000 hysterectomy and myomectomy procedures are done using laparoscopic morcellator extraction procedures. The procedure becomes cumbersome when the size of the uterus is big and thus restricts successful vaginal removal of large specimens. The power morcellators have been used to do rapid division of large myomas into fragments, which can be retrieved by small port site incisions. Because of high prevalence of symptomatic myoma (40%–60%) in reproductive age group who are not prepared for hysterectomy the procedure is adequately utilised in myoma surgery.[2]

TYPES OF MORCELLATORS

In gynaecology three types of morcellation procedures are used. Vaginal cold knife morcellation can be performed during laparoscopic or vaginal hysterectomy for large uterus; hysteroscopic morcellation of intracavity fibroids can be performed, but the controversy is over laparoscopic power morcellation (LPM) of specimens at myomectomy or hysterectomy[5,6] In the laparoscopic technique, most of the surgeons use power morcellators, shredding the enlarged tissue and retrieve it in piecemeal.

■ COMPLICATIONS OF LAPAROSCOPIC MORCELLATION

The complications arising from this procedure maybe fatal. Immediate complications are almost due to its fast rotating blade, inability to see the tip of the morcellator or due to inexperience of the surgeon. Delayed complications are either due to intra-abdominal spread of an undetected malignancy or due to some rare conditions.

Immediate complication (Direct Injury)

Despite the well-established benefits of power morcellation during laparoscopy, the intraoperative injuries are often fatal when the instrument is not used with caution. According to the manufacturer and user facility device experience (MAUDE) database, injuries to intestine, major vessels, kidney, ureter, bladder and even diaphragm have been reported using power morcellators.[7] Though the injuries are rare, it is recommended to have control over the instrument and never lose the morcellators tip out of sight, while performing the procedure in adequately distended abdomen.

Upstaging or Worsening of Leiomyosarcoma

It is difficult to determine the exact risk of undetected uterine malignancy in a patient undergoing a planned myomectomy. There are a few case reports of adverse surgical outcomes in the form of seeding of sarcomatous tissue at a distant site.[9,10] Uterine leiomyosarcomas (LMS) is a rare, but highly aggressive uterine malignancy. There is a wide variation in the incidence of LMS in the literature ranging between 1 in 360 and 1 in 7400 procedures making it difficult to estimate the exact prevalence of undetected LMS in a planned laparoscopic myomectomy.[11] Due to deep involvement of myometrium, in 20% to 30% cases of LMS, preoperative curettage misses the disease and only a full histopathological specimen is required to reach the concluding diagnosis.[12] 5 year overall survival after detection of high grade LMS ranges from 17% to 55%, which increases up to 83% if an 'en bloc' removal of locally confined LMS has been done.[13] Intact removal of specimen is not possible, if power morcellator is used and there is a risk of upstaging of LMS due to microscopic dissemination of tissues during morcellation.

Parasitic Fibroid

The increasing number of case reports of parasitic fibroids after the use of laparoscopic morcellation has contributed to the development of an iatrogenic theory. It has been reported that seeding of residual tissue fragments after morcellation can further lead to the development of parasitic fibroids in the peritoneal cavity.[14] The overall incidence of parasitic fibroids after laparoscopic surgery with the use of morcellation is reported to be between 0.12% and 0.9%.[15–18] Due to its rarity, it is hypothesised that prolonged exposure to steroid hormones (e.g. hormone replacement therapy) could be a risk factor for the development of parasitic fibroids. Incidence of parasitic fibroid is not associated with increased mortality, but the condition is frequently inoperable and therefore much more difficult to manage than the original disease.[19]

Missing the Diagnosis

Using the morcellator, removal of an intact specimen is not possible, which leads to confusion in interpreting the final histopathology examination. The amount of tissue retrieved are often distorted anatomically, making the pathologist's job difficult. Detailed interpretation of gross examination, margins, surface involvement, adjacency to surrounding structures is not possible due to distortion of the histopathological specimen.[20] This could lead to delayed diagnosis and difficulty in staging (e.g. endometrial carcinoma and leiomyosarcoma), causing unnecessary treatment delay. The nature of the specimen received by the pathology laboratory after morcellation of leiomyomas makes evaluation for malignancy, and in particular leiomyosarcoma, difficult.

The gross appearance is so altered that sampling of an area that if intact may have been deemed suspect may not occur.[21] In addition, often pathologists resample a specimen if they are concerned, and submit additional sections for analysis. In a morcellated specimen, there is no way to know whether you are resampling the same 'myoma'. Histologic features that define leiomyosarcoma include coagulative necrosis, haemorrhage, atypia, mitotic activity and lack of circumscription. It is difficult to assess these in small fragments, in particular lack of circumscription. Morcellation poses challenges for the pathologist who evaluates the specimen. In as much as the endometrial cavity often cannot be identified, Tam et al,[22] suggest that instilling dye into the uterine cavity before the procedure is helpful.

Endometriosis

Theories of endometriosis development include lymphatic or vascular dissemination, retrograde menstruation, and metaplasia of coelomic epithelium. Uterine morcellation may disseminate endometrial implants and result in endometriosis, in a manner similar in mechanism to the theory of implanted retrograde menstruation. Endometriosis has developed in morcellator incisions[23] and in the pelvis.[24] Sepilian and Della

Badia[24] noted that there was no endometriosis appreciated at the original surgery in their case, refuting worsening of preexisting endometriosis.

Long-term Complications of Morcellation

May include dissemination of both benign and malignant disease (leiomyoma, diffuse peritoneal leiomyomatosis, leiomyosarcoma, endometrial stromal sarcoma, endometriosis, endometrial carcinoma, adenomyosis and adenomyomatosis), leading to morbidity and rarely to death. Unexpected malignancy is a real, but rare complication associated with uterine morcellation performed to treat presumed benign disease. This rare but possible complication must be conveyed as part of the informed consent process in patients at low risk who are candidates for a morcellation procedure. Future directions might include creation of a registry of patients requiring repeat operation because of recurrent peritoneal nodules after morcellation, to better assess the risk of this complication.

■ CURRENT CONTROVERSY OVER POWER MORCELLATION

Recent media attention on a highly publicized case of disseminated leiomyosarcoma after laparoscopic hysterectomy utilising power morcellator was the reason behind scrutinizing this procedure. USFDA issued a warning on use of laparoscopic power morcellators in a statement on April 17, 2014 saying not to use LPM in suspected or known uterine malignancy. If laparoscopic power morcellation is performed in women with unsuspected uterine sarcoma, there is a risk that the procedure will spread the cancerous tissue within the abdomen and pelvis, significantly worsening the patient's likelihood of long-term survival. For this reason, and because there is no reliable method for predicting whether a woman with fibroids may have a uterine sarcoma, the FDA discourages the use of LPM during hysterectomy or myomectomy for uterine fibroids. FDA clearly states that usage of LPM should be individualised, after a careful benefit-risk evaluation. If laparoscopic power morcellation is considered as the best therapeutic option for an individual, the health care provider should

1. Inform patients that their fibroid(s) may contain unexpected cancerous tissue and that power morcellation may spread the cancer, significantly worsening their prognosis.
2. Be aware that some clinicians and medical institutions now advocate using a specimen 'bag' during morcellation in an attempt to contain the uterine tissue and minimize the risk of spread in the abdomen and pelvis.

Responding to the USFDA, American Association of Gynaecologic Laparoscopists (AAGL) issued a statement On July 11, 2014 stating that the risk of death from abdominal hysterectomy is slightly higher than from laparoscopic hysterectomy with power morcellation including LMS and potential dissemination.[25] Measuring the effectiveness and benefits of LPM, AAGL clearly mentioned that the procedure needs to be improved not abandoned and full benefit of the procedure can be obtained only by preoperative screening and selecting appropriate cases.

On November 24, 2014 USFDA issued a fresh warning against the use of LPMs in the majority of women undergoing myomectomy or hysterectomy for treatment of fibroids. Limiting the patients for whom laparoscopic morcellators are indicated, the strong warning on the risk of spreading unsuspected cancer and the recommendation that doctors share this information directly with their patients, are part of FDA guidance to manufacturers of morcellators.[26] The guidance strongly urges these manufacturers to include this new information in their product labels.

But following the April 2014 FDA safety communication, regarding power morcellation, the cases of minimally invasive myomectomy decreased with consequent increase in hospital stay and the potential complications of open surgery.[27]

In January 2016, a group of 49 physicians led by William H Parker wrote a commentary disagreeing with the USFDA view. While FDA estimated the risk of occult LMS as 1 in 458, this group reanalysed the data and estimated the risk as 1 in 1550.[28]

However, a recent cohort study of 34,728 women who underwent hysterectomies preformed for leiomyomas found the incidence of occult uterine sarcoma as 1 of 278, and the incidence of leiomyosarcoma as 1 of 429.[29]

The American College of Obstetricians and Gynaecologists (ACOG) issued a recent statement, which states "Without question, morcellation of an undiagnosed sarcoma can disseminate malignant tissue". However, by allowing some women to avoid the higher morbidity and mortality associated with open abdominal surgery, morcellation can also save lives. It further states "as a result of the continuing conversation about morcellation, obstetrician-gynecologists are better able to evaluate each individual woman's risk of an undiagnosed sarcoma, and to counsel her to receive the right approach for her own unique medical needs."[30]

■ WAY FORWARD

Considering the risks of conventional open surgery and the benefits of MIS for women, we cannot abandon a procedure which has more benefits than risks if utilised properly. Meticulous preoperative investigations, adequate counselling, safe surgical practices like in-bag morcellation and overall triaging the women who will actually get the benefit of MIS should be considered.

Preoperative Investigations

Appropriate preoperative screening is required to get the maximum benefit of the procedure without causing any harm to the patient. Apart from routine investigations, following tests are more specific in suspecting the adverse outcomes of laparoscopic myomectomy cases where surgeon should be cautious using laparoscopic morcellation procedure.

Imaging

Ultrasound/Magnetic Resonance Imaging

The characteristic imaging findings of LMS either in ultrasound (USG) or magnetic resonance imaging (MRI) is 31 a large > 8 cm, solitary, heterogeneous, oval-shaped, highly vascularised, irregular, myometrial tumour with central necrosis/degenerative cystic changes and absence of calcifications.[32,33] MR imaging is superior to computed tomography (CT) scan to delineate the extent and to evaluate the tissue characteristics of the lesion. Characteristic features of sarcomatous tissue on T2 weighted sequences of MRI may help evaluating tumour extension in the uterus and in differentiating between a leiomyoma and a LMS.[34]

Positron Emission Tomography (PET) Scan

The uptake of fludeoxyglucose (FDG) in a fibroid is associated with the oestrogen status, cellularity and the presence of malignancy. Studies shown accuracy of deoxyfluorothymidine (FLT) or alphafluorobeta-estradiol (FES) in distinguishing LMS from fibroids are superior to FDG (93% vs 81%), which is more commonly used during PET scan.[35]

Tumour Markers

Lactate Dehydrogenase (LDH)

Evidence suggests that the level of lactate dehydrogenase isoenzyme 3 is elevated in patients of LMS compared to benign tumours.[36] More cross sectional studies are required in evaluating LDH as a differentiating tumour marker between benign and malignant disease.

CA 125

In a series of 42 consecutive LMS, the values of preoperative serum CA125 were significantly higher in the uterine LMS group than those in the uterine leiomyoma group. However, there was significant overlapping of preoperative serum CA125 between the uterine leiomyoma group and early-stage uterine LMS, which limits the clinical use.[37]

Histopathology

Histopathology is the 'gold standard' for differentiating between benign and malignant tumours. The differentiating features are based on mitotic activity, cellular atypia and necrosis. High mitotic activity (> 10/high power field), loss of differentiation, altered nucleus cytoplasmic ratio is suggestive of malignant transformation of tissue.

As leiomyosarcomas arises within the smooth muscle, preoperative dilatation and curettage followed by biopsy is of limited value. The role of image-guided needle biopsies is not completely clear. No data are found on the possible spread of sarcoma cells by multiple puncturing of the sarcoma. Multiple trans abdominal biopsies and frozen section before proceeding with morcellation without any adverse outcome has also been reported in literature.[38]

■ CONTAINED MORCELLATION

Various studies suggests that the development of safer morcellation techniques in the abdominal cavity by technical innovation, including in-bag morcellation, has the potential to avoid many of the reported morcellation complications. The concept of in bag morcellation is innovative. Though various in-bag morcellation preocedures have been reported 39 there are risks such as spillage from the content of the bag in the abdomen especially if the bag leaks. In the near future we should see rapid improvement in the design and variety of bags. In the currently available bags, the laparoscope and the morcellator go into the bag and morcellation is performed inside the bag. The Morsafe bag is getting popular in India (Figs 27.1 to 27.3). The studies so far on usage of in bag morcellation are mainly done in 'in vitro' set up. We do require more prospective trials to evaluate the risk benefit ratio of the morcellation procedure (Figs 27.4A and B).

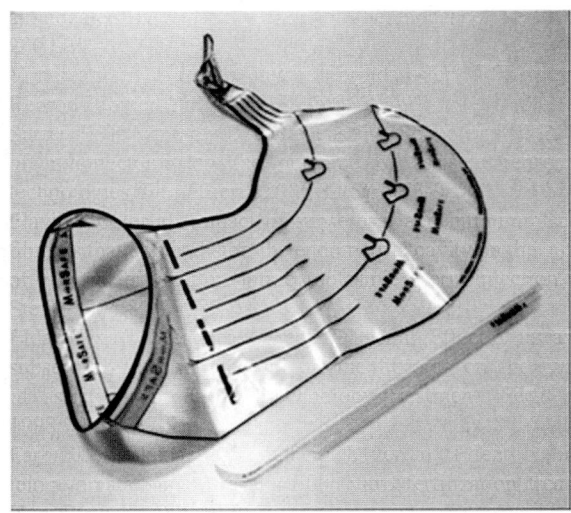

Fig. 27.1: The Morsafe bag

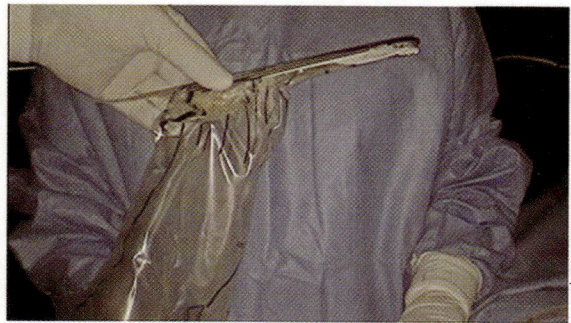

Fig. 27.2: Morsafe bag with the introducer

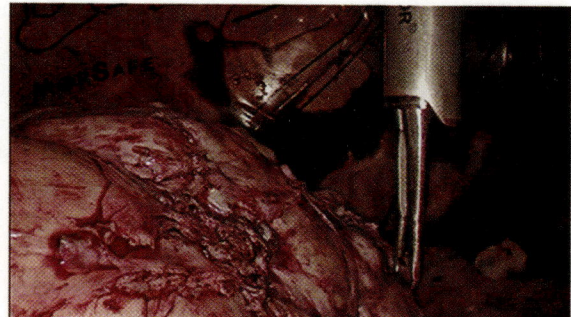

Fig. 27.3: Laparoscopic power morcellator being used inside a morsafe bag

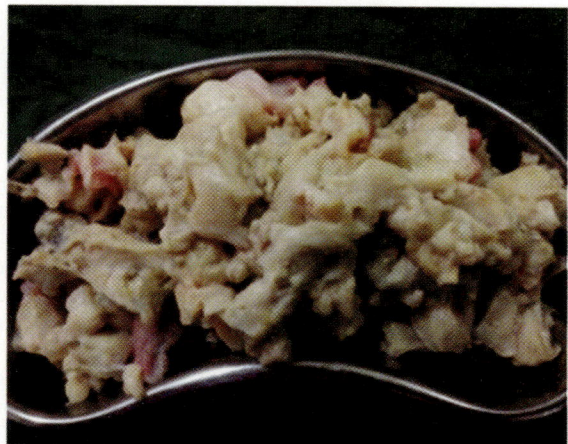

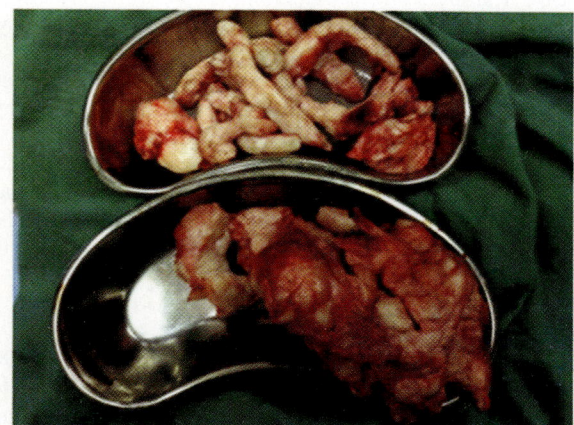

Figs 27.4A and B: Pieces of fibroid made after use of morcellator

CONCLUSION

The recent FDA communication discouraging use of power morcellators has reopened discussion about optimal management of large pelvic masses by minimally invasive techniques. The exact incidence of de novo pathology as well as the incidence of uterine malignancy post morcellation is largely unknown due to lack of appropriate prospective studies. Balance between gain in quality of life and inadvertent dissemination of a worse pathological condition must qualify advances in minimally invasive surgery. The elimination of power morcellation would result in increasing number of open surgical procedureswith its consequent morbidity and mortality especially in the elderly and obese women. However, the risk benefit ratio of uncontained power morcellation has to be assessed before it can be recommended. Current best practice should include proper counselling, adequate preoperative work up and in-bag morcellation in high risk cases. Future directions will only be provided if and when we have better quality studies estimating the risk of occult mailignancy in myoma, the real risk of upstaging of LMS and technological advances in contained morcellation. Minimally invasive myomectomies offering in bag morcellation. Reducing accidental spread of uterine malignancies while preserving the benefits of MIS, requires more studies on patient preferences, in bag morcellation and alternative methods of tissue extraction.

REFERENCES

1. Anupama R, Ahmad SZ, Kuriakose S, et al. Disseminated peritoneal leiomyosarcomas after laparoscopic "myomectomy" and morcellation. J Minim Invasive Gynecol. 2011;18(3):386-9.
2. Anupama R, Ahmad SZ, Kuriakose S, et al. Disseminated peritoneal leiomyosarcomas after laparoscopic "myomectomy" and morcellation. J Minim Invasive Gynecol. 2011;18(3):386-9.
3. Zimmermann A, Bernuit D, Gerlinger C, et al. Prevalence, symptoms and management of uterine fibroids: an international internet-based survey of 21,746 women. BMC women's health. 2012;12:16
4. Warren L, Ladapo JA, Borah BJ, et al. Open abdominal versus laparoscopic and vaginal hysterectomy: analysis of a large United States payer measuring quality and cost of care. J Minim Invasive Gynecol. 2009;16(5):581-8.
5. Sarah Cohen and James A Greenberg. Hysteroscopic Morcellation for Treating Intrauterine Pathology, Rev Obstet Gynecol. 2011;4(2):73-80.
6. Lieng M, Istre O, Qvigstad E. Treatment of endometrial polyps: a systematic review. Acta Obstet Gynecol Scand. 2010;89:992-1002.

7. Milad MP, Sokol E. Laparoscopic morcellator-related injuries. Am J Assoc Gynecol Laparosc. 2003;10(3):383-5.

8. Milad MP, Milad EA. Laparoscopic morcellator-related complications. J Minim Invasive Gynecol. 2014;21(3):486-91.

9. Seidman MA, Oduyebo T, Muto MG, et al. "Peritoneal Dissemination Complicating Morcellation of Uterine Mesenchymal Neoplasms". PLoS ONE 7 (11): e50058.

10. Della BC, Karini H. Endometrial stromal sarcoma diagnosed after uterine morcellation in laparoscopic supracervical hysterectomy. J Minim Invasive Gynecol. 2010;17(6):791-3.

11. Lurain JR, Piver MS. Uterine sarcomas: clinical features and management. In: Coppleson X, Monagham J, Morrow P, Tattersall M (Eds). Gynecologic oncology. London: Chruchill Livingstone. 1992. pp. 827-40.

12. Della BC, Karini H. Endometrial stromal sarcoma diagnosed after uterine morcellation in laparoscopic supracervical hysterectomy. J Minim Invasive Gynecol. 2010;17(6):791-3.

13. Einstein MH, Barakat RR, Chi DS, et al. Management of uterine malignancy found incidentally after supracervical hysterectomy or uterine morcellation for presumed benign disease. Int J Gynecol Cancer. 2008;18(5):1065-70.

14. Cucinella G, Granese R, Calagna G, et al. Parasitic myomas after laparoscopic surgery: an emerging complication in the use of morcellator? Description of four cases. Fertil Steril. 2011;96(2):e90–e96. doi: 10.1016/j.fertnstert. 2011.05.095.

15. Nezhat C, Kho K. Iatrogenic myomas: new class of myomas? J Minim Invasive Gynecol. 2010;17(5):544-50.

16. Donnez O, Jadoul P, Squifflet J, et al. A series of 3190 laparoscopic hysterectomies for benign disease from 1990 to 2006: evaluation of complications compared with vaginal and abdominal procedures. BJOG. 2009;116(4):492-500.

17. Cucinella G, Granese R, Calagna G, et al. Parasitic myomas after laparoscopic surgery: an emerging complication in the use of morcellator? Description of four cases. Fertil Steril. 2011;96(2):e90-e96.

18. Leren V, Langebrekke A, Qvigstad E. Parasitic leiomyomas after laparoscopic surgery with morcellation. Acta Obstet Gynecol Scand. 2012;91(10):1233-6.

19. Ordulu Z, Dal CP, Chong WW, et al. Disseminated peritoneal leiomyomatosis after laparoscopic supracervical hysterectomy with characteristic molecular cytogenetic findings of uterine leiomyoma. Genes Chromosome Cancer. 2010;49(12):1152-60.

20. Senapati S, Tu FF, Magrina JF. Power morcellators: a review of current practice and assessment of risk. Am J Obstet Gynecol. 2015;212(1):18-23.

21. RekhaW, Amita M, Sudeep G, et al. Unexpected complication of uterine myoma morcellation. Aust N Z J Obstet Gynaecol. 2005;45:248-58.

22. Tam T, Harkins G, Caldwell T, et al. Endometrial dye instillation: a novel approach to histopathologic evaluation of morcellated hysterectomy specimens. JMIG. 2013;20:667-71.

23. Brown RL. Iatrogenic endometriosis caused by uterine morcellation during a supracervical hysterectomy. Obstet Gynecol. 2004;103:583.

24. Sepilian V, Della Badia C. Iatrogenic endometriosis caused by uterine morcellation during a supracervical hysterectomy. Obstet Gynecol. 2003;102:1125-7.

25. Brown J. AAGL advancing minimally invasive gynecology worldwide: statement to the FDA on power morcellation. J Minim Invasive Gynecol. 2014;21(6):970-1.

26. Linda a. Johnson (November 24, 2014). "FDA strengthens warning on device linked to cancer". AP Business Writer. Retrieved November 24, 2014. FDA strengthens warning on gynecologic surgical device linked to spreading cancer inside women.

27. ACOG Statement on FDA Regulation of Morcellation; http://www.acog.org/About-ACOG/News-Room/Statements/2015/ACOG-Statement-on-FDA-Regulation-of-Morcellation, accessed on 12th January, 2016.

28. Troy Brown, Leading Physicians Refute FDA Warning on Morcellation; Medscape Medical News, http://www.medscape.com/viewarticle/855654#vp_2, accessed on 12th January, 2016

29. Parker WH, Kaunitz AM, Pritts EA, et al. U.S. Food and Drug Administration's guidance regarding morcellation of leiomyomas: well-intentioned, but is it harmful for women?. Obstet Gynecol. 2016;127:18-22.

30. Parker WH, Kaunitz AM, Pritts EA, et al. U.S. Food and Drug Administration's guidance regarding morcellation of leiomyomas: well-intentioned, but is it harmful for women?. Obstet Gynecol. 2016;127:29.

31. Fukunishi H, Funaki K, Ikuma K, et al. Unsuspected uterine leiomyosarcoma: magnetic resonance imaging findings before and after focused ultrasound surgery. Int J Gynecol Cancer. 2007;17(3):724-8.

32. Pattani SJ, Kier R, Deal R, et al. MRI of uterine leiomyosarcoma. Magn Reson Imaging. 1995; 3(2):331-3.

33. Takemori M, Nishimura R, Sugimura K. Magnetic resonance imaging of uterine leiomyosarcoma. Arch Gynecol Obstet. 1992;251(4):215-8.

34. Zhang HJ, Zhan FH, Li YJ, et al. Fluorodeoxyglucose positron emission tomography/computed tomography and magnetic resonance imaging of uterine leiomyosarcomas: 2 cases report. Chin Med J (Engl). 2011;124(14):2237-40.

35. Yoshida Y, Kiyono Y, Tsujikawa T, et al. Additional value of 16 alpha-[18F] fluoro-17 beta-oestradiol PET for differential diagnosis between uterine sarcoma and leiomyoma in patients with positive or equivocal findings on [18F] fluorodeoxyglucose PET. Eur J Nucl Med Mol Imaging. 2011;38(10):1824-31.

36. Goto A, Takeuchi S, Sugimura K, et al. Usefulness of Gd-DTPA contrast-enhanced dynamic MRI and serum determination of LDH and its isozymes in the differential diagnosis of leiomyosarcoma from degenerated leiomyoma of the uterus. Int J Gynecol Cancer. 2002;12(4):354-61.

37. Juang CM, Yen MS, Horng HC, et al. Potential role of preoperative serum CA125 for the differential diagnosis between uterine leiomyoma and uterine leiomyosarcoma. Eur J Gynaecol Oncol. 2006;27(4):370-4.

38. Tulandi T, Ferenczy A. Biopsy of uterine leiomyomata and frozen sections before laparoscopic morcellation. J Minim Invasive Gynecol. 2014;14:10.

39. McKenna JB, Kanade T, Choi S, et al. The Sydney Contained In Bag Morcellation Technique. J Minim Invasive Gynecol. 2014;15:S1553-4650(14)00351-3.

CHAPTER 28

Recent Advances in Management of Fibroids

● Shwetha Pramodh

■ PHARMACOLOGICAL TREATMENT (Table 28.1)

Selective Progesterone Receptor Modulator

Selective progesterone receptor modulators (SPRMs) are a class of drug with both agonist and antagonist activity. They have the potential to exhibit beneficial effects of progestins and progesterone antagonists, without their drawbacks.

Mechanism of Action

SPRMs have both agonist and antagonist role; agonist on the endometrium, breast and ovary, partial agonist on the myometrium of pregnant uterus and antagonist in the myometrium of the fibroid tissue. Their action is via the progesterone receptors (PR), which exist as two isofroms, i.e. PR-A and PR-B. Proliferation of endometrium is primarily via PR-B receptors. The SPRMs cause atrophy of the endometrium, leading to amenorrhea by direct inhibitory effect on the endometrium.

Asoprisnil has been tested in clinical trials demonstrating high tissue selectivity and binds to progesterone receptors with a 3-fold greater affinity than progesterone.[1] Phase 1 studies confirmed that suppression of menstruation induced by asoprisnil was reversible, while having variable effects on ovulation.[2] In phase 2 multicentre double-blind placebo controlled studies efficacy and safety of three doses (5, 10 and 25 mg and placebo) were compared in 129 women over 12 weeks. Asoprisinil has demonstrated dose-dependent reduction in the uterine and fibroid volumes. Also, a dose-dependent decrease in menorrhagia scores in women with

Table 28.1: Recent advances in management of fibroids (contents)

Category	Groups	Product
Pharmacological treatment (drugs)	1. SPRMS 2. Nano carriers 3. GnRH analogues	Asoprisnil Atrigel, regel, liquogel
Surgical treatment	1. Robotic myomectomy 2. Hysteroscopic morcellation 3. Laser ablation 4. Radiofrequency Ablation	Da Vinci system Nd-YAG laser (under MRI guidance) The Acessa system (Halt medical; Brentwood, CA) (percutaneous laparoscopic guidance)
Uterine artery embolisation (UAE)		Ex Ablate 2000 (In Sightec Ltd, Haifa, Israel)
MRgFUS		
Gene therapy	1. Dominant- negative oestrogen receptor (delivered via an adenovirus) 2. Adenovirus herpes simplex virus thymidine kinase-ganciclovir (Ad-HSV-TK/GCV)	Ultrasound guided/ endoscope guided injection

menorrhagia at baseline was observed. Amenorrhoea rates increased with the dose (28.1% with 5 mg, 64.3% with 10 mg and 83.3% with 25 mg), however with no associated increase in the rates of unscheduled bleeding in all three dose groups. The other observed effects were significant reduction in bloating and pelvic pressure, which was observed in the 10 mg and 25 mg groups. In comparison with placebo, all three treatment groups demonstrated an improvement in haemoglobin levels, with no significant adverse effects recorded.[3,4]

Ulipristal and its acetate analogue are progesterone receptor antagonists and were developed as SPRMs. Ulipristal has minimal antiglucocorticoid effects and is under investigation for use in symptomatic fibroids. Significant reduction (P = 0.01 and P = 0.04) in fibroid volume and related symptoms have been reported over placebo in small in vitro studies and small randomized trials involving ulipristal with no reported adverse effects.[5] In a randomized controlled trial for 13 weeks, ulipristal acetate administered to women with symptomatic fibroids, menometrorrhagia, and anaemia, controlled excessive bleeding with associated reduction in fibroid volume.[6] Studies have also used total fibroid volume change as assessed by magnetic resonance imaging (MRI) as primary outcome measure for success of ulipristal therapy.[7] Ulipristal acetate is currently in phase 3 clinical trial.

Another SPRM, telepristone with significant progesterone antagonist activity and low antiglucocorticoid activity is undergoing investigations. Telepristone is being developed for use in the treatment of uterine fibroids and endometriosis as an antiprogestin. In clinical trials, telepristone has demonstrated fibroid volume reduction by up to 40% with significant decrease in vaginal bleeding. In one study, telepristone was reported to induce apoptosis in fibroid cells[8] however other studies did not report similar effects.[9,10] The United States (US) Food Drug Association (FDA) has placed a hold on telepristone clinical development in August 2009 as there is an associated liver enzyme elevation with drug treatment.

Adverse Effects

All the SPRMs investigated till date have demonstrated a good safety profile and are well tolerated. The common and self-limiting adverse events reported for asoprisnil in clinical trials are headache and abdominal pain. Abdominal pain, headache, nausea, bleeding and unusual tiredness are some of the adverse events observed with ulipristal, while uterine bleeding was observed in clinical trials with telepristone.

Novel Therapies Enabled by Smart Nanocarriers

The evolution of nano-carriers that are designed to deliver and protect drug therapeutics is now able to provide new options for drug delivery. The nano-carriers are considered for therapeutic agents such as antifibrotic, aromatase inhibitors, progestins, etc. With advances in guided-ultrasound technology, it is now feasible to precisely visualize and generate a drug depot inside the fibroid tissue by local injection-utilizing nanocarriers.[11]

Under guided-ultrasound, physicians inject the therapy into the fibroid mass in an outpatient setting. With this procedure, loss of drug concentration due to diffusion and distribution into surrounding tissue is avoided. This procedure also prolongs drug release and delays inactivation thereby avoiding repeated injection. Following nanocarriers are under investigation and development:

1. Atrigel is a combination of water-insoluble biodegradable polymer (e.g. polylactic-coglycolic acid, PLGA) dissolved in a biocompatible, water-miscible organic solvent (e.g. N-methyl-2-pyrrolidone, NMP).[12]
2. ReGel is a triblock copolymer formed from poly lactide-co-glycolide (PLGA) and polyethylene glycol in repetitions of PLGA-PEG-PLGA or PEG-PLGA-PEG.[12]
3. LiquoGel is a tetrameric copolymer derived by thermogelling N-isopropylacrylamide; a biodegrading macromer of polylactic acid and 2-hydroxyethyl methacrylate; hydrophilic acrylic acid (to maintain solubility of decomposition products); and multifunctional hyperbranched polyglycerol to covalently attached drugs.[13]

Gonadotrophin-releasing Hormone Analogues

Gonadotrophin-releasing hormone agonists (GnRHa) are synthetic derivatives of the natural hypothalamic neuropeptide gonadotrophin-releasing hormone. The agonists are released in pulses and stimulate the pituitary gland to release the follicle-stimulating hormone (FSH) and leutenizing hormone (LH). Production of oestrogen and progesterone by the ovary are regulated by FSH and LH in turn. GnRHa peptides are commercially available as long-acting injectable depot formulations. GnRHa suppress oestrogen creating a menopause-like state and are currently used to prevent bleeding during surgical procedures in women with symptomatic fibroids. Long-term use of GnRHa is associated with adverse effects such as osteoporosis, vaginal dryness, impotence, reduced breast size, emotional instability, depression, hair loss, and musculoskeletal stiffness.[14]

In contrary, GnRH antagonist are formed by alterations in position 2 and/or 3 and compete with endogenous GnRH for pituitary-binding sites. The first generation antagonists were hydrophilic, contained replacements for His at position 2 and for Trp at position 3 and were associated with anaphylactic reactions. With the evolution of third generation antagonists such as cetrorelix and ganirelix the anaphylactic reactions were eliminated. Short half-life of the antagonists and the non-availability of depot formulations is one of the major limitations resulting in the need of repetitive dosing in fibroid treatment.[15] The next generation GnRH antagonists, degarelix and ozarelix are currently being evaluated as depot preparations in late stage clinical development.

The flare-up effect present with GnRHa is not present with GnRH antagonist treatment thus providing greater advantage. Unlike GnRHa, the antagonists suppress pituitary gonadotropins immediately thereby allowing flexibility in the degree of pituitary-gonadal suppression. Rapid and predictable recovery of the pituitary-gonadal axis following discontinuation of GnRH antagonist is the added advantage.[16] Few randomized controlled trials evaluating the effect of GnRH antagonists exist for fibroids; however observational studies on small numbers of patients suggest beneficial effects.[17,18] Daily treatment with ganirelix resulted in rapid reduction of the fibroid and uterine volume in premenopausal women with minor side effects.[19] Engel et al, studied the effect of different doses of cetrorelix with a 4-week treatment regimen prior to surgery in patients with uterine fibroids. The study involved 109 premenopausal women randomized to placebo and different cetrorelix dosing regimens. Significant response in reduction of fibroid volume versus placebo (p < 0.05) occurred in the 4*10 mg group (42.3% versus 11.1%).[20] If longer-acting GnRH antagonists become available, pretreatment with GnRH antagonists should be preferred over GnRH agonists prior to surgery.

■ LAPAROSCOPIC (HYSTEROSCOPIC) PROCEDURES

Myomectomy (Da Vinci)

Myomectomy is the surgical removal of fibroids from the uterus. It allows the uterus to be left in place and also increases the chance of pregnancy in some women. Myomectomy is the preferred treatment for fibroids in women who want to become pregnant. The traditional abdominal myomectomy is associated with several risk factors such as blood loss, infection and are now limited in practice.

In 2004, Advincula and colleagues first introduced the robot-assisted myomectomy, which was established to be safe and reproducible surgical approach to uterine fibroids.[21] In April 2005, US FDA approved the da Vinci surgical system for gynaecologic applications. The instrument has 7 degrees of freedom: 3 degrees provided by the robotic arms (insertion, pitch, yaw) and 4 degrees from the 'wristed' instruments (pitch, yaw, roll, and grip).[22] Single fibroids smaller than 15 cm and with fewer than 15 fibroids in total are ideally suited for robotic myomectomy.

Advincula and colleagues in 2007, compared short-term surgical outcomes and costs of robot-assisted and open myomectomy. Significantly decreased blood loss, complication rates and length of stay was observed in patients undergoing robot-assisted laparoscopic myomectomy. However, the operative times were significantly longer with professional charges and hospital charges of approximately $13,000.[23] Bedient CE et al, in 2009 retrospectively compared

81 patients undergoing robotic (n = 40) and laparoscopic (n = 41) myomectomy. The study observed no significant differences in operating time, blood loss, intraoperative or postoperative complications, hospital stay more than 2 days, readmissions or symptom resolution between the two groups.[24]

Hysteroscopic Morcellation

Hysteroscopic morcellator is a mechanical cutting device used to reduce the tumour into small chips and consequently evacuating these chips out of the uterine cavity by aspiration. Hysteroscopic morcellation aims to remove fibroids during a single insertion of a hysteroscope into the uterus. Morcellation reduces the risk of traumatic injury to the uterus and inadvertent fluid overload associated with traditional procedures.

In 2005, Emanuel MH retrospectively compared 200 patients with fibroids; 28 hysteroscopic morcellation versus 172 transcervical resection using a resectoscope. The study reported that all patients were symptom free at 3-month follow-up. The study also reported a mean operating times of 16 minutes vs 42 minutes and mean fluid deficits of 660 mL vs 742 mL for hysteroscopic morcellation and transcervical resection respectively.[25] A RCT by Van Dongen in 2008 compared the use of conventional resectoscopy with hysteroscopic morcellation in 60 patients. The study reported mean operating times of 11 and 17 minutes, respectively (P = 0.008) and mean total fluid deficits of 409 mL and 545 mL for hysteroscopic morcellation and conventional resectoscopy respectively (P = 0.224).[26] Another study by Hamerlynck in 2010 with 37 patients reported mean equipment installation time as 8.7 minutes, mean operating time as 18.2 minutes, and median fluid deficit as 440 mL.[27] Hysteroscopic morcellation is considered as a fast, safe and easy technique for removal of smaller fibroids (Fig. 28.1).

■ LASER ABLATION

The technique involves use of the neodymium:yttrium-aluminium garnet (Nd:YAG) laser to coagulate the fibroid. Under magnetic resonance-image guidance needles are inserted, percutaneously after local anaesthesia, into the centre of the targeted uterine fibroid. Laser fibres are then inserted through the centre of each of the needles into the targeted fibroid. A thermal mapping sequence is then used to depict the extent of the heated tissue in the target area during the procedure.

A study in 1999 and 2000 in 12 patients indicated 37.5% decrease in fibroid volume at 3 month follow-up in 7 patients. Patients also reported subjective improvement in symptoms.[28,29] A study by Hindley et al (2002) in 66 patients with symptomatic fibroids indicated 31% reduction in fibroid volume in 47 patients at 3 months follow-up, 41% reduction in fibroid volume at 1 year follow-up in 24 patients and 6/20

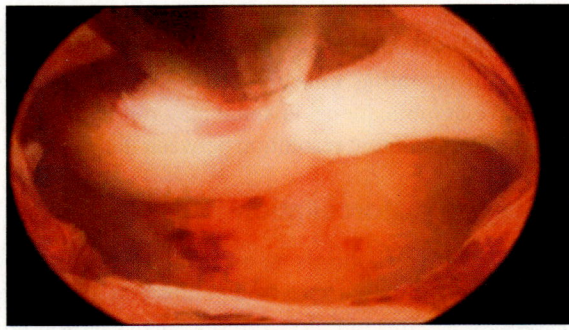

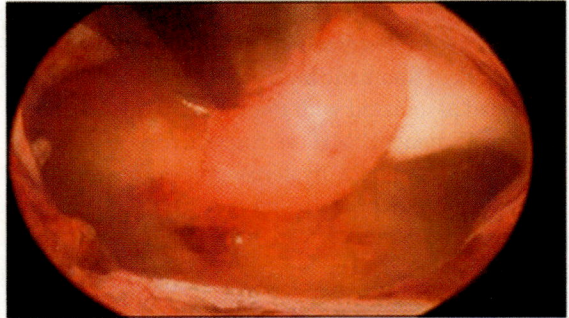

Fig. 28.1: Hysteroscopic morcellation of submucous

patients had a substantial increase at 12 months.[30] The results of all case series is summarised in Table 28.2. Laser ablation is a minimally invasive approach offering an alternative to surgery for women with fibroids, however longer follow-up is required to ascertain maximal fibroid shrinkage and to compare outcome with traditional surgery (Table 28.2).

■ RADIOFREQUENCY ABLATION

The Acessa™ System (Halt Medical; Brentwood, CA) was cleared for marketing by the US FDA in 2012. It is indicated for percutaneous laparoscopic coagulation and ablation of soft tissue and treatment of symptomatic uterine fibroids under laparoscopic ultrasound guidance.

In 2014, Brucker et al published an industry-sponsored RCT comparing radiofrequency ablation to laparoscopic myomectomy. The study included 51 premenopausal women with symptomatic uterine fibroids less than 10 cm in any diameter. The primary study outcome of non-inferiority was met; mean time to hospital discharge was 10.0 ± 5.5 hours in the radiofrequency ablation group and 29.9 ± 14.2 hours in the myomectomy group31. Similar uncontrolled case series was initially published in 2013 by Chudnoff et al. It included 135 premenopausal women with 6 or fewer treatable fibroids and no single fibroid larger than 7 cm. The study evaluated change in the volume of menstrual bleeding and the surgical reintervention rate after 12 months. In the study, 53 of 127 women experienced at least a 50% reduction in the volume of menstrual bleeding and most women experienced a decrease in menstrual bleeding at 12 months.[32] 3-year outcomes were reported by 104/135 women who participated in the study. Eleven women had hysterectomies, 2 had myomectomies, and 1 had uterine artery embolisation (UAE).[33] Radiofrequency ablation provides a safe and shorter operative and postoperative involvement for patients with fibroids. The procedure is also associated with less intraoperative blood loss, allows treatment of a greater number of fibroids without myometrial incisions, and less fatigue.

Table 28.2: Summary of efficacy and safety findings from case series on laser ablation

Authors and date		Hindley et al (2002)[30]	Law et al 1999 and Law and Regan 2000[28,29]
Study details		Case series: 66 patients with symptomatic fibroids	Case series: 12 patients symptomatic fibroids who had not responded to medical management Mean ablation was 15 minutes
Key efficacy findings	Fibroids-volume reduction	3 month follow-up (47 pts) fibroid volume had decreased by 31% 1 year follow-up (24 pts) fibroid volume had decreased by 41% 6/20 patients had a substantial increase at 12 months	3 month follow-up (7 pts) fibroid volume decreased by 37.5% Women reported subjective improvement in symptoms Four women went on to have subsequent surgery
	Menstrual blood loss	8 patients Post treatment 121.2 mL 3 months 81.2 mL	Not reported
	Menorrhagia outcomes questionnaire (MOQ) 35/37	Compared to a historical group undergoing hysterectomy patients undergoing MRI laser ablation reported a worse total outcome score	Not reported
Key safety findings	Adverse events and concomitant medication	3 patients required antibiotic therapy for urinary tract infections 2 patients sustained minor skin burns	No complications were reported 2 patients experienced vaginal bleeding

CRYOABLATION (CRYOMYOLYSIS)

Cryomyolysis uses gas-cooled cryoprobes, which operate on the Joule-Thompson principle, in which pressurized gas is expanded through a small orifice to produce cooling. During surgery, the inserted cryoprobe reaches a temperature of less than −90°C, creating an elliptical ice ball around the probe after 8–10 minutes with a transverse diameter of 3–4 cm and a length of 5–7 cm in the fibroid. A temperature of −20°C causes sclerohyaline degeneration of the fibroid. At the leading edge of the ice ball the tissue is not destroyed as the temperature is 0°C–2°C.

In 1998, Zreik and colleagues published a prospective pilot study with 14 patients, where patients were given a GnRHa before the procedure to reduce the size of the fibroid. Cryomyolysis maintained or slightly reduced the post-GnRH uterine size.[34]

In a study involving 10 premenopausal women, 8 patients were free of symptoms and two had improved after 3 months of cryoablation. Progressive shrinkage of the treated fibroid was observed during follow-up with a 22.2% reduction after 1 month, 37.5% after 3 months and 52.6% after 6 months. After cryoablation a significant reduction in central blood flow of the fibroid was observed.[35] Interpretation of these studies is limited due to their small size and lack of a comparison group (Figs 28.2 and 28.3).

UTERINE ARTERY EMBOLISATION

The first report of embolisation for symptomatic fibroids was published in 1995.[36] The procedure is performed under sedation and involves percutaneous insertion of an angiography catheter via femoral artery into the ipsilateral or the contralateral uterine artery. Polyvinyl alcohol particles 300–500 μm in size are injected into the vessel until blood flow ceases. Angiography is useful for comprehensive assessment of the anatomy of the internal iliac artery, its pattern of division, and its branches.[37–39] Doppler ultrasonography,

contrast material-enhanced magnetic resonance imaging, and magnetic resonance angiography also may be useful for evaluation of the arterial supply to the fibroid tumour before embolisation.[38]

As a standard, the usual angiographic end point is complete occlusion of the uterine arteries indicated by stasis of contrast material.[40–43] This endpoint is for embolisation performed with non-spherical polyvinyl alcohol particles. With the advent of microsphere embolisation different angiographic endpoints are investigated. The main uterine artery is spared as the target of embolisation with microsphere embolisation is the perifibroid arterial plexus. With calibrated microspheres, embolisation is stopped when the fibroid branch arteries are occluded, despite the antegrade flow presence in the main uterine artery.[44] Uterine artery embolisation (UAE) has gained popularity as an alternative treatment to myomectomy and hysterectomy. It has been shown to be safe and effective when compared with hysterectomy, has fewer complications and a shorter hospital stay.[45]

The multi-centre RCT 'EMMY' (EMbolisation versus HysterectoMY) evaluated health-related quality of life outcomes for hysterectomy and UAE for up to 24 months. These were related to mental and physical health, urinary function and overall patient satisfaction. The results from this study concluded that patients who underwent hysterectomy were more satisfied with the treatment received than women who underwent UAE. No other differences were observed.[46]

In another retrospective multi-centre cohort study 'HOPEFUL' (Hysterectomy Or Percutaneous Embolisation For Uterine Leiomyomata) hysterectomy and UAE were assessed for efficacy, safety, and cost-effectiveness. This study concluded that complications and cost were lower in the UAE group.[47] In a randomised study by Edward et al, comparing UAE with hysterectomy for symptomatic uterine fibroids faster recovery time was reported, however associated with the risk of treatment failure in 9% to 20% of cases.[48] Studies have reported permanent loss of ovarian function after UAE

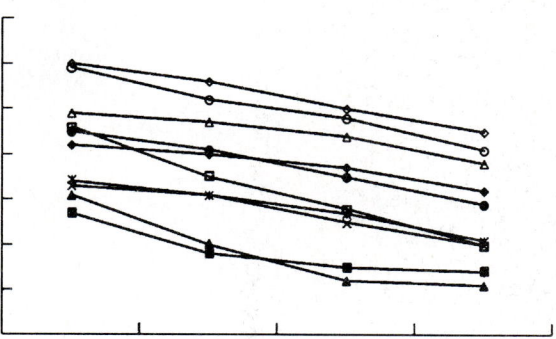

Fig. 28.2: Graph showing reduction in diameter over time for each of the ten fibroids treated by cryomyolysis[35]

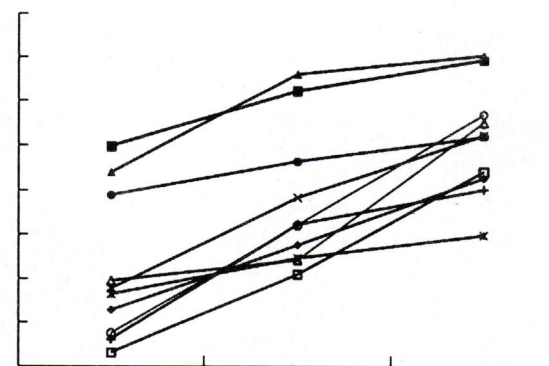

Fig. 28.3: Graph showing percentage volume reduction over time for each of the ten fibroids treated by cryomyolysis[35]

in women aged over 45, and impaired ovarian function in younger patients.[49] A long-term efficacy and complications study in UAE after 5 to 7 years has shown a satisfaction rate of 88% in women wishing to avoid hysterectomy.[50,51]

■ NON-INVASIVE TREATMENT: MR-GUIDED FOCUSED ULTRASOUND SURGERY

The ExAblate 2000 (InSightec Ltd., Haifa, Israel) is the first device to combine magnetic resonance imaging (MRI) with high-intensity focused ultrasound (MRgFUS) to destroy tumours non-invasively, approved by the FDA in 2004. MRgFUS uses high-intensity focused ultrasonic waves to destroy (ablate) the fibroids under real-time monitoring of the treated tissue. This is done as an outpatient procedure and patients remain conscious, however sedated and feeling no pain. It does not require general anaesthesia and recovery time is also significantly reduced compared with surgical alternatives. Although relatively new, this treatment option will give a subset of women a treatment choice that gives them fast recovery with limited side effects. In contrast to the more diffuse necrosis caused by UAE, the targeting ability of high-intensity focused ultrasound produces few adverse effects. Currently this procedure is FDA approved for premenopausal women with symptomatic uterine fibroids who are not planning for future pregnancy.

The safety and efficacy of this technique was further evaluated by Stewart et al, in a multicentre trial involving 55 women with symptomatic fibroids.[52] The same group further evaluated the procedure in 109 patients and reported that 71% of women reached the targeted symptom reduction at 6 months, and 51% reached this at 12 months.[53] Other studies have also reported similar results.[54,55]

Data from studies demonstrated few serious adverse effects related to MRgFUS. Skin burns, secondary to poor coupling from hair and scars on the skin and nerve damage are the only device-related adverse events reported following MRgFUS.[54] Other rare adverse events are damage to adjacent organs, such as bowel perforation.[56] A prospective registry maintained by the device manufacturer, reported 54 pregnancies in 51 women occurring after MRgFUS. The mean time to conception was 8 months after treatment with live births in 41% of women. Spontaneous abortion was reported in 28%, elective pregnancy termination in 11% and ongoing pregnancies beyond 20 gestational weeks in 20% women. Vaginal delivery rate was 64% with mean birth weight of 3.3 kg.[57] In addition to direct medical benefits, the economic impact of MRgFUS was important to note. The mean time of return to work after MRgFUS was approximately 1 day, compared with 13 days after uterine artery ablation and approximately 6 weeks after abdominal myomectomy or hysterectomy (Table 28.3).[58]

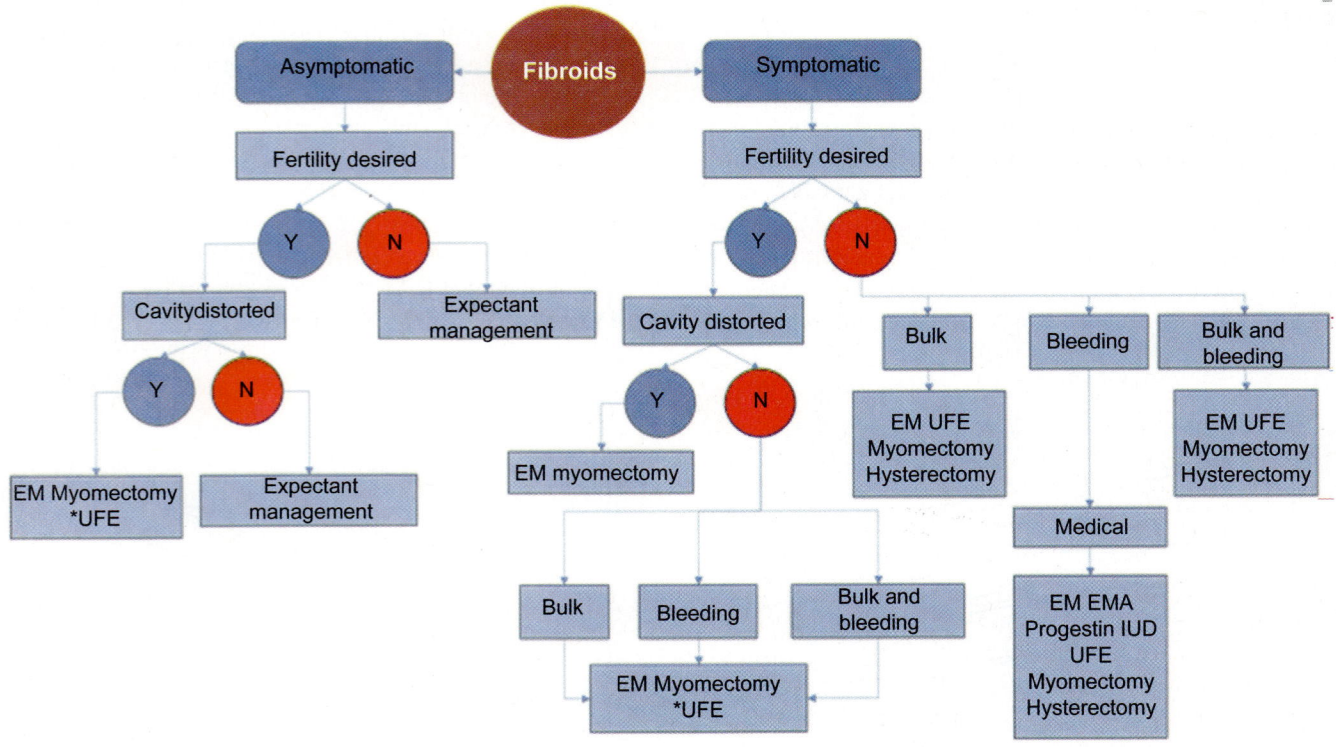

Fig. 28.4: Goldberg fibroid treatment algorithm. EM, expectant management (no treatment); EMA, endometrial ablation; UFE, uterine fibroid embolisation; * Relatively contra-indicated (Source:http://www.einstein.edu/fibroid-centre/fibroid-algorithm/).

Table 28.3: Summary of treatment options for fibroids. **Depending on how the surgery is done (Fig. 28.4)

	Description	Advantages	Disadvantages
Hormone treatment	Medications reduce bleeding and decrease fibroid tumour size	No procedure necessary Preserves uterus	Can cause menopause-like symptoms and bone loss. Symptoms return when treatment stops.
MR-guided focused ultrasound (MRgFUS)	Ultrasound waves penetrate the abdominal wall and heat fibroid tissue, causing the tumour to shrink.	No incision. 1 to 2 day recovery with minimal discomfort. Preserves uterus.	Procedure can take several hours. Usually only appropriate for small fibroids near the surface of the uterus. Insurance may not cover. Fibroids may recur, requiring additional procedures.
Uterine fibroid embolisation (UFE)	Nonsurgical procedure to block blood flow to fibroids, causing them to shrink. Performed by an interventional radiologist.	Very small incision; no general anaesthesia required. One week recovery. Few major complications. Preserves uterus.	Mild fatigue and low grade fever may occur, but can be treated and typically pass quickly. Fibroids may recur, requiring additional procedures.
Endometrial ablation	Removal of the lining of the uterus to reduce bleeding. Can only be used in presence of submucosal fibroids	Can effectively control bleeding. Preserves uterus.	May not be possible, depending on location or size of fibroids. Will not reduce symptoms related to fibroid bulk. Abnormal uterine bleeding may recur, requiring additional procedures.
Myomectomy • Hysteroscopic • Laparoscopic, including robotic • Abdominal	Surgical removal of fibroid tumours	Relieves symptoms and preserves uterus. Currently the only procedure recommended for fertility.	Risks associated with surgery and general anaesthesia. Two day to six week recovery.** Fibroids may recur, requiring additional procedures. May not be recommended depending on location, size, and number of fibroids.
Hysterectomy • Vaginal • Laparoscopic, including robotic • Abdominal	Surgical removal of the uterus	Permanently relieves symptoms.	Loss of fertility. Risks associated with surgery and general anaesthesia. Two to six week recovery.** Hormonal changes if ovaries are removed. Longer-term side effects have been reported.

GENE THERAPY

Gene therapy means delivery of genetic material to target cells for achieving therapeutic benefits by either interfering with a certain gene's function, restoring lost function or initiating a new function. For successful gene therapy, certain criteria must be fulfilled; a vehicle to deliver the therapeutic gene to the right target cells must exist and once gene delivery to target cells has been achieved, the expression of the therapeutic gene at right levels in the target tissue must be achieved. Predominantly, the delivery and expression of the therapeutic gene must not be lethal to the patient or the environment. Uterine fibroid is a preferred target for gene therapy as it is localised and well contained in the uterus within a fibrous capsules. Fibroids allow targeting the viral load by direct ultrasound-guided or endoscope-mediated intra-tumour injection. Alternatively, the viral vector delivery to the fibroid is achieved by transarterial injection through a uterine artery catheter threaded to the artery feeding the fibroid.

Several evidences suggest the down-regulation of apoptotic mechanisms in fibroid cells compared with normal myometrium.[59] Gene therapy of fibroids therefore focusses on activating the apoptosis mechanism by both either extrinsic or intrinsic pathways. This can be achieved by delivering apoptosis-inducing ligands, such as tumour-necrosing factor (TNF), TNF-related apoptosis-inducing ligand (TRAIL) and FasL. Alternatively apoptosis can also be achieved by delivering proapoptotic members of the Bcl-2 family, such as Bax or active caspase molecules. Growth of fibroid is driven by angiogenesis, which in turn is regulated by growth factors such as basic fibroblast growth factor (bFGF), vascular endothelial growth factor (VEGF) and platelet-derived endothelial growth factor (PDGF).[60–63] Apoptosis-inducing ligands and angiogenic factors thus are potential gene-therapy candidates.

Dominant-negative oestrogen receptor (delivered via an adenovirus) and adenovirus herpes simplex virus thymidine kinase-ganciclovir (Ad-HSV-TK/GCV) are currently the two approaches considered for inducing apoptosis and eventually shrinking the fibroid. These approaches are being considered as the basis for future clinical trials.[64] A study evaluating Ad-HSV-TK/GCV mediated 'bystander effect' demonstrated 48.6% (human) and 65.6% (rat) cell death occurring when 5% of the fibroid cells were transfected with the pNGVL1-TK vector. Based on the 16.7% and 39.8% transfection efficiency, 0.84% and 1.9% of the cells were expected to express thymidine kinase as determined by the reporter gene assay in human and rat fibroid cells, respectively.[65]

Gene therapy is a potential treatment strategy for treatment of women with uterine fibroids, either alone or in combination with existing treatment modalities.

■ REFERENCES

1. Brahma PK, Martel KM, Christman GM. Future directions in myoma research. Obstet Gynecol Clin North Am. 2006;33:199-224.

2. Chwalisz K, Elger W, Stickler T Mattia-Goldberg C, et al. The effects of 1-month administration of asoprisnil (J867), a selective progesterone receptor modulator, in healthy premenopausal women. Hum Reprod. 2005;20:1090-99.

3. Chwalisz K, Lamar Parker R, Williamson S. Treatment of uterine leiomyomas with the novel selective progesterone receptor modulator (SPRM). J Soc Gynecol Investig. 2003;10:636.

4. Chwalisz K, Larsen L, McCrary K. Effects of the novel selective progesterone receptor modulator (SPRM) asoprisinil on bleeding patterns in subjects with leiomyomata. J Soc Gynecol Investig. 2004;11:728.

5. Rodriguez MI, Warden M, Darney PD. Intrauterine progestins, progesterone antagonists, and receptor modulators: A review of gynecologic applications. Am. J. Obstet. Gynecol. 2010;202(5):420-8.

6. Donnez J, Tatarchuk TF, Bouchard P, et al. Ulipristal acetate versus placebo for fibroid treatment before surgery. N. Engl. J. Med. 2012;366(5):409-20.

7. Nieman LK, Blocker W, Nansel T, et al. Efficacy and tolerability of cdb-2914 treatment for symptomatic uterine fibroids: A randomized, double-blind, placebo-controlled, phase IIb study. Fertil Steril. 2011;95(2):767-9.

8. Luo X, Yin P, Coon V JS, et al. The selective progesterone receptor modulator cdb4124 inhibits proliferation and induces apoptosis in uterine leiomyoma cells. Fertil Steril. 2010;93(8):2668-73.

9. Roeder H, Jayes F, Feng L, et al. Cdb-4124 does not cause apoptosis in cultured fibroid cells. Reproductive Sciences. 2011;18(9):850-7.

10. Wade HE, Kobayashi S, Eaton ML, et al. Multimodal regulation of e2f1 gene expression by progestins. Mol. Cell. Biol. 2010;30(8):1866-77.

11. Wikland M, Blad S, Bungum L, et al. A randomized controlled study comparing pain experience between a newly designed needle with a thin tip and a standard needle for oocyte aspiration. Hum. Reprod. 2011;26(6):1377-83.

12. Wright, JC, et al. In situ forming systems (depots). In: Wright, JC, Burgess DJ (Eds). Long acting injections and implants. New York: Springer US. 2012. pp. 153-66.

13. Taylor DK, Jayes FL, House AJ, et al. Temperature-responsive biocompatible copolymers incorporating hyperbranched polyglycerols for adjustable functionality. J. Funct. Biomater. 2011;2(3):173-94.

14. Parsanezhad M, et al. Medical management of uterine fibroids. Current Obstetrics and Gynecology Reports. 2012:1-8.

15. Sabry M, Al-Hendy A. Innovative oral treatments of uterine leiomyoma. Obstetrics and Gynecology International. 2012.

16. The Ganerelix Dose Finding Study Group. A double blind, randomized, dose finding study to assess the efficacy of the gonadotropin-releasing hormone antagonist gaverelix (Org 37462) to prevent premature luteinizing hormone surge in women undergoing ovarian stimulation with recombinant follicle stimulating hormone (Puregon). Hum Reprod. 1998;13:3023-31.

17. Kettel LM, Murphy AA, Morales AJ, et al. Rapid regression of uterine leiomyomas in response to daily administration of gonadotropin-releasing hormone antagonist. Fertil Steril. 1993;60:642-6.

18. Gonzalez-Barcena D, Alvarez RB, Ochoa EP, et al. Treatment of uterine leiomyomas with luteinizing hormone-releasing hormone antagonist Cetrorelix. Hum Reprod. 1997;12:2028-35.

19. Flierman PA, Oberye' JJ, van der Hulst VP, et al. Rapid reduction of leiomyoma volume during treatment with the GnRH antagonist ganirelix. Br J Obstet Gynaecol. 2005;112:638-42.

20. Engel, Jörg B, Audebert A, et al. Presurgical short term treatment of uterine fibroids with different doses of cetrorelix acetate: A double-blind, placebo-controlled multicenter study Eur J Obstet Gynecol Reprod Biol. 134(2):225-32.

21. Advincula AP, Song A, Burke W, et al. Preliminary experience with robot-assisted laparoscopic myomectomy. J Am Assoc Gynecol Laparosc. 2004;11:511-8.

22. Visco AG, Advincula AP. Robotic gynecologic surgery. Obstet Gynecol. 2008;112:1369-84.

23. Advincula AP, Xu X, Goudeau S 4th, et al. Robot-assisted laparoscopic myomectomy versus abdominal myomectomy: a comparison of shortterm surgical outcomes and immediate costs. J Minim Invasive Gynecol. 2007;14:698-705.

24. Bedient CE, Magrina JF, Noble BN, et al. Comparison of robotic and laparoscopic myomectomy. Am J Obstet Gynecol. 2009;201:566.e1-5.

25. Emanuel MH, Wamsteker K. The Intra Uterine Morcellator: a new hysteroscopic operating technique to remove intrauterine polyps and myomas. J Minim Invasive Gynecol. 2005;12(1):62-6.

26. van Dongen H, Emanuel MH, Wolterbeek R, et al. Hysteroscopic morcellator for removal of intrauterine polyps and myomas: a randomized controlled pilot study among residents in training. J Minim Invasive Gynecol. 2008;15(4):466-712.

27. Hamerlynck T, Dietz V, Schoot BC. Clinical implementation of the hysteroscopic morcellator for removal of intrauterine myomas and polyps. A retrospective descriptive study. Gynecol Surg. 2011;8(2):193-6.

28. Law P, Gedroyc WM, Regan L. Magnetic resonance-guided percutaneous laser ablation of uterine fibroids. J Magn Reson Imaging. 2000;12(4):565-70.

29. Law P, Gedroyc WM, Regan L. Magnetic-resonance-guided percutaneous laser ablation of uterine fibroids. Lancet. 1999;354:2049-50.

30. Hindley JT, Law PA, Hickey M, et al. Clinical outcomes following percutaneous magnetic resonance image guided laser ablation of symptomatic uterine fibroids. Hum Reprod. 2002;17(10):2737-41.

31. Brucker SY, Hahn M, Kraemer D, et al. Laparoscopic radiofrequency volumetric thermal ablation of fibroids versus laparoscopic myomectomy. Int J Gynaecol Obstet. 2014;125(3):261-5.

32. Chudnoff SG, Berman JM, Levine DJ, et al. Outpatient procedure for the treatment and relief of symptomatic uterine myomas. Obstet Gynecol. 2013;121(5):1075-82.

33. Berman JM, Guido RS, Garza Leal JG, et al. Three-Year Outcome of the Halt Trial: A Prospective Analysis of Radiofrequency Volumetric Thermal Ablation of Myomas. J Minim Invasive Gynecol. 2014;21(5):767-74.

34. Zreik TG, Rutherford TJ, Palter SF, et al. Cryomyolysis, a new procedure for the conservative treatment of uterine fibroids. J Am Assoc Gynecol Laparosc. 1998;5(1):33-8.

35. Exacoustos C, Zupi E, Marconi D, et al. Ultrasound-assisted laparoscopic cryomyolysis: two- and three-dimensional findings before, during and after treatment. Ultrasound Obstet Gynecol. 2005;25:393-400.

36. Ravina JH, Herbreteau D, Ciraru-Vigneron N, et al. Arterial embolization to treat uterine myomata. Lancet. 1995;346:671-2.

37. Gomez-Jorge J, Keyoung A, Levy EB, et al. Uterine artery anatomy relevant to uterine leiomyomata embolization. Cardiovasc Intervent Radiol. 2003;26:522-7.

38. Merland JJ, Chiras J. Vascular territories. In Merland JJ, Chiras J (Eds). Arteriography of the pelvis. Berlin, Germany: Springer-Verlag. 1981. pp. 69-72.

39. Pelage JP, Le Dref O, Beregi JP, et al. Limited uterine artery embolization with trisacryl gelatin microspheres for uterine fibroids. J Vasc Interv Radiol. 2003;14:15-20.

40. Ravina JH, Herbreteau D, Ciraru-Vigneron N, et al. Arterial embolisation to treat myomata. Lancet. 1995;346(8976):671-2.

41. Spies JB, Ascher SA, Roth AR, et al. Uterine artery embolization for leiomyomata. Obstet Gynecol. 2001;98:29-34.

42. Walker WJ, Pelage JP. Uterine artery embolization for symptomatic fibroids: clinical results in 400 women with imaging follow-up. BJOG. 2002;109:1262-72.

43. Pron G, Bennett J, Common A, et al. The Ontario uterine fibroid embolization trial: uterine fibroid reduction and symptom relief after uterine artery embolization for fibroids. Fertil Steril. 2003;79:120-7.

44. Farrer-Brown G, Beilby JO, Tarbit MH. The vascular patterns of myomatous uteri. J Obstet Gynaecol Br Common. 1970;77:967-75.

45. Pinto I, Chimeno P, Romo A, et al. Uterine fibroids: uterine artery embolization versus abdominal hysterectomy for treatment—a prospective, randomized, and controlled clinical trial. Radiology. 2003;226:425-31.

46. Hehenkamp WJ, Volkers NA, Birnie E, et al. Symptomatic uterine fibroids: treatment with uterine artery embolization or hysterectomy-results from the randomized clinical Embolisation versus Hysterectomy (EMMY) Trial. Radiology. 2008;246:823-32.

47. Hirst A, Dutton S, Wu O. A multi-centre retrospective cohort study comparing the efficacy, safety and cost-effectiveness of hysterectomy and uterine artery embolisation for the treatment of symptomatic uterine fibroids. The HOPEFUL study. Health Technol Assess. 2008;12:1-248.

48. Edwards RD, Moss JG, Lumsden MA, et al. Committee of the Randomised Trial of Embolization versus Surgical Treatment for Fibroids: Uterine-artery embolization versus surgery for symptomatic uterine fibroids. N Engl J Med. 2007;356:360-70.

49. Hehenkamp WJ, Volkers NA, Broekmans FJ, et al. Loss of ovarian reserve after uterine artery embolization: a randomized comparison with hysterectomy. Hum Reprod. 2007;22:1996-2005.

50. Davis BJ, Haneke KE, Miner K, et al: The fibroid growth study: determinants of therapeutic intervention. J Women's Health. 2009;18:725-32.

51. Walker WJ, Barton-Smith P. Long-term follow up of uterine artery embolisation–an effective alternative in the treatment of fibroids. BJOG. 2006;113:464-8.

52. Stewart EA, Gedroyc WM, Tempany CM, et al. Focused ultrasound treatment of uterine fibroid tumors: safety and feasibility of a noninvasive thermoablative technique. Am J Obstet Gynecol. 2003;189:48-54.

53. Stewart EA, Rabinovici J, Tempany CM, et al. Clinical outcomes of focused ultrasound surgery for the treatment of uterine fibroids. Fertil Steril. 2006;85(1):22-9.

54. Hindley J, Gedroyc WM, Regan L, et al. MRI guidance of focused ultrasound therapy of uterine fibroids: early results. AJR Am J Roentgenol. 2004;183(6):1713-9.

55. Fennessy FM, Tempany CM, McDannold NJ So MJ, et al. Uterine leiomyomas: MR imaging-guided focused ultrasound surgery--results of different treatment protocols. Radiology. 2007;243(3):885-93.

56. Hesley GK, Gorny KR, Henrichsen TL, et al. A clinical review of focused ultrasound ablation with magnetic resonance guidance: an option for treating uterine fibroids. Ultrasound Q. 2008;24(2):131-9.

57. Rabinovici J, David M, Fukunishi H, et al. Pregnancy outcome after magnetic resonance-guided focused ultrasound surgery (MRgFUS) for conservative treatment of uterine fibroids. Fertil Steril. 2010;93(1):199-209.

58. Pron G, Mocarski E, Bennett J, et al. Tolerance, hospital stay, and recovery after uterine artery embolization for fibroids: the Ontario Uterine Fibroid Embolization Trial. J Vasc Interv Radiol. 2003;14:1243-50.

59. Hoffman PJ, Milliken DB, Gregg LC, et al. Molecular characterization of uterine fibroids and its implication for underlying mechanisms of pathogenesis. Fertil Steril. 2004;82:639-49.

60. Niu H, Simari RD, Zimmermann EM, et al. Nonviral vector-mediated thymidine kinase gene transfer and ganciclovir treatment in leiomyoma cells. Obstet Gynecol. 1998;91:735-40.

61. Al-Hendy A1, Salama S. Gene therapy and uterine leiomyoma: a review. Hum Reprod Update. 2006;12(4):385-400.

62. Hyder SM, Huang JC, Nawaz Z, et al. Regulation of vascular endothelial growth factor expression by estrogens and progestins. Environ Health Perspect. 2000;108:785-90.

63. Gentry CC, Okolo SO, Fong LF, et al. Quantification of vascular endothelial growth factor-A in leiomyomas and adjacent myometrium. Clin Sci (Colch). 2001;101:691-5.

64. Hong T, Shimada Y, Uchida S, et al. Expression of angiogenic factors and apoptotic factors in leiomyosarcoma and leiomyoma. Int J Mol Med. 2001;8(2):141-8.

65. Di Lieto A, De Falco M, Pollio F, Mansueto G, et al. Clinical response, vascular change, and angiogenesis in gonadotropin-releasing hormone analogue-treated women with uterine myomas. J Soc Gynecol Invest. 2005;12(2):123-8.

CHAPTER 29

Robotic-assisted Myomectomy

● Sabhyata Gupta

Myomas are benign, monoclonal smooth muscle tumours of the myometrium. They are the most common pelvic neoplasm, with an 80% incidence among women. Although only 25% of women are affected by symptoms like pelvic pain, pressure, heavy menses, recurrent pregnancy loss and infertility, it remains the leading indication for hysterectomy and a common women's health concern.[1,2] Treatment alternatives include medical management with oral contraceptives, non-steroidal anti-inflammatory medications or gonadotropin-releasing hormone (GnRH) agonists. Additional conservative options are uterine artery embolisation, MRI-guided high frequency ultrasound and radiofrequency ablation. Myomectomy remains the appropriate option for women affected by symptoms who desire uterine preservation and future fertility.

Myomectomy has traditionally been performed by laparotomy. Although laparotomy seems advantageous for the surgeon with depth perception and tactile feedback, the large abdominal incision, prolonged hospitalisation, increased postoperative analgesic requirements and higher morbidity are disadvantages for the patient. Interest in minimally invasive gynaecology has been increasing over the last few decades. Laparoscopic myomectomy was first reported in 1979.[3] This technique has been performed safely and has consistently demonstrated advantages such as decreased blood loss, shorter hospital stay, less postoperative disability and comparable complications to abdominal myomectomy. Clinical outcomes for fertility and obstetrical outcomes are also comparable to abdominal myomectomy.[4] The American College of Obstetricians and Gynecologists and the American Association of Gynecologic Laparoscopists have confirmed the advantages of laparoscopy over laparotomy. Today many cases of intramural and subserous fibroids are managed with laparoscopic myomectomy and selected cases of submucosal myomas are managed with hysteroscopic myomectomy.

Instrumentation, complex disease and steep learning curves are often cited as obstacles to minimally invasive surgery. Other limitations of conventional laparoscopy include counterintuitive hand movement (fulcrum effect), an unsteady two- or three-dimensional visual field, and limited degrees of instrument motion as well as ergonomic difficulty and tremor amplification.[5]

The emergence of robotic technology provides a means to overcome the limitations of conventional laparoscopy through the use of 3-dimensional imaging and more dexterous and precise instruments. Currently, the da Vinci surgical system is the only robotic system that is approved by the Food Drug Administration (FDA). It received clearance for use in gynecologic procedures in 2005. As robotic technology has gained popularity in the various surgical specialties, studies comparing laparoscopic vs robotic performance in laboratory drills have emerged. These studies demonstrate improved accuracy, fewer errors, a shorter learning curve, and faster intracorporeal suturing and knot tying.[6] These attributes of robotic assistance provide a means of performing traditional open surgery via minimally invasive methods. Current studies clearly demonstrate the feasibility and safety of applying robotics to the entire spectrum of gynecologic procedures including hysterectomy, myomectomy, sacrocolpoplexy, gynecologic cancer staging and tubal reanastomosis. Studies have demonstrated improved surgical outcomes (decreased blood loss, shorter length of stay, decreased pain and earlier return to activities) with robotic surgery when compared with an abdominal route.[7]

Laparoscopic myomectomy is surgically challenging and requires considerable training and expertise. The ability to enucleate myomas and adequately perform a multilayered closure, the associated learning curve, concern about uterine rupture and the risk of recurrence, which seems to be higher after laparoscopic myomectomy compared with laparotomy, may explain the reluctance to shift to a laparoscopic approach.[8] The emergence of robotic technology has allowed patients who typically would have undergone laparotomy in the past to now undergo minimally invasive myomectomy.[9,10] The use of robotic assistance greatly facilitates a surgeon's ability to perform the crucial steps in a myomectomy including meticulous dissection and skilled suturing and thus expands the scope of eligible patients. Robotic assistance helps to remove myomas and suture the uterine defect in odd locations as well. Lack of equivalent haptic feedback, inability to apply torque and extended operative time are challenges that surgeons encounter when performing robotic assisted myomectomy. Comparison of outcomes for laparoscopic and robotic-assisted laparoscopic myomectomy has demonstrated comparable clinical outcomes for blood loss, hospital stay and complications despite longer robotic operative times.[11,12]

Robotic-assisted myomectomies are performed under general anaesthesia with a standard 4–5 port approach. All patients are placed in a low dorsal lithotomy position with arms padded and tucked at their sides. Four-five trocars are typically used after pneumoperitoneum is obtained. A 12-mm supraumbilical or umbilical camera port (depending on the size of the uterus), and two or three lower quadrant ancillary 8-mm ports are mounted to the robotic arms. A precise bipolar forceps, a monopolar scissors and a single tooth tenaculum are used as the instruments. If need be, even robotic harmonic instrument can be used. An additional 5-mm accessory port is inserted laterally for the suction-irrigation device. This could be a 12-mm port, which facilitates introduction of suture and a tissue morcellator. The patient is placed in steep trendelenburg position and the each trocar is attached to the assigned robotic arm. The robot can be docked using central or side docking.

Side docking (Fig. 29.1) is preferred as most patients receive an intrauterine manipulator to better mobilize the uterus. Operative field survey is performed, after which a diluted solution of vasopressin may be infiltrated into the myometrium surrounding the myoma as an adjunct for haemostasis.[13]

The myoma's visceral peritoneum is incised by Hot Shears scissors, proceeding in depth into the correct plane under the myometrium till the myoma capsule is identified and the myoma surface is exposed.

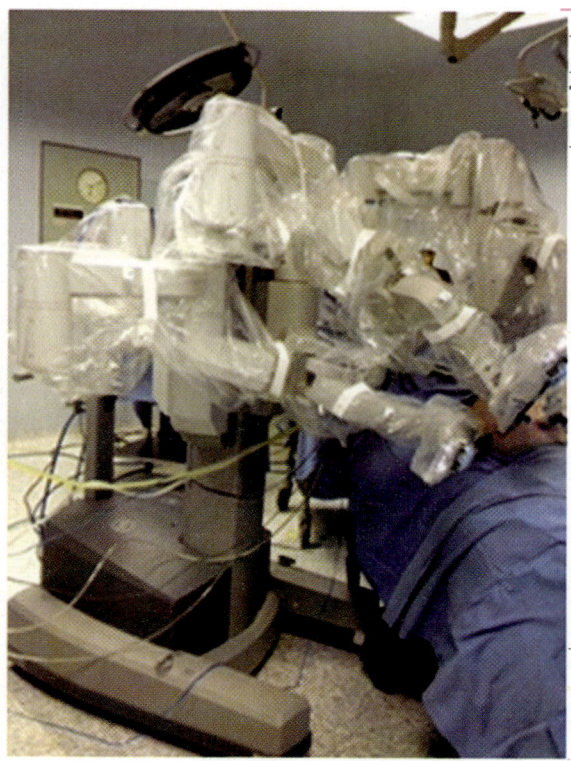

Fig. 29.1: Side docking

Monopolar scissors are used to free the base of the myoma and haemostasis is achieved by low-wattage bipolar forceps. Goal is to minimize the trauma and decrease the blood loss. If need be, even robotic harmonic instruments are then changed to needle drivers.

Myometrium closure is performed in multiple layers of 0 vicryl or barbed Vloc running suture and covered with baseball type suture (Fig. 29.2).

If the uterine cavity is opened, deep myometrial sutures are employed to the edges. All suturing is done intracorporally. The specimen is removed via morcellation. An adhesion/haemostatic prophylaxis measure can be employed. Chromopertubation is performed to check for tubal patency when deep intramural myomas are removed in patients with infertility.

The earliest published series of robot-assisted laparoscopic myomectomy was from Advincula et al. In their series of 35 patients, mean (SD) myoma weight was 223.2 (244.1) g (95% confidence interval, 135-310.6). The mean number of myomas removed was 1.6 (range, 1-5), and the mean diameter was 7.9+/-3.9 cm (95%CI, 6.6-9.1). Mean estimated blood loss was 169 (198.7) mL (95% CI, 201.6-260.0). Mean operating time was 230.8 (83) minutes (95% CI, 201-260.0). Median length of stay for these patients was 1 day. Total conversion rate was 8.6%, comparable to other published studies of conventional

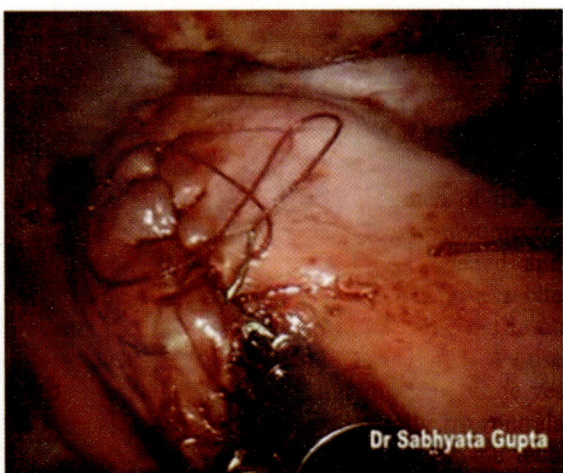

Fig. 29.2: Closure of myometrium

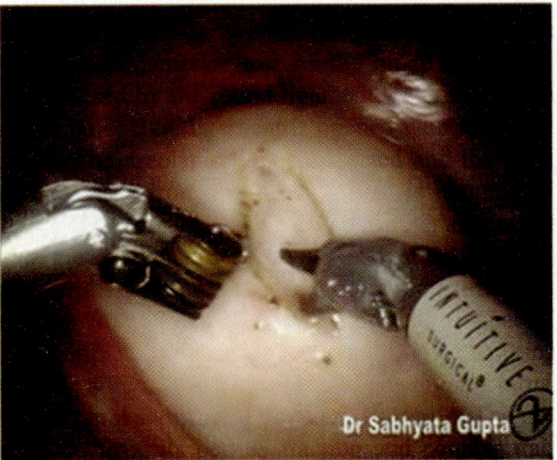

Fig. 29.3: The fibroid is secured by a robotic tenaculum to perform the traction necessary for its enucleation

laparoscopic myomectomy with ranges from 0% through 28.7%. Two of the reported conversions were secondary to an absence of tactile feedback, which made enucleation of myomas difficult (Figs 29.3 and 29.4).[14]

The largest comparative study to date of robotic myomectomy compared with the standard approach to laparotomy is also by Advincula et al. 58 patients with symptomatic fibroids were studied in a retrospective case-matched analysis with 29 patients in each arm. Noteworthy findings were decreased estimated blood loss (mean, 195.69 mL) and length of stay (mean, 1.48 days). Both these differences were statistically significant at p < 0.5. Complication rates were also lower in the robotic group. Operative time was longer in the robotic group (mean, 231.38 minutes).[13]

Given the limited tactile sensation appreciated during robotic-assisted myomectomy, accurate preoperative fibroid mapping is essential. The sensitivity to detect uterine fibroids has been reported to be 2-fold greater with magnetic resonance imaging compared with transvaginal ultrasonography (80% vs 40%). A study by Griffin et al hypothesized that small intramural myomas, not visible laparoscopically but palpable abdominally may be missed during robotic surgery. The conclusion was that patients undergoing robotic-assisted myomectomy had a higher residual fibroid burden (5 times greater) outcome compared with patients undergoing abdominal myomectomy when measured by ultrasonography 12 weeks after surgery. This difference was most evident in patients who had large uteri, large surgical specimens and prolonged operative times.[15]

Recent literature on neurofibres and neuropeptides in the fibroid pseudocapsule suggest new horizon in endoscopic gynecological surgery. This fibroid pseudocapsule is composed of a neurovascular network rich in neurofibres similar to the neurovascular bundle surrounding a prostate. Gentle uterine leiomyoma detachment from the pseudocapsule

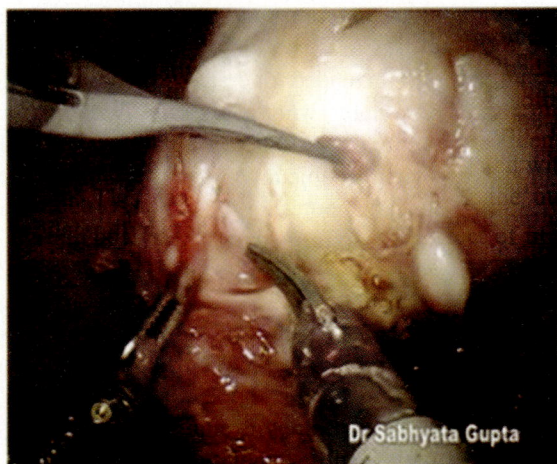

Fig. 29.4: Fibroid being enucleated

neurovasscular bundle has allowed a reduction in uterine bleeding and uterine musculature trauma with sparing of the pseudocapsule neuropeptide fibres. The intracapsular fibroid nerve-sparing micro surgery with robotic magnification preserves the neurovascular bundle and neurotransmitters surrounding fibroids. This maximizes uterine healing and restoration of myometrium for potential future fertility and minimizes risk of uterine rupture during pregnancy or labour.[16]

The pregnancy outcomes following robotic-assisted myomectomies are similar to the open surgery. Pitter et al, studied these outcomes, reporting 92 deliveries out of 107 patients studied with only 1 uterine rupture.[17] Successful term pregnancies after robotic myomectomy have also been reported.[18]

In future comprehensive evaluation with larger sample sizes answering the pertinent questions of uterine rupture and pregnancy rates are needed. Long term surgical outcomes and more accurate cost-benefit analysis are warranted.

REFERENCES

1. Laughlin S K, Stewart EA. Uterine Leiomyomas; individualizing the approach to a heterogeneous condition. Obstet Gynecol. 2011;117(2):396-403.
2. Agdi M, Tulandi T. Minimally Invasive approach for Myomectomy. Semin repord Med. 2010;28(3):228-34.
3. Semm K. New Methods of pelviscopy (gynecologic laparoscopy) for myomectomy, ovariectomy, Tubectomy and adnectomy. Endoscopy. 1979;11(2):85-93.
4. Gobern J, Rosemeyer CJ, Barter J, et al. Comparison of Robotic, Laparoscopic and Abdominal myomectomy in a community hospital. Journal of the society of Laparoendoscopic surgeons. (2013)17:116-20.
5. Stylopoulos N, Rattner D. Robotics and ergonomics. Surg Clin North Am. 2003;83:1-12.
6. Magrina JF. Robotic surgery in Gynecolgoy. Eur J Gynaecol Oncol. 2007;28:77-82.
7. Patzkowsky KE, Sawsan As-Sanie, Smorgick N, et al. Perioperative outcomes of Robotic versus laparoscopic hysterectomy for benign disease. Journal of the society of Laparoendoscopic surgeons. (2013)17:100-6.
8. Doribot V, Dubuisson JB, Chapron C, et al. Recurrence of leiomyomata after laparoscopic myomectomy. J Am Assoc Gynecol Laparosc. 2001;8:495-500.
9. Barakat EE, Bedaiway MA, Zimberg S, et al. Robotic-assisted Laparoscopic and abdominal myomectomy; a comparison of surgical outcomes. Obstet Gynecol. 2011;117(2Pt1):256-65.
10. Nash K, Feinglass J, Zei C, et al. Robotic assisted laparoscopic myomectomy versus abdominal myomectomy: a comparative analysis of surgical outcomes and costs. Arch Gynecol Obstet. 2012;285(2):435-40.
11. Bedient CE, Magrina JF, Noble BN, et al. Comparison of Robotic and Laparoscopic myomectomy. Am J Obstet Gynecol. 2009;201(6):566.e1-5.
12. Nezhat C, Lavie O, Hsu S, et al. Robotic-assisted Laparoscopic myomectomy compared with standard laparoscopic myomectomy- a retrospective matched control study. Fertil Steril. 2009;91(2):556-9.
13. Arnold P. Advincula, Xiao Xu, et al. Robotic Assisted Laparoscopic myomectomy versus abdominal myomectomy: A comparison of short-term surgical outcomes and immediate costs. Journal of Minimally Invasive Gynecology. 2007;14:698-705.
14. Advincula AP, Song A, Burke W, et al. Preliminary experience with robot-assisted laparoscopic myomectomy. J Am Assoc Gynecol Laparosc. 2004;11:511-8.
15. Griffin L, Feinglass J, Garret A, et al. Postoperative outcomes after Robotic versus abdominal myomectomy. Journal of the society of Laparoendoscopic surgeons. 2013;17:407-13.
16. Tinelli A, Malvasi A, Mettler L, et al. Surgical management of neurovascular bundle in uterine fibroid pseudocapsule . Journal of the society of Laparoendoscopic surgeons. 2012;16:119-29.
17. Pitter MC, Gargiulo AR, Bonaventura LM, et al. Pregnancy outcomes following robot-assited myomectomy. Hum Reprod. 2013;28:99-108.
18. Bocca S, Stadtmauer L, Oehninger S. Uncomplicated full term pregnancy after da Vinci-assisted laparoscopic myomectomy. Reprod Biomed Online. 2007;14:246-9.

SECTION 6

Others

CHAPTER 30

Iatrogenic Fibroids

● Chaithra TM

The prevalence of minimally invasive surgery has led to a new type of parasitic myoma—the iatrogenic parasitic myoma.[1,2] In some papers, this kind of myoma is called disseminated peritoneal leiomyomatosis (DPL).[3–5] This suggests a subset of DPL that is secondary to transcoelomic dissemination of a primary uterine leiomyoma rather than a de novo peritoneal metaplasia.[6]

In the minimally invasive procedures, the removal of different sizes of myoma through small wounds requires fragmenting the myomas in the abdominal cavity. However, this morcellation process may disseminate viable myoma particles in the abdominal cavity. In rare instances, minute myoma particles may survive and become implanted into tissue. In the past 10 years, the incidence of iatrogenic parasitic myomas has increased because of the increased use of minimally invasive surgery. Iatrogenic parasitic myoma nevertheless remains a rare late complication with an incidence of < 1% (Fig. 30.1). Iatrogenic fibroids are classified as:

1. Iatrogenic parasitic fibroid.
2. Disseminated peritoneal leiomyomatosis.

The most common symptoms are pain, mass sensation and deep dyspareunia. Most of parasitic myomas are asymptomatic. From the literature review, most (78%) patients received laparoscopic myomectomy with morcellation for their first surgery, and there were often multiple lesions with varying sizes (range, 0.8–30 cm).

Parasitic myoma occurred at various sites, including the port site, intestines, peritoneum and omentum in the abdominal cavity (Fig. 30.2). These sites are also the dependent part of the abdominal cavity and receive abundant blood supply, which suggests seeding of myometrial tissues during morcellation1. The interval between the initial surgery and the second surgery ranged from 2 to 108 months (on average, 47.2 months).

A few cases of disseminated leiomyomas have also been reported after abdominal hysterectomy,[8–10] which suggests that factors other than morcellation may be responsible for the recurrence.

Relationship to hormonal stimulation is supported by oestrogen and progesterone receptors in the lesions and by the occurrence of cases in an increased hormonal milieu such as pregnancy, oral contraceptive use, hormone replacement therapy, tamoxifen administration, oestrogen-secreting tumours, ovarian stimulation.[4]

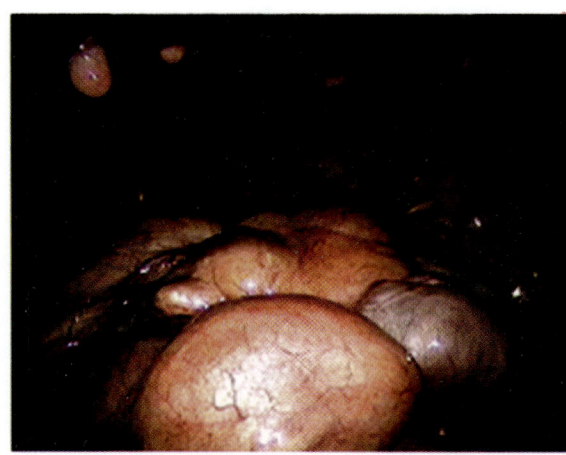

Fig. 30.1: Diffuse peritoneal leiomatosis

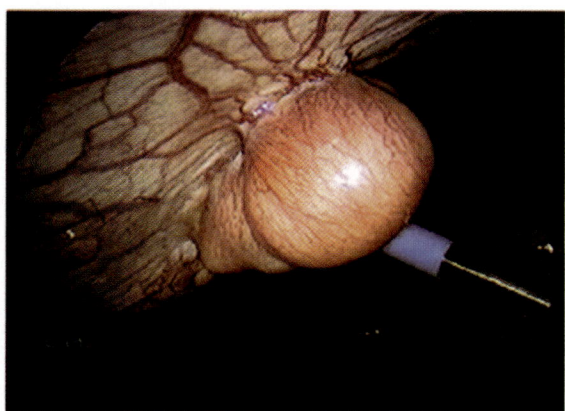

Fig. 30.2: Morcellator site parasitic fibroid

■ PREVENTION

Minute fragments of myoma tissue will be produced if the morcellator is not sufficiently sharp, which can be easily missed and left in the abdomen, and may become implanted into peritoneal or omental tissue. Therefore, it is imperative to ensure that the morcellator is sufficiently sharp. For fragile myomas, the fragments can be collected into an endobag and removed completely. If morcellation is performed after the enucleation of multiple myomas, specimens may be missed and remain in the abdomen because of the Trendelenburg position, especially when the myomas are small. Therefore, in situ morcellation, careful removal of remnants and vigorous irrigation with normal saline with a concomitant change in position may decrease the incidence of retained myoma tissue in the abdomen during surgery (Fig. 30.3).[11–13]

At the end of surgery, long-term follow-up is likewise recommended to detect the occurrence of parasitic myoma even in menopausal patients because of the potential of malignancy. For patients with suspected malignant myomas, a total abdominal hysterectomy is recommended. If malignancy is an incidental finding in laparoscopic myomectomy, complete cancer staging surgery is mandatory (Bos 30.1).

Box 30.1: Prevention of parasitic iatrogenic myoma

Prevention of parasitic iatrogenic myoma
Morcellator should be adequately sharp
Morcellation inside the endobag
Removing bits of myomas thoroughly then and there
Vigorous irrigation of pelvis in reverse trendlenberg position with normal saline with a concomitant change in position may decrease the incidence of retained myoma
Keep a check on all the myomas enucleated
Use the morcellator with least scattering effect

■ MANAGEMENT

Surgical treatment for symptomatic lesions and role of GnRH agonists in their treatment have to be further evaluated. Leren et al[14] have reported a case of intestinal perforation during surgery for parasitic myomas measuring 5 cm. Aust et al[15] have reported a case of parasitic myoma resembling ovarian malignancy in which surgery was performed by a gynecologic oncologist. Extensive and complicated surgery may be required for parasitic myomas. Patients should be informed about this extensive surgery (Table 30.1).

Case 1

Iatrogenic parasitic fibroid (Fig. 30.4) from anterior wall of rectum presented as chronic constipation, presenting 18 months after a total laparoscopic hysterectomy for multiple fibroid uterus. This surgery was done with gastroenterologist assistance and went on for 5 hours due to retroperitoneal location of fibroid and adhesions.

Case 2

44 year lady presented with acute urinary retention to emergency department, following total abdominal hysterectomy and left salpingophorectomy for 28 weeks size fibroid uterus with chocolate cyst. On examination she had 16

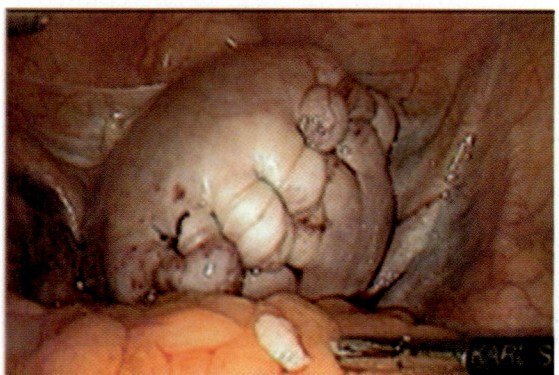

Fig. 30.3: Piece of fibroid, which can give rise to parasitic fibroid

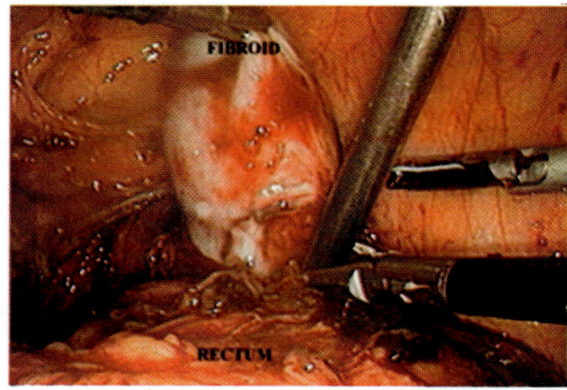

Fig. 30.4: Iatrogenic fibroid

Table 30.1: Review of the literature of parasitic myoma after surgery

Study	No. of cases	Diagnosis	First operation	Morcellation	Interval (mo)	Signs and symptoms	Second operation	M (no.)	M size (cm)	Location	Histology
Ostrzenski, 1997[3]	1	Uterine leiomyoma particle growing	LM	Yes	2	Mass	Lapa	1	1	Port site	Leiomyoma
Hutchins and Reinoehl, 1998[7]	1	Retained myoma	LASH	Yes	1	Abdominal pain	Lapa	5	4	Liver, gallbladder	Leiomyoma
Rajab et al, 2000[17]	1	DPL	TAH + BSO	Yes	24	Abdominal distension	Lapa	m	12	CDS, suprapubic, small bowel, liver	Multiple leiomyomatosis disseminata
Sharma et al, 2004[18]	1	DPL with malignant change	TAH	Unknown	84	Abdominal swelling	Lapa	m	7	Omentum, mesentery	Leiomyosarcoma arising in leiomyomatosis peritonealis disseminata
LaCoursiere et al, 2005	1	Retained myoma	TLH	Yes	10	Dyspareunia, dysuria, and pelvic pain	LM	4	4	Abdomen and pelvis	Leiomyoma-cervical tissue
Donnez et al, 2006[11]	1	Iatrogenic peritoneal adenomyoma	LASH + BSO	Yes	60	Pelvic pain, dyspareunia	LM	1	4	CDS	Adenomyosis
Paul and Koshy, 2006[19]	1	Multiple peritoneal parasitic myomas	LM	Yes	30	None	LM	3	2	Port site, fundus, right paracolic gutter	Leiomyoma
Sinha et al, 2007[2]	2	Postlaparoscopic hysterectomy myomas	LM/TLH	Yes	12, 36	Pain, mass	LM	2, 3	10, 15	Sigmoid colon serosa, lateral pelvic wall, CDS, diaphragm dome	Leiomyoma
Takeda et al, 2007	1	Parasitic peritoneal leiomyosis	LM (in situ)	Yes	72	Mass	LM	5	6	Omentum, round ligament, pelvic sidewall, CDS	Leiomyoma
Moon et al, 2008	1	Parasitic leiomyoma	LM	Yes	36	Mass	Lapa	1	3	Port site	Leiomyoma

Contd...

Contd...

Study											
Kumar et al, 2008	1	DPL	LM	Yes	11	Abdominal distension	Lapa	6	30	Omentum, colon	Leiomyoma
Epstein et al, 2009	1	Parasitic myoma	LM	Yes	18	Pelvic pain	LM	2	8	Omentum, sigmoid colon	Leiomyoma
Thian et al, 2009[6]	1	DPL	LM	Yes	29	Mass	Lapa	>50	15	Omentum, colon, abdominal wound	Leiomyoma
Wada-Hiraike et al, 2009	1	Aberrant myoma	LAM	Scalpel	54	Mass	Lapa	1	15	Previous operation site	Leiomyoma
Kho et al, 2009	9	Parasitic myoma	6 LM, 1 TAH, 2 M	8: 6 LSC and 2 Lapa	75	Pain, menorrhagia, dyspareunia, pelvic pressure		(3; all are LM)		Pelvis (14/15), GI tract (6/15), upper abdomen (1/15)	Leiomyoma
Al-Talib and Tulandi, 2010[4]	1	DPL	LASH	Yes	84	Mass	Lapa	16	9	Abdomen and pelvis	
Larrain et al, 2010	4	Iatrogenic parasitic myoma	2 LM, 2 TLH	Yes	99	Pain, vaginal mass	3 LM, TVM	4	4–7	Pelvis, vagina, CDS	Leiomyoma
Payyapilly et al, 2010[12]	1	Iatrogenic Parasitic myoma	LAM	Scalpel	36	Infertility	LM				
Pezzuto et al, 2010	2	Bowel leiomyoma	2 LM	Yes	132	None	LAVH, M	3	3,5	Intestine	Leiomyoma
Cucinella et al, 2011[20]	4	Parasitic myoma	LM, TAH	Yes	####, ####	Mass, pain, dyspareunia	LM	1,2, 3,5	1.8,3. 5,6,6		Leiomyoma
Current report[21]	1	Parasitic myoma	LM	Yes	87	Mass	LM	2	6	Small intestine, left tube	Cellular leiomyoma

BSO = bilateral salpingoophorectmy; CDS = cul-de-sac; DPL = disseminated peritoneal leiomyomatosis; GI = gastrointestinal; LAM = laparoscopic-assisted myomectomy; Lapa = laparotomy; LASH = laparoscopic subtotal hysterectomy; LAVH = laparoscopic-assisted vaginal hysterectomy; LM = laparoscopic myomectomy; LSC = laparoscope; m = multiple; M = myomectomy; TAH = transabdominal hysterectomy; TLH = total laparoscopic hysterectomy; TVM = transvaginal myomectomy.

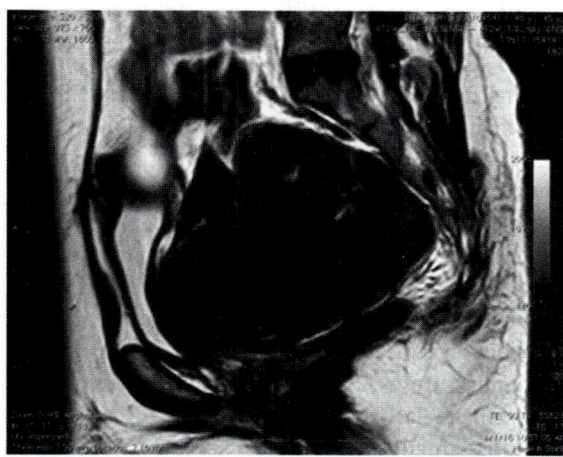

Fig. 30.5: Multiplanar MRI images of a 45-year-old female who has undergone hysterectomy 2 years back. Midline sagittal T2WI through pelvis, showing hypointense well defined solid mass lesion with lobulated outline, filling nearly the pelvis, displacing the small bowel loops, compressing the urinary bladder and neck of bladder, consistent with recurrent fibroid.

weeks size mass and on magnetic resonance imaging (MRI) (Fig. 30.5) a fibroid filling nearly the pelvis and displacing the bowel loops, compressing the urinary bladder and neck of bladder was seen and was removed laparoscopically.

◼ REFERENCES

1. Williams LJ, Pavlick FJ. Leiomyomatosis peritonealis disseminata: two case reports and a review of the medical literature. Cancer. 1980;45:1726-33.
2. Sinha R, Sundaram M, Mahajan C, et al. Multiple leiomyomas after laparoscopic hysterectomy: report of two cases. J Minim Invasive Gynecol. 2007;14:123-7.
3. Ostrzenski A. Uterine leiomyoma particle growing in an abdominal wall incision after laparoscopic retrieval. Obstet Gynecol. 1997;89:853-4.
4. Al-Talib A, Tulandi T. Pathophysiology and possible iatrogenic cause of leiomyomatosis Peritonealis disseminata. Gynecol Obstet Invest. 2010;69:239-44.
5. Willson JR, Peale AR. Multiple peritoneal leiomyomas associated with a granulose cell tumor of the ovary. Am J Obstet Gynecol. 1952;64:204-8.
6. Thian YL, Tan KH, Kwek JW, et al. Leiomyomatosis peritonealis disseminata and subcutaneous myomada rare complication of laparoscopic myomectomy. Abdom Imaging. 2009;34:235-8.
7. Hutchins FL, Reinoehl EM. Retained myoma after laparoscopic supra-cervical hysterectomy with morcellation. J Am Assoc Gynecol Laparosc. 1998;5:293-5.
8. Chang WC, Chou LY, Chang DY, et al. Simultaneous laparoscopic uterine artery ligation and laparoscopic myomectomy for symptomatic uterine myomas with and without in situ morcellation. Hum Reprod. 2011;26:1735-40.
9. Chen SY, Huang SC, Sheu BC, et al. Simultaneous enucleation and in situ morcellation of myomas in laparoscopic myomectomy. Taiwan J Obstet Gynecol. 2009;49:279-84.
10. Chang WC, Huang PS, Wang PH, et al. Comparison of laparoscopic myomectomy using in situ morcellation with and without uterine artery ligation for treatment of symptomatic myomas. J Minim Invasive Gynecol. 2012;19:715-21.
11. Donnez O, Jadoul P, Squifflet J, et al. Iatrogenic peritoneal adenomyoma after laparoscopic subtotal hysterectomy and uterine morcellation. Fertil Steril. 2006;86:1511-2.
12. Payyapilly PG, Naik S, Borisa R, et al. Laparoscopic removal of multiple parasitic myomas adherent to the bowel. J Gynecol Surg. 2010;26:73-7.
13. Nezhat C, Kho K. Iatrogenic myomas: new class of myomas? J Minim Invasive Gynecol. 2010;17:544-50.
14. Leren V, Langebrekke A, Qvigstad E. Parasitic leiomyomas after laparoscopic surgery with morcellation. Acta Obstet Gynecol Scand. 2012;91:1233-6.
15. Aust T, Gale P, Cario G, et al. Bowel resection for iatrogenic parasitic fibroids with preoperative investigations suggestive of malignancy. Fertil Steril. 2011;96:e1-3.
16. PS Huang, et al. Taiwanese Journal of Obstetrics & Gynecology. 2014;53:392-6.
17. KE Rajab, AN Aradi, BN Datta. Post-menopausal leiomyomatosis peritonealis disseminate.Int J Gynaecol Obstet. 2000;68:271-2.
18. P Sharma, KU Chaturvedi, R Gupta, et al. Leiomyomatosis peritonealis disseminata with malignant change in a post-menopausal woman. Gynecol Oncol. 2004;95:742-5.
19. PG Paul, AK Koshy. Multiple peritoneal parasitic myomas after laparoscopic myomectomy and morcellation. Fertil Steril. 2006;85:492-3.
20. Cucinella R, Granese G, Calagna E, et al. Parasitic myomas after laparoscopic surgery: an emerging complication in the use of morcellator? Description of four cases.Fertil Steril. 2011;96:e90-e96.
21. Ramesh B, Sharma Pooja, Gunge Dipti. Abdominal wall parasitic myoma following electromechanical morcellation. The Journal of Obstetrics and Gynecology of India. 2014;64):S73-S75.

CHAPTER 31

Rare Forms of Fibroids

● Rachana Ghanti

■ INTRODUCTION

Leiomyomas are the most common tumours of the uterus. They are responsible for about 1/3rd of hospital admissions to gynaecology department. Growth of leiomyoma is dependent on oestrogen production. The tumour thrives during the period of greatest ovarian activity. Continuous oestrogen secretion especially when uninterrupted by pregnancy and lactation is thought to be the most important risk factor in development of myomata. After menopause, with regression of ovarian oestrogen secretion, growth of leiomyoma usually ceases.

■ TYPICAL SYMPTOMS OF UTERINE MYOMAS

The symptoms of this disease are mainly related to the physical changes in the pelvic organs arising from the onset of this tumour and may present in women of any age, but usually in women between menarche and menopause. When a female of reproductive age presents with symptoms like menorrhagia, dysmenorrhoea, giddiness, pallor, dyspnoea, urinary frequency and constipation, it may be common to quickly assume a diagnosis of uterine fibroids. On the other hand, some unusual or atypical symptoms like acute abdominal pain, and pain between periods or internal bleeding do occur in patients with a well-established diagnosis of uterine fibroids that may be ignored, leading to a misdiagnosis and further delay in medical management (Table 31.1).

Compression Symptoms

The symptoms related to myomas are primarily those of physical changes to the pelvic organs due to the presence of an enlarging mass.[1–3] Pelvic heaviness or a dull aching sensation, increased urinary frequency and urgency can also develop, especially when these tumours arise from the anterior wall of the uterus. In addition, these symptoms might worsen with the onset of menses, thereby aggravating menses-related symptoms.[3]

Table 31.1: Typical and atypical symptoms of fibroids

Typical symptoms	Atypical symptoms
Menorrhagia	Rectal symptoms—constipation-Tenesmus
Pain	Urinary symptoms—urinary retention, haematuria, others
Dysmenorrhoea	Abdominal symptoms
Infertility	Respiratory symptoms—dyspnoea, chest pain
Pressure symptoms	Pruritus
	Hiccup or internal bleeding
	Vaginal protruding mass/uterine inversion
	Deep dyspareunia

Menses-related Symptoms

Abnormal menstruation, including excess or prolonged bleeding, is believed to be the most common symptom and is experienced by about 30% of women with myomas. However, the most common menses-related symptom is menorrhagia. Other symptoms of anaemia, including pallor, fainting, dyspnoea, and fatigue might result from massive blood loss whenever menses begins, and could worsen during menses.

Pain-related Symptoms

About one-third of women with myomas experience pelvic pain. Dysmenorrhoea seems less common in this group.

■ ATYPICAL SYMPTOMS OF UTERINE MYOMAS

Uncommon Compression-related Symptoms

The masses arising from the posterior wall might cause rectal symptoms like tenesmus, back pain or constipation, though they appear to be less common. These symptoms might worsen when menses comes and can aggravate the symptoms related to menses. Flank pain, especially on the right side, is an atypical symptom of the uterine myoma, and is due to compression of the ureter, although its incidence is far below our expectation.

Transient relief after lying on the opposite side might be reliable evidence of the existence of this compression.[4]

Cardiac Symptoms

Chest pain might occur in a rare condition known as intravenous leiomyomatosis.[5] Benign smooth muscle fibres invade the venous channels of the pelvis and, even though they grow slowly, they might grow into the vena cava and right heart and cause these unusual symptoms.

Abdominal Symptoms

Abdominal symptoms mimicking pelvic carcinomatosis multiple pelvic growths with various compression symptoms with or without ascites will raise the suspicion of pelvic carcinomatosis. However, another rare benign condition, leiomyomatosis peritonealis disseminata (LPD), which is caused by the direct seeding of myomatous cells on the surface of the peritoneum, could be the possible diagnosis. It is believed that LPD is associated with recent pregnancy or previous operation for myoma using a morcellator.[6,7]

Respiratory Symptoms

Dyspnoea with pleural effusion, pelvic mass and ascites mimicking Meigs syndrome is another rare carcinoma-like presentation of this disease. Leiomyoma arising from the uterus,[8] ovary[9] or fallopian tube[10] might be the only diagnosis.

Pruritus

Pruritus with multiple raised skin lesions on the limbs is unusual and is the only symptom of piloleiomyoma.[11] However, the coexistence of uterine myoma and cutaneous leiomyoma nodules might be the initial symptom of piloleiomyoma. Renal evaluation should be done first in cases of piloleiomyoma, before conservative follow-up is recommended, because piloleiomyoma is often accompanied with renal carcinoma.

Hiccup or Internal Bleeding

Unusual symptoms like hiccup or internal bleeding might result from a subserosal myoma with rapid growth. While the former might be irritation of the vagus or phrenic nerve and deserve a more thorough evaluation before operation. The latter might be due to rupture of superficial vessels and deserve prompt diagnosis and emergency management.

Vaginal Protruding Mass or Uterine Inversion

Sometimes submucous myoma induces uterine inversion, which results in haemorrhage. If this rapid growth occurs in a menopausal woman, then malignant change must be highly suspected, and imaging might help to distinguish benign and malignant uterine masses.

Urinary Symptoms

Uterine fibroid can atypically present with haematuria and ureteric colic, and cause extrinsic ureteral obstruction. Although the uterine fibroid is the most common benign tumour of the female upper genital tract and the one most likely to cause ureteral obstruction in females,[5] it rarely obstructs the ureter.

■ RARE VARIETIES

Broad Ligament Fibroid

Broad ligament is a very uncommon site for presentation of leiomyoma. On account of their size and nature (pedunculated or sessile), clinically leiomyomas may present variably (Figs 31.1A and B).

On developing a long tenacious stalk, the subserosal leiomyoma may become a wandering or migrating leiomyoma. Occasionally, such masses become adherent to the surrounding structures such as broad ligament or omentum or retroperitoneal connective tissue, where they receive auxiliary blood supply and lose their original attachment to the uterus. They are then called parasitic leiomyoma. On histological evaluation, they exhibit features similar to those of their uterine counterparts.

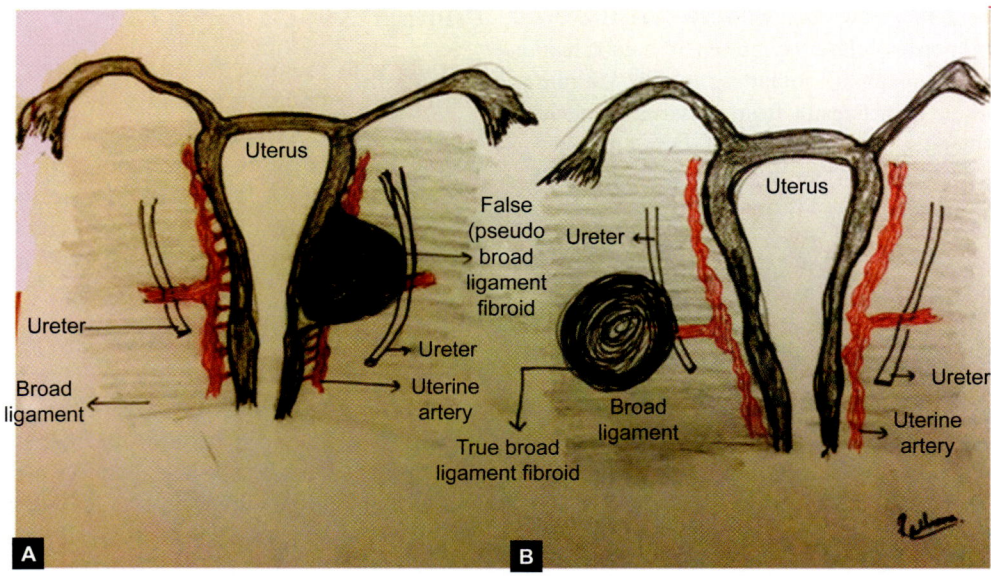

Figs 31.1A and B: A. Pseudo broad ligament fibroid—note the relation of ureter, lateral and below the fibroid; **B.** True broad ligament fibroid—the ureter is usually medial and below or above the fibroid.

Patients usually present with lower abdominal pain, mass per abdomen or pelvic mass. Paraovarian leiomyoma can present as inguinal masses or acute abdomen. Rarely, pedunculated leiomyoma undergo torsion and present with acute abdomen. Giant fibroids are known to arise from the uterus, but occasionally from the broad ligament. Sometimes broad ligament leiomyoma may be associated with massive ascites and bilateral pleural effusion (Table 31.2).

Table 31.2: Difference between true and pseudo broad ligament fibroid

True broad ligament fibroid	False broad ligament fibroid
Arises from mesenchymal remnants of broad ligament or smooth muscle in intima media of blood vessels	Arises from lateral wall of uterus or supravaginal cervix
No pseudocapsule	Has a pseudocapsule
Does not have any connection with the uterus	Has a pedicle connecting it to the uterus, usually broad
Ureter can lie anywhere, above, below, medial or lateral to the fibroid	Ureter always lies below and lateral to the fibroid

Key point—always stay within the pseudocapsule while dissecting the fibroid (enucleation) to prevent ureteric injury.

(Kindly refer to videos for the demonstration of broad ligament myomectomy).

Retroperitoneal Fibroids

Incidence

The incidence is quite low, and it is even lower for those extending to or originating in the abdomen. 73% of these are located in the pelvis. Most of the published case reports diagnosed the cases clinically as retroperitoneal growths with high suspicion of malignancy without suspecting their leiomyomatous nature.

Origin

Poliquin and coworkers observed a 40% association of retroperitoneal leiomyomas with uterine counterparts or a history of hysterectomy due to uterine leiomyomata. Zaitoon suggested the parasitic theory for such tumour growth, while Stutterecker et al, claimed that müllerian cell rests or smooth muscle cells in the retroperitoneal vessels wall are the putative origin. Kho and Nezhat proposed an 'iatrogenic' origin for such growths, while analyzing a case series of extrauterine leiomyomata, mostly of retroperitoneal or intraperitoneal location with no visible connection to the uterus. They found out that 83% of their case series had previous abdominal operations, and 67% had myomectomies, most of them via laparoscopy with morcellation. Thorough radiographic imaging of sonographically diagnosed leiomyomata is important, especially for those which are large in size or present in an uncommon location. The exact aetiology is still an unexplored issue that merits more investigation.

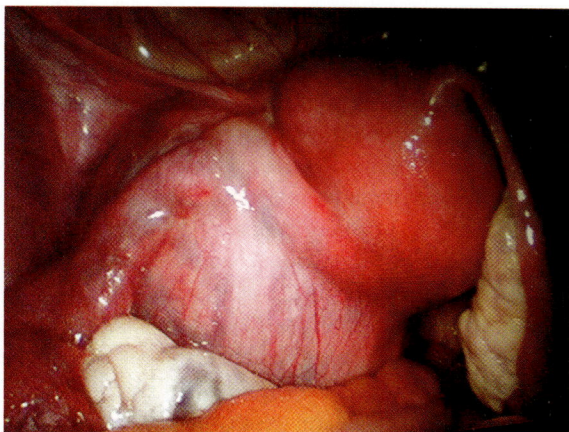

Fig. 31.2: Image of vaginal wall fibroid

Vaginal Wall Fibroids (Fig. 31.2)

Incidence

Leiomyomas in female genital tract are common in the uterus and to some extent in the cervix followed by the round ligament, uterosacral ligament, ovary and inguinal canal. Occurrence in vagina is very rare. Vaginal leiomyomas are commonly seen in the age group ranging from 35 to 50 years and are reported to be more common among caucasian women. They usually occur as single, well-circumscribed mass arising from the midline anterior wall and less commonly, from the posterior and lateral walls. They may be asymptomatic, but depending on the site of occurrence, they can give rise to varying symptoms including lower abdominal pain, low back pain, vaginal bleeding, dyspareunia, frequency of micturition, dysuria or other features of urinary obstruction. These tumours can be intramural or pedunculated and solid as well as cystic. Usually these tumours are single, benign and slow growing but sarcomatous transformation has been reported.

Diagnosis

Preoperatively, diagnosis by ultrasonography may be difficult, but magnetic resonance imaging usually clinches the diagnosis. In magnetic resonance imaging (MRI), they appear as well-demarcated solid masses of low signal intensity in T1- and T2-weighted images, with homogenous contrast enhancement, while leiomyosarcomas and other vaginal malignancies show characteristic high T2 signal intensity with irregular and heterogeneous areas of necrosis or haemorrhage. However, histopathological confirmation is the gold standard of diagnosis and also beneficial to rule out any possible focus of malignancy.

Treatment

Surgical removal of the tumour through vaginal approach, preferably with urethral catheterisation to protect the urethra during surgery, is usually the treatment of choice. In case of large tumours, however, an abdominoperineal approach is preferred.

Bizarre Leiomyoma

An unusual atypical smooth muscle tumour was first described in the stomach by Martin and associates in 1960. Variously called bizarre leiomyoma, leiomyoblastoma, clear-cell leiomyoma, and plexiform tumourlet, these atypical smooth tumours probably all belong together.

Histologically, the characteristic feature is the mixture of rounded polygonal cells and multinucleated giant cells present in epithelioid clear-cell and plexiform patterns.

Clinically, in the uterus most of these tumours are benign. They may rarely exhibit malignant potential. Epithelioid neoplasm's having more than five mitotic figures per 10 high-power fields should be called epithelioid leiomyosarcomas and that the term epithelioid leiomyoma should be applied when there is a lower level of mitotic activity.

Treatment

Although combination therapy (surgery plus radiation therapy or chemotherapy) may not be indicated for a patient with an epithelioid leiomyoma, follow-up should be considered essential, as emphasized by Klunder and colleagues.

Intravenous Leiomyomatosis

An unusual benign form of leiomyomata uteri, it was first recognized at the turn of the 20th century and has been reported sporadically since then.

The characteristic feature being the extension of the polypoid intravascular projections into the veins of the parametrium and broad ligaments. Although there may be some difficulty in distinguishing such lesions from low-grade sarcoma, they are distinctly different histologically from stromatosis uteri because the intravenous plugs are mainly smooth muscle in origin. In 1966, Edwards and Peacock collected 32 cases of intravenous leiomyomatosis in which approximately 50% of the cases, the intravenous tumour was confined to the parametrium; in 75%, it extended no further than the veins of the broad ligament, which suggested that the severed intravenous extensions are probably incapable of independent parasitic existence and remain dormant after removal of the uterus.

Total surgical excision of the tumour should be attempted for successful therapy. Incomplete resection has a tendency of recurrence. This tumour behaves clinically like a benign neoplasm, although its worm-like extensions may involve uterine, vaginal, ovarian and iliac veins. The uterine veins in the broad ligaments are the most common sites of extension.

The mitotic index is quite low, with the most active lesions showing only one mitosis per 15 high-power fields.

Extension of benign leiomyomatosis up to vena cava and into the right atrium has been reported in several cases, with a fatal outcome in some. Several recent cases requiring open-heart surgery to remove the intracardiac tumour thrombosis have been successful and without recurrence. All reported cases occurred in women.

Both intravenous leiomyomatosis and benign metastasizing leiomyoma have been reported to metastasize to the lung. Oophorectomy may be indicated in patients with these conditions, again because of the possibility that these tumours may be oestrogen dependent or that oestrogens may have the ability to stimulate their development, whether in a uterine or extrauterine location and whether they appear to be endothelial or mesenchymal in origin.

The possibility of metastases from a histologically benign uterine leiomyoma may occur, which is usually settled by finding a sarcomatous component in the leiomyoma or by finding evidence of intravenous leiomyomatosis.

Treatment

The recommended treatment consists of surgical removal with castration and little or no oestrogen replacement.

Leiomyomatosis Peritonealis Disseminata

Leiomyomatosis peritonealis disseminata is sometimes confused with intravenous leiomyomatosis. However, only subperitoneal surfaces of the uterus and other pelvic and abdominal viscera are involved with leiomyomatosis peritonealis disseminata, and invasion of the lumen of blood vessels does not occur. Most commonly occurs in patients in the reproductive years who often had large uterine leiomyomata and were usually pregnant or taking oral contraceptives. The condition is likely to be confused with a disseminated intra-abdominal malignancy, but it is entirely benign histologically and clinically.

It may be due to prolonged and continuous stimulation of subperitoneal decidua by either endogenous or exogenous oestrogen or progesterone is important in the pathogenesis of this condition.

Treatment

Although the cell of origin of this tumour is still controversial, the tumour is benign, and the acceptable treatment to date is total abdominal hysterectomy and bilateral salpingo-oophorectomy. If this tumour occurs in the omentum, an omentectomy should also be performed to define more clearly the histologic nature of the lesion.

Ovarian leiomyoma

A primary leiomyoma of the ovary is a very rare case and approximately 70 cases are reported in the literature, since Sangalli first described this tumour in 1862. The size of primary ovarian leiomyoma was usually < 3 cm. Most of these tumours are unilateral. Interestingly, most of the bilateral cases are diagnosed in young patients. The oldest age reported in a bilateral case is 35 years. Usually the presentation of ovarian leiomyoma occurs in the premenopausal, childbearing years. This is also the common age for developing uterine leiomyoma. However, postmenopausal patients represent approximately 16% of cases (Figs 31.3A to C).

Ovarian leiomyomas are mainly asymptomatic and are discovered accidentally during imaging or operation for uterine leiomyoma or other pathologies. A rare presentation was reported by Kurai et al, who reported leiomyoma of the ovary presented with Meigs syndrome, which disappeared after removal of the ovary. Other rare presentations have included lower abdominal mass, ascites with hydrothorax, ascites with polymyositis, ascites with elevated CA125 or even hydronephrosis as a consequence of its huge size. Ovarian leiomyoma is often misdiagnosed preoperatively as pedunculated uterine myoma, ovarian fibroma or even ovarian endometrioma.

The histogenesis of ovarian leiomyoma is not well-known. Some theories hypothesize that the tumour may originate from hilar blood vessels, smooth muscle metaplasia of ovarian stroma, or smooth muscle-like theca externa cells. Its association with uterine leiomyoma may suggest that they share the same mechanisms of development. This theory is explained by the rapid growth of such tumours during pregnancy and their positivity for oestrogen and/or progesterone receptors. Tomas et al, have suggested that ovarian leiomyoma could arise from smooth muscle metaplasia of endometriotic stroma, or it could be derived from myofibroblasts that originate from metaplastic ovarian stromal cells present in the rim of the endometriotic cyst especially if the tumour was associated with endometriosis or endometriotic cysts. The presence of normal ovarian tissue beside the tumour confirms the ovarian origin of the tumour and excludes tumours of other origins, such as leiomyoma of broad ligament or a subserous leiomyoma that grew large and lost its attachments to the uterus (wandering leiomyoma). Despite its rarity, leiomyosarcoma, which has a characteristic microscopic appearance, should also be considered in the differential diagnosis.

Apart from leiomyoma there are other ovarian tumours that show a spindle cell microscopic appearance. Fibroma is the most common ovarian spindle cell neoplasm, but other neoplasms of the sex cord-stromal group may contain spindle

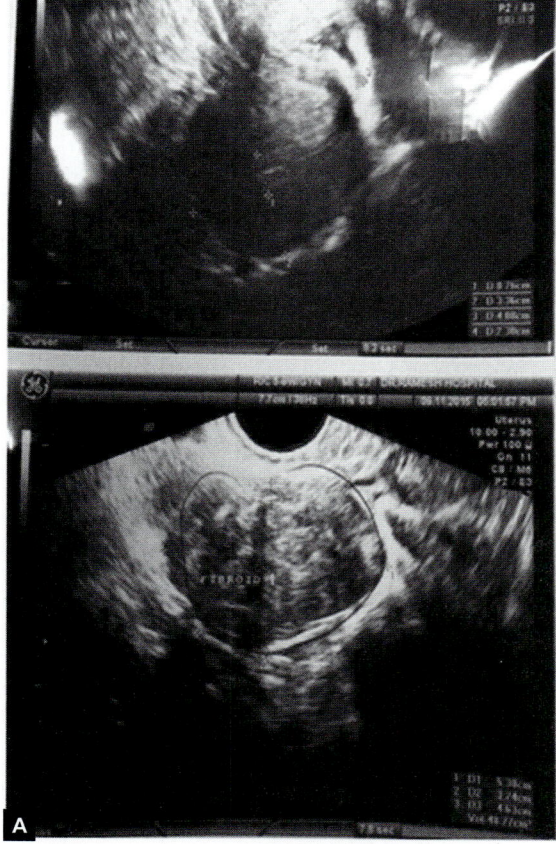

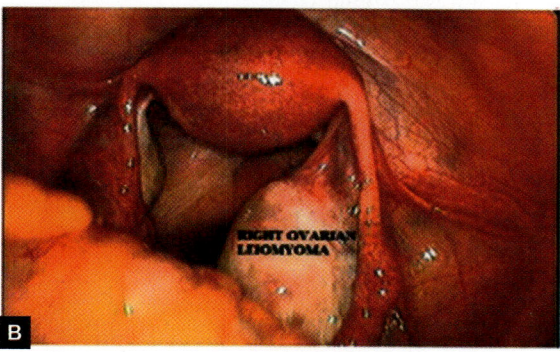

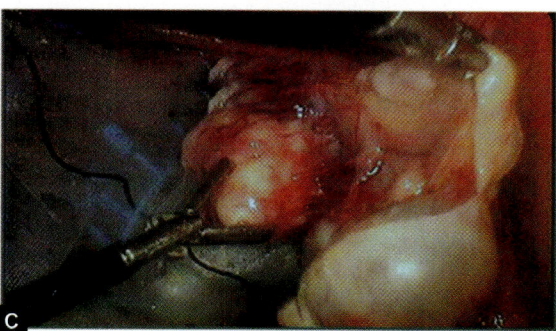

Figs 31.3A to C: A. USG showing ovarian fibroid; **B.** Laparoscopic view of ovarian leiomyoma seen separately from the uterus along with right ovarian endometriotic cyst; **C.** Resection of the tumour completely inside the endobag.

cells and the differential diagnoses may include thecoma, granulosa cell tumour, Sertoli-Leydig cell tumour, sclerosing stromal tumour, and signet-ring stromal tumour.

To confirm the diagnosis and rule out the differential diagnosis the immunohistochemical staining with desmin, inhibin, and α-smooth muscle actin (α-SMA) or histochemical staining with Masson's trichrome should be done. The leiomyoma's cells will be stained with Masson's trichrome, desmin, and α-SMA.

Desmin can be helpful especially, in distinction between leiomyomas and fibromatous tumours because desmin shows diffuse positivity in leiomyomas, whereas fibromatous tumours are typically negative or only focally positive. Ovarian leiomyomas must be also differentiated from leiomyosarcoma, but due to the rarity of these tumours histologic features of malignancy have not been well defined. The literature has reported that many patients with ovarian leiomyomas are nulligravidas. This suggests that oestrogen may play a role in the development of ovarian leiomyomas. A common surgical approach to ovarian leiomyomas in middle-aged to elderly patients is hysterectomy in conjunction with bilateral salpingo-oophorectomy. For bilateral ovarian leiomyomas, bilateral oophorectomy is often required. Wei et al, reported a case in which pedunculated unilateral ovarian leiomyoma and ovarian preservation were possible. In the present case, we performed laparoscopic excision of the tumour with endometriotic cystectomy.

All cases of ovarian leiomyomas demonstrated an excellent prognosis without recurrence despite the active mitosis observed in the tumour. Therefore the surgeon should make an effort to perform less invasive surgery, particularly in young women, to preserve fertility. In conclusion, it is difficult to diagnose ovarian leiomyomas accurately due to their rarity and diagnostic difficulties. However, because primary ovarian leiomyomas occur in young women, the nature of the tumour is typically benign, prognosis is excellent and recurrence is rare, surgeons should consider ovary-preserving surgery as a first choice in surgical management.

A 28-year-old patient presented with infertility and pain abdomen. On USG the mass looked like subserosal fibroid.

We have reported this case in Int J Reprod Contracept obstet Gynecol 2016; 5(3): 927-932 under the title - An uncommon entity of primary ovarian fibroid: A case report.

■ OTHER CLINICAL MANIFESTATIONS

1. Less than 0.5% of women with leiomyomas develop myomatous erythrocytosis syndrome. This may result from excessive erythropoietin production by the kidneys or by the leiomyomas themselves (Kohama, 2000; Yokoyama, 2003). In either case, red cell mass returns to normal following hysterectomy.

20 Leiomyomas occasionally may cause pseudo-Meigs syndrome. Traditionally, Meigs syndrome consists of ascites and pleural effusions that accompany benign ovarian fibromas. However, any pelvic tumour including large, cystic leiomyomas or other benign ovarian cysts can cause this. The presumed aetiology stems from discordancy between the arterial supply to and the venous and lymphatic drainage from leiomyomas. Resolution of ascites and hydrothorax follows hysterectomy.

CONCLUSION

Rare forms are extremely rare and often misdiagnosed. Hence, proper diagnosis and treatment is essential.

REFERENCES

1. Gupta S, Jose J, Manyonda I. Clinical presentation of fibroids. Best Pract Res Clin Obstet Gynaecol. 2008;22:615-26.
2. Cheng MH, Chao HT, Wang PH. Medical treatment for uterine myomas. Taiwan J Obstet Gynecol. 2008;47:18-23.
3. Horng HC, Wen KC, Su WH, et al. Review of myomectomy. Taiwan J Obstet Gynecol. 2012;51:7-11.
4. Wu KY, Yen CF, Huang KG. Obstructive uropathy with acute pyelonephritis induced by a voluminous postmenopausal uterine leiomyoma. Taiwan J Obstet Gynecol. 2009;48:82-3.
5. Lou YF, Shi XP, Song ZZ. Intravenous leiomyomatosis of the uterus with extension to the right heart. Cardiovasc Ultrasound. 2011;9:25.
6. Karasahin KE, Gezginc K, Ulubay M, et al. Disseminated peritoneal leiomyomatosis. Taiwan J Obstet Gynecol. 2008;47:123-5.
7. Cucinella G, Granese R, Calagna G, et al. Parasitic myomas after laparoscopic surgery: an emerging complication in the use of morcellator? Description of four cases. Fertil Steril. 2011;96:e90-6.
8. Hsu WCTP, Chow SN, Huang SC. Pseudo-Meigs' syndrome with degenerative uterine leiomyoma in pregnancy. Taiwan J Obstet Gynecol. 2004;43:161-4.
9. Hsiao CH, Wang HC, Chang SL. Ovarian leiomyoma in a pregnant woman. Taiwan J Obstet Gynecol. 2007;46:311-3.
10. Yang CC, Wen KC, Chen P, et al. Primary leiomyoma of the fallopian tube: preoperative ultrasound findings. J Chin Med Assoc. 2007;70:80-3.
11. Hsiao CH, Wang HC, Chang SL. Ovarian leiomyoma in a pregnant woman. Taiwan J Obstet Gynecol. 2007;46:311-3.

CHAPTER 32

Leiomyosarcoma of the Uterus

● Varsha Rangaraj

■ INTRODUCTION

Uterine sarcomas are a rare and aggressive form of uterine carcinoma. Compared to the more common endometrial carcinomas, uterine sarcomas are more aggressive and have a poorer prognosis.

Most cases of uterine leiomyosarcomas (ULMS) are diagnosed postoperatively as they present as benign leiomyomas clinically. In laparoscopy specimens have to be removed from the abdominal cavity through the trocar opening or the vaginal outlet. When specimens are too large to pass through these they have to be reduced. Power morcellator was being used for this purpose. In April 2014, Food and Drug Administration (FDA) issued a press release discouraging the use of power morcellation during hysterectomy or myomectomy for uterine fibroids due to potential upstaging of uterine sarcoma.[1] This was following an incident where a routine laparoscopic hysterectomy for presumed fibroids revealed occult leiomyosarcoma during pathology examination. The patient further had extensive metastasis, which was thought to have been the result of power morcellation.

Presently 'in-bag' morcellation is investigated as it may possibly prevent morcellation complications.[2]

It is therefore very important for us as laparoscopic surgeons to know how this group of carcinoma presents, the clinical course, management and outcome so we can offer wise choices and advice to our patients.

■ INCIDENCE

Uterine leiomyosarcomas are rare smooth muscle tumours accounting for approximately 1% of patients with uterine cancer[3] with an estimated annual incidence of 0.64 per 100,000 women.[4]

The estimated incidence of occult leiomyosarcoma in patients having surgery for presumed leiomyomata is between 1:200 and 1:11005,[6] with the FDA quoting a risk of 1 in 350 based on its comprehensive review of the literature (Table 32.1).

Uterine leiomyosarcomas are neoplasms of high metastatic potential with 5 year overall survival rates varying between 17% and 55%.[7,8]

Table 32.1: Risk factors for uterine sarcoma

Age	Mean age at diagnosis is 60 years
Race	Two fold higher incidence of leiomyosarcoma in black race
Pelvic irradiation	Strong association especially with carcinosarcoma
Tamoxifen use	Prolonged tamoxifen exposure for 5 years or more
History of childhood retinoblastoma	Higher risk for sarcomas in general, including uterine sarcoma
Hereditary leiomyomatosis and renal cell carcinoma (HLRCC) syndrome	Rare autosomal dominant syndrome. Association of HLRCC and uterine sarcomas often seen in younger women.

AGE GROUP

About 40 to 60 years of age, though rarely seen in women below 40 years.

CLINICAL FEATURES

Abnormal vaginal bleeding and pelvic or abdominal pain is the most common presentation. Amount of bleeding ranges from spotting to menorrhagia and is often associated with foul-smelling vaginal discharge.

Some less common symptoms are weight loss, weakness, lethargy and fever.[10,11] Pelvic examination usually reveals uterus enlarged, sometimes tumour is seen prolapsing through the cervical os and into the vaginal canal. Diagnosis is usually made after surgery based on histopathology so many patients present with advanced disease.

Benign leiomyomas and uterine leiomyosarcomas often coexist in the same uterus, but are genetically distinct entities. Uterine leiomyosarcomas are less common and not hormonally driven.

Leiomyomas are usually multiple, variable size, firm, whorled surface, white in colour, haemorrhage and necrosis less common whereas leiomyosarcomas are often solitary, large > 10 cm, have a soft fleshy cut surface, yellow in colour with haemorrhage and necrosis usually present.

The belief that the risk of uterine leiomyosarcomas is high among women with a 'rapidly growing ' uterus or leiomyoma was proved false in a study of 1322 women admitted to two community hospitals for hysterectomy or myomectomy. Fibroids rarely, if ever, degenerate into uterine leiomyosarcomas.[12]

CLASSIFICATION

The Gynecologic Oncology Group (GOG) divides uterine sarcomas into five categories:
1. Mixed homologous mullerian sarcoma.
2. Mixed heterologous mullerian sarcoma.
3. Leiomyosarcoma.
4. Endometrial stromal sarcoma.
5. Others.

A study on the expression of particular markers in gynaecological cancers (p53, epidermal growth factor, platelet derived growth factor) in tissue samples of patients who had uterine leiomyosarcomas or benign leiomyomas showed significant and molecular differences between benign and malignant smooth muscle tumours of the uterus. Study also showed a prognostic interrelationship between expression of p53 and stage in ULMS.[14]

SMOOTH MUSCLE TUMOURS OF UNCERTAIN MALIGNANT POTENTIAL

A subset of smooth muscle tumours which are not easily classified based on the criteria are called Smooth muscle tumours of uncertain malignant potential (STUMP). There are not enough studies to determine if proliferation index or p53 stains along with basic criteria of mitoses, necrosis and cytologic atypia can help understand the malignant potential of STUMP lesions. However, definitive diagnosis of sarcoma is never based on these stains alone15,16.

Some tumours formerly classified as STUMP have been assigned to the leiomyoma category and should be distinguished from their sarcomatous counterparts. These tumours are mitotically active, cellular, epitheloid, myxoid and atypical tumours.

Mitotically active leiomyomas: Occur in pre-menopausal women, have the typical macroscopic and histologic appearance of a leiomyoma with exception that they have > 5 mf/hpf.

Cellular leiomyomas: Are hypercellular, lack tumour cell necrosis, cytologic atypia and mitotic figures.

Epitheloid leiomyomas: Are yellow or gray and may contain visible areas of haemorrhage and necrosis, usually solitary and softer than usual leiomyoma.

Myxoid leiomyomas: Have myxoid material separating the tumour cells. They are soft and translucent with circumscribed margins with neither cytologic atypia nor mitotic figures.

Atypical leiomyoma: Lack all the other components with the exception of atypia and have little recurrence potential.

Diagnosis

Patients with abnormal uterine bleeding or a suspicious uterine lesion should undergo endometrial sampling. Imaging studies and clinical findings are not specific for ULMS versus other uterine tumours.

Ultrasound examination, magnetic resonance imaging (MRI) or computed tomography (CT) do not distinguish between sarcoma, leiomyoma, endometrial cancer, lymphoma, intravenous leiomyomatosis or adenomyosis (Table 32.2).[17]

Role of MRI in Diagnosis

Usefulness of MRI is being evaluated. A study has been reported where MRI of 12 patients (9 with pathologically proven LMS and three with STUMP) were analysed with another group with benign leiomyoma, with some exceptions the authors concluded that more than 50% of high signal on T2-weighted images and the presence of any small high—signal areas on T1-weighted images with unenhanced pockets were considered MRI suggestive for STUMPS and LMS.[18]

Table 32.2: Diagnostic criteria for LMS (Adapted from 2003 WHO guidelines)[13]

	Standard smooth muscle differentiation	Epithelioid differentiation	Myxoid differentiation
Histology	Cigar=shaped spindled cells with scanty to abundant eosinophilic cytoplasm	Rounded cells with central nuclei and clear to eosinophilic cytoplasm	Spindle-shaped cells set within an abundant myxoid matrix
Criteria for LMS	Any coagulative tumour cell necrosis In the absence of tumour cell necrosis, the diagnosis required diffuse, moderate-to-severe cytological atypia and a mitotic index of > 10 mf/10 hpf*.If the mitotic index is < 10 mf/10 hpf, chance of recurrence is low (less than 2%–3%) In the absence of coagulative tumour cell necrosis and significant atypia, a high mitotic index is compatible with a benign clinical course	Any coagulative tumour cell necrosis In the absence of tumour cell necrosis, the diagnosis requires diffuse, moderate-to-severe cytological atypia and a mitotic index of > 5 mf/10 hpf	Any coagulative tumour cell necrosis In the absence of tumour cell necrosis, the diagnosis requires diffuse, moderate-to-severe cytological atypia and a mitotic index of > 5 mf/10 hpf
*mf/hpf = mitotic figures/high power fields			

PET Scan

Positron emission tomography (PET) has a place in diagnosis of presumed fibroids. In PET scanning, a radionuclide (tracer) on a biologically active molecule is visualised. In imaging of fibroids, usually fluodeoxyglucose (FDG) is used, but other molecules, such as deoxyfluorothymidine (FLT) or alphafluorobeta – estradiol (FES) have been reported. The uptake of FDG in a fibroid is associated with oestrogen status, cellularity and the presence of malignancy.[19] FES may be more accurate in distinguishing LMS from fibroids than FDG, with an accuracy of respectively 93% and 81%.[20]

Serum Markers (LDH and CA125)

The total LDH and LDH isozyme type 3 were elevated in patients with LMS compared to degenerated leiomyomas.[21]

Elevated CA125 have been reported in patients with LMS, especially in advanced stage LMS.[22]

Needle Biopsies

Transcervical or transabdominal needle biopsy may prove of help in differentiating between LMS and a fibroid, although no data are available on spread of tumour cells caused by the biopsy needle.[23]

Staging

Staging is based on surgical not clinical findings. Extensive local growth is a hallmark of ULMS and spread occur by local, lymphatic and haematogenous routes. Metastasis to lung is common. If diagnosis of ULMS is known preoperatively, chest imaging is necessary to evaluate for metastatic disease.

Uterine leiomyosarcoma was staged using the FIGO system for endometrial cancers. The new FIGO system takes into consideration tumour size disregarding myometrial and cervical involvement (Table 32.3).

Table 32.3: The International Federation of Gynaecology and Obstetrics (FIGO) Staging of ULMS

Stage	Definition
1	Tumour limited to uterus
1A	< 5 cm
1B	> 5 cm
2	Tumour extends to the pelvis
2A	Adnexal involvement
2B	Tumour extends to extrauterine pelvic tissue
3	Tumour invades abdominal tissues
3A	One site
3B	More than one site
3C	Metastasis to pelvic and/or para-aortic lymph nodes
4	Distant disease
4A	Tumour invades bladder and /or rectum
4B	Other distant metastasis

The surgery involves peritoneal washings for cytology, extrafascial total abdominal hysterectomy, bilateral salpingo-oophrectomy, removal of enlarged lymph nodes and biopsy of any suspicious areas. Some oncologists recommend omentectomy and pelvic and para-aortic lymph node sampling.

In laparoscopic hysterectomy for fibroids, endobags that are specifically designed for contained morcellation should be used. Contained laparoscopic morcellation involves an endobag inflated with carbon dioxide with the camera and morcellator placed into the inflated bag, allowing for contained morcellation under direct visualisation without tissue spillage.

■ TREATMENT FOR LOCALISED DISEASE

Surgical Treatment

At a minimum, surgical treatment of a patient with a ULMS of the uterus should include a total hysterectomy and removal of the cervix.

Adjuvant Radiotherapy

Benefit of postoperative adjuvant radiotherapy (RT) in ULMS is unclear. In a study by the European organisation for Research and Treatment of Cancer (EORTC) patients with uterine sarcoma including ULMS were given pelvic external beam radiation. Report suggested a lower rate of local recurrence in the irradiated group but no improvement in overall survival.[24]

A major obstacle with ULMS is that even if pelvic control is achieved, the majority of women develop distant extra abdominal metastases.[25]

Guidelines from the National Comprehensive Cancer Network (NCCN) suggest that adjuvant RT can be considered for all women with resected stage 1 or stage 2 ULMS. For stage 3 ULMS with positive lymph nodes, the NCCN recommends consideration of adjuvant chemotherapy and pelvic RT, vaginal brachytherapy, and/or adjuvant chemotherapy.[26]

The use of RT needs to be balanced with the negative effects of therapy. Short term or immediate side effects include vaginal bleeding, vaginal discharge, skin reactions, hair loss, urinary problems, diarrhea and pain. Long-term side effects include changes in bowel/bladder function and sexual function.

Adjuvant Chemotherapy

No prospective studies are available that focus on patients with ULMS and there is no definitive evidence that adjuvant chemotherapy improves overall survival. Therefore it cannot be recommended as the standard of care and should be considered in individual circumstances.

Neoadjuvant chemotherapy can be used to improve respectability of advanced disease in the appropriate setting. The data is limited, at best.[27,28]

■ TREATMENT FOR RECURRENT, ADVANCED OR METASTATIC DISEASE

Surgery

Recurrent ULMS is diagnosed by the new development of symptoms. Most relapses occur in the pelvis, followed by the lung and abdomen. Bone and brain metastases are uncommon. Surgical resection should be considered in patients with localised single foci recurrences, either local or metastatic.[29] With regard to radiofrequency ablation (RFA) and video-assisted thoracic surgery (VATS), there is limited literature on sarcomas and more studies are needed prior to recommendations.[30–32]

Chemotherapy

Single agent doxorubicin has been shown to be an effective drug for advanced ULMS.[33,34]

The combination of gemcitabine and docetaxel is the most effective chemotherapy regimen for ULMS patients with advanced disease described to date.[35,36]

Some uterine tumours respond to hormonal therapy because they express oestrogen and/or progesterone receptors. However this is not the case in ULMS and adjuvant hormonal therapy is not recommended for any stage of ULMS.

Chemotherapy is palliative and should be used to relieve symptoms. Considering there is no survival benefit with the current chemotherapeutic options, toxicity versus symptom management should be evaluated on a case by case basis with full informed consent.

■ CONCLUSION

Uterine leiomyosarcomas are rare tumours with a limited body of literature to help guide treatment. The issue on sarcoma risk in patients scheduled for fibroid morcellation should be clarified. More data needs to be collected to estimate the risk of sarcoma in individual patients with presumed fibroids, based on epidemiological data from the patient and diagnostic tests such as imaging. Technical innovation, such as in-bag morcellation, should enable safe morcellation of intra-abdominal specimens. Patient care should be individualised. Informed consent should be taken from all patients before laparoscopic surgery for fibroids with the best available evidence and options for the patient. Further investigation is needed to improve the treatment options for our patients with this disease.

■ REFERENCES

1. FDA. FDA discourages use of laparoscopic power morcellation for removal of uterus or uterine fibroids. Food Drug Adm. 2014;17:4.
2. Brölmann H, Tanos V, Grimbizis G, et al. Options on fibroid morcellation: a literature review. Gynecological Surgery. 2015;12(1):3-15.
3. Norris HJ, Zaloudek CJ. Mesenchymal tumors of the uterus. In: Blaustein A (Ed). Pathology of the female genital tract. New York: Springer. 1982. p. 352.
4. Harlow BL, Weis NS, Lofton S. The epidemiology of sarcoma of the uterus. J Natl Cancer Inst. 1986;76:399.
5. Kho KA, Nezhat CH. Evaluating the risks of electric uterine morcellation. JAMA. 2014;311(19):905-6.
6. Leung F, Terzibachian JJ. Re: "The impact of tumor morcellation during surgery on the prognosis of patients with apparently early uterine leiomyosarcoma". Gynecol Oncol. 2012;124(1):172-3.
7. Lurain JR, PiverMS . Uterine sarcomas: clinical features and management. In: Coppleson X, Monagham J, Morrow P,

Tattersall M (Eds) Gynecologic oncology. Churchill Livingstone, London. 1992. pp. 827-40.

8. Ng JS, Han A, Chew SH, et al. A clinicopathologic study of uterine smooth muscle tumours of uncertain malignant potential (STUMP). Ann Acad Med Singap. 2010;39(8):625-8.

9. AAGL Practice Report: Morcellation During Uterine Tissue Extraction. J Minim Invasive Gynecol. 2014;21(4):517-30.

10. Van Dinh T, Woodruff JO. Leiomyosarcoma of the uterus. Am J Obstet Gynecol. 1982;144:817.

11. Schwartz Z, Dgani R, Lancet M, et al. Uterine Sarcoma in Israel: a study of 104 cases. Gynecol Oncol. 1985;20:354.

12. Parker WH, Fu YS, Berek JS. Uterine sarcoma in patients operated on for presumed leiomyoma and rapidly growing leiomyoma. Obstet Gynecol. 1994;83:414.

13. World Health Organization Classification of Tumours: Pathology and Genetics, Pathology and Genetics of Tumours of the Breast and Female Genital Organs. IARC Press, France, 2003.

14. Anderson SE, Nonaka D, Chuai S, et al. P53, epidermal growth factor, and platelet-derived growth factor in uterine leiomyosarcoma and leiomyomas. Intl J Gynecol Cancer. 2006;16:849-53.

15. Layfield LJ, Liu K, Dodge R, et al. Uterine smooth muscle tumors: utility of classification by proliferation, ploidy, and prognostic markers versus traditional histopathology. Arch Pathol Laboratory Med. 2000;124(2):221-7.

16. Mittal K, Demopoulos RI. MIB-1 (Ki-67), p53, estrogen receptor, and progesterone receptor expression in uterine smooth muscle tumors. Hum Pathology. 2001;32(9):984-7.

17. Rha SE, Byun JY, Jung SE, et al. CT and MRI of uterine sarcoma and their mimickers. Am J Roentgenol. 2003;181:1369.

18. Tanaka YO, Nishida M, Tsunoda H, et al. Smooth muscle tumors of uncertain malignant potential and leiomyosarcomas of the uterus: MR findings. J. Magnetic Resonance Imaging. 2004;20(6): 998-1007.

19. Zhang HJ, Zhan FH, Li YJ, et al. Fluorodeoxyglucose positron emission tomography/computed tomography and magnetic resonance imaging of uterine Leiomyosarcomas: 2 cases report. Chin Med J (Engl). 2011;124(14): 2237-40.

20. Yoshida Y, Kiyono Y, Tsujikawa T, et al. Additional value of 16 alpha-[18F] fluoro-17 beta-oestradiol PET for differential diagnosis between uterine sarcoma and leiomyoma in patients with positive or equivocal findings on [18F] fluorodeoxyglucose PET. Eur J Nucl Med Mol Imaging. 2011;38 (10):1824-31.

21. Goto A, Takeuchi S, Sugimura K, et al. Usefulness of Gd-DTPA contrast-enhanced dynamic MRI and serum determination of LDH and its isozymes in the differential diagnosis of leiomyosarcoma from degenerated leiomyoma of the uterus. Int J. Gynecol Cancer. 2002;12(4):354-61.

22. Juang CM, Yen MS, Horng HC, et al. Potential role of preoperative serum CA125 for the differential diagnosis between uterine leiomyoma and uterine leiomyosarcoma. Eur J Gynaecol Oncol. 2006;27(4):370-4.

23. Kawamura N, Ichimura T, Ito F, et al .Transcervical needle biopsy for the differential diagnosis between uterine sarcoma and leiomyoma. Int J Gynecol Cancer. 2002;94(6):1713-20.

24. Reed NS, Mangioni C, Malmstrom H, et al. First results of a randomized trial comparing radiotherapy versus observation postoperatively in patients with uterine sarcomas. An EORTCGCG study (abstract) Int J Gynecol Cancer. 2003;13:4.

25. Major FJ, Blessing RA, Silverberg SG, et al. Prognostic factors in early-stage uterine sarcoma. A Gynecologic Oncology Group study. Cancer. 1993;71:1702.

26. The NCCN Guidelines Uterine Cancer. Clinical Practice Guidelines in Oncology (version V.2.2006). www.nccn.org.

27. Bodner K, Bodner-Adler B, Kimberger O, et al. Evaluating prognostic parameters in women with uterine leiomyosarcoma. A clinicopathologic study. J Reprod Med. 2003;48:95.

28. Dinh TA, Oliva EA, Fuller AF, et al. The treatment of uterine leiomyosarcoma. Results form a 10-year experience (1990-1999) at the Massachusetts General Hospital. Gynecol Oncol. 2004;92:648.

29. Guintoli RL, Metzinger DS, DiMarco CS, et al. Retrospective review of 208 patients with leiomyosarcoma of the uterus: prognostic indicators, surgical management and adjuvant therapy. Gynecol Oncol. 2003;89:460.

30. Ambrogi MC, Lucchi M, Dini P, et al. Percutaneous radiofrequency ablation of lung tumours: results in the mid term. Eur J Cardiothoracic Surgery. 2006;30:177.

31. Lin JC, Wiechmann RJ, Szwerc MF, et al. Diagnostic and therapeutic video-assisted thoracic surgery resection of pulmonary metastases. Surgery. 1999;216:636.

32. Lawes D, Chopada A, Gilliams A, et al. Radiofrequency ablation as a cytoreductive strategy for hepatic metastasis from breast cancer. Ann R Coll Surg England. 2006;88:639.

33. Kanjeekal S, Chambers A, Fung MF, et al. Systemic therapy for advanced uterine sarcoma: a systematic review of the literature. Gynecol Oncol. 2005;97:624.

34. Sutton GP, Blessing JA, Hanjani R, et al. Phase II evaluation of liposomal doxorubicin (Doxil) in recurrent or advanced leiomyosarcoma of the uterus: a Gynecology Oncology Group study. Gynecol Oncol. 2005;96:749.

35. Sutton GP, Blessing JA, Barrett RJ, et al. Phase II trial of ifosfamide and mesna in leiomyosarcoma of the uterus: a Gynecologic Oncology Group Study. Am J Obstet Gynecol. 1992;166:556.

36. Sutton GP, Blessing JA, Malfetano JH. Ifosamide and doxorubicin in the treatment of advanced leiomyosarcomas of the uterus: a Gynecologic Oncology Group study. Gynecol Oncol. 1996;62:226.

CHAPTER 33

Management of Huge Fibroid

● Dipti Gunge

Uterine leiomyomas are the most common benign tumours of the female pelvis, which consist of benign smooth muscle surrounded by a pseudocapsule and extracellular matrix with compressed muscle fibres.

Almost 50% of myomas are found incidentally without symptoms and only about 25% are symptomatic for laparoscopic management of huge fibroid one of the major concerns is the high degree of technical difficulty; large uterus occupying whole of the pelvis with difficulty in mobilising and manipulating uterus, thus restricting surgeons vision to the surrounding anatomic structures and impairing to find correct surgical planes and spaces (Fig. 33.1).

Above technical issues can be overcome by adequate training and acquisition of expertise in minimally invasive surgery. In this chapter we will be discussing about difficulties faced and modifications in surgical techniques like high epigastric port placement,[1] preoperative gonadotropin-releasing hormone (GnRH) agonist treatment[2] and specimen retrieval to suit our needs for successful surgery in such cases.

Patients with large submucosal and intramural fibroids commonly present with menorrhagia, menometrorrhagia, pelvic pain, backache, subfertility, repeated pregnancy loss and dyspareunia. Large subserosal fibroids usually presents with pressure symptoms like frequency or retention of urine, sometimes hesitancy, constipation and rectal pain (Fig. 33.2). Rarely patient might be asymptomatic.

■ INVESTIGATIONS

Fibroid mapping is the most important factor preoperatively in laparoscopic myomectomy. Large myomas may be best imaged with a combination of transabdominal and transvaginal sonography. Evaluation of pressure symptoms on urinary system is most important in huge fibroids. One should look for hydronephrosis, hydroureter due to fibroid compression.

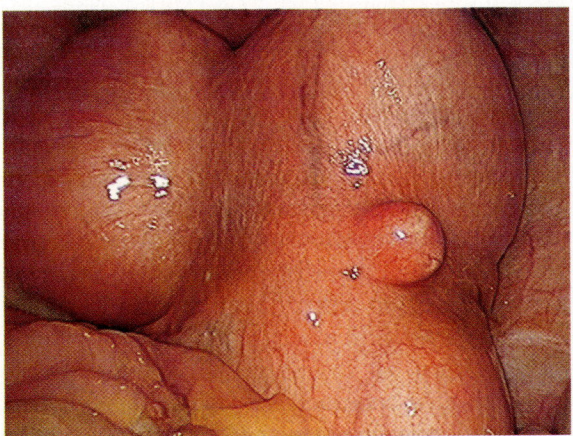

Fig. 33.1: Multiple fibroid uterus (28 weeks size)

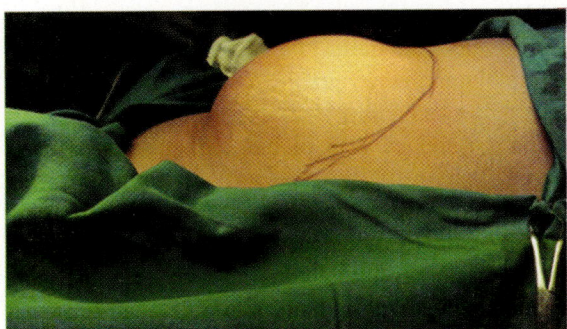

Fig. 33.2: 28 weeks size multiple fibroids

Magnetic resonance imaging (MRI) is an excellent method to evaluate the size, position and number of uterine myomas and is the best modality for exact evaluation of submucous myoma penetration into the myometrium.[3] MRI has been used for more accurate myoma 'mapping' as well as for differentiation of pedunculated myomas from adnexal masses.

MANAGEMENT

The treatment of huge leiomyomas for women who have completed childbearing has been, in the vast majority of cases, hysterectomy. Myomectomy is the 'gold standard' for treatment for women who want to retain fertility.

The route of surgery is influenced by location and size of leiomyomas, prior medical and surgical history, concomitant pathology, patient preference, desire for future fertility and the surgeon's experience. There are different modes of myomectomy surgery:

1. Abdominal myomectomy.
2. Laparoscopic myomectomy.

Abdominal Myomectomy

Certainly, for those women in the reproductive age group wanting to maintain fertility, myomectomy remains the 'gold standard'. Abdominal myomectomy, however, is associated with significant morbidity including excessive blood loss, a high rate of blood transfusions, infection and postoperative adhesions.[4] There are varying opinions regarding the feasibility and outcome of laparoscopic myomectomy especially of large myomas.

Laparoscopic Myomectomy

Operative laparoscopy of huge fibroids has a limitation of the operative field, inadequate angle of approach for the laparoscopic instruments, increased blood loss and operative time is increased.

PREOPERATIVE PREPARATION

One should ensure that for laparoscopy in cases of the large myomas the bowel loops must be empty at the time of the procedure. Bowel preparation with peglac can be done. Few surgeons prefer to keep patient on liquid diet for 2 days before the procedure. Antithromboembolic prophylaxis measures must be included as low-molecular-weight heparin subcutaneous injection and sequential compression devices.

The two major concerns in laparoscopic large myoma excision is myoma bed closure and tissue retrival through small incision. Now we will be discussing steps to overcome above technical issues.

Trocar Placement

In laparoscopic myomectomy for huge fibroids the placement of trocars is most important factor for secured operative visibility, free handling the instrument smoothly without being hindered by the large uterus, specimen retrieval , and decreasing intraoperative blood loss.

The Palmer's point[5] (a point 3 cm below the left costal margin in the midclavicular line) is a safe zone, which is devoid of major adhesions and a safe entry point (Fig. 33.3). In huge uterus, the Veress and the 5-mm port may be placed at the Palmer point except in patients with splenomegaly. A 5-mm telescope is introduced through this port and the uterus with the adnexa is evaluated. One important pre-requisite for Palmer's point entry is to deflate the stomach completely using nasogastric tube. The 10-mm port is inserted under vision at the midline supraumbilical site or higher depending on the size of the uterus. Entry under vision avoids damage to major vessels directly beneath the insertion site and the port can be placed at a variable point depending on the size of the uterus. This helps the surgeon to obtain a good operative field, which allows smooth manipulation of the instruments above the uterus.

Port placement at correct site is important in cases of large myoma excision. Surgeon has to modify port placement depending on surgeon's choice of ipsilateral or contralateral suturing, morcellation site and to get adequate space to

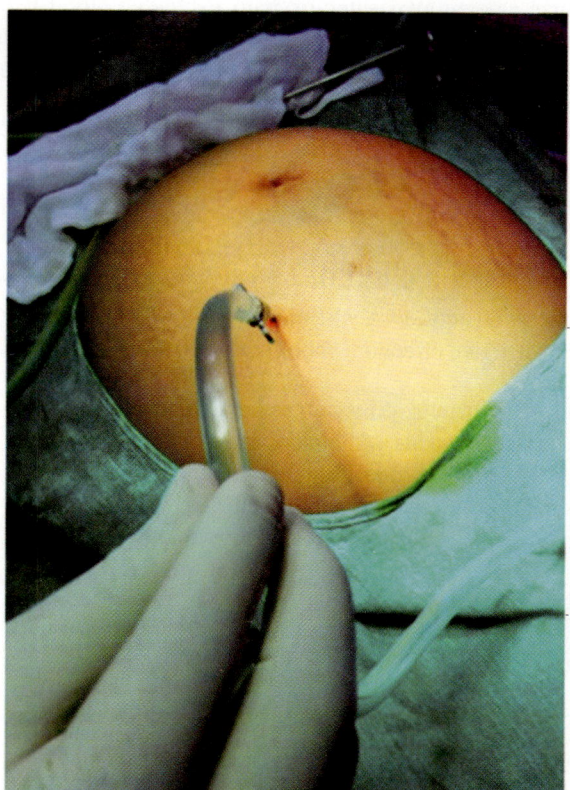

Fig. 33.3: Palmar's point (Veress needle entry)

operate, avoid collision of instruments and adequate vision for proper dissection. Primary trocar 10mm should be placed supraumbilically above the uterine height for proper visualisation of surrounding structures and to prevent the tangling of instruments during surgery (Fig. 33.4). Preferably use 30 degree 10 mm telescope to assess the size and position of the large myomas from various angles as vision may get obscured with a 0 degree telescope and for planning of lateral ports. The level of placement of the accessory ports is tailored to the size, position and number of fibroids—varies from the level of anterior iliac spine till supraumbilicus. All trocars should be in 'safe zone', which consists of the intersecting area 2 cm above a line drawn transversely between the right and left anterior superioriliac spine and within 1 cm of the midline and out of the ellipses of the ilioinguinal and iliohypogastric nerves to avoid potential injury to the ilioinguinal and iliohypogastric nerves and the inferior epigastric arteris.[5]

Preferably two accessory ports should be placed in the upper quadrants above the uterine height to ensure an unobstructed passage above the fundus of the uterus mainly left lateral upper quadrant, right lateral upper quadrant and left lateral lower quadrant.

■ PREVENTION OF INTRAOPERATIVE BLOOD LOSS

Myomas are vascular tumours with exclusive blood supply from uterine arteries. Large myomas are highly vascular leading to increased blood loss during myomectomy, which can be prevented by:
1. Vasopressin injection.
2. Uterine artery ligation.
3. Preoperative use of GnRH analogues injection.

Vasopressin Injection

Vasopresssin acts as a chemical tourniquet with a strong vasoconstrictive effect on smooth muscle. Vasopressin diluted

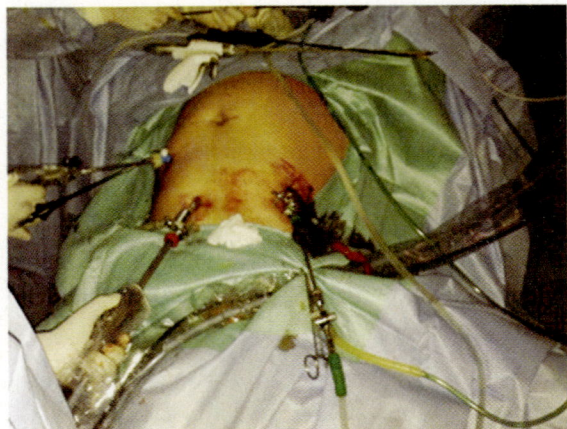

Fig. 33.4: Primary port and secondary trocars position

at a concentration of 10 U in 100 mL of saline solution and is infiltrated at several points beneath the pseudocapsule of fibroid. It constricts the capsular flow and reduces blood loss. The amount of vasopressin to be infiltrated varies from 200 to 400 mL depending on fibroid size, in larger myomas injecting large amount of vasopressin can be detrimental. As large myomas can cause increased blood loss during myomectomy, however the effect of vasopressin lasts less as its half life is 24.1 minute, and in large myomas, other methods are needed to decrease blood loss.[6]

Uterine Artery Ligation

Laparoscopic ligation of uterine arteries combined with myomectomy, devascularizes the myoma and successfully reduces intraoperative blood loss. As per Burbank's 'transient uterine ischaemia' theory post uterine vessel occlusion, both myometrial and myoma bed vessels are occluded by clotting resulting in ischaemic necrosis in myoma, but not in myometrium , further leading to shrinkage of myoma.[7] Most of the cases of large myomas can be devascularised prior to myomectomy by laparoscopic intracorporeal suturing of uterine arteries by anterior or posterior approach depending on location of fibroid. In cases of lower uterine segment or cervical fibroids, uterine artery can be ligated at its origin from anterior division of internal iliac artery.[8] The additional advantage of UAL is it shrinks small fibroids and prevent the recurrence of fibroids. Technically it might be difficult to ligate uterine artery in large myoma as anatomy might be distorted, however with adequate training and good surgical skills it can be achieved.

Preoperative Use of GnRH Analogues Injection

Use of GnRH analogues leads to shrinkage of both fibroids and uterus as fibroids are oestrogen-dependent tumours and thus it relieves symptoms such as pain and pressure from the pelvic mass.[9] 3 to 6 months use of GnRH analogues before myomectomy and hysterectomy will result in 36% and 77% of shrinkage of fibroids size , most of it ususally occurs in the first 3 months further associated with shorter operative time and decreased intraoperative bleeding.[10–12]

However, laparoscopic myomectomy with pretreatment of GnRH analogues is associated with obliteration of the psuedocapsule resulting in increased difficulty in myoma enucleation because of degeneration of the myoma.[13,14] The benefits of pretreatment with GnRH agonist is mainly in huge myoma surgery as it leads to correction of anaemia, decrease in intraoperative blood loss and improved postoperative haemoglobin. The unwanted effects mainly vasomotor symptoms mood swings, insomnia, headaches and vaginal dryness and reduction in bone mineral density (BMD) are due to hypoestrogenic state. However in cases of laparoscopic myomectomy for multiple fibroids there is increased risk of myoma recurrence secondary to missing of shrunken small myomas due to GnRH analogues.[15]

◼ UTERINE MANIPULATION

Appropriate manipulation of the uterus with means of a uterine manipulator with blades that reach up to the fundus is of utmost importance. In cases of large and huge myomas its difficult to manipulate the uterus with uterine manipulator, however once the myoma screw is inserted into the myoma, manipulation becomes much easier.

Myoma screw is one of the best instrument to manipulate the huge uterus laparoscopically during TLH. During TLH, important is cutting of the uterosacral ligament before hand rather than just pushing the uterus upwards as in sunrise technique to prevent ureteric injury.

In myoma screw, all the force acts at cervico vaginal junction to lateralise the ureter, while in uterine manipulators most of the force acts at infravaginal portion of the cervix. Ideal myoma screw for uterine manipulation should be rod like with tapered and rimmed at the end which facilitates manipulation and less chance of slipping of myoma screw. Myoma screw should be mostly placed in right lateral port as per surgeons convenience. Depending on the size of the uterus, myoma screw, postion varies. In normal size uterus it should be applied between two round ligaments. In large uterus, myoma screw should be attached close to the round ligament and then pull the uterus. The position of myoma screw varies depending on the steps of the surgery. If head end of the patient is considered as 12 O'clock position, 11 O'clock pull with myoma screw will make left corneal structures prominent for dissection (Fig. 33.5). Pull at 9 O'cock will facilitate dissection of posterior leaf of broad ligament, uterosacral ligament and vaginal attachment of cervix. 6 O'clock myoma screw push will make anterior bladder peritoneum prominent and easy to dissect along with counter traction to push uterus down will help further.

Advantages

1. As per literature , right ureter at high risk of injury to prevent it fix myoma screw at right round ligament and lift such that corneal structures should come beyond the midline.
2. Large size uterus can be manipulated with myoma screw attaching close to the fundus posteriorly.
3. Cutting uterosacral ligament before hand facilitates longer vaginal length postoperative.

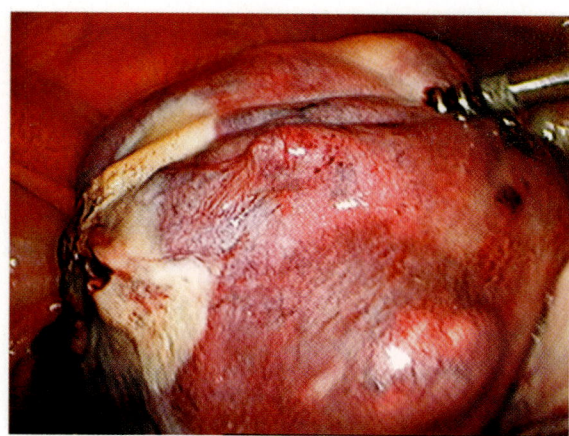

Fig. 33.5: Myoma screw for uterine manipulation

Disadvantage

1. Extra 5 mm port required.
2. After removing myoma screw, it can bleed especially in large size uterus. Bleeding can be controlled by bipolar coagulation.

◼ MYOMA ENUCLEATION

In large myoma enucleation, we need few modifications in the standard technique to reduce the technical difficulty in the push-pull maneuvers due to limited space. Bilateral uterine artery ligation should be done to devascularise the large myoma. As intrauterine vessels run in horizontal direction, so one should prefer an horizontal incision as associated with less bleeding and should be made on the most prominent part of the convex surface of the uterus instead of base of the myoma as in smaller fibroids.[16] The myoma capsule is opened with harmonic ultracision or with monopolar hook or bipolar scissors as per surgeons preference. Incision size should be appropriate to the fibroid size to avoid unnecessary struggle for enucleation in the smaller size. Enucleation is made along the cleavage plane dissecting myoma by traction with 5 mm myoma screw and countertraction on the cervix with a tenaculum (Fig. 33.6).

In large posterior uterine wall myoma surgeon should trace the course of ureter and sacral uterine ligament attachment to assess the relation of uterine arteries. In large myomas seldom difficult to delinate the boundaries, in such cases broad ligament is opened with an anterior approach. In cases of intraligamentous or broad ligament huge myomas one should observe the course of the ureter and uterine vessels before taking incision on anterior or posterior leaf of the broad ligament depending on the myoma location. Large cervical fibroid distorts pelvic anatomy with displacement of surrounding organs as bladder, ureter and uterine blood vessel. To minimize the risk of damaging surrounding organs

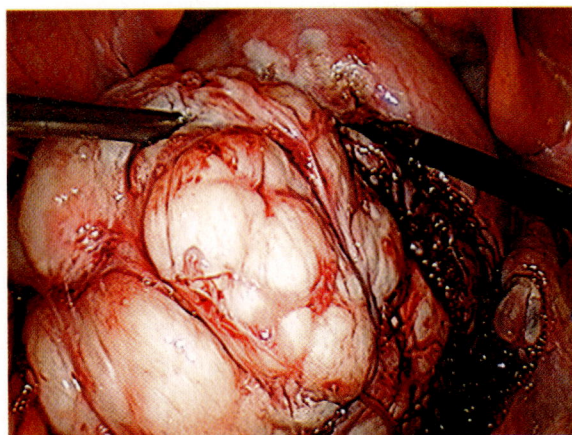

Fig. 33.6: Huge myoma enucleation

the incision should be places as lateral as possible to the uteine corpus.[17] For large subserosal myomas the incision should be 2 to 3 cm distal to the junction between the myoma and the uterus for easy closure of defect and to avoid electrosurgical damage to the myometrium.

■ IN SITU MORCELLATION

In conventional laparoscopic myomectomy, we do morcellation after enucleation which might be technically difficult in cases of large myoma with limited space for traction and large myomas are often soft due to degenerative changes making traction-countertraction difficult with myoma screw. An modified technique 'in situ morcellation' can be used in which morcellation is performed when myoma is still attached to the uterus with an advantage of increased operative space with better panoramic view and optimum movement of instruments.[18,19]

During in situ morcellation enucleate the fibroid up to half of its circumference. The upper left lateral 5 mm port then convert into a 15-mm port for the insertion of the 15-mm serrated-edge electromechanical morcellator. With the traumatic claw forceps of the morcellator, myoma should be held and progressively morcellate strips of myoma away from the base under vision to prevent damage to the uterine wall.

As uterine size is reduced with morcellation, additional space is created for the optimum movement of the instruments. The traction maintained on the myoma by the claw forceps, countertraction by grasping the wound margin and cervical pull with the help of the tenaculum held by the assistant causes progressive enucleation of the myoma from its base in the uterine wall. As the volume of myoma is decreased, its capsule collapses and compresses snugly over the myoma. The redundant pseudocapsule can be morcellated for precise reconstruction of the uterine wall. Intraoperative haemorrhage can be controlled by subcapsular injection of

vasopressin,[20] bilateral ligation of the uterine artery[21,22] and bipolar coagulation. This technique combines enucleation and morcellation, which is very useful for large myoma with advantages as mentioned below;

1. Reduces operative time mainly in myomas more than 10 cm and multiple myomas.
2. Progressive morcellation increases operative space in the pelvic cavity for optimum movement of the instruments.
3. Minimizes the risk of missing small myomas as in cases of multiple myomas.
4. Avoids the struggle with myoma screw in large degenerated myomas as in ISM myoma spontaneously bulges out from pseudocapsule.
5. It facilitates enucleation of dense myomas after use of GnRH analogues.

ISM requires experience with adequate training to use morcellator as it carries the risk of catastrophic vascular or visceral injuries. If exit point is not seen there is always risk of the injury to uterus, fallopian tubes and ovaries. The morcellator blade should be moved like a peeling of an apple, both entry and exit point must be under constant vision to prevent inadvertent damage to the pelvic structures. The camera assistant should be well trained to use 30 degree foreoblique telescope for panaromic view. In cases of very deep intramural large myomas surgeon has to be very cautious about inadvertent injury to endometrium during morcellation.[23]

■ MYOMA BED SUTURING IN LARGE MYOMAS

The gold standard of myometrial closure is obliteration of the dead space by multi-layered closure with interrupted intracorporeal sutures with 1-0 polyglactin in single or multilayer depending on the defect in the uterine wall (Figs 33.7A and B). Surgeon should be careful to exclude endometrium from the suture line if uterine cavity was opened. Nowadays, absorbable, unidirectional barbed suture (V-Loc, Covidien) is used for multilayer closure of the myoma bed by haemostatic baseball stitch fashion to minimize suture exposure and subsequent adhesions. The a davantages of using absorbable barbed suture to surgeons are elimination of knot tying, shorter closure time and better tension distribution throughout the wound.[24]

■ MINILAPAROTOMY MYOMECTOMY

Laparoscopic-assisted myomectomy and minilaparotomy myomectomy have also been suggested as viable alternatives especially in the case of large myomas. Minilaparotomy incision is a safe alternative to myomectomy by laparotomy. It is technically less difficult to perform than laparoscopic myomectomy, allows better closure of the uterine defect, and may require less time to perform.[25] Hysterectomy in huge

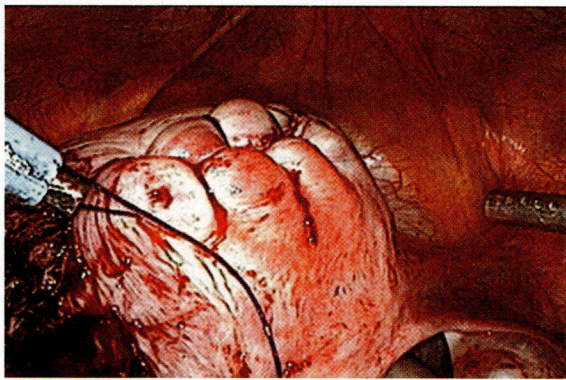

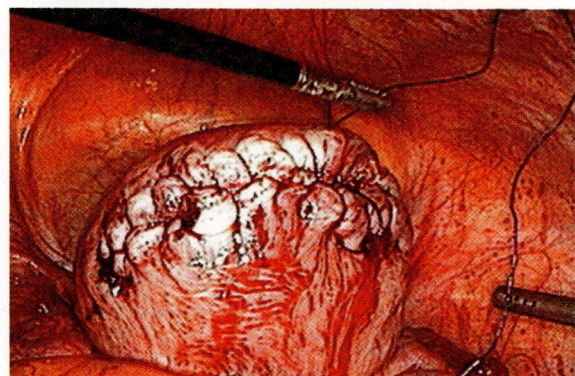

Figs 33.7A and B: Myoma bed baseball suturing—second layer closure

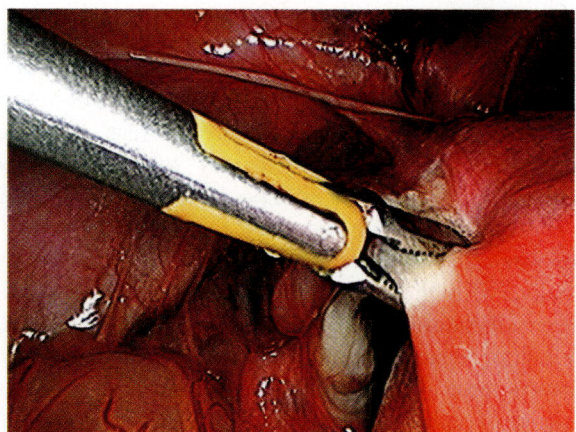

Fig. 33.8: Coagulation of ovarian ligament

fibroids—hysterectomy is the most common surgery in patients with huge fibroid and route of surgery depending on surgeons preference as per surgical skill and experience as laparotomy , laparoscopy or vaginally. In past, majority of cases were operated by laparotomy via midline incision,[26] but recent advances in minimal invasive surgery has made laparoscopic hysterectomy very feasible and safe technique in cases of huge myoma with evident benefits for the patient.[27] Size, shape and mobility of the uterus and associated pathologies remain the limiting factors for performing laparoscopic hysterectomy.

In cases of TLH for huge myoma, the port placement is generally as described above, primary port should be placed supraumbilically for visualisation and proper traction angles with instruments. Lateral tilt of operative table by 20 to 35 degree to contralateral side facilitates exposure of the vascular pedicle mainly infundibulopelvic ligament and uterine vessels (Fig. 33.8). Myoma spiral is used as a good manipulator and can be placed at different locations as per surgeons preference. In huge uterus or cases of multiple fibroids for TLH, first complete devascularisation of uterus by uterine artery ligation has been described to reduce blood loss in such cases.[28]

Later, in cases of multiple myomas or pedunculated fibroids, intraoperative myomectomy allows better access to the vascular pedicles and facilitates to identify correct operative plane in pelvis by increasing operative space. In cases of huge cervical or posterior wall myoma, ureter should be traced at the pelvic brim. The ureter can then be followed to the cardinal web (the infundibulopelvic ligament is taken as soon as the ureter is separated from it if the ovary is to be taken), and the uterine vessel can usually be easily found at this level coming off the hypogastric artery (internal iliac artery) lateral to the ureter and clipped. An alternative anterior approach has been described utilizing retrograde tracking of the umbilical ligament (RUL).[29] Once the vascular pedicles are controlled, careful uterine reduction will allow the remaining dissection of the posterior cul-de-sac.

■ SPECIMEN RETRIEVAL IN A HUGE UTERUS

Normal to bulky sized uterus can be removed vaginally in routine TLH ,but huge uterus requires special techniques for its retrieval via morcellation. As specimen retrival impacts significantly on operative time, surgeon's skill and is not without complications, usually resulting from seeding of tissue particles in the peritoneum.[30] Preoperative assessment of likelihood of benignity is essential in huge uterus as morcellation is needed for specimen retrieval. Other parameters also should be assessed preoperatively like uterine mobility, vaginal width and body mass index to plan route of tissue retrieval. In present scenario electromechanical morcellation has become controversial, but these can be diminished by alternative techniques, instrumentation, and skill of the surgeon. A number of techniques exist to facilitate reduction of the bulky uterus such as morcellation (power morcellator or manual morcellation), coring and bisection.

Vaginal Retrieval Methods for Huge Uterus

1. Mechanical morcellation.
2. Vaginal paper roll technique.
3. Use of alexis retraction system.
4. Bowel bag technique.
5. Helical incision technique.

Mechanical Morcellation

Mechanical morcellation by scalpel can be done via vaginal or abdominal route has a role in today's controversial scenario for use of power morcellator for fear of spread of leiomyosarcoma (Fig. 33.9). Various studies have found no difference in infection rate, postoperative pain, hospital stay and return to work compared to patients in whom the uterus was removed after hand morcellation abdominally or vaginally.[31] Bisection is the most frequently used technique to retrieve the uterus through the vagina. Cervix is grasped by volsellum or tenaculum bilaterally and the uterus is bisected in antero-posterior direction with knife with progressive reposition of volsellum till the fundus. Bisection of uterus is one of the important technique, which is used in NDVH, LAVH as well as TLH. In a few cases complete bisection is required so that one half of the uterus could be delivered out into the vagina. Another method commonly used in large uterus is Lash procedure in which coring of uterine wall is done by cutting specimen circumferentially few mm at a time with constant traction on the cervix. In Lash technique long elongated uterine specimen is retrieved with progressive incision with peeling and rotating clockwise on specimen at higher level till fundus is delivered.

Paper Roll Technique

This technique has been described for large uteri to retrieve them vaginally and uterus can be reconstructed easily after retrieval and that helps the pathologist for evaluation of specimen.[32] In this technique, cervix is lifted with 2 large vulsellum forceps toward the 12 O'clock position and slightly to the left so that under direct vision, maximum uterine tissue can be cut. Two Heaney's retractor are placed at 2 O'clock and 10 O'clock position. Incision is begun at the 6 O'clock position and is directed toward the left Heaney retractor at approximately the 10 O'clock position. At the same time, the uterus is pulled down toward the floor during the cut, enabling complete monitoring of the entire cutting process. A minor degree of constant clockwise rotation during traction, especially toward the end of a cut, can be useful, and may

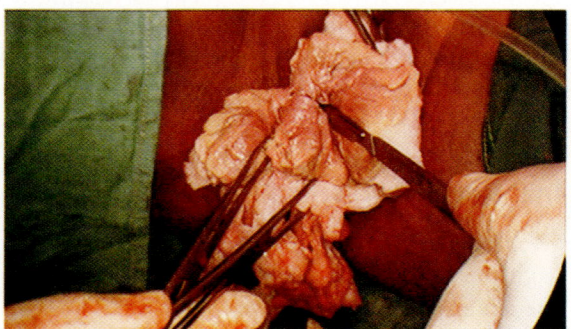

Fig. 33.9: Vaginal mechanical morcellation with knife

result in spontaneous rotation of the remaining uterus and new presentation of tissue for the subsequent cut.

On many occasions, the uterus will keep rolling and enable complete removal of the uterus (like unwinding a roll of paper). If the uterus gets stuck, uterus can be repositioned into a space that allows for new descent and further cuts to be made. This part may be similar to the Lash procedure as described earlier. The authors found that a single direction of pull can result in only small advancement of the uterus, whereas constant changing of the position of the remaining uterus through rolling enables more outward presentation of the uterus for a new cut. Nearly all large uteri can be morcellated using this technique with adequate expertise and experience.

Alexis Retraction System

Vaginal application of the Alexis retraction device allows for safe, easy removal of large myomatous uteri. Alexis wound retraction system (Applied Medical, Rancho Santa Margarita, CA), is a disposable self-retaining retractor that consists of a flexible polymer membrane in the shape of a cylinder attached to two semi rigid polymer rings on each end and is available in various sizes. This was designed initially for retracting during abdominal surgeries, as it is atraumatic ring can be used vaginal wall retraction, while removing large uterine specimen. Studies have suggested its use in surgeries that require manipulation through a small incision and possible anti-infective properties.[33] Once complete detachment of uterus occurs laparoscopically, this retractor is placed in the vagina. One ring is pushed inside and it lies in cul-de-sac and the other ring outside to form a uniform, circumferential orifice that distributes the retraction force evenly throughout the vaginal vault and proceeded with mechanical morcellation. Alex retraction system is particularly helpful in cases of narrow vagina where exposure is very difficult. It is also helpful in cases with high body mass index (BMI) and prevents vaginal lacerations, tears and bruising caused by the vaginal wall retractors. Most important advantage is it works as self-retaining retractor and reduces the need for assistance.

Bowel Bag Technique

Dr Heaton developed the bowel bag technique for pelvic mass isolation. In this technique, after the hysterectomy is completed extrafascially, with the uterus intact, a bowel bag is inserted into the abdomen via the vagina, and the uterus is maneuvered into it. The mouth of the bag is then brought out through the vagina, and the uterus is morcellated vaginally with retractors placed inside the bag in the vagina in the same manner as they would be placed for a vaginal hysterectomy. This technique was developed by Dr Heaton to prevent intra-abdominal contamination with a potentially malignant mass.[34]

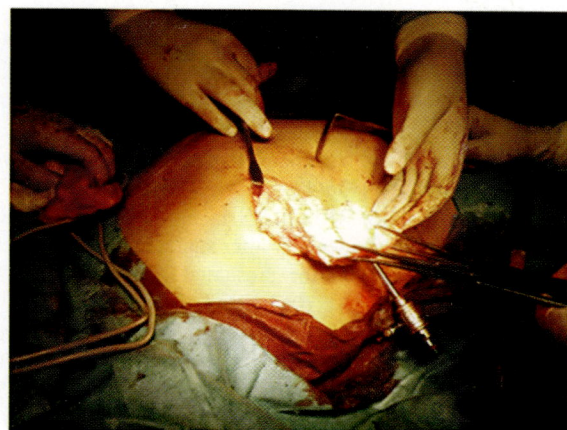

Fig. 33.10: Mechanical morcellation by extending port incision

Helical Incision Technique

In this technique, 2 vaginal retractors, 1 at the front and 1 at the back are used, which entails pulling the uterus forward during cutting and then rotating the entire uterus clockwise to enable a new incision. The helical technique includes cutting the uterine specimen in a transverse or spiral manner, with a further cut to follow the aided rotation of the remaining specimen within the pelvis. In cases in which the vagina is narrow, the ends of the large retractors could sometimes hold back a large uterus and prevent it from further descent.[35]

Abdominal Specimen Retrieval

1. Power morcellator—controversial.
2. Morcellation in an endobag.
3. Myomectomy followed by hysterectomy.
4. By extending one of the ports and doing manual morcellation (Fig. 33.10).

■ MORCELLATION IN ENDOBAG

Recent advances in minimal invasive surgery has put forth lot of litigations on use of power morcellator, so nowadays to increase patients safety endobag morcellation is recommended. Preoperatively proper counselling and well informed consent is mandatory for use of power morcellator. Various endobags are available commercially according to specimen size and different techniques to insert endobag, trocars and morcellator.

■ REFERENCES

1. Lee YS. Benefits of high epigastric port placement for removing the very larg uterus. J Am Assoc Gynecol Laparosc. 2001;8:425-8.
2. Seracchioli R, Venturoli S, Colombo FM, et al. GnRH agonist treatment before total laparoscopic hysterectomy for large uteri. J Am Assoc Gynecol Laparosc. 2003;10:316-9.
3. Dueholm M, Lundorf E, Hansen ES, et al. Evaluation of the uterine cavity with magnetic resonance imaging, transvaginal sonography, hysterosonographic examination, and diagnostic hysteroscopy. Fertil Steril. 2001;76:350-7.
4. Berkeley AS, DeCherney AH, Polon ML. Abdominal myomectomy and subsequent infertility. Surg Gynecol and Obstet. 1983;156:391-422.
5. Whiteside JL, Barber MD, Walters MD, et al. Anatomy of ilioinguinal and iliohypogastric nerves in relation to trocar placement and low transverse incisions. Am J Obstet Gynecol. 2003;189:1574-8.
6. Baumann G, Dingman JF. Distribution, blood transport, and degradation of antidiuretic hormone in man. J Clin Invest. 1976;57:1109-16.
7. Burbank F, Hutchins Jr FL. Uterine artery occlusion by embolization or surgery for treatment of fibroids: A unifying hypothesis – transient uterine ischaemia. J Am Assos Gynaecol Laparosc. 2000:7;S1-49.
8. R Sinha, M Sundaram, C Mahajan, et al. Laparoscopic myomectomy with uterine artery ligation. Review article and comparative analysis .Journal of Gynaecological Endoscopy and Surgery. 2011 Volume -2 / issue-1 / Jan-June.
9. Lethaby A, Vollenhoven B. Fibroids (uterine myomatosis, leiomyomas). Clin Evid 2005 Dec;(14):2264–82.
10. van Leusden HA, Dogterom AA. Rapid reduction of uterine leiomyomas with monthly injections of D-Trp6-GnRH. Gynecol Endocrinol 1988;2: 45–51.
11. Matta WH, Stabile I, Shaw RW, Campbell S. Doppler assessment of uterine blood flow changes in patients with fibroids receiving the gonadotropin- releasing hormone agonist buserelin. Fertil Steril 1988;49:1083–5.
12. Hackenberg R, Gesenhues T, Deichert U, Duda V, Schmidt-Rhode P, Schulz KD. The response of uterine fibroids to GnRH-agonist treatment can be predicted in most cases after one month. Eur J Obstet Gynecol Reprod Biol 1992;45:125–9.
13. Lethaby A, Vollenhoven B, Sowter M. Pre-operative GnRH analogue therapy before hysterectomy or myomectomy for uterine fibroids. Cochrane Database Syst Rev. 2001;(2):000547.
14. Friedman AJ, Garfield JM, Rein MS, et al. A randomized, placebo controlled, double-blind study evaluating leuprolide acetate depot treatment before myomectomy. Fertil Steril. 1989;52:728–749.
15. Friedman AJ, Juneau-Norcross M, Rein MS. Adverse effects of leuprolide acetate depot treatment. Fertil Steril. 1993;59:448-450.
16. Dubuisson JB, Chapron C, Fauconnier A, et al. Laparoscopic myomectomy and myolysis. Curr Opin Obstet Gynecol. 1997;9:233-8.
17. Shozo Matsuoka, MD*, Iwaho Kikuchi, MD, Mari Kitade, MD et al ; Strategy for Laparoscopic Cervical Myomectomy . Journal of Minimally Invasive Gynecology. 2010;17:301-5.
18. Sinha R, Hegde A, Warty N, et al. Laparoscopic myomectomy: enucleation of the myoma by morcellation while it is attached to the uterus. J Minim Invasive Gynecol. 2005;12:284-9.
19. Torng PL, Hwang JS, Huang SC, et al. Effect of simultaneous morcellation in situ on operative time during laparoscopic myomectomy. Hum Reprod. 2008;23:2220-6.
20. Frederick J, Fletcher H, Simeon D, et al. Intramyometrial vasopressin as a haemostatic agent during myomectomy. Br J Obstet Gynaecol. 1994;101:435-7.

21. Alborzi S, Ghannadan E, Alborzi M. A comparison of combined laparoscopic uterine artery ligation and myomectomy versus laparoscopic myomectomy in treatment of symptomatic myoma. Fertil Steril. 2009;92:742-7.

22. Sinha R, Sundaram M, Lakhotia S, et al. Cervical myomectomy with uterine artery ligation at its origin. J Minim Invasive Gynecol. 2009;16:604-8.

23. Rakesh Sinha, Aparna Hegde, Neeta Warty, and Chaitali Mahajan. Laparoscopic myomectomy: Enucleation of the myoma by morcellation while it is attached to the uterus. Journal of Minimally Invasive Gynecology. 2005;12:284-9.

24. James Robinson and Gaby Moawad. Ins and outs of straight-stick laparoscopic myomectomy. OBG Management. 2012;24(9).

25. Nezhat C, Nezhat F, Bess O. Laparoscopically assisted myomectomy: a report of a new technique in 57 cases. Intl J Fertil Menop Stud. 1994;39:39-44.

26. Davies A, Hart R, Magos A, et al. Hysterectomy: surgical route and complications. Eur J Obstet Gynecol Reprod Biol. 2002; 104:148-151.

27. Boike G, Efstrand E, DePriore G, et al. Laparoscopically assisted vaginal hysterectomy in a university hospital: report of 82 cases and comparison with abdominal and vaginal hysterectomy. Am J Obstet Gynecol. 1993;68:1690-701.

28. Andrea Fiaccavento, Stefano Landi, Fabrizio Barbieri, et al. Total laparoscopic hysterectomy in cases of very large uteri: A retrospective comparative study. Journal of Minimally Invasive Gynecology. 2007;14:559-63.

29. Horace Roman, Joel Zanati, Ludovic Friederich, et al. Laparoscopic Hysterectomy of Large Uteri With Uterine Artery Coagulation at Its Origin. JSLS. 2008;12:25-9.

30. Chang WC, Torng PL, Huang SC, et al. Laparoscopic-assisted vaginal hysterectomy with uterine artery ligation through retrograde umbilical ligament tracking. J Minim Invasive Gynecol. 2005;12(4):336-42.

31. Einstein MH, Barakat RR, Chi DS, et al. Management of uterine malignancy found incidentally after supracervical hysterectomy or uterine morcellation for presumed benign disease. Int J Gynecol Cancer. 2008;18:1065-70.

32. Virk KS. Womencare of Williamsburg, Williamsburg, Virginia. First 2 Cases of Hand Morcellattion When the Morcellator Failed. Journal of Minimally Invasive Gynecology. 2013;20:S133-S181.

33. Wu Shun Felix Wong, Tat Choi Eric Lee, Chi Eung Danforn Lim. Novel Vaginal "Paper Roll" Uterine Morcellation Technique for Removal of Large (500 g) Uterus. Journal of Minimally Invasive Gynecology. 2010;17(3).

34. Horiuchi T, Tanishima H, Tamagowa K, et al. Randomized, controlled investigation of the anti-infective properties of the Alexis Retractor/ Protector of incision sites. J Trauma. 2007; 62:212-215). (Magrina JF. Self-retaining retractor for vaginal operations. J Gynecol Surg. 1991;7:33-6.

35. Walid MS, Heaton RL. Use of bowel bags in gynecologic laparoscopy. Arch Gynecol Obstet. 2009;279(5):777-9.

36. Lin Y-S. New helical incision for removal of large uteri during laparoscopic-assisted vaginal hysterectomy. JAmAssoc Gynecol Laparosc. 2004;11:519-24.

CHAPTER 34

Perioperative Management of High-risk Patients Undergoing Major Laparoscopic Surgery

● MK Pathanjali Prasanna, B Narayanan, VK Ramachandran

■ INTRODUCTION

In 25% to 30% of women, fibroids are diagnosed. Myomas are the most common solid benign tumours of the female genital tract. The treatment options range from medical management, hysteroscopy, laparoscopic myomectomy, robotic-assisted laparoscopic myomectomy, open myomectomy to hysterectomy. Laparoscopic hysterectomy is done for various reasons such as endometrial cancer, cervical cancer and ovarian cancer and can be simple hysterectomy to more complicated procedures such as lymph node removal and pelvic exenteration.

The leading causes of intensive care unit (ICU) admission in postoperative gynaecology patients are haemorrhage, infection and cardiorespiratory failure, and in these patients the 6-month mortality is 26%.[1] The mortality of high risk patients undergoing elective procedures is 5% and emergency procedures is more than 30%.[2] The overall mortality of high risk patients admitted with cancer to intensive therapy unit (ITU) is 47%, whereas the mortality of patients with gynaecological tumours admitted to ITU is just 17% indicating the advances in surgical, anaesthetic and intensive care practice.[3] These include targeted exercise ('prehabilitation'), optimisation of fluid and inotropic therapy, selection of surgical and anaesthetic personnel of appropriate seniority, and appropriate use of critical care facilities. However, allocation of such resources relies on recognition of 'at risk and high risk' patients.

■ HIGH RISK GYNAECOLOGIC PATIENT

Preoperative assessment of the patient helps in recognizing 'at risk' patients, quantifying the risk and helps in planning adequate postoperative care. Most gynaecological procedures are considered 'low risk' whereas laparoscopic surgery is intermediate to high risk surgery. Preoperative assessment should follow general principles paying particular attention to general risk factors such as increased age, smoking, obesity and disease factors such as size of the tumour and spread to distant organs. The paraneoplastic syndromes depicted by ovarian tumours such as cerebellar degeneration, retinopathy, nephrotic syndrome and caudaequina syndrome and uterine cancer such as hypercalcemia, retinopathy, peripheral neuropathy, encephalitis, myelitis and dermatomyositis should also be borne in mind.

Patients are graded as per the American Society of Anesthesiologists (ASA) score grading 1 to 5 based on an anaesthesiologist's subjective assessment of the severity of comorbidities, which however the system lacks discriminatory power. Lee's revised cardiac risk index (RCRI)[4] is currently the most prominent tool to stratify patients into risk categories for postoperative cardiac complications (Table 34.1). Some tools, for example, the Physiological and Operative Severity Score for the enumeration of Mortality and Morbidity (POSSuM) score, incorporate variable weighting, whereby the factors that have the strongest association with poor outcome count the most.

Table 34.1: Lee class and risk of major cardiac complication

Points	Class	Risk (%)
0	I	0.4
1	II	0.9
2	III	6.6
≥ 3	IV	11

Each predictor adds one point to the final score and is associated with a Lee class and incidence of major cardiac complications (cardiac death, myocardial infarction, pulmonary oedema, complete heart block and cardiac arrest) as indicated:

1. High-risk surgery (intraperitoneal, intrathoracic or suprainguinal vascular procedures).
2. Ischaemic heart disease.
3. History of congestive cardiac failure.
4. History of cerebrovascular disease.
5. Insulin therapy for diabetes mellitus.
6. Preoperative creatinine level < 176 μmollitre.[1]

■ COMPLICATIONS OF LAPAROSCOPIC MYOMECTOMY AND HYSTERECTOMY

The complications result from:

1. Patient factors (obesity, intra-abdominal spread of cancer resulting in adhesions, ascites, bowel obstruction/perforation and cardiorespiratory disorders)
2. Laparoscopic surgery.
3. Patient positioning and neuropathic injuries.
4. Complications specific to procedures.

Patient Factors

Obesity

Among Obese patients undergoing laparoscopic hysterectomies, about 40% of laparoscopic hysterectomies happen in morbidly obese (BMI > 40) and 19.6% occur in super obese patients (BMI > 50).[5] Perioperative management of obese surgical patients is beyond the scope of this chapter, but general considerations are given below (Box 34.1).[6]

1. Every hospital should nominate an anaesthetic lead for obesity.
2. Operating lists should include the patients weight and body mass index (BMI) (obesity surgery mortality risk stratification score OS-MRS > 4–5 done by consultant level anaesthetist.
3. Experienced anaesthetic and surgical staff should manage obese patients.
4. Additional specialised equipment is necessary.
5. Central obesity and metabolic syndrome should be identified as risk factors.

Box 34.1: Equipment needed to manage obese patients

Ward equipment
Specialised electrically operated beds that can raise a patient to standing without the need for manual handling with pressure-relieving mattresses
Suitable bathrooms with floor-mounted toilets, suitable commodes
Large blood pressure measuring cuffs
Extra large gowns
Suitably sized compression stockings and intermittent compression devices
Larger chairs, wheelchairs and trolleys, all marked with the maximal recommended weight
Scales capable of weighing up to 300 kg
On-site blood gas analysis
Continuous positive airway pressure or high-flow oxygen delivery device for the post-anaesthesia care unit
Patient hoist or other moving device (may be shared with other departments)
Theatre equipment
Bariatric operating table, able to incorporate armboards and table extensions, attachments for positioning such as leg supports for the lithotomy position, and shoulder and foot supports
Gel pads and padding for pressure points
Wide velcro strapping to secure the patient to the operating table
Ramping device/pillows
Raised step for the anaesthesiologist
Large tourniquets
Readily available difficult airway equipment
Anaesthetic ventilator capable of positive end-expiratory pressure and various pressure modalities
Portable ultrasound machine
Hover-mattress or slide sheet
Long spinal and epidural needles
Long arterial lines if femoral access is necessary
Neuromuscular blockade monitor
Depth of anaesthesia monitoring to minimise residual sedation

6. Sleep-disordered breathing and its consequences should always be considered in the obese.
7. Anaesthetising the patient in the operating theatre with adequate positioning equipment should be considered.
8. Regional anaesthesia is recommended, but is often technically difficult and may often be impossible to achieve.
9. A robust airway strategy must be planned and discussed, as desaturation occurs quickly in the obese patient and airway management can be difficult. A neck circumference > 60 cm at the level of Adam's apple predicts 35% risk of difficult intubation.

10. Use of the ramped or sitting position is recommended as an aid to induction and recovery.
11. Drug dosing should generally be based upon lean body weight and titrated to effect, rather than dosed to total body weight.
12. Caution is required with the use of long-acting opioids and sedatives.
13. Neuromuscular monitoring should always be used whenever neuromuscular blocking drugs are used.
14. Depth of anaesthesia monitoring should be considered, especially when total intravenous anaesthesia is used in conjunction with neuromuscular blocking drugs.
15. Full monitoring instituted in post anaesthesia care unit. O_2 therapy is given to maintain saturations equivalent to preoperative levels. CPAP instituted immediately if used in preoperative period. Ongoing hypoventilation will require level 2 ICU. Patient can be discharged to the ward if routine discharge criteria are met, no periods of apnea or hypoventilation for at least an hour and arterial O_2 concentration return to preoperative levels with or without O_2 supplementation.
16. Appropriate prophylaxis against venous thromboembolism (VTE) and early mobilisation are recommended since the incidence of venous thromboembolism is increased in the obese. The mainstay of VTE prophylaxis in obesity is pharmacological, with the criteria for pharmacological prophylaxis including prolonged immobilisation; total theatre time > 90 min; age > 60 years; BMI > 30 kg^{m-2}; cancer; dehydration and a family history of VTE.
17. Postoperative intensive care support should be considered, but is determined more by comorbidities and surgery than by obesity on its own. If admitted to critical care requiring mechanical ventilation, tidal volumes of 5–7 mL/Kg are calculated based on ideal body weight with peak pressure to be limited to < 35 cm H_2O. Tracheostomies are performed early. Levels of drugs are monitored routinely and early hypocaloric diets instituted. Cardio pulmonary resuscitation will possess a challenge in this group of patients.

Other Factors

Patients with stage 3 or 4 ovarian cancer has 89% incidence of ascites. Extensive spread may make the surgery long and complicated. Cardiorespiratory assessment should be done early in the preoperative period to decide the postoperative plan and location of care. Adequate postoperative pain control with low thoracic epidural analgesia for extensive hysterectomies improves patient outcome. Gabapentin 250 mg to 500 mg orally 1 hour preoperatively as a one off dose or continued three times a day for 4 days are followed in lot of hospitals with good results. Perioperative gabapentin reduces postoperative pain and opioid requirements and may reduce

the incidence of vomiting, pruritis and urinary retention, but increases the risk of sedation (which would need individual patient titration) in the postoperative patient. However, they are not very effective analgesics on their own and hence need to be used in a multimodal approach with other drugs.

Laparoscopic Surgery

The risks and benefits of laparoscopic surgeries are detailed in Table 34.2.

Table 34.2: Risks and benefits of laparoscopic surgeries

Benefits	Risks
Reduced wound infection	Visceral and vascular damage
Faster recovery	Complications associated with extremes of positioning
Reduced morbidity	Acute kidney injury
Reduced pain	Cardiocerebral vascular insufficiency
	Pulmonary atelectasis
	Venous gas embolism
	'Well leg compartment syndrome'

Complications associated from pneumoperitoneum rarely occur, although pneumothorax, mediastinal emphysema and diaphragmatic rupture may result from high insufflation pressures. Vascular absorption of CO_2 gas may also cause an acidosis or even be fatal, as with gas emboli. Not uncommonly, patients may experience subcutaneous emphysema and crepitus may be noted upon examination. Referred shoulder pain originates from diaphragmatic irritation from gas, blood or fluid. These minor side effects generally resolve within 24 hours, but can be concerning to the patient.

Reported complications in gynecologic laparoscopy range from 0.1% to 10%, with over 50% of injuries occurring at the time of entry and 20% to 25% not recognized until the postoperative period. The incidence of entry access injury has been reported as 5 to 30 occurrences per 100,000 procedures, with bowel and retroperitoneal vascular injuries comprising almost 76% of all injuries.[7] Almost half of small and large bowel injuries went unrecognized for at least 24 hours, with most of the injuries recognized as patients' experienced increasing abdominal pain, fever and prolonged ileus. Vascular injury is less common in laparoscopy but certainly occurs and can have significant morbidity and mortality. The iliac artery is the most common site of vascular injury, involving 19% of all laparoscopic injuries. Injury to the iliac vein or other retroperitoneal veins constitute 9% of vascular injuries during laparoscopy.[7] Although the aorta and inferior vena cava are the vessels most commonly injured in fatal occurrences, fortunately, large vessel injury comprises a very small percentage of all laparoscopic injuries, with the aorta and inferior vena cava injured in just 6% and 4% of total injuries, respectively. So vigilance in the postoperative period regarding the above complications is necessary.

Several risk factors increase the complication rate of laparoscopy. Patients with a significant surgical history including one or more laparotomies or abdominal wall hernias are at risk for significant adhesive disease, especially involving the anterior abdominal wall. Those patients with a history of intra-abdominal disease including pelvic inflammatory disease, endometriosis or diverticulitis are also at an inherently higher risk of complications secondary to adhesive disease. Other risk factors involved with laparoscopy may include very large pelvic masses, bowel distention, cardiopulmonary disease and obesity. The surgeon's laparoscopic experience may play a role in the rate of complications and learning curve of approximately 30 procedures for TLH is recognized.[8]

Other complications such as injuries to urinary tract, which is suspected by the presence of blood in the urinary catheter and increasing serum creatinine, large abdominal wall haematomas, wound infections and sepsis may warrant prolonged postoperative care.

Patient Positioning and Neuropathic Injuries

Either supine or modified lithotomy position (if uterine manipulation is required) is advisable, with the patient's arms flexed over the chest.

Although the Trendelenburg position is not frequently associated with stasis of blood in the extremities, the lithotomy position with general anaesthesia and use of muscle relaxants may increase the predisposition to deep venous thrombosis (DVT). Graded compression stockings, sequential compression device and subcutaneous low-molecular-weight heparin together reduce the incidence of DVT by almost 75%.[9]

In steep Trendelenburg position (25°–40°) with pneumoperitoneum as can occur with prolonged robotic surgeries, Badaway et al, reported an incidence of intraoperative hypercapnia (ETCO$_2$ > 5 mm Hg) in 18% of their series of 133 patients undergoing robotic hysterectomy. Their incidence of significant intraoperative hypoxemia (SpO$_2$ < 90%) was less than 4%.[10]

Edema of the face can be seen, along with conjunctival edema. Corneal abrasions are associated with gynecological laparoscopy.[11] This edema can push the patient's upper and lower eyelids apart, causing desiccation and abrasion of the cornea, even when the eyes are taped closed. A horizontal line across the cornea is seen on ophthalmic examination postoperatively. Steep Trendelenburg with increased intra-abdominal pressure from insufflation raises intragastric pressure, and passive aspiration of stomach fluid into the patient's eye.[12]

Furthermore, of concern to the anesthesiologist is the possibility of edema of the supraglottic airway structures,

namely the vocal cords, arytenoids and epiglottis.[13] The lower extremities may be hypo perfused in steep Trendelenburg and cases of postoperative rhabdomyolysis have been reported.[14] A situation such as this would be made worse by overly-tight table straps and improper positioning of leg holders (which can also cause peroneal and femoral nerve damage).[15] Femoral vein blood flow is decreased by pneumoperitoneum.[16] Proper care should be taken to protect pressure points and to prevent neuropathic injuries. Padding of the arms and access to the drips, and arterial line will depend on the patient's body habitus and availability of equipment; arms may be wrapped by the side, tucked on chest, or placed on arm boards. The precise position may be guided by surgical need for adequate operative access. In open procedures, we would place the patient's arms out on arm boards, while in lithotomy head down position for laparoscopic procedures, arms are wrapped by the patient's side, aiding surgery, frequently making anaesthetic access a challenge.

Complications Specific to Procedures

The average time for Laparoscopic myomectomy is 113 minutes,[17] total abdominal hysterectomy is 98 minutes and laparascopy assisted vaginal hysterectomy is 144 minutes.[18] robotic-assisted surgeries take a long time depending on the skill of the operator. The average blood loss for these surgeries is less than 200 mL,[19] but with complicated surgeries with multiple patient comorbidities, intraoperative and postoperative management would require invasive monitoring.

Laparoscopic Myomectomy

Laparoscopic myomectomy has resulted in significant advantages to the patients in medical, social and economic terms with shorter recovery time and less postoperative time and equal comparable results with open myomectomy. Specific concerns for the anesthesiologist are as follows:

Vasopressin: Before incising the myometrium covering the myoma, a 10 cc solution of vasopressin or diluted adrenaline (1/100) is frequently injected into the tissue layers, to make tissue ischemia easier and better delineate the cleavage plane and the pseudocapsule. As it is a potent systemic vasoconstrictor, it often causes hypertension and bradycardia. It has a plasma half life of 10 to 20 minutes. Care should be taken to infiltrate a dilute solution with haemodynamic monitoring. To avoid unwanted surges in blood pressure, Nitroglycerine, which is a vasodilator can be given in small aliquots. Care should be taken to prevent myocardial ischemia during injection of vasopressin.

Intra-operative and postoperative hypothermia: Prolonged laparoscopy under general anaesthesia or combined general and regional anaesthesia induces hypothermia, despite reduced bowel exposure during laparoscopic surgery. Using a closed circuit with low flows that give warm humidified gases, warm intravenous fluids and a thermoflator reduces postoperative hypothermia and analgesia requirement.

Analgesia: Pain varies and depends upon the length of surgery, intra-abdominal pressure, and the amount of dissection involved. Multimodal analgesia with a single preoperative dose of dexamethasone has lead to the introduction of 'dexamethasone-induced postoperative pain reduction' theory, due to its strong anti-inflammatory properties. Although analgesic mechanism of dexamethasone is still unclear, it seems that a decrease in cyclooxygenase and lipoxygenase production, via inhibition of peripheral phospholipase, plays a main role.[20] High-dose intravenous paracetamol 1 g 4 times a day with non-steroidal anti-inflammatory drugs (NSAIDs) with local anaesthetic infiltration at the port sites is sufficient. Epidural analgesia is a good option if the surgical dissection is extensive and if the patient is admitted in hospital for at least 2 to 3 days. It has various advantages like decreasing movement related pain, reduced incidence of DVT, improving respiratory mechanics, decreased stress response due to surgery thus facilitating bowel movement, all of which will aid in a smooth and early recovery.

Transverse abdominus plane block which has to be done bilaterally using the ultrasound is another option which can give pain relief from 18 to 24 hours.

Delirium: Postoperative confusion has been studied in patients over the age of 60 undergoing gynaeoncology surgery. Delirium occurred in 17.5% of patients, more commonly in the elderly and those with hypoalbuminemia, associated comorbidities, postoperative blood transfusion and immobility.[21]

PONV: Risk factors for PONV should be identified before operation. Preventive strategies aimed at decreasing the baseline risk such as the use of intraoperative regional analgesia, the avoidance of volatile agents or nitrous oxide, and use of antiemetic drugs should be applied. Additional treatment in the postoperative period should include serotonin antagonists, dexamethasone and dopamine antagonists. Aprepitant is a new agent, licensed for chemotherapy-induced nausea and vomiting, and has been used as an oral dose before operation in PONV prevention. It is as effective as the other classes of antiemetics.[22]

Laparascopic Hysterectomy

1. The RCT of 2616 patients treated by laparoscopic or abdominal hysterectomy reported no significant difference in the rate of intraoperative complications (10% [160/1682] vs 8% [69/909], p = 0.106), but significantly fewer postoperative complications after laparoscopic compared with abdominal hysterectomy (14% [240/1682] vs 21% [191/909], p < 0.00123).

2. The RCT of 2616 patients and the non-randomized comparative study of 309 patients reported intraoperative complications of bowel injury (2% [37/1682] and less than 1% [1/165]), vascular injury (4% [75/1682] and 1% [2/165]), bladder injury (1% [21/1682 and 2/165]) and ureter injury (less than 1% [14/1682 and 1/165]) among patients treated by laparoscopic hysterectomy.[23]

3. Antibiotic prophylaxis should be administered at induction of anaesthesia. In prolonged procedures, a repeat dose needs to be considered. The choice of antibiotic should follow local protocols.

4. Thromboprophylaxis can be either mechanical or pharmacological, which includes graded compression stockings or elastic stockings, intermittent pneumatic compression (IPC) devices, low-dose-unfractionated heparin (LDUH), low-molecular-weight heparin (LMWH), fondaparinux, aspirin, inferior vena cava (IVC) filters and surveillance with venous compression ultrasonography (VCU) have all been used to prevent venous thromboembolism (VTE).

The following risk stratification is a simple classification to identify the high risk group. In high-risk patients, a combined regimen of medical and mechanical prophylaxis may improve clinical efficacy, although there is limited evidence in gynecologic patients. Extrapolation from the general surgery literature suggests a significant benefit from a combined regimen.[24,25] Since there are no guidelines formulated specifically for laparoscopic procedures. The American College of Obstetricians and Gynecologists (ACOG) recommends that, until more evidence is accumulated, patients undergoing laparoscopic surgery should be stratified by risk category and should receive prophylaxis similar to that provided to patients undergoing laparotomy (Table 24.3).[26]

Table 34.4: Traditional risk classification for gynecologic surgery[27]

Risk level	Definition
Low	Surgery lasting < 30 minutes in patients < 40 years with no additional risk factors
Moderate	Surgery lasting < 30 minutes in patients with additional risk factors; surgery lasting < 30 minutes in patients aged 40–60 years with no additional risk factors; major surgery in patients < 40 years with no additional risk factors
High	Surgery lasting < 30 minutes in patients >60 years or with additional risk factors; major surgery in patients > 40 years or with additional risk factors
Highest	Major surgery in patients > 60 years plus prior VTE, cancer or molecular hypercoagulable state

Overall risk of deep vein thrombosis (DVT) is 7% to 45%, and is associated with fatal embolism in 1%.[28] Thromboembolic events may be the presenting feature of cancer and hence may complicate surgical planning.

5. Postoperative analgesia should be a continuation of the intraoperative analgesia using a multimodal approach where possible. Standard pain management after laparoscopic or open hysterectomy includes PCA using opioids with subsequent conversion to oral controlled-release oxycodone. Procedure-specific postoperative pain management website (http://www.postoppain.org) has issued recommendations for abdominal hysterectomies. In patients with high risk of developing significant postoperative pain, epidural analgesia is recommended. Chronic pain after abdominal hysterectomy ranges in incidence between 5% and 32%. These studies also included benign conditions and endometriosis patients. The surgical process is responsible for 22% of chronic pain overall. Various approaches in hysterectomy (laparoscopic or open) are not associated with an increased incidence of chronic pain development. Important contributing factors include poorly controlled pre- or postoperative pain and anxiety.

CONCLUSION

Entry-level bowel injuries are the commonest cause of mortality in gynecologic laparoscopic surgeries. It is found that even patients with advanced cardiorespiratory problems, other organ failure such as renal, gastrointestinal, sepsis are more common than cardiac problems. Thorough preoperative assessment and selection of patients, appropriate intraoperative care including monitoring, careful positioning, adequate anaesthesia and post operative care involving prompt recognition of complications and management are essential for reducing mortality and morbidity following laparoscopic gynecological surgeries.

REFERENCES

1. Heinonen S, Tyrvainen E, Penttinen J, et al. Need for critical care in gynaecology: a population based analysis. Crit Care. 2002;6:371-5.
2. National Confidential Enquiry into Patient Outcome and Death. Knowing the risk. A review of the peri-operative care of surgical patients. 2011.
3. Namendys-Silva SA, Gonzáles-Herrera MO, Texcocano-Becerra J, et al. Outcomes of critically ill gynaecological cancers admitted to intensive care unit. Am J Hosp Palliat Care. 2013;30:7-11.
4. Lee TH, Marcantonio ER, Mangione CM, et al. Derivation and prospective validation of a simple index for prediction of cardiac risk of major noncardiac surgery. Circulation. 1999;100:1043-9.
5. Giugale LE, Di Santo N, Smolkin ME, et al. Beyond mere obesity: effect of increasing obesity classifications on hysterectomy outcomes for uterine cancer/hysperplasia. GynecolOncol. 2012;127:326-31.
6. Anaesthesia; Volume 70, Issue 7, pages 859–876, July 2015.
7. Chandler JG, Corson SL, Way LW. Three spectra of laparoscopic entry access injuries. J Am Coll Surg. 2001;192(4):478-90.
8. Tunitsky E, Citil A, Ayaz R, et al. Does surgical volume influence short-term outcomes of laparoscopic hysterectomy?.American Journal of Obstetrics and Gynecology. 2010/07. 203(1):24e1-24e6.
9. Manju Sinha and Sheetal Chiplonkar. Anesthesia Concerns in Laparoscopic Myomectomy Gynecol Endosc Surg. 2011;2(1):18-20.
10. Badaway M, Beique F, Al-Halal H, et al. Anesthesia considerations for robotic surgery in gynecologic oncology. J Robot Surg. 2011;5:235-9.
11. Kim K, Kim HJ, No JH, et al. Increased risk for post-operative corneal injuries in patients who undergo laparoscopic gynecologic surgery. ActaAnaesthesiol Scand. 2012;56:504-6.
12. J Thomas McLarney and Gregory L Rose. Anaesthetic Implications of Robotic Gynecologic SurgeryJ Gynecol Endosc Surg. 2011;2(2):75-8.
13. Phong SV, Koh LK. Anaesthesia for robotic-assisted radical prostatectomy: Considerations for laparoscopy in the Trendelenburg position. Anaesth Intensive Care. 2007;35:281-5.
14. Galyon SW, Richards KA, Pettus JA, et al. Three-limb compartment syndrome and rhabdomyolysis after robotic cystoprostatectomy. J ClinAnesth. 2011;23:75-8.
15. Olympio MA. Anaesthetic considerations for robotic urologic surgery. In: Hemel AK, Menon M, editors. Robotics in Genitourinary Surgery. London: Springer-Verlag Limited. 2011. pp. 79-95.
16. O'Malley C, Cunningham AJ. Physiologic changes during laparoscopy. AnesthesiolClin North America. 2001;19:1-19.
17. Shushan A1, Mohamed H, Magos AL. How long does laparoscopic surgery really take? Lessons learned from 1000 operative laparoscopies. Hum Reprod. 1999;14(1):39-43.
18. James E Carter, Jisun Ryoo, Amy Katz. Laparoscopic-Assisted Vaginal Hysterectomy:A Case Control Comparative Study With Total Abdominal Hysterectomy. J Amer Assoc Gynecol Laparosc. 1997;1:259-62.
19. A Perino, G Cucinella, R Venezia, et al. Total laparoscopic hysterectomy versus total abdominal hysterectomy: an assessment of the learning curve in a prospective randomized study. Human Reproduction. 1999;14(12):2996-9.
20. Callery MP. Preoperative steroids for laparoscopic surgery. Ann Surg. 2003;238(5):661–2. doi: 10.1097/01 sla.0000094391.39418.8e. [PMC free article] [PubMed] [Cross Ref]
21. McAlpine JN, Hodgson EJ, Abramowitz S, et al. The incidence and risk factors associated with postoperative delirium in geriatric patients undergoing surgery for suspected gynaecologic malignancies. GynecolOncol. 2008;109:296-302.
22. McAlpine JN, Hodgson EJ, Abramowitz S, et al. The incidence and risk factors associated with postoperative delirium in

geriatric patients undergoing surgery for suspected gynaecologic malignancies. GynecolOncol. 2008;109:296-302.

23. Laparoscopic hysterectomy (including laparoscopic total hysterectomy and laparoscopically assisted vaginal hysterectomy) for endometrial cancer. NICE interventional procedure guidance [IPG356]; Published September 2010.

24. Agnelli G, Piovella F, Buoncristiani P, et al. Enoxaparin plus compression stockings compared with compression stockings alone in the prevention of venous thromboembolism after elective neurosurgery. N Engl J Med. 1998;339:80-5.

25. Wille-Jorgensen P, Rasmussen MS, Andersen BR, et al. Heparins and mechanical methods for thromboprophylaxis in colorectal surgery. Cochrane Database of Systematic Reviews 2004, Issue 1. Art. No.: CD001217. DOI: 10.1002/14651858.CD001217.

26. ACOG Practice Bulletin No. 84: Prevention of deep vein thrombosis and pulmonary embolism. Obstet Gynecol. 2007;110(2 Pt 1):429-40.

27. Modified from ACOG Practice Bulletin No. 84: Prevention of deep vein thrombosis and pulmonary embolism. Obstet Gynecol. 2007;110(2 Pt 1):429-40.

28. Gadducci A, Cosio S, Spirito N, et al. The perioperative management of patients with gynaecological cancer undergoing major surgery: A debated clinical challenge. Clin Rev Oncol Hematol. 2010;73:126-40.

CHAPTER 35

Vaginal Hysterectomy in Fibroids

● Pooja Sharma Dimri

The vaginal route of hysterectomy has an important role in the management of benign gynecological pathologies even in the era of laparoscopic surgery. In the age of laparoscopic hysterectomy, vaginal hysterectomy (VH) still retains its place and utility in the armamentarium of the gynecologist because of its use of a natural orifice, low morbidity and fast recovery and low cost. VH is the signature surgery of a gynecologist and must be judiciously performed for carefully chosen patients. Traditionally, VH is performed for cases of uterine descent. But it is also useful in cases of benign pathology with non-descent of the uterus. According to a recent systematic review, as compared to abdominal hysterectomies the advantages of vaginal hysterectomies are significantly speedier return to normal activities, shorter duration of hospital stay, and fewer unspecified infections or febrile episodes.[1]

The main aim of laparoscopic hysterectomy (TLH) was to replace abdominal hysterectomy (AH), which was associated with high morbidity, increased blood loss and long postoperative recovery. The advent of laparoscopy started the question on choice of type of hysterectomy. But it was not meant to be an alternative to vaginal hysterectomy, which by itself a least invasive approach. The route of hysterectomy should be chosen keeping in mind the benefit to the patient and not the surgeon. In case of uterovaginal prolapse, vaginal hysterectomy is the route of choice. The question arises in case of non-descent uterus with benign conditions like fibroid/dysfunctional uterine bleeding and adenomyosis. Vaginal hysterectomy is not only feasible for normal sized uteri, but also for bigger uteri including those with fibroids. Uterine myoma should not be considered a contraindication

for vaginal hysterectomy. Also, it should be remembered that no step, which is done laparoscopically, i.e. ligating the upper pedicle, bladder dissection or uterine artery ligation makes the vaginal part of the surgery any simpler. The most important factors determining the feasibility of hysterectomy by vaginal approach is the access, which is dependent on the subpubic arch and size of uterus if access is restricted. In the absence of pelvic pathology, every woman has sufficient descent to initiate vaginal hysterectomy and once the uterosacral and cardinal ligaments are divided, progressive descent occurs. In case the access is limited, vaginal hysterectomy is going to be difficult especially in case of big uterus and fibroid uterus. In this case, a laparoscopic hysterectomy in trained hands will be a better suited minimal access technique.

■ ROUTE OF HYSTERECTOMY: WHAT DOES EVIDENCE SAY?

The 2009 Cochrane Database Systemic Review, which included only randomized controlled trials, comparing one surgical approach of hysterectomy with another and looked at the most beneficial and least harmful surgical approach to hysterectomy for women with benign gynecological conditions. Evidence concludes that no benefits accrue from TLH when compared with VH. TLH is accompanied by disadvantages of increased operation time—operation theatre occupancy and higher complication rate. The conclusion drawn from all the parameters in this study is that VH should be performed in preference to AH where possible and where VH is not possible, TLH may avoid the need for AH.[2] Donnez et al, presented a series of 3190 laparoscopic hysterectomies for benign disease from 1990 to 2006, wherein complications of TLH/LAVH were compared with those of AH and VH. The authors concluded that in experienced hands, TLH is safe, cost-effective, and without any increase in major complication rates.

However, when VH can be performed safely, the laparoscopic method does not come into consideration. In other words, TLH can replace AH. Remarkably, they reduced the incidence of AH to a paltry 3.8%.[3] A prospective observational multicenter study was undertaken in France and 12 out of 15 university hospitals participated in it. The aim was to evaluate complications and the routes of hysterectomy for benign pathology. The results showed that the vaginal route is being increasingly used for hysterectomy in France and is the route of choice for benign disorders.[4] The evaluate hysterectomy study, a multicenter randomized trial showed TLH was associated with a significantly higher risk of major complications and took longer time than AH.[5] The value (vaginal, abdominal, laparoscopic uterine extirpation) study was conducted in UK to study about various routes of hysterectomy. 37,298 cases were reported which is estimated to reflect about 45% of hysterectomies performed during the studied period.

The proportions of women having abdominal, vaginal or laparoscopically assisted hysterectomy were 67%, 30% and 3%, respectively. Laparoscopic hysterectomy accounted for only a small number (7.6%) and the remainder were performed vaginally (18.4%). The preferred method of removing the uterus is mainly determined by the preference of the surgeon and his or her training and experience in a particular technique.[6] In the USA, a country where litigation is very common, the American College of Obstetricians and Gynecologists (ACOG) recommends the use of laparoscopy to assist vaginal surgery, i.e. by LAVH in case of adhesiolysis, pelvic endometriosis, difficult oophorectomy, fibroid that complicates VH and when evaluation of abdominal/pelvic cavity is warranted to avoid opening the abdomen. It also means that in absence of the above complications/situations, hysterectomy can be completed vaginally. Cost, theatre occupancy, and complications somehow reduce the credibility and advantages of use of the laparoscope.[7] Vaginal hysterectomy is considered least invasive and cost-effective surgical method of surgical removal of the uterus.[8]

In spite of its clear advantages, gynecologists do not prefer vaginal hysterectomy as the preferred mode of removal of uterus removal. Only 20% to 25% hysterectomies are performed vaginally. The main issue is lack of skill and adequate training among gynecologists. Therefore, any condition that increases the technical difficulty like nulliparity,

history of previous surgery, existence of adnexal disease and large uterus may lead to rejection of vaginal hysterectomy as a viable option. But with regular training and skill development, these may not be considered as contraindications to vaginal hysterectomy.[6,9–11] With adequate vaginal access, technical skill and good uterine mobility, vaginal hysterectomy can easily be achieved. The main supports of the uterus, the uterosacral and cardinal ligaments, situated in close proximity to the vaginal vault can be easily divided to produce descent. Multiparity, lax tissues due to poor involution following multiple deliveries and lesser tissue tensile strength give a lot of comfort to vaginal surgeon even in the presence of significant uterine enlargement. The other important reason for the lower proportion of hysterectomies performed vaginally is the presence of uterine enlargement with leiomyomas, one of the most common indications.

However, big and bulky uteri can be dealt with by techniques like bisection, myomectomy, wedge debulking and intramyometrial coring (morcellation). There are various studies bulky uteri up to 20 weeks size pregnant uterus have been removed vaginally without undue rise in incidence of complications, blood loss, operative time or hospital stay.

■ FACTORS AFFECTING VAGINAL HYSTERECTOMY IN UTERINE MYOMA (Box 35.2)

Vaginal Access

As discussed earlier, the limiting factor to successful performance of vaginal hysterectomy is the access of the vagina is the access to the vagina. Access may be restricted in cases of nulliparity. The important factors governing vaginal access are angle of the pubic arch and the breadth of the vaginal apex. A subpubic angle greater than 90 degrees generally will allow easy access to the uterus and to insert instruments. The other factor is breadth of the vaginal apex, which should be at least more than 3 cm to allow anterior and posterior accessibility as well as visualisation of uterine vessels laterally. Both the pubic arch and vaginal apex can be assessed at the preoperative visit in the outpatient department. In case of a narrow introitus a midline episiotomy incision can be given to widen the entry and facilitate the procedure. Fixed or self-retaining retractors can also improve the exposure along with good anaesthesia and proper lighting. Another factor considered to be important is uterine descent. Descent is measured relative to ischial spines. Usually descent 1 cm below the ischial spine is considered adequate for vaginal hysterectomy. But even in absence of descent, vaginal hysterectomy is feasible if access is there. Examination under anaesthesia may be useful in determining the choice of route.

Box 35.2: Factors determining vaginal hysterectomy in fibroid uterus

Vaginal Access
Pubic arch/vaginal apex/descent
Size and shape of the uterus
Volume of uterus/size and number of fibroids/lateral fibro
Presence of extra-uterine pathology
Pelvic adhesions/endometriosis/large adnexal mass
Debulking the uterus
Medical methods/mechanical reduction in size
Use of energy source like ERBE BiClamp (BiClamp VIO system ceramic, insulated, angled 18°, smooth)
Skill and experience of the surgeon

Size, Site and Shape of Uterus

Large uterine size is a deterrent to most surgeons for performing vaginal hysterectomy. Traditionally, uterine size is assessed by bimanual examination and is expressed corresponding to weeks of gestation. In case of multiple fibroids, laterally enlarged uterus and obese patient the assessment of uterine size is not accurate and uterine volume is a better indicator to determine feasibility of surgery. In case of uterus more than 200 cm^3 volume or 8 to 10 weeks size uterine volume should be determined preoperatively. Uterine volume can be determined by ultrasound assessment and is a better assessment then size alone for debulking. Relying on fundal height alone may lead to unexpected difficulty during surgery as uterine volumes can grossly vary in uteri corresponding to the same fundal height.[12,13] It is to be remembered that the cut off for size and volume increases with surgeon skill and experience. The evaluation of uterine shape, mobility and number and location of fibroids is also as important. Big fibroids in the cervix and lower uterine segment can make colpotomy difficult. Large lateral fibroids interfere with the side accessibility. It is difficult to secure the uterine vessels in these cases and also to reach the uterine upper pedicle (cornual structures). Any fibroid that does not allow uterine descent is a contraindication to hysterectomy.

A uterine size of 16 weeks or 400 cm^3 may be tackled by an average vaginal surgeon. When the uterine size exceeds 16 weeks or 400 cm^3 a skilled surgeon with greater experience in debulking is the key. A trial of vaginal hysterectomy is warranted in uterine size greater than 16 weeks with informed consent for laparoscopic or abdominal hysterectomy taken from the patient preoperatively. A uterus with size greater than 20 to 24 weeks or 600 to 800 cm^3 are better dealt with abdominally preferably by laparoscopic route.

Reduction in Size of Uterus/Debulking

Debulking of fibroid or uterus is an important step in the performance of a vaginal hysterectomy. Good technique of debulking is essential in uterine size greater than 400 cm^3 or corresponding to 16 week of gestation size. A preoperative administration of gonadotropin-releasing hormone (GnRH) agonists can lead to reduction in size of fibroid and uterus and make vaginal hysterectomy feasible. The size can be reduced from 25% to 50% after 3 months course of GnRH agonists. This not only reduces the size, making the surgery easier, but also gives time to improve the haemoglobin in anemic patients by reducing blood loss. Debulking becomes necessary when all accessible tissue has been cut and no further descent is possible for the delivery of uterus from anterior or posterior space. A uterus more than 12 to 14 weeks in size or 250 to 350 cm^3 volume will invariably require debulking.[14] Total size of the uterus, total uterine volume and access to the myoma for debulking are important considerations.

Transvaginal uterine morcellation can be used for debulking the uterus during vaginal hysterectomy. This obviates the main concern of vaginal delivery of a large uterus with fibroids by the vaginal route. The various methods of mechanical morcellation are haemisection of the uterus, myometrial coring and myomectomy to reduce the size of the uterus (Box 35.2).

Box 35.2: Methods of uterine debulking during vaginal hysterectomy

Bisection
Wedge resection
Intramyometrial coring
Myomectomy

Presence of Extrauterine Pathology

Another important consideration is concomitant presence of disease outside the uterus. This includes presence of pelvic adhesions, endometriosis and large adnexal masses. Vaginal route may be contraindicated in case of extensive pelvic pathology. In case of suspicion of pelvic disease in a woman otherwise fit for vaginal hysterectomy, a diagnostic laparoscopy can be performed to assess the feasibility for hysterectomy and even procedures like adhesiolysis can be done to facilitate it.

Surgeon Factors

The skill and capability of the surgeon is an important consideration in performance of a difficult hysterectomy. The development of skill requires adequate training and experience.

DEBULKING OF UTERUS IN VAGINAL HYSTERECTOMY

Debulking the fibroid or large uterus is the essential requisite in performance of a hysterectomy for a fibroid uterus. Debulking requires a certain degree of training and skill to perform to avoid injury and complications. Before debulking a detailed sonographic assessment of the uterus including, uterine dimensions and uterine volume, number, site and size of fibroids, distance of myoma from internal os, endometrial surface and fundus and differentiation from adenomyosis. The angle between lateral cervix and uterine border can be used to assess the feasibility of vaginal hysterectomy. If the angle is less than or equal to 90 degrees, vaginal hysterectomy is contraindicated (Fig. 35.1).[15]

Also a careful assessment of adnexa should be done. Debulking should be done only after the uterine vessels are secured. Bladder should be empty and catheterized. The bladder anteriorly and the rectum posteriorly should be protected by two Sim's specula or retractors. The debulking process involves continues traction on the cervix to bring the uterus nearer to the operator. The principle is to convert the transverse bulk of the uterus into a longitudinal cylinder, which can be delivered vaginally. The operator should be aware that uterine fibroids can cause distortion of the anatomy and the course of ureter and uterine artery may vary in these cases. During debulking injury to the vaginal wall should also be prevented. The full description of vaginal hysterectomy is beyond the scope of this chapter. We will discuss the various methods of debulking the uterus in the following section.

Uterine Bisection (Figs 35.2A and B)

In this traction is applied to the cervix and it is pulled towards the operator. Then it is incised anteriorly and posteriorly. Care should be taken to always retract bladder anteriorly and rectum posteriorly using retractors. The incision is extended

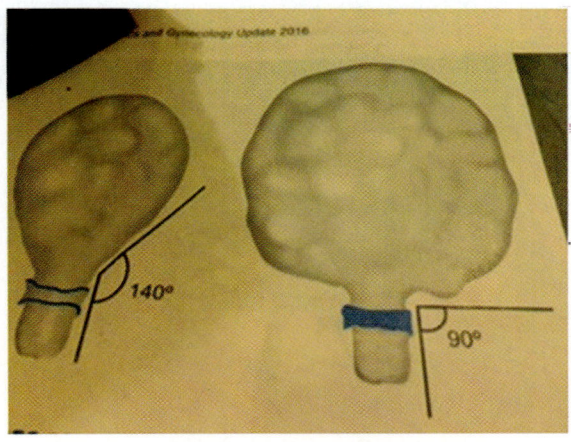

Fig. 35.1: Angle between cervix and lateral border of uterus

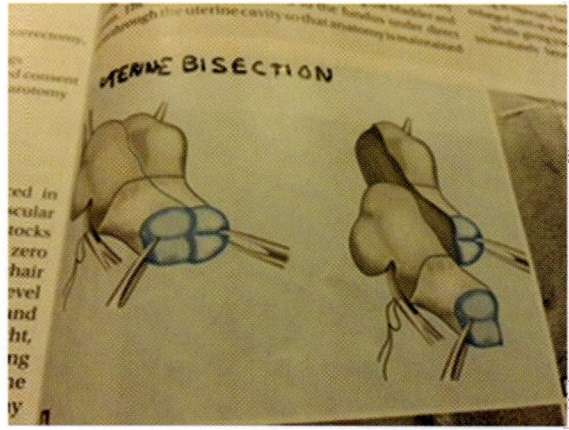

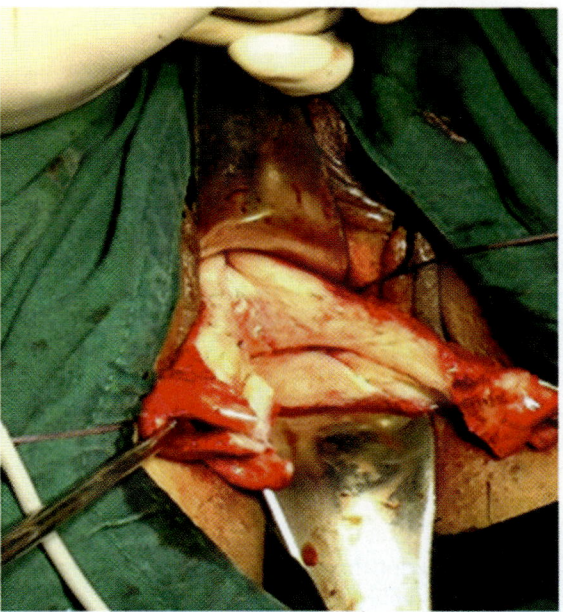

Figs 35.2A and B: A. Bisection; B. Uterine bisection in progress

upwards till the uterine fundus under vision. One half of the uterine specimen is pushed inside to create space for the opposite adnexal pedicle. It improves the exposure and the upper pedicles can be clamped and divided easily.

Intramyometrial Coring (Fig. 35.3)

This process was described by Lash for removing globularly enlarged uteri especially in patients with a narrow subpubic arch. In this method traction is given to the cervix and the outer myometrial tissue present immediately below the serosa, parallel to the uterine cavity is circumferentially incised with a scalpel. It is usually begun at the isthmic area. This process is continued till the fundus is delivered.[16]

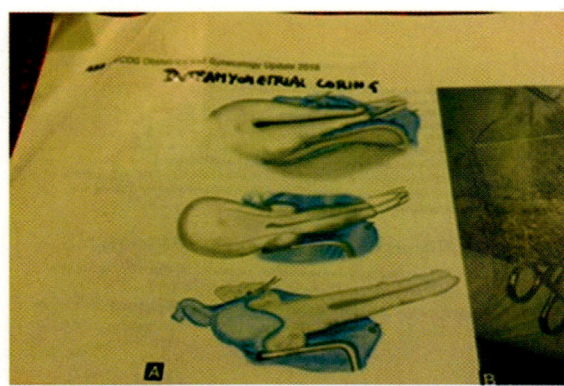

Fig. 35.3: Intramyometrial coring

Wedge Resection (Figs 35.4A and B)

Wedge resection is useful in grossly enlarged uteri with adenomyosis. Wedge resection is done symmetrically around the midline to avoid lateral deviation towards one adnexa. Strong clamps are used to hold the uterus and a long handled scalpel is used to create triangular wedges of tissues. Coring incisions can be made from partially created wedges. Cervical wedge resection can be done for grossly enlarged cervix.

Myomectomy (Figs 35.5A to E)

Myomas can be enucleated or mechanically morcellated during vaginal hysterectomy. Smaller fibroids can be enucleated completely, but larger ones may require morcellation. This process can majorly debulk the uterus and make vaginal hysterectomy feasible. Submucous myoma should be removed first followed by lateral wall fibroids and then fundal fibroids at the end. Posterior myomas may be easier to remove than anterior ones. Sometimes large cervical myomas may interfere with colpotomy, so they have to be enucleated before one can proceed. The easiest to deal with is a posterior wall cervical fibroid and the least desirable is a large lateral wall cervical fibroid. As long as the total uterine volume and/or size does not contraindicate the vaginal route for hysterectomy, a cervical fibroid should not deter the gynecologist. A cervical polyp or a large submucous myomatous polyp that extrudes from the cervical canal or arising from the cervical lip, fills the vagina partly or wholly and obscures speculum examination, is often subjected to AH. Prima facie speculum findings in such a case will suggest that the vaginal route is not possible; at the same time the laparoscope is not helpful for the submucous polyp protruding from the cervix and seen at the vaginal end. High anterior and fundal myomas are difficult to access and enucleate.

Core Enucleation

Doyen used a coring tube to remove cylindrical columns of tissue from centre of large solid myomas. This method is also used for resecting thick myometrium. The cutting of the tube is pressed into the centre of the tissue and advanced to depth of 3 to 4 cm by rotation. The coring tube is removed and the cylinder of tissue is held and excised.[17]

■ FACILITATING VAGINAL HYSTERECTOMY IN FIBROIDS: OTHER INTERVENTIONS

Infiltration with Saline and Vasoconstrictors

Saline infiltration with or without vasoconstrictor solutions like vasopressin or adrenaline may be used during anterior or posterior dissection and during enucleation of fibroids. This benefit in two ways. It helps to create a plane for dissection and also helps in haemostasis. It should be remembered that the patient should be evaluated for any contraindications to these drugs. Also the anesthetist should be informed beforehand.

Increasing Exposure

In case of narrow vagina and introitus a midline episiotomy may facilitate the exposure and increase the space for the operator to work with.

Preventing Injuries

As discussed earlier the bladder and rectum should be protected from an inadvertent injury by debulking in between

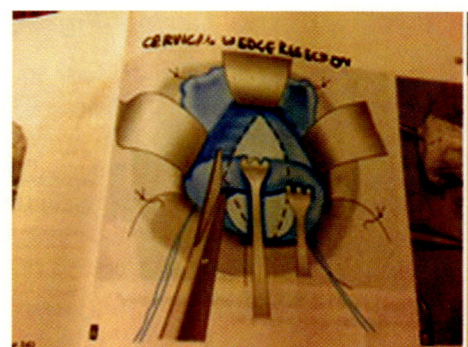
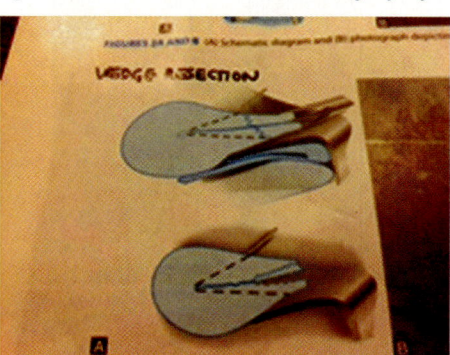

Figs 35.4A and B: **A.** Wedge resection; **B.** Cervical wedge resection.

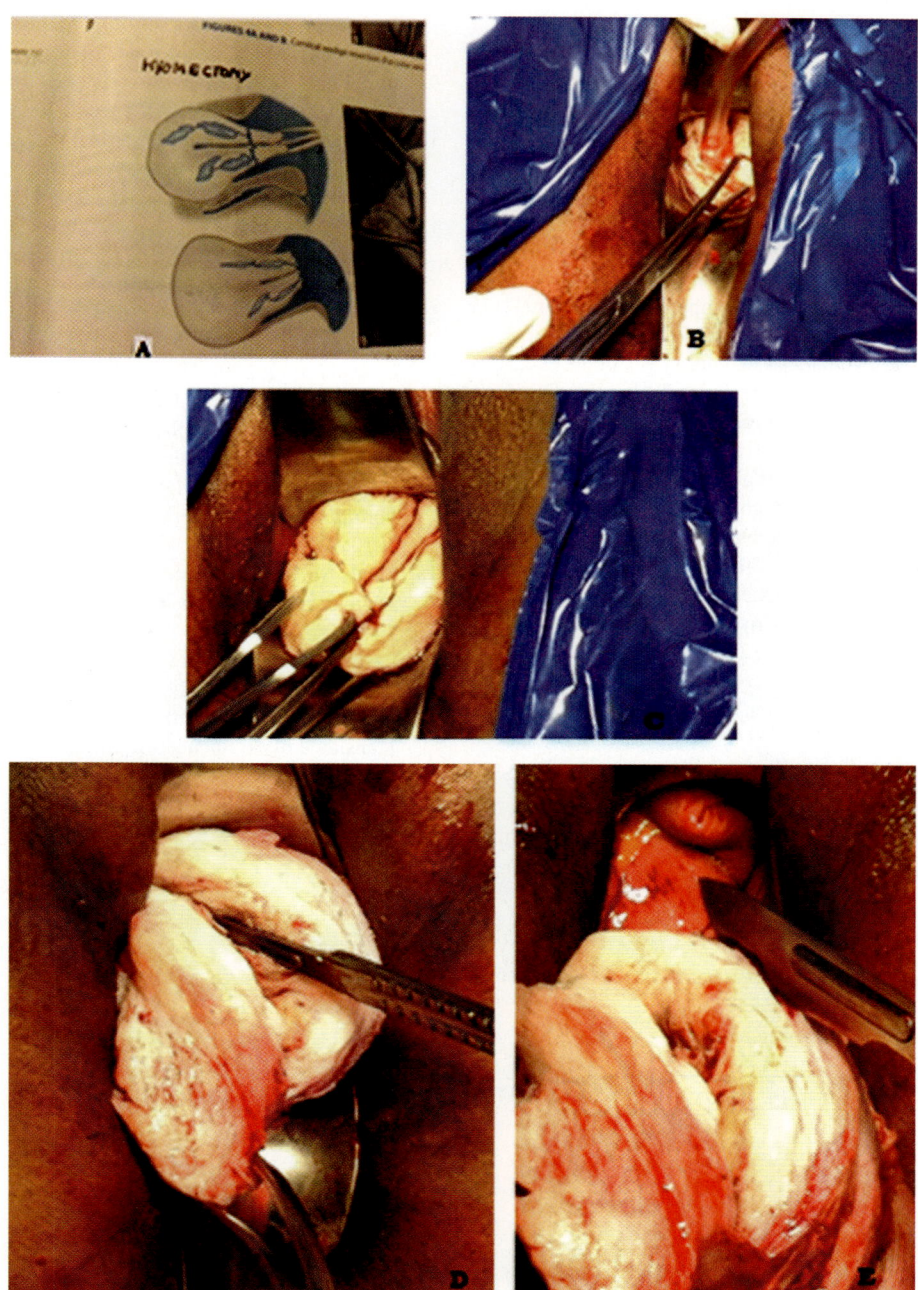

Figs 35.5A to E: A. Myomectomy; **B.** Myoma held with tenaculum; **C.** Myoma pulled out to make it prominent; **D and E.** Myoma morcellation for debulking.

two retractors. Potential omental or bowel adhesions to the uterus should also be kept in mind. Digital palpation and adequate retraction should be used. If adhesions are present, sharp dissection with scissors should be done.

Vaginal hysterectomy is the signature surgery of the gynecologist. It is the least invasive method of performing a hysterectomy as it utilizes a natural orifice and has advantages of lower morbidity, hospital stay and cost. The mere presence of fibroid should not be considered as a contraindication to vaginal hysterectomy. Careful selection of cases, skilled and experienced surgeon and debulking the uterus will allow successful and safe performance of vaginal hysterectomy in fibroids imparting benefits to the patients.

■ REFERENCES

1. Johnson N, Barlow D, Lethaby A, et al. Methods of hysterectomy: systematic review and meta-analysis of randomised controlled trials. BMJ. 2005;330:1478.
2. Nieboer TE, Johnson N, Lethaby A, et al. Surgical approach to hysterectomy for benign gynaecological disease. Cochrane Database Syst Rev. 2009;8(3):CD003677.
3. Donnez O, Jadoul P, Squifflet J, et al. A series of 3190 laparoscopic hysterectomies for benign disease from 1990 to 2006: evaluation of complications compared with vaginal and abdominal procedures. BJOG. 2009;116:492-500.
4. David-Montefiore E, Rouzier R, Chapron C, et al. Surgical routes and complications of hysterectomy for benign disorders: a prospective observational study in French university hospitals. Hum Reprod. 2007;22(1):260-5.
5. Garry R, Fountain J, Mason S, et al. The eVALuate study: two parallel randomized trials, one comparing laparoscopic with abdominal hysterectomy, and the other comparing laparoscopic with vaginal hysterectomy. BMJ. 2004;328:129.
6. Maresh MJ, Metcalfe MA, Mcpherson K, et al. The VALUE national hysterectomy study: description of the patients and their surgery. BJOG. 2002;109(3):302-12.
7. Appropriate use of laparoscopically assisted vaginal hysterectomy (Committee Opinion). Compendium of selected publication. Washington DC (USA): The American College of Obstetricians and Gynecologists Women's Health Care Physicians. 2006. pp. 13-14.
8. Richardson RE, Bournas N, Magos AL. Is laparoscopic hysterectomy a waste of time? Lancet. 1995;345:36-41.
9. Farquhar CM, Steiner CA. Hysterectomy rates in the United States 1990-1997. Obstet Gynecol. 2002;99:229-34.
10. Doucette RC, Sharp HT, Alder SC. Challenging generally accepted contraindications to vaginal hysterectomy. Am J Obstet Gynecol. 2001;184:1386-9. Discussion 1390-1.
11. Paparella P, Sizzi O, Rossetti A, et al. Vaginal hysterectomy in generally considered contraindications to vaginal surgery. Arch Gynecol Obstet. 2004;270:104-9.
12. Sheth SS. Preoperative sonographic estimation of uterine volume: An aid to determine the route of hysterectomy. J Gynecol Surg. 2002;18:13-22.
13. Agostini A, Bretelle F, Cravello L, et al. Vaginal hysterectomy in nulliparous women without prolapse: a prospective comparative study. BJOG. 2003;110:515-8.
14. Quinlan D, Quinlan DK. Vaginal Hysterectomy in enlarged fibroid uterus: a report of 85 cases. J Obstet Gynecol Can. 2010;32(10):980-3.
15. Sheth SS. Uterine fibroids. In. Sheth SS, Studd JWW (Eds). Vaginal Hysterectomy. London: Martin Dunitz Ltd. 2012. pp. 79-94.
16. Lash AF. A method for reducing the size of the uterus in vaginal hysterectomy. Am J Obstet Gynecol. 1941;42:452-9.
17. Doyen E. Surgical therapeutics and operative technique. Translated by H. Spencer-Browne. London Bailliree, Tindal and Cox; 1920.

Index